P9-DNL-377

3 6274 00074504 1

THE ENCYCLOPEDIA OF

AUTOIMMUNE DISEASES

THE ENCYCLOPEDIA OF

AUTOIMMUNE
DISEASES

Dana K. Cassell

Noel Rose, M.D., Ph.D.
Director, Johns Hopkins
Center for Autoimmune
Disease Research

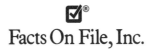

Facts On File, Inc.

The Encyclopedia of Autoimmune Diseases

Facts On File, Inc.
132 West 31st Street
New York NY 10001

Library of Congress Cataloging-in-Publication Data

Cassell, Dana K.
The encyclopedia of autoimmune diseases / Dana Cassell, Noel Rose.
p. cm.—(The Facts On File library of health and living)
Includes bibliographical references and index.
ISBN 0-8160-4340-X
1. Autoimmune diseases—Encyclopedias. I. Rose, Noel R. II. Title. III. Series.
RC600 .C37 2002
616.97'8'003—dc21   2002002029

Facts On File books are available at special discounts when purchased in bulk quantities for businesses, associations, institutions, or sales promotions. Please call our Special Sales Department in New York at (212) 967-8800 or (800) 322-8755.

You can find Facts On File on the World Wide Web at http://www.factsonfile.com

Text and cover design by Cathy Rincon
Illustrations by Dale Williams

Printed in the United States of America

VB FOF 10 9 8 7 6 5 4 3 2 1

This book is printed on acid-free paper.

CONTENTS

FOREWORD

The Commonality of the Autoimmune Diseases

Not many years ago, the idea of an encyclopedia of autoimmune diseases would have been inconceivable. The reason is not that there were no autoimmune diseases; in fact, they have been with us from time immemorial. It is rather because we were not in the habit of thinking of the autoimmune diseases as a group. The explanation is quite understandable. The autoimmune diseases, which result from the pathological effects of a misguided, self-directed immune response, can affect essentially any site in the body. There is an autoimmune disease of the skin, brain, heart, liver, lung, kidney, joints, and so forth. The clinical presentation of the disease depends upon its location, and, therefore, it varies greatly from one disease to another. Equally important, the treatment of the different autoimmune diseases falls to different medical specialists, who are usually arranged according to the organ system with which they are concerned. Thus, particular autoimmune diseases are cared for by physicians specializing in dermatology, neurology, cardiology, gastroenterology, nephrology, rheumatology, etc. There was, in the past, very little reason or incentive for bringing these disparate disorders together into a single category.

A transformation occurred toward the end of the 20th century when medical scientists began to find that there is a remarkable commonality among these diseases. First, the misguided immune response causes, or at least contributes significantly, to the progression of the disease. Our newer knowledge of the immune response, acquired from basic research, has allowed us to understand a great deal more about the factors that normally regulate the immune response and where they might go wrong. We now realize that autoimmunity (an immune response directed to oneself) is actually quite common. This concept violated some of the most basic early tenets of immunology and took some time to be accepted. Although most autoimmune responses are limited and harmless, sometimes an immune response to oneself goes too far and produces the type of injury we recognize as autoimmune disease.

The Incidence of Autoimmune Disease

The autoimmune diseases are among the leading causes of illness in the United States. They are, in general, chronic disabling conditions requiring lifelong care, and several of them, if not correctly diagnosed and appropriately treated, can cause death. In fact, the autoimmune diseases as a group are among the leading causes of death in women under the age of 65 in the United States. It has been estimated by the National Institutes of Health that between 5 percent and 8 percent of the population of the United States suffer from an autoimmune disease; this translates into 14 million to 22 million people. These are, however, only rough estimates, since relatively few reliable studies of the incidence have been carried out on specific autoimmune diseases. To place these estimates in context, it might help to mention that in the United States in 1997, cancer of all sites occurred in a slightly fewer than 9 million people, and the number of cases of heart disease in 1996 in the United States was a little more than 2 million. Thus, the autoimmune diseases, collectively, are among the top-three categories of disease in the United States.

The Burden of Autoimmune Disease

Because of the chronic nature of most autoimmune diseases, their burden is greatly amplified. Moreover, the disease affects not only the patient but also the family and other caregivers. The economic impact of these diseases in the United States in terms of expenses of treatment, missed time at work, and missed opportunities has been estimated to cost the nation more than $100 billion a year.

The autoimmune diseases represent a special burden to women. Estimates suggest that about 75 percent of cases occur in women. Some of the most prominent autoimmune diseases, such as lupus and multiple sclerosis, strike women during the early adult years when the greatest demands are placed upon them in the form of child bearing, child rearing, and initiating a professional career. The basis of this female bias is still not well understood, but it probably represents a confluence of several factors, including the role played by sex-related hormones, such as estrogen and prolactin. Yet, the autoimmune diseases are not confined to any particular age. Type 1 diabetes and juvenile rheumatoid arthritis are devastating illnesses of childhood. Among the elderly, the autoimmune thyroid diseases, chronic (Hashimoto's) thyroiditis and Graves' disease, present special problems. Low thyroid functions that follow chronic thyroiditis may be responsible for many of the symptoms of chronic fatigue, depression, brittle hair, coarse skin, and weight gain that we associate with aging. A special burden for women is the occurrence of post-partum autoimmunity. Although a number of autoimmune diseases, such as rheumatoid arthritis and Graves' disease may remit during pregnancy, they will often return with even greater severity after delivery. There is reason to suggest that post-partum thyroiditis accounts for a significant proportion of post-partum depression with all of its debilitating manifestation in new mothers.

The Causes of Autoimmune Disease

Understanding the cause of autoimmune diseases is important for a number of reasons. The information will help to develop earlier diagnoses, design better treatments, and, most important, devise novel strategies for prevention. To establish the cause of disease, we are dependent for the most part on animal models in which it is possible to dissect the individual components of the immune response in order to identify the particular steps where errors have occurred. It may be that something alters the molecules in our own bodies and the immune system mistakes them for foreign ones. Perhaps an invading microorganism is so similar to something in our own bodies that the immune response to the pathogen crosses over and injures ourselves. Sometimes the regulators that normally limit the immune response and keep it under control are crippled. These basic mechanisms and related ones underlie all of the autoimmune disorders and justify studying them together in the research laboratory.

Studies of both humans and animal models have shown that an important hereditary component plays a role in the autoimmune diseases. In contrast to classical inherited diseases, such as sickle-cell anemia, however, the autoimmune diseases are not caused by the mutation in a single gene. Typically, a large number of genes is involved, perhaps as many as 20 or 30, each of which produces subtle changes in immune function. In combination, they promote the disease process. This complexity makes genetic analysis difficult.

The genes regulating the immune response have been the topic of a great deal of research. The primary control of the immune system is vested in the genes of the major histocompatibility complex (MHC), a family of genes that regulates the interaction between cells, including cells of the immune system. MHC genes, then, determine what the immune system actually recognizes, as well as affecting the vigor of reaction. In humans, the MHC genes are referred to as HLA, and the particular HLA profile of a person allows us to predict, to some degree, the susceptibility to an autoimmune disease and sometimes the likely response to treatment.

Many non-MHC genes also contribute to susceptibility to autoimmune disease. In general, the more of such genes one inherits, the more likely it is that an autoimmune disease develops. Some of the genes appear to favor the development of a particular autoimmune disease or of another autoimmune disease of the same organ. For example, we often come upon thyroiditis and Graves' disease, two diseases of the thyroid gland, in members of the same family. Other susceptibility genes convey a predilection for a larger group of disorders, such as of the endocrine organs. Thus, patients with Type 1 diabetes are at higher risk for developing thyroid disease. Finally, some traits seem to heighten susceptibility to autoimmune diseases generally. It is, therefore, common to see clusters of autoimmune diseases where the same individual may have more than one autoimmune disorder, or where multiple autoimmune diseases may occur in the same family. Two members of the family may have the same autoimmune disease or a different one.

Classifying the genes that confer susceptibility to autoimmune disease has proved to be a difficult task, but has been greatly advanced by recent genomic research. Investigations that have solved the entire human and mouse genomes have revealed new opportunities to identify susceptibility genes outside of the major histocompatibility complex. They often turn out to be genes that modulate the immune response or make the target organ more vulnerable to autoimmune attack.

Evidence for the role of genetic factors in autoimmune diseases in humans derives mainly from studies comparing identical (monozygotic) twins with nonidentical (dizygotic) twins. As a general rule, it appears that about a fifth to a half of the risk of developing an autoimmune disease is inherited. This figure suggests that more than half of the susceptibility is caused by some environmental factor. We must remember, however, that the immune system itself is highly variable and that a certain randomness is built into immune responses, so that even genetically identical individuals are not immunologically identical. Nevertheless, it is clear that external agents from the environment interact with the genetic predisposition to trigger autoimmune disease in many instances.

A number of examples shows that the onset of an autoimmune disease can clearly be associated with some environmental exposure. The best studied agents are certain drugs that can produce a lupuslike illness in a small proportion of genetically susceptible patients. This form of disease, however, usually disappears when the drug is discontinued. Infectious agents are likely inducers of chronic autoimmune disease. A good example is rheumatic heart disease that follows repeated infection by the common beta-hemolytic streptococcus. It is actually possible to prevent rheumatic heart disease by perennial treatment with antibiotics to avoid recurrent streptococcal infection in children who have had rheumatic fever. Many other microorganisms have been incriminated as inducers of autoimmune disease. They include the agents of Lyme disease, *Chlamydia* infection, and gastrointestinal disorders associated with *Salmonella*. Recently, streptococcal infections have been implicated in a type of pediatric autoimmune neuropsychiatric disorder.

The agents most commonly associated with autoimmune diseases have been the viruses. A strong case can be made that herpes simplex viruses cause an autoimmune disease of the eye, called stromal keratitis. Coxsackie-B viruses have been incriminated in autoimmune myocarditis and Type 1 diabetes, and EB virus in rheumatoid arthritis and lupus. Analyzing the mechanisms by which these agents induce autoimmune disease has been a fascinating recent chapter of research. A few examples of dietary factors and environmental pollutants have been related to an autoimmune disease. Excessive iodine in the diet may be important in explaining the rising incidence of autoimmune thyroid disease in certain countries. Workers who are exposed to silica seem to have a higher incidence of the disease scleroderma. Several industrial chemicals have been implicated as possible triggers of autoimmune disease in genetically predisposed individuals, although hard and fast evidence that they actually cause disease is still lacking. Even our commonly used vaccines have been considered as possible triggers of autoimmune disease, but careful research has not yet supported the claim.

Treatment of Autoimmune Disease

Recently, the tempo of therapeutic research has increased perceptibly. Although no wholesale cures are yet available, improved treatments are now emerging regularly. Many of these newer treatments are applicable to more than one autoimmune disease. This commonality is another valid reason why the medical investigator increasingly considers the autoimmune diseases as representing a fundamental issue much as he or she thinks of treatments for the many types of cancer jointly as a general problem.

Our present therapeutic approaches to the autoimmune diseases can be broadly classified into two types. The first mode of treatment is to correct the immune-mediated defect. This strategy is more effective if the disease affects a single organ. If, for example, we are dealing with an overactive thyroid, as found in Graves' disease, the gland can be removed surgically or down-regulated medically. Radioactive iodine, which is taken up specifically by the thyroid gland, is a very effective means of dampening an overactive thyroid. On the other hand, if the autoimmune response has damaged or destroyed an organ, its function can sometimes be partially replaced; for example, synthetic thyroid hormone will reconstitute most of the functions of a normal thyroid gland, and insulin is useful for restoring the loss of the insulin-producing beta cells of the pancreatic islets. Myasthenia gravis can usually be effectively treated by overcoming the specific block at the nerve-muscle junction induced by an autoantibody to the acetylcholine receptor, using especially designed drugs to protect acetylcholine. In general, these treatments are lifelong but require careful medical management. Moreover, they apply only when the autoimmune damage is highly targeted.

In cases where the immune-mediated injury is more general, another approach is required. It involves blunting the entire immune response. This may be done by using drugs that damage the metabolism of the active immune cells, such as methotrexate. Other drugs reduce the inflammatory response. A common example of such drugs are the steroids, such as prednisone. Although often highly effective and even life-saving, these drugs are hazardous because they can reduce the immune defenses of the patient and often have broad general side effects on vital body functions.

There is a great deal of interest in developing new, better focused, and more enduring therapies. One possibility is to attack the immune system cells responsible for immune responses. Some of these cells bear particular markers on their surface, called CD3 or CD4. Monoclonal antibodies directed to these cell surface molecules will undercut the autoimmune response. However, they often have unwanted effects on the immune system generally. Therefore, newer research efforts are directed toward identifying the small populations of immune cells actually responsible for the damaging autoimmune response. We know that the key immune cells, T cells, recognize a particular antigen through receptors on the cell surface. One approach, therefore, is to develop reagents that specifically interact with this cell surface recognition structure. These reagents are monoclonal antibodies that may be tailored specifically for this receptor and will kill the rogue T cell. Counterfeit antigens may block the receptor and prevent it from reacting with the autoantigens of the body. A drug of this type, glatiramer, is being used to treat some forms of multiple sclerosis. T cells recognize an antigen only if it is presented by the MHC. Another strategy is to disable the particular MHC that is required for presentation of the autoantigen. These approaches all have in common the problem that the autoantigen inciting disease must be clearly identified. Unfortunately, this is now possible in relatively few diseases. The reason is that autoimmune responses tend to spread to adjacent antigens after the disease process begins. Compared to experimental animals, it is difficult to trace the initiating antigen in human patients, who present themselves only after the disease has advanced to a clinically significant level.

A practical strategy for present purposes, therefore, is to inactivate the inflammatory mediators generated by the autoantigen-specific T cells that cause the autoimmune disease. Very successful treatments based on inhibitors of specific cell products, called cytokines, have had a great impact on current therapy. For example, agents that block the cytokine, tumor necrosis factor-alpha, have been successful in treating some patients with rheumatoid arthritis, inflammatory bowel disease, and other autoimmune diseases. They offer the promise that new approaches of this sort will be successful.

Prevention of Autoimmune Disease

All investigators agree that the ultimate goal in caring for patients with autoimmune disease is prevention. Only then can irreversible damage to vital organs be avoided. The way forward is clear. We must know who is at high risk for developing an autoimmune disease. Studies of the genetic traits that confer heightened susceptibility will provide this information. The Human Genome Project has now made this goal feasible. Next, we must identify the environmental trigger, since experience has taught us that even genetically at-risk individuals do not develop disease if they can avoid the inciting agent. Thus, patients with celiac disease can prevent symptoms by adopting a strict gluten-free diet. If avoidance of the environmental trigger is not feasible, one option is early intervention; that is, treatment before the disease is fully under way. Such a treatment must necessarily have minimal or no side effects. For that purpose, we would call upon our increasing knowledge of the specific T cell that is the root cause of almost all autoimmune diseases. The strategy of targeting the T-cell receptor or its counterpart MHC has been described previously. Another idea is to delete or inactivate the T cell by administering the incriminated antigen by mouth. A novel concept that is receiving much attention recently is the injection of the antigen in a manner that deviates a harmful autoimmune

response to a harmless one. Surely, we have only begun to think of ways in which we can control autoimmunity by learning to understand the biologic laws that govern the immune response.

A Final Word

From the point of view of the patient, there are persuasive reasons for linking the autoimmune diseases. Common genes contribute to the susceptibility to multiple autoimmune reactions. Thus, the autoimmune diseases often cluster so that a patient with one autoimmune disease shows increased risk of another autoimmune disorder. Several members of a family may share a proclivity to autoimmune disease, although it may not be manifest as the same illness. It is, therefore, of great importance that the patient recognize the autoimmune nature of the ailment at a very early point in time and that the physician caring for the patient be fully apprised of the situation.

It is past time to assemble a single volume summarizing the many autoimmune diseases and present our current understanding of this group of diseases in language that the average person understands. I am pleased to welcome this encyclopedia as a tribute to the many investigators seeking to understand autoimmune disease and the many courageous patients suffering from one of these diseases.

—Noel R. Rose, M.D., Ph.D.
Professor of Pathology
Professor of Molecular
Microbiology & Immunology
Director, Johns Hopkins Center
for Autoimmune Disease Research
Johns Hopkins University

ACKNOWLEDGMENTS

No work of this size could be completed without assistance from many sources. Of particular help in today's world is the wonderful World Wide Web, with its vast treasure trove of information, sources, statistics, and explanations. The National Library of Medicine, the various National Institutes of Health, Health Canada, and the many disease-specific organizations all maintain excellent repositories of information invaluable to researchers. Hidden behind those endless waves of Web pages are real people who gather and post that information for the use of the medical community, patients, researchers, and the general public. Without all that work being done behind the scenes, this book would have been much more difficult to write.

And a special thanks to Vicki DeLalla, who spent many hours helping mine that information on the Web. Her combination of computer savvy and medical training certainly facilitated the completion of the project.

Finally, a note of appreciation to Jim Chambers, my editor, without whose suggestions and input this book would not have been nearly so comprehensive.

—Dana K. Cassell

INTRODUCTION

Any family can be struck by one or more of the nearly 100 autoimmune diseases. Traditionally looked at as individual diseases rather than collectively, autoimmune diseases have long been considered rare. Indeed, a few of the individual diseases are rare. But together, they affect up to 22 million Americans—8 percent of the population, or one in five people—including as many as 17 million American women. They also strike children, teenagers, men, and senior citizens.

The following are examples of how likely it is for any family—your family—to be directly affected by an autoimmune disease:

- Approximately 2 percent of the U.S. population, or more than 4.5 million people, will have alopecia areata at some point in their lives.
- An estimated 16 to 18 million people are infected with Chagas' disease (mostly in South America); of those infected, 50,000 will die each year.
- Fibromyalgia affects 3 million to 6 million Americans. It primarily occurs in women of childbearing age, but children, the elderly, and men can also be affected.
- Peripheral neuropathy affects 2 million people in the United States, most commonly those of middle age and the elderly.
- Psoriasis affects about 5.5 million Americans.
- Scientists estimate that about 2.1 million people have rheumatoid arthritis.
- Estimates are that 2 million to 4 million Americans have Sjögren's syndrome.
- The number of Americans diagnosed with systemic lupus erythematosus (SLE) is estimated at 1 million.

- About 1 percent to 2 percent of the world's population, or 40 million to 50 million people, have vitiligo. In the United States, 2 million to 5 million people have the disorder.

In an analysis of published journal articles about 24 autoimmune diseases and U.S. Census data, researchers from Johns Hopkins University estimated in 1997 that 8,511,845 persons in the United States, or approximately 1 in 31 Americans, was at that time afflicted with one of the 24 diseases. From the incidence data, it was estimated that approximately 1,186,015 new cases of these 24 autoimmune diseases occur in the United States every five years.

Any numbers such as these are likely low; not all instances of autoimmune disease are correctly diagnosed or reported. In addition, the researchers concluded, because many autoimmune diseases are infrequently studied by epidemiologists, the total burden of disease is surely greater than these estimates.

Also, some autoimmune diseases occur more frequently in certain minority populations. For example, lupus is more common in African-American and Hispanic women than in Caucasian women of European ancestry. Rheumatoid arthritis and scleroderma affect a higher percentage of residents in some Native American communities than in the general U.S. population. It is critical that all people, many of whom fall into one or more populations targeted by at least one autoimmune disease, be aware of the risks and outlooks for themselves, their families, and coworkers.

The Seriousness of Autoimmune Diseases

The social, economic, and health impact from autoimmune diseases is far-reaching and extends not only to family but also to employers, coworkers, and friends. Autoimmune diseases make up the fifth-leading cause of death among women aged 15 to 44. Also, autoimmune diseases are often chronic, requiring lifelong care. They present a significant disease problem in the United States, Canada, and many other countries.

Following are a few examples of what autoimmune diseases are costing the U.S. government:

- Insulin dependent diabetes mellitus (IDDM) costs the U.S. Medicare program more than $2 billion per year just for renal dialysis.
- Psoriasis costs the nation between $2 billion and $3 billion each year.
- The direct medical costs of rheumatoid arthritis approach $5 billion annually, with nearly 70 percent of these costs attributable to hospitalizations and home nursing care.

Overall, autoimmune conditions cost an estimated $100 billion a year in health care expenditures in the United States. But autoimmune costs spread beyond direct medical expenses for Medicare, Medicaid, insurance companies, and individuals. In industrialized societies, autoimmune diseases are serious medical problems because of their chronic and disabling effects. Autoimmunity is the fourth leading cause of disability among women overall.

As one example, lost productivity costs due to rheumatoid arthritis approach $20 billion annually, and rheumatoid arthritis patients lose, on average, 50 percent of potential earnings, with approximately 50 percent of patients being unable to work within 10 years of onset. The lifetime indirect costs of rheumatoid arthritis are similar to those for stroke or coronary artery disease.

In another example, about one in five lupus sufferers is disabled and receives disability payments. Because people are often disabled by lupus at a very young age, the economic impact of lupus on the federal treasury is several billion dollars annually.

The Enigma of Autoimmune Diseases

Because the average person—even the average medical practitioner—does not truly understand autoimmune diseases, oftentimes they are misdiagnosed—at least initially—causing the sufferers unnecessary pain, incapacitation, and frustration until the specific autoimmune disease is finally determined. Addressing a 1997 AARDA conference, an official of the National Institutes of Health called autoimmune diseases the "least investigated, most difficult to diagnose, and physically and emotionally most painful diseases that face Americans today."

One recent newspaper headline for a story describing autoimmune diseases read: "Old Illnesses, Strange Clues." Because they are "odd," autoimmune diseases can be difficult for the patient and her (or his) family to comprehend or cope with. Diagnosis of an autoimmune disease often has a profound impact on the patient's family—not only due to the pain and suffering from the disease itself, but also from the stress, uncertainty, even depression, of dealing with a chronic illness they know little about.

The medical community is still trying to solve the puzzle of autoimmune diseases. According to the American Association of Autoimmune and Related Diseases (AARDA), it takes an average of seven years and five doctors before most autoimmune diseases are properly diagnosed. In an AARDA survey of autoimmune disease patients, "many were incorrectly diagnosed with a variety of conditions that have no specific blood test to confirm the diagnosis. Many were told that their symptoms were in their heads or that they were under too much stress. Further, the survey revealed that 45 percent of autoimmune disease patients had been labeled hypochondriacs in the earliest stages of their illnesses."

The reason for this enigma certainly cannot be attributed to the "newness" of autoimmune diseases. As Dr. Rose has explained in the foreword, they have been with us a very long time. For example, articles describing lupus symptoms date back to Hippocrates himself, according to Daniel J. Wallace, M.D., author of The Lupus Book (New York: Oxford University Press, 2000). Considered only a skin disease in the mid-1800s, the first writings on how lupus affected kidney, heart, and lung tissues appeared during the 1920s and 1930s. Wallace notes that "until 1948, there were no effective treatments for lupus except for local skin salves or aspirin."

Multiple sclerosis (MS) also has a long history. From descriptions written as long ago as the Middle Ages, medical historians have identified people who undoubtedly had MS. According to Loren A. Rolak, M.D. ("MS: An Historical Perspective," National Multiple Sclerosis Society, 1996), MS has always been with us. "Once the scientific method took hold in medicine, MS was among the first disease to be described scientifically. The 19th-century doctors did not understand what they saw and recorded, but drawings from autopsies done as early as 1838 clearly show what we today recognize as MS."

Yet, other autoimmune diseases appear to have shorter histories. Rheumatoid arthritis (RA) has been thought to be of comparatively recent, New World origin. According to Danish author P. Halberg, no convincing descriptions of the lesions of RA can be found in the medical literature before 1800, although nonmedical literature, the visual arts, and paleopathological observations before 1800 revealed finger abnormalities suggestive of RA. But many authorities disregard those interpretations. Recent paleopathological observations of skeletons from 1000 to 3000 B.C.E. in the United States have shown convincing bone erosions compatible with RA, suggesting that rheumatoid arthritis may be an old disease in the New World and may have been transferred to the Old World after the time of Columbus.

Other autoimmune diseases have been recognized as such even more recently. Autoimmune lymphoproliferative syndrome (ALPS), for example, was discovered in 1995 by a team of doctors and scientists at the National Institutes of Health (NIH).

Among the reasons given for the difficulty in diagnosing autoimmune diseases have been the multiple causes, overlapping symptoms common to many other diseases, and perplexing waxing and waning of these symptoms.

- All of the autoimmune diseases show evidence of a genetic predisposition. Yet none of them are "inherited." But they are more common in some families than in others—much as cancer is. And they can be triggered by several environmental factors.
- Common autoimmune disease symptoms such as fatigue, headaches, fever, rashes, and painful joints overlap with many other diseases, extending the diagnosis process.
- Many of these symptoms "flare up" then subside or disappear altogether, leading to frustration for the patient who is trying to "get across" to family and physician what is happening in her body, as well as for the doctor who is attempting to pinpoint a cause for symptoms that may not present the same at each examination.

The Promises of Autoimmune Research

Because they affect so many women, autoimmune diseases have been moved to the top of the national women's research agenda by the National Institutes of Health (NIH). Various autoimmune research initiatives at NIH now number the greatest in history, according to Vivian W. Pinn, M.D., director of NIH's Office of Research on Women's Health (ORWH), and were spurred by a $30 million NIH appropriation in 1999.

Other research initiatives have followed. For example, in February 2002, the National Institute of Arthritis and Musculoskeletal and Skin Diseases (NIAMS) at the NIH announced funding for 10 new research grants on scleroderma. The grants, totaling more than $2 million per year, included both basic and clinical research studies. Also, NIAMS and its partners recently funded 15 new fibromyalgia projects totaling more than $3.6 million.

More local attention is also being given to autoimmune diseases. Florida announced in early 2002 that it would become the first state to offer screening to determine an infant's lifetime probability of developing IDDM. Funded by a $10 million grant from the American Diabetes Association, the program was scheduled to launch within the year. Then in March 2002, scientists at the Pacific Northwest Research Institute in Seattle announced they had begun testing the blood samples of 32,000

Washington children to see if they carry a genetic marker for juvenile diabetes.

Research scientists have only recently reported promising inroads in the areas of genetics and female reproductive connections to autoimmunity. Other areas in which investigators are concentrating include studies of the immune system during the progression of an autoimmune disease, the role of infectious agents in autoimmune diseases, of animal models of autoimmune diseases, and the effects of therapeutic intervention on the immune system in an autoimmune disease.

Within This Book

This encyclopedia is divided into two basic sections: first is the A-to-Z main body; second is the Appendixes. Within the alphabetical body of the book, you will find medical terms related to autoimmunity that will help explain immune response and the relationships of the various diseases, sociological terms that point out the ramifications of autoimmune disease, and each of the 80-plus autoimmune and autoimmune-related diseases.

Each disease listing provides a description and overview of its prevalence, seriousness, and demographics, followed by suspected causes, the disease's clinical features, possible complications, and treatment strategies. Any terms used within a listing that have their own separate listings are designated by small capital letters so that you can quickly and easily find expanded information. Also, many listings end with references to articles and books on the topic for further study.

The appendixes includes organizations and groups that offer information and support (arranged by disease), Internet websites for various diseases, bibliographies of books and articles (arranged first on autoimmune diseases generally, followed by individual diseases), patient research registries, and National Institutes of Health research initiatives, among other lists and charts. Overall, you will find a comprehensive overview of autoimmune diseases, with in-depth treatment of individual diseases, in an easy-to-access format, and with plenty of assistance on where to go next for additional information on those diseases of particular significance to you.

ENTRIES A–Z

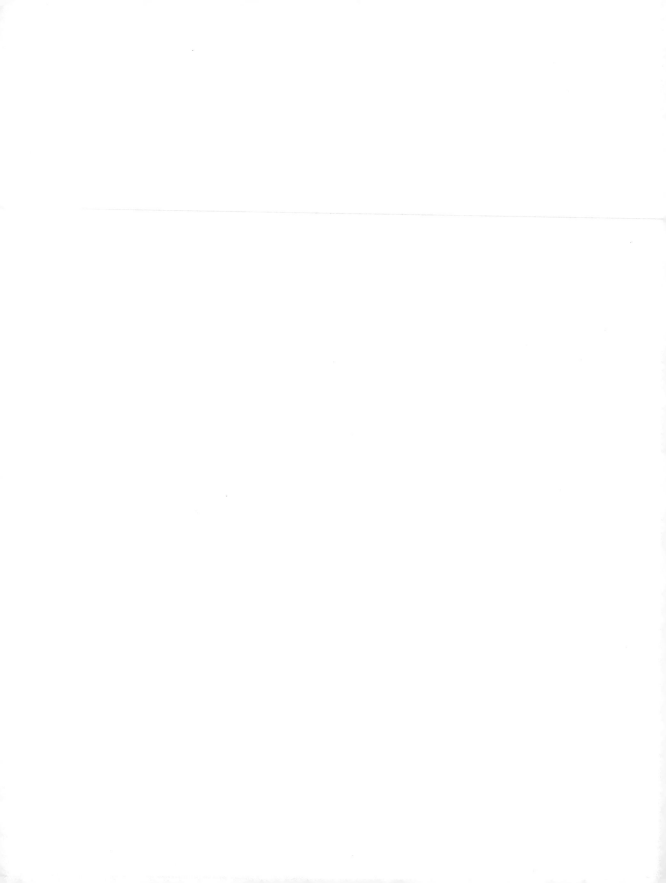

absolute risk Risk of having a disease, or the rate at which a disease occurs in a defined population over a specified time period. Absolute risk can be expressed either as the number of cases per a specified number of persons—most commonly in 100,000—or as a cumulative risk up to a particular age—such as one in eight lifetime risk for non-Hispanic white women. In statistical comparisons when evaluating disease risks, absolute risk is the actual number of persons in two groups of people, exposed and unexposed, who acquired the disease. If the incidence of a disease is one in 1,000, then the absolute risk is one in 1,000 or 0.1 percent.

acquired immunity See IMMUNITY.

acquired immunodeficiency syndrome See AIDS.

active immunity Immunity produced by the body in response to stimulation by a disease-causing organism (naturally acquired active immunity) or by a vaccine (artificially acquired active immunity).

acute-phase proteins These are a group of plasma proteins, many of which are produced by the liver, whose plasma concentrations rise by 25 percent or more during certain inflammatory disorders. Because of this known response, acute-phase proteins play a major role in determining the presence and intensity of inflammation. The best-known of the acute-phase proteins is C-reactive protein (CRP). The level of CRP in blood plasma can rise as high as 1,000-fold with inflammation. Conditions that commonly lead to significant changes in CRP include infection, trauma, surgery, burns, inflammatory conditions, and advanced cancer. Moderate changes occur after strenuous exercise, heatstroke, and childbirth. Small changes occur after psychological stress and in several psychiatric illnesses. An increase in C-reactive protein, however, does not point to only one specific disease.

Addison, Thomas (1793–1860) An eminent London physician of the 19th century. Born in Longbenton, Northumberland, near Newcastle, he graduated from the University of Edinburgh (M.D.) in 1815, became assistant physician at Guy's Hospital in London in 1824, and full physician in 1837. Addison earned a reputation as an outstanding doctor, teacher, and researcher. His thorough examinations and uncanny diagnoses have been described as legendary. In 1839, he wrote *Elements of the Practice of Medicine* with Richard Bright. His most important research centered on pneumonia, tuberculosis, and the effects of glandular deficiencies on human disease—specifically the disease of the suprarenal (adrenal) glands known as ADDISON'S DISEASE. Prior to his research paper in 1855, that condition had been thought to be caused only by tuberculosis, but Addison recognized it as any form of disease of the adrenal glands or adrenal cortex deficiency. He also was the first to describe "Addison's anemia," known today as PERNICIOUS ANEMIA.

Addison's disease An uncommon chronic, progressive endocrine or hormonal disorder that affects about one in 100,000 people. No accurate statistics on the incidence of the disease exist in the United States. Comparisons with a London study projected about 8,600 cases in the United States, but experts consider that number to be low. It occurs in all age groups and afflicts men and women equally. The disease is characterized by weight loss, muscle weakness, fatigue, low blood pressure, and sometimes darkening of the skin in both exposed and nonexposed parts of the body. Although not curable, the disease is treatable once correctly diagnosed.

Addison's disease occurs when the adrenal glands do not produce enough of the hormone cortisol and, in some cases, the hormone aldosterone. For this reason, the disease is sometimes called chronic adrenal insufficiency, or hypocortisolism.

Cortisol is normally produced by the adrenal glands, located just above each kidney. It belongs to a vital class of hormones called glucocorticoids, which affect almost every organ and tissue in the body and thus are necessary for the maintenance of life. Scientists think that cortisol has possibly hundreds of effects in the body. Cortisol's primary function is to help the body respond to stress. Among its other vital tasks, cortisol helps maintain blood pressure and cardiovascular function, helps slow the immune system's inflammatory response, helps balance the effects of insulin in breaking sugar for energy, and helps regulate the metabolism of proteins, carbohydrates, and fats.

Because cortisol is so vital to health, the amount of cortisol produced by the adrenals is precisely balanced. Like many other hormones, cortisol is regulated by the brain's hypothalamus and the pituitary gland, a bean-sized organ at the base of the brain. First, the hypothalamus sends "releasing hormones" to the pituitary gland. The pituitary responds by secreting other hormones that regulate growth, thyroid and adrenal function, and sex hormones such as estrogen and testosterone. One of the pituitary's main functions is to secrete ACTH (adrenocorticotropin), a hormone that stimulates the adrenal glands. When the adrenals receive the pituitary's signal in the form of ACTH, they respond by producing cortisol. To complete the cycle, cortisol then signals the pituitary to lower secretion of ACTH.

Aldosterone belongs to a class of hormones called mineralocorticoids, also produced by the adrenal glands. It helps maintain blood pressure and both water and salt balance in the body by helping the kidney retain sodium and excrete potassium. When aldosterone production falls too low, the kidneys are not able to regulate salt and water balance, causing blood volume and blood pressure to drop.

Failure to produce adequate levels of cortisol, or adrenal insufficiency, can occur for different reasons. The problem may be due to a disorder of the adrenal glands themselves (primary adrenal insufficiency) or to inadequate secretion of ACTH by the pituitary gland (secondary adrenal insufficiency).

Primary Adrenal Insufficiency or Autoimmune Addison's Disease

Most cases of Addison's disease are caused by the gradual destruction of the adrenal cortex, the outer layer of the adrenal glands, by the body's own immune system. About 70 percent of reported cases of Addison's disease are due to autoimmune disorders in which the immune system attacks the cells of the adrenal cortex and slowly destroys them. Adrenal insufficiency occurs when at least 90 percent of the adrenal cortex has been destroyed, a process that can take months or years. As a result, often both glucocorticoid and mineralocorticoid hormones are lacking. Sometimes only the adrenal gland is affected, as in idiopathic adrenal insufficiency; sometimes other glands also are affected, as in the polyendocrine deficiency syndrome.

The polyendocrine deficiency syndrome is classified into two separate forms, referred to as type I and type II. Type I occurs in children. Adrenal insufficiency may be accompanied by underactive parathyroid glands, slow sexual development, pernicious anemia, chronic candida infections, chronic active hepatitis, and, in very rare cases, hair loss. Type II, often called Schmidt's syndrome, usually afflicts young adults. Features of type II may include an underactive thyroid gland, slow sexual development, and diabetes mellitus. About 10 percent of patients with type II have vitiligo, or loss of pigment, on areas of the skin. Scientists think that the polyendocrine deficiency syndrome is inherited because frequently more than one family member tends to have one or more endocrine deficiencies.

Tuberculosis (TB) accounts for about 20 percent of cases of primary adrenal insufficiency in developed countries. When adrenal insufficiency was first identified by Dr. THOMAS ADDISON in 1849, TB was found during autopsies in 70 to 90 percent of cases. As the treatment for TB improved, however, the incidence of adrenal insufficiency due to TB of the adrenal glands has greatly decreased.

Less common causes of primary adrenal insufficiency are chronic infections, mainly fungal infections; cancer cells spreading from other parts of the body to the adrenal glands; amyloidosis; and surgical removal of the adrenal glands. Very rarely, primary adrenal insufficiency can result from hemorrhaging of the adrenal glands because of shock.

Secondary Adrenal Insufficiency

This form of Addison's disease can be traced to a lack of ACTH, which causes a drop in the adrenal glands' production of cortisol but not aldosterone. A temporary form of secondary adrenal insufficiency may occur when a person who has been receiving a glucocorticoid hormone such as prednisone for a long time abruptly stops or interrupts taking the medication. Glucocorticoid hormones, which are often used to treat inflammatory illnesses like rheumatoid arthritis, asthma, or ulcerative colitis, block the release of both corticotropin-releasing hormone (CRH) and ACTH. Normally, CRH instructs the pituitary gland to release ACTH. If CRH levels drop, the pituitary is not stimulated to release ACTH, and the adrenals then fail to secrete sufficient levels of cortisol.

Another cause of secondary adrenal insufficiency is the surgical removal of benign, or noncancerous, ACTH-producing tumors of the pituitary gland (Cushing's disease). In this case, the source of ACTH is suddenly removed, and replacement hormone must be taken until normal ACTH and cortisol production resumes. Less commonly, adrenal insufficiency occurs when the pituitary gland either decreases in size of stops producing ACTH. This can result from tumors or infections of the area, loss of blood flow to the pituitary, radiation for the treatment of pituitary tumors, or surgical removal of parts of the hypothalamus or the pituitary gland during neurosurgery of these areas.

Clinical Features

The symptoms of adrenal insufficiency usually develop gradually and steadily grow worse. Chronic fatigue and muscle weakness, loss of appetite, and weight loss are characteristic of the disease. Nausea,

vomiting, and diarrhea occur in about 50 percent of cases. Blood pressure is low and falls further when standing, causing dizziness or fainting. Skin changes also are common in Addison's disease, with areas of hyperpigmentation, or dark tanning, covering both exposed and nonexposed parts of the body. This darkening of the skin usually occurs in patches and is most visible on scars; skin folds; pressure points such as the elbows, knees, knuckles, and toes; lips; and mucous membranes.

Addison's disease can cause emotional shifts, especially irritability and depression. Because of salt loss, craving of salty foods also is common. Hypoglycemia, or low blood sugar, is more severe in children than in adults. In women, menstrual periods may become irregular or stop.

Because the symptoms progress slowly, they are usually ignored until a stressful event like an illness or an accident causes them to become worse. This is called an addisonian crisis, or acute adrenal insufficiency. In most patients, symptoms are severe enough to seek medical treatment before a crisis occurs. However, in about 25 percent of patients, symptoms first appear during an addisonian crisis, which is considered a medical emergency. Symptoms of an addisonian crisis include sudden, penetrating pain in the lower back, abdomen, or legs and severe vomiting and diarrhea, followed by dehydration, low blood pressure, and loss of consciousness. If left untreated, an addisonian crisis can be fatal.

Diagnosis

In its early stages, adrenal insufficiency can be difficult to diagnose. In addition, because of its rarity, some doctors have never seen a case. In most cases, though, a review of a patient's medical history based on the symptoms, especially the dark tanning of the skin, will lead a doctor to suspect Addison's disease.

A diagnosis of Addison's disease is made by biochemical laboratory tests. The aim of these tests is first to determine whether there are insufficient levels of cortisol and then to establish the cause. X-ray exams of the adrenal and pituitary glands are also useful in helping to establish the cause.

ACTH stimulation test This is the most specific test for diagnosing Addison's disease. In this test, blood and/or urine cortisol levels are measured before and after a synthetic form of ACTH is given by injection. In the so-called short, or rapid, ACTH test, cortisol measurement in blood is repeated 30 to 60 minutes after an intravenous ACTH injection. The normal response after an injection of ACTH is a rise in blood and urine cortisol levels. Patients with either form of adrenal insufficiency respond poorly or do not respond at all.

When the response to the short ACTH test is abnormal, a "long" ACTH stimulation test is required to determine the cause of adrenal insufficiency. In this test, synthetic ACTH is injected either intravenously or intramuscularly over a 48- to 72-hour period, and blood and/or urine cortisol are measured the day before and during the two to three days of the injection. Patients with primary adrenal insufficiency do not produce cortisol during the 48- to 72-hour period; however, patients with secondary adrenal insufficiency have adequate responses to the test on the second or third day.

In patients suspected of having an addisonian crisis, the doctor must begin treatment with injections of salt, fluids, and glucocorticoid hormones immediately. Although a reliable diagnosis is not possible while the patient is being treated, measurement of blood ACTH and cortisol during the crisis and before glucocorticoids are given is sufficient to make the diagnosis. Once the crisis is controlled and medication has been stopped, the doctor will delay further testing for up to one month to obtain an accurate diagnosis.

Insulin-induced hypoglycemia test A reliable test to determine how the hypothalamus, pituitary, and adrenal glands respond to stress is the insulin-induced hypoglycemia test. In this test, blood is drawn to measure the blood glucose and cortisol levels, followed by an injection of fast-acting insulin. Blood glucose and cortisol levels are measured again at 30, 45, and 90 minutes after the insulin injection. The normal response is for blood glucose levels to fall and cortisol levels to rise.

Other tests Once a diagnosis of primary adrenal insufficiency has been made, X-ray exams of the abdomen may be taken to see if the adrenals have any signs of calcium deposits. Calcium deposits may indicate TB. A tuberculin skin test also may be used.

If secondary adrenal insufficiency is the cause, doctors may use different imaging tools to reveal the size and shape of the pituitary gland. The most common is the CT scan, which produces a series of X-ray pictures giving a cross-sectional image of a body part. The function of the pituitary and its ability to produce other hormones are also tested.

Complications

Patients with chronic adrenal insufficiency who need surgery with general anesthesia are treated with injections of hydrocortisone, saline, and glucose. Injections begin on the evening before surgery and continue until the patient is fully awake and able to take medication by mouth. The dosage is adjusted until reaching the maintenance dosage given before surgery.

Women with primary adrenal insufficiency who become pregnant are treated with standard replacement therapy. If nausea and vomiting in early pregnancy interfere with oral medication, injections of the hormone may be necessary. During delivery, treatment is similar to that of patients needing surgery. Following delivery, the dose is gradually tapered and the usual maintenance doses of hydrocortisone and fludrocortisone acetate by mouth are not reached until about 10 days after childbirth.

Treatment

Once fatal, Addison's disease is now treated by replacing, or substituting, the hormones that the adrenal glands are not making. Cortisol is replaced orally with hydrocortisone tablets, a synthetic glucocorticoid, taken once or twice a day. If aldosterone is also deficient, it is replaced with oral doses of a mineralocorticoid, called fludrocortisone acetate (Florinef), which is taken once a day. Patients receiving aldosterone replacement therapy are usually advised by a doctor to increase their salt intake. Because patients with secondary adrenal insufficiency normally maintain aldosterone production, they do not require aldosterone replacement therapy. The doses of each of these medications are adjusted to meet the needs of individual patients.

During an addisonian crisis, low blood pressure, low blood sugar, and high levels of potassium can be life threatening. Standard therapy involves intravenous injections of hydrocortisone, saline (salt water), and dextrose (sugar). This treatment usually brings rapid improvement. When the patient can take fluids and medications by mouth, the amount of hydrocortisone is decreased until a maintenance dose is achieved. If aldosterone is deficient, maintenance therapy also includes oral doses of fludrocortisone acetate.

Although treatment is lifelong and daily, an "Addisonian" (as people with this disease are called) who faithfully takes properly dosed medication can expect to live a normal life with no physical restrictions. Regular monitoring by a physician will assure proper dosage of medicine and should prevent addisonian crises. Because of the importance of monitoring medication during other medical emergencies, physicians strongly advise Addisonians to wear medical identification bracelets or necklaces in order to alert emergency personnel of their condition and to carry a medical emergency card explaining what should be done if the person is unconscious or otherwise unable to communicate. See also CHRONIC FATIGUE SYNDROME.

Corrigan, Eileen K. "Addison's Disease." NIDDK Office of Health Research Reports, National Institutes of Health. Available online. URL: http://www.niddk.nih.gov/health/endo/pubs/addison/addison.htm. Posted on 12 February 1998.
Erickson, Q. L., E. J. Faleski, M. K. Koops, and D. M. Elston. "Addison's Disease: The Potentially Life-Threatening Tan." *Cutis* 66, no. 1 (2000): 72–74.
Margulies, Paul. "Addison's Disease: The Facts You Need to Know," National Adrenal Disease Foundation. Available online. URL: http://www.medhelp.org/nadf/nadf3.htm. Downloaded on 12 July 2002.

adolescents with autoimmune diseases Several autoimmune diseases either especially target adolescents or present special problems for adolescents who suffer from them:

- ANKYLOSING SPONDYLITIS can strike young people in their teens. However, because this age group is typically active in sports, the early symptoms of back pain or joint aches are sometimes erroneously blamed on athletic activity or injuries.

- Adolescents do suffer from CHRONIC FATIGUE SYNDROME (CFS), but little is known about its incidence among this age group. What has been stressed regarding CFS in adolescents is the importance of dealing with the unique problems of chronically ill teens, such as their interactions with family members, teachers, friends, and other students. With some adolescents, particular attention sometimes needs to be given to the impact of fatiguing illness on concentration, memory, and organization, with a close monitoring of academic attendance and performance. At times, specific educational needs need to be addressed as well as the student's physical needs. Personality assessment may assist in determining coping abilities and whether there is a coexisting affective disorder requiring treatment.

- CROHN'S DISEASE, a chronic inflammatory disease that can affect any part of the gastrointestinal tract, afflicts some 50,000 Americans and is most common in adolescents and young adults.

- Thyroid enlargement in adolescents is most frequently caused by HASHIMOTO'S THYROIDITIS (autoimmune thyroiditis), which has a prevalence of 1.2 percent in adolescence aged 11 to 18 years as reported in studies in the United States and western Europe.

- Primary IGA NEPHROPATHY is an autoimmune kidney disease marked by IgA glomerulonephritis due to the glomerular immune deposit formation in the kidney. IgA nephropathy usually occurs in adolescents or young adults between the ages of 15 and 35.

- INSULIN-DEPENDENT DIABETES mellitus (IDDM), or Type 1 diabetes, in children and adolescents is more prevalent than any other severe chronic pediatric disease. An estimated 100,000 to 127,000 cases occur in children and adolescents under the age of 19. Not only is IDDM a challenge to treat, but adolescents find it especially difficult to live with. The physical and psychological changes the body goes through during the four to eight years of maturation during adolescence often make glucose control difficult. Then the daily constraints of insulin treatment often clash with the adolescent's fundamental drive for freedom and self-sufficiency. Dr. Challener further illustrated how diabetes can intrude upon normal adolescence by listing possible interferences for the following adolescent psychological and developmental changes:

1. Physical and sexual maturation—delayed sexual maturation, small stature, invasion of privacy by frequent examinations.
2. Conformity with peer group—meals must be eaten on time, receiving injections and blood tests.
3. Self-image—"hypos" expose the adolescent as different.
4. Self-esteem—defective body image.
5. Independence from parents—parental overconcern, battles over diabetes.
6. Economic independence—increasing of insurance premiums, discrimination by employers.

Adolescents with diabetes are also at a much higher risk for the life-threatening ketoacidosis because they are less likely to comply with insulin therapy. The challenge for health care providers, then, is to set treatment regimes for adolescent IDDM patients that are realistic and attainable for their short attention spans while offering encouragement and motivation.

In agreement, the Oklahoma School Diabetes Plan states, "Many adolescent issues stem from the need to fit in or not appear to be different from peers. Fearing rejection, the adolescent may attempt to hide the fact that he/she has diabetes. In some instances, DENIAL may lead to a deliberate rejection of components of self-management, which may result in poor disease control. Other issues that may interfere with the successful management of diabetes in adolescents include weight awareness and/or body image, particularly with females, as well as DEPRESSION, which is related to self-image or disease management."

- Juvenile rheumatoid arthritis (JRA) causes joint inflammation and stiffness in children under the age of 16 (see JUVENILE ARTHRITIS). Adolescents often outgrow JRA; however, the disease can affect bone development in the growing child. Inflammation causes redness, swelling, warmth, and soreness in the joints, although many children with JRA do not complain of joint pain. Any joint can be affected, and inflammation may limit the mobility of affected joints. JRA affects the entire family, who must cope with the special challenges of this disease. JRA can strain a child's participation in social and after-school activities and make schoolwork more difficult.

- The majority of cases of RHEUMATIC FEVER occur in children, adolescents, and young adults, with the peak age of incidence between five and 15 years.

- Adolescents, who tend to focus heavily on how they look to their peers can be devastated by widespread VITILIGO. The resultant white patches of skin appearing on various parts of their bodies can lead to embarrassment for anyone, but especially for image-conscious adolescents.

Challener, Jill. "Managing Diabetes in Children and Adolescents." *Professional Care of Mother & Child* 9 no. 1 (1999): 11–13.

Plotnick, Leslie, and Randi Henderson. *Clinical Management of the Child and Teenager with Diabetes.* Baltimore, Md.: The Johns Hopkins University Press, 1998.

"Recommendations for Management of Diabetes for Children in School," Oklahoma Department of Health. Available online. URL: www.health.state.ok.us/chds/comanche/Services/School-Diabetes%20Plan.htm. Downloaded 12 July 2002.

Williams, C. "Gender, Adolescence and the Management of Diabetes." *Journal of Advanced Nursing* 30, no. 5 (November 1999): 1160–1166.

African Americans with autoimmune diseases
Some autoimmune diseases occur more frequently in certain minority populations, including African Americans; others occur less frequently.

- ALLERGIC ASTHMA is a growing concern throughout the United States but especially among inner-city African Americans. In a 1993 study among children and young adults, African Americans were three to four times more likely than Caucasians to be hospitalized for asthma and were four to six times more likely to die from asthma. To identify factors responsible for the higher incidence of asthma among inner-city children, the National Institute of Allergy and Infectious Diseases (NIAID) held the National Cooperative Inner-City Asthma Study (1991–94) of 1,528 children and their families. Asthma risk factors found to be present in these urban families included high levels of indoor allergens, especially cockroach allergen, and high levels of nitrogen dioxide, a respiratory irritant produced by inadequately vented stoves and heating appliances. In addition, researchers funded by NIAID have identified genetic changes in interleukin-4 (IL-4) and IL-13, immune-signaling molecules involved in asthma and allergic response, that correlates with asthma severity. This change appears to be much more common among African Americans than among Caucasians.

- A small number of African Americans have INSULIN-DEPENDENT DIABETES mellitus (IDDM), or Type 1 diabetes. The prevalence rate in African-American children aged 15 and younger is about half the prevalence rate in Caucasian American children of the same age. Researchers tend to agree that genetics probably make Type 1 diabetes more common among children with European ancestry. In fact, African-American children with some European ancestry have a slightly higher prevalence of Type 1 diabetes. However, compared with Caucasian Americans, African Americans experience higher rates of three diabetes complications—blindness, kidney failure, and amputations.

- MULTIPLE SCLEROSIS (MS) has always been considered a Caucasian disease, with Caucasians more than twice as likely to develop the incurable, degenerative nerve disease. In June 2000, the Consortium of Multiple Sclerosis Centers/North American Research Committee on MS released demographic information showing 14,420 (89.0 percent) non-Hispanic Caucasians with MS, while only 818 were African Americans (5.1 percent). Now, though, researchers are saying that part of the reason for the disproportion may be that African Americans are not always diagnosed. Because doctors are not expecting to see MS in a non-Caucasian patient, it will get missed far more frequently than it will in Caucasian patients. Instead of coordinating the various symptoms into an MS pattern, doctors treating African-American patients will tend to treat those same symptoms as isolated instances.

- Systemic SCLERODERMA affects more women of African-American than European descent.

- African-American women are the number one target of SYSTEMIC LUPUS ERYTHEMATOSUS (SLE), with the prevalence, incidence, and mortality rates of the disease three times higher in African-American women than in Caucasian women. The reason for this disparity is unknown, with researchers still searching for the answers. No genetic predisposition has been found to be stronger in African Americans than in Caucasians, and lupus is relatively uncommon in West and Central Africa. A serious complication in treatment of lupus among African-American women is their tendency not to be knowledgeable about the disease and their generally nonchalant attitude about health care, relying on home remedies more than professional medical attention. With this in mind, Health and Human Services Secretary Louis Sullivan, M.D., announced in late 1991 a new booklet, "What Black Women Should Know About Lupus," produced by the National Institute of Arthritis and Musculoskeletal and Skin Diseases. A copy is available by writing Lupus Booklet, Box AMS, 9000 Rockville Pike, Bethesda, MD 20892.

- VITILIGO, which leads to the loss of skin pigment, does not strike any particular race or culture more than any other, but it is more noticeable among African Americans. These vitiligo patients have reported psychological problems in dealing with the spreading white patches of skin, which strike at the very core of their identity.

"Asthma: A Concern for Minority Populations," URL: http://www.BlackHealthCare.com/BHC/Asthma/Description.asp. Downloaded 2000.

"Diabetes in African Americans?" URL: http://www.BlackHealthCare.com/BHC/Diabetes/Description.asp. Downloaded 2000.

Zisner, Naome. "Multiple Sclerosis Is Shifting Gears to African-Americans." *The Medical Herald* 13, no. 12 (January 2002): 1, 31.

aging and autoimmune diseases Autoimmune diseases generally peak in middle age and are less common in elderly persons, contrary to what might be expected because of current knowledge about decreased tolerance to self with age. On the other hand, autoantibodies (see AUTOANTIBODY) do increase with age and may play a role in some of the degenerative diseases of aging. However, several autoimmune diseases do have particular ramifications for older people:

- BULLOUS PEMPHIGOID typically occurs in middle-aged or elderly persons.

- CELIAC DISEASE is being increasingly recognized in older people. It has a peak incidence in the fourth decade in women and the sixth and seventh decades in men.

- CICATRICIAL PEMPHIGOID is predominantly a disease of the elderly, most often occurring between 60 and 80 years of age.

- COLD AGGLUTININ DISEASE most commonly affects elderly persons.

- According to Chau and Edelman, "Lean elderly diabetic patients may even display features of autoimmune changes normally attributed to younger Type 1 diabetic patients. Islet cell antibodies and marked insulin deficiency are increasingly seen in lean elderly diabetic patients. Thus, it is important to remember that both Type 1 (insulin-dependent) and type 2 (non-insulin-dependent) diabetes occur in the elderly."

- HASHIMOTO'S (chronic lymphoid) THYROIDITIS is more prevalent in women than in men, and its incidence increases with age, especially in women after age 40.

- MÉNIÈRE'S DISEASE occurs more frequently in males than in females, with the onset usually after the age of 50.

- NEUTROPENIA has a higher incidence rate among elderly individuals than younger people.

- PERIPHERAL NEUROPATHY most commonly affects those of middle age and the elderly.

- POLYMYALGIA RHEUMATICA is fairly common and generally occurs in people 50 years of age and

older, with 70 the average age at onset. Women are affected two times more frequently than men, and the condition occurs predominantly in Caucasians.

- SJÖGREN'S SYNDROME affects especially older women and is often associated with RHEUMATOID ARTHRITIS, which generally starts between the ages of 20 and 50 but is occurring with increasing frequency in older people.

- TEMPORAL ARTERITIS is almost unheard of in people under 50 years of age. Among people over 50, it strikes about one person in 1,000. It is at least 10 times as common in those over 80 years of age as in those between 50 and 59 years of age. Temporal arteritis is twice as common in women as in men.

Chau, Diane, and Steven V. Edelman. "Clinical Management of Diabetes in the Elderly: Practical Pointers." *Clinical Diabetes* 19, no. 4 (April 2001): 172–175.
Michel, Jean-Pierre, and Jacques Proust. "Aging and the Immune System," in *The Merck Manual of Geriatrics*. Whitehouse Station, N.J.: Merck & Co., 2000, pp. 1,351–1,359.

agranulocytes Nongranular leukocytes (white blood cells). The agranulocytes include the monocytes and the lymphocytes.

AIDS Acquired immunodeficiency syndrome, AIDS applies to the most advanced stages of infection with the human immunodeficiency virus (HIV). AIDS was first reported in the United States in 1981 and has since become a major worldwide epidemic that affects tens of millions of people. The majority of people with AIDS are between the ages of 15 and 44, poor, heterosexual, and live in developing nations in Africa and Asia.

More than 700,000 cases of AIDS have been reported in the United States since 1981, and as many as 900,000 Americans may be infected with HIV. AIDS is the leading cause of death among Americans between the ages of 25 and 44. The epidemic is growing most rapidly among minority populations and is a leading killer of African-American males. According to the U.S. Centers for Disease Control and Prevention (CDC), AIDS affects nearly seven times more African Americans than non-Hispanic Caucasians and three times more Hispanics than non-Hispanic Caucasians.

People diagnosed with AIDS may get life-threatening diseases called opportunistic infections, which are caused by microbes such as viruses or bacteria that usually do not make healthy people sick.

The CDC developed official criteria for the definition of AIDS and is responsible for tracking the spread of AIDS in the United States. The CDC's definition of AIDS includes all HIV-infected people who have fewer than 200 CD4+ T cells per cubic millimeter of blood. (Healthy adults usually have CD4+ T cell counts of 1,000 or more.) In addition, the definition includes 26 clinical conditions that affect people with advanced HIV disease. Most of these conditions are opportunistic infections that generally do not affect healthy people. In people with AIDS, these infections are often severe and sometimes fatal because the immune system is so ravaged by HIV that the body cannot fight off certain bacteria, viruses, fungi, parasites, and other microbes.

Many people are so debilitated by the symptoms of AIDS that they cannot hold steady employment or do household chores. Other people with AIDS may experience phases of intense life-threatening illness followed by phases in which they function normally.

A small number of people (fewer than 50) first infected with HIV 10 or more years ago have not developed symptoms of AIDS. Scientists are trying to determine what factors may account for their lack of progression to AIDS, such as particular characteristics of their immune systems, whether they were infected with a less aggressive strain of the virus, or if their genes may protect them from the effects of HIV. Scientists hope that understanding the body's natural method of control may lead to ideas for protective HIV vaccines and use of vaccines to prevent the disease from progressing.

Causes

AIDS is caused by the human immunodeficiency virus (HIV). By killing or damaging cells of the body's immune system, HIV progressively destroys the body's ability to fight infections and certain cancers. A person most frequently contracts HIV through sexual intercourse with a person who has the virus, a blood transfusion from a donor who has the virus, or sharing drug needles with a person who has the virus.

Clinical Features

Symptoms of opportunistic infections common in people with AIDS include coughing and shortness of breath, seizures and lack of coordination, difficult or painful swallowing, mental symptoms such as confusion and forgetfulness, severe and persistent diarrhea, fever, vision loss, nausea, abdominal cramps and vomiting, weight loss and extreme fatigue, severe headaches, and coma.

Children with AIDS may get the same opportunistic infections as do adults with the disease. In addition, they also have severe forms of the bacterial infections all children may get, such as conjunctivitis (pinkeye), ear infections, and tonsillitis. Children may grow slowly or be sick a lot.

During the course of HIV infection, most people experience a gradual decline in the number of CD4+ T cells, although some may have abrupt and dramatic drops in their CD4+ T cell counts. A person with CD4+ T cells above 200 may experience some of the early symptoms of HIV disease. Others may have no symptoms even though their CD4+ T cell count is below 200.

As the immune system deteriorates, a variety of complications start to take over. For many people, their first sign of infection is large lymph nodes or "swollen glands" that may be enlarged for more than three months. Other symptoms often experienced months to years before the onset of AIDS include lack of energy, weight loss, frequent fevers and sweats, persistent or frequent yeast infections (oral or vaginal), persistent skin rashes or flaky skin, pelvic inflammatory disease in women that does not respond to treatment, and short-term memory loss. Some people develop frequent and severe herpes infections that cause mouth, genital, or anal sores or develop a painful nerve disease called shingles.

Complications

People with AIDS are particularly prone to developing various cancers, especially those caused by viruses such as Kaposi's sarcoma and cervical cancer or cancers of the immune system known as lymphomas. These cancers are usually more aggressive and difficult to treat in people with AIDS. Signs of Kaposi's sarcoma in light-skinned people are round brown, reddish, or purple spots that develop in the skin or in the mouth. In dark-skinned people, the spots are more pigmented.

Treatment

When AIDS first surfaced in the United States, there were no medicines to combat the underlying immune deficiency and few treatments existed for the opportunistic diseases that resulted. Over the past 10 years, however, researchers have developed drugs to fight both HIV infection and its associated infections and cancers.

The U.S. Food and Drug Administration (FDA) has approved a number of drugs for treating HIV infection. The first group of drugs used to treat HIV infection, called nucleoside reverse transcriptase (RT) inhibitors, interrupts an early stage of the virus from making copies of itself. Included in this class of drugs (called nucleoside analogs) are AZT (also known as zidovudine or ZDV), ddC (zalcitabine), ddI (dideoxyinosine), d4T (stavudine), and 3TC (lamivudine). These drugs may slow the spread of HIV in the body and delay the onset of opportunistic infections.

Doctors also prescribe nonnucleoside reverse transcriptase inhibitors (NNRTIs), such as delvaridine (Rescriptor), nevirapine (Viramune), and efravirenz (Sustiva), in combination with other antiretroviral drugs.

More recently, the FDA has approved a second class of drugs for treating HIV infection. These drugs, called protease inhibitors, interrupt virus replication at a later step in the virus's life cycle. They include ritonavir (Norvir), saquinivir (Invirase), indinavir (Crixivan), amprenivir (Agenerase), nelfinavir (Viracept), and lopinavir (Kaletra). Because HIV can become resistant to any of these drugs, health care providers must use a combination treatment to suppress the virus effectively.

Currently available antiretroviral drugs do not cure people of HIV infection or AIDS, however, and they all have side effects that can be severe. Some of the nucleoside RT inhibitors may cause a depletion of red or white blood cells, especially when taken in the later stages of the disease. Some may also cause an inflammation of the pancreas and painful nerve damage. There have been reports of complications and other severe reactions, including death, attributed to some of the antiretroviral nucleoside analogs when used alone or in combination. Therefore, health care experts recommend that people on antiretroviral therapy be routinely seen and followed up by their providers.

The most common side effects associated with protease inhibitors include nausea, diarrhea, and other gastrointestinal symptoms. In addition, protease inhibitors can interact with other drugs, resulting in serious side effects.

Researchers have credited highly active antiretroviral therapy, or HAART, as being a major factor in reducing the number of deaths from AIDS in this country by 47 percent in 1997. HAART is a treatment regimen that uses a combination of reverse transcriptase inhibitors and protease inhibitors to treat patients. Patients who are newly infected with HIV as well as AIDS patients can take the combination.

Although HAART is not a cure for AIDS, it has greatly improved the health of many people with AIDS. It also reduces the amount of virus circulating in the blood to nearly undetectable levels. Researchers have shown that HAART cannot eradicate HIV entirely from the body, however. HIV remains present, lurking in hiding places such as the lymph nodes, the brain, the testes, and the retina of the eye, even in patients who have been treated.

A number of drugs are available to help treat opportunistic infections to which people with HIV are especially prone. These drugs include foscarnet and ganciclovir to treat cytomegalovirus eye infections, fluconazole to treat yeast and other fungal infections, trimethoprim/sulfamethoxazole (TMP/SMX) or pentamidine to treat *Pneumocystis carinii* pneumonia (PCP).

In addition to antiretroviral therapy, physicians treat adults with HIV whose CD4+ T cell counts drop below 200 to prevent the occurrence of PCP, which is one of the most common and deadly opportunistic infections associated with HIV. They give children PCP preventive therapy when their CD4+ T cell counts drop to levels considered below normal for their age group. Regardless of their CD4+ T cell counts, HIV-infected children and adults who have survived an episode of PCP take drugs for the rest of their lives to prevent a recurrence of the pneumonia.

HIV-infected individuals who develop Kaposi's sarcoma or other cancers are treated with radiation, chemotherapy, or injections of alpha interferon, a genetically engineered, naturally occurring protein.

Alcamo, Edward I. *AIDS in the Modern World.* Malden, Mass.: Blackwell Publishing, 2002.

Altman, Lawrence K. "The Doctor's World: The AIDS Questions That Linger," *New York Times* 30 January 2001, Section F, Page 1, Column 1.

Sande, Merle A., and Paul Volberding, eds. *The Medical Management of AIDS.* Philadelphia: W. B. Saunders Co., 1999.

Stine, Gerald J. *AIDS Update 2001: An Annual Overview of Acquired Immune Deficiency Syndrome.* Upper Saddle River, N.J.: Prentice Hall College Division, 2000.

AIDS research   Researchers supported by the National Institute of Allergy and Infectious Diseases (NIAID) are conducting numerous studies on HIV infection, including developing and testing HIV vaccines and new therapies for the disease and some of its associated conditions. Investigators are testing 29 HIV vaccines in people and are developing or testing many drugs for HIV infection or AIDS-associated opportunistic infections. NIAID-supported investigators also continue to trace how the disease progresses in different people.

Researchers are also investigating exactly how HIV damages the immune system. Recent advances in this area include using the body's own antibodies to slow down the replication of HIV. The natural ability to fight off HIV is lost early in the infection process (or retained longer by some individuals who have slow progression of disease). Researchers are trying to learn how this response is lost and how to restore it by therapy.

Scientists are also investigating and testing chemical barriers, such as topical microbicides, that people can use in the vagina or in the rectum during sex to prevent HIV transmission. They are also looking at other ways to prevent transmission, such as controlling sexually transmitted diseases and modifying people's behavior, as well as ways to prevent transmission from mother to child.

Grady, Denise. "AIDS at 20: Scientists Shifting Strategies in Quest for an AIDS Vaccine," *New York Times,* 5 June 2001, Section F, Page 1, Column 1.

Alaska Natives and autoimmune diseases   In a study conducted by the Alaska Native Medical Center, Anchorage, and presented in 1998, the prevalence in Alaska Natives of autoimmune hepatitis (AIH) was 41.3 per 100,000, and the prevalence of PRIMARY BILIARY CIRRHOSIS (PBC) was 13.4 per 100,000. This rate of AIH is more than twice as high as and this rate of PBC is as high as previously reported in other populations.

The Alaska Native Medical Center also maintains a database for their clients with arthritis around the state, most of whom are Alaska Natives. Rheumatoid arthritis is more prevalent among the Inupiat of the North Slope area and the Tlingit of Southeast Alaska but not among other groups. However, the Yupik, who share common ancestry with the Inupiat, have prevalence rates within the same range as the general United States population. The prevalence of SYSTEMIC LUPUS ERYTHEMATOSUS is also elevated among the Tlingit. (See HEPATITIS [AUTOIMMUNE].)

alcohol, effects on autoimmune diseases   Abuse of alcohol can weaken the immune system, and some scientists believe it may play some role in autoimmune diseases. However, PRIMARY BILIARY CIRRHOSIS (PBC), a slow-acting, chronic autoimmune liver disease, is not alcohol related. Like most chronic liver diseases, though, PBC can impair the capacity of the liver to break down toxic drugs and chemicals. These include prescribed and over-the-counter medicines, alcohol, and even foods. CARDIOMYOPATHY, a disease of the heart muscle, has been linked to alcohol because alcohol has a direct suppressant effect on the heart. Dilated cardiomyopathy can be caused by chronic, excessive consumption of alcohol, particularly in combination with dietary deficiencies. Although no scientific evidence has tied alcohol directly to FIBROMYALGIA, many fibromyalgia patients have expressed an intolerance for it. Similarly, INTERSTITIAL CYSTITIS

(IC) patients and their doctors have reported a possible connection between alcohol and bladder irritation and inflammation. Doctors have also suggested that abstaining from alcohol may soften and spread out the attacks of MÉNIÈRE'S DISEASE.

allergen A substance that can cause an allergic reaction. In some people, the immune system recognizes allergens as "dangerous," but in most people, allergens cause no harm. For those allergic people, airborne allergens (in the form of mold, dander, pollen, and so on) enter their eyes, nose, and lungs where the allergens provoke the immune system to react.

When an allergic person first comes into contact with an allergen, the immune system treats the allergen as an invader and mobilizes to attack. The immune system does this by generating large amounts of a type of antibody (a disease-fighting protein) called immunoglobin E, or IgE. Each IgE antibody is specific for one particular allergenic (allergy-producing) substance. In the case of pollen allergy, the antibody is specific for each type of pollen: one type of antibody may be produced to react against oak pollen and another against ragweed pollen, for example. Other common allergens include certain contactants (such as chemicals and plants), drugs (such as antibiotics and serums), foods (such as milk, chocolate, strawberries, and wheat), infectious agents (such as bacteria, viruses, and animal parasites), and physical agents (such as heat, light, friction, and radiation).

allergic asthma Also called bronchial asthma, allergic asthma is an inflammatory disorder of the lungs characterized by recurring bouts of coughing, wheezing, and difficulty breathing that occur when the small breathing tubes in the lungs narrow and fill up with sticky mucus. Allergies are involved in many cases of asthma, especially in children. Allergic asthma affects about 3 million children (8 to 12 percent of all children) and 7 million adults in the United States at a cost estimated at $6.2 billion a year. About 90 percent of children and 50 percent to 70 percent of adults who have asthma have allergic asthma. Although asthma usually begins in childhood and half of those affected will outgrow it

by adolescence, it can also occur for the first time at any age. There is often an allergic background and a tendency for asthma to run in families. The National Institute of Allergy and Infectious Diseases estimates that asthma incidence has increased 75 percent in the United States since 1980 for reasons that are not fully understood. Asthma-related hospitalizations have also increased 20 percent in recent years despite more aggressive treatment. Asthma affects an estimated 17 million Americans.

Symptoms develop when an environmental allergen, such as pollen or animal dander, is breathed into the lungs. The body recognizes it as a foreign substance and produces special antibodies to fight this invader. The antibody involved in asthma is known as IgE (called immunoglobulin E). These IgE molecules are special because IgE is the only class of antibody that attaches tightly to the body's mast cells, which are tissue cells, and to basophils, which are blood cells. When the allergen next encounters its specific IgE, it attaches to the antibody like a key fitting into a lock, signaling the cell to which the IgE is attached to release (and in some cases to produce) powerful inflammatory chemicals like histamine, cytokines, and leukotrienes. These chemicals act on tissues in various parts of the body, such as the respiratory system, and cause the symptoms of allergy.

Asthma can be disabling and can sometimes be fatal. If wheezing and shortness of breath accompany allergy symptoms, it is a signal that the bronchial tubes have also become involved, indicating the need for medical attention.

Though death from asthma is relatively rare, it is becoming more frequent. Asthma mortality in the United States declined by nearly 8 percent per year during the 1970s. However, by 1977, the trend reversed, and the number of deaths due to asthma began to climb steadily, increasing about 6 percent per year. Asthma killed 1,674 Americans in 1977. However, by 1991, the death rate had risen to 5,106 (from 0.8 to 2.0 per 100,000 people). Although most asthmatics who die of the disease are over 50 years old, rates of asthma death have increased in almost all age groups.

Although some evidence suggests that asthma's death toll could be leveling off, the rising rate of hospital admissions and emergency room and doctor's office visits for asthma suggests that the disease is actually becoming more severe. Between 1965 and 1983, hospitalization rates for asthma increased by 50 percent in adults and over 200 percent in children. Approximately 4.5 percent more children were hospitalized for asthma each year from 1979 to 1987.

Causes

The exact cause of allergic asthma is unknown. Children with an asthmatic parent are much more likely to become asthmatic themselves, indicating a probable important genetic role in the disease. Some people have an underlying predisposition. There is strong evidence that exposure to allergens in early life increases the risk of developing asthma.

Some researchers theorize that the decline in serious infectious diseases may be a factor in the increase in allergic asthma. They speculate that an underutilized immune system may overreact to lesser threats or irritants, inappropriately producing antibody molecules that result in a release of histamines and other inflammatory substances in the lungs. Other researchers implicate the increased time youngsters spend indoors—and their resulting exposure to the carpeting and other allergen catchers that people in developed nations surround themselves with.

What is known more clearly is that dust mites (which are living creatures that produce droppings that contain a highly allergenic protein), cockroaches, molds, pollens, and domesticated animals produce some of the allergens known to trigger asthma attacks. A study is now under way to determine the roles of other key environmental agents in asthma, both in bringing on respiratory crises and initiating the illness in the first place. The research is being supported jointly by scientists at the National Institute of Environmental Health Sciences and the National Institute of Allergy and Infectious Diseases, two divisions of the National Institutes of Health.

Clinical Features

Asthma attacks may last only a few minutes or for several days. An episode can be mild or a painful struggle to breathe. When the symptoms are apparently caused by an allergy because the patient's medical history indicates that the symptoms recur at the same time each year, a seasonal allergen (like pollen) is likely involved. Allergists (physicians specializing in the diagnosis and treatment of allergies) recognize the patterns of potential allergens common during local seasons and the association between these patterns and symptoms. The medical history suggests which allergens are the likely culprits. Also, the mucous membranes will often appear swollen and pale or bluish in persons with allergic conditions.

Complications

Asthma patients exposed to tobacco smoke have been known to have decreased levels of pulmonary function and increased need for medication. Asthma sufferers have also been shown to have increased prevalence of aspirin sensitivity as they have grown older or suffered from greater severity asthma. Also, viral respiratory infections can exacerbate asthma, particularly in children under the age of 10. For this reason, annual influenza vaccinations are usually recommended for patients with persistent asthma.

Chronic lung disease, including asthma, increases osteoporosis risk. In one study, men with asthma or chronic obstructive pulmonary disease (COPD) were found to have a five times greater risk for osteoporosis than healthy men. The risk was nine times greater in those who used inhaled or used oral glucocorticoid medications. The study did not track bone density in women with asthma, but it is believed that menopausal women face an even higher risk than men.

Treatment

As yet, there is no real cure for asthma. The drugs used to treat it either prevent the occurrence of an attack or control asthma symptoms by reducing the frequency and severity of attacks and reversing airflow obstruction.

Asthma medications are categorized into two general classes: *long-term-control* medications taken daily on a long-term basis to control persistent asthma and *quick-relief* medications taken to provide prompt reversal of acute airflow obstruction and relief of accompanying bronchoconstriction. Long-term-control medications include corticosteroids, cromolyn sodium and nedocromil, beta2-agonists, methylxanthines, and the newer leukotriene modifiers. Quick-relief medications include short-acting inhaled beta2-agonists, anticholinergics, systemic steroids, and corticosteroids.

Antihistamines, the mainstay of allergy treatment, are available over-the-counter and by prescription. These medications work by blocking the effects of histamines, the chemicals that cause many allergy symptoms. Some antihistamines can be sedating. Corticosteroid nasal sprays are often recommended to reduce nasal inflammation and the accompanying congestion, sneezing, and runny nose. Another treatment option is a decongestant, which helps to dry up tissues in the nasal passages and reduce the swelling that causes nasal stuffiness.

If symptoms are severe or chronic, an allergist may suggest a series of allergy shots. These injections contain tiny amounts of the substance to which a person is allergic. If given regularly, they gradually desensitize the body to the offending allergens.

Friebele, Elaine. "The Attack of Asthma." *Environmental Health Perspectives* 104, no. 1 (January 1996): 22–25.

National Heart, Lung, and Blood Institute, *Practical Guide for the Diagnosis and Management of Asthma.* Based on the Expert Panel Report 2: *Guidelines for the Diagnosis and Management of Asthma.* NIH Publication No. 97-4053, October 1997.

National Institute of Environmental Health Sciences, *Asthma and Its Environmental Triggers: Scientists Take a Practical New Look at a Familiar Illness.* NIEHS Fact Sheet #9, July 1997.

allergic reaction   An adverse immune system response to a specific substance (allergen) to which a person is exposed.

allergic rhinitis   An inflammation of the mucous membranes lining the nose, caused by an allergy to pollen, dander, or other airborne particles. Allergic rhinitis is commonly known as "hay fever." This is a misnomer because hay does not cause allergic rhinitis, and no fever is involved. Allergic rhinitis results in a combination of symptoms affecting the eyes and nasal passages. These symptoms are caused by an allergic reaction to pollen and a variety of other allergens. Allergic rhinitis may occur only during certain seasons or persist year-round.

Allergic rhinitis that lasts all year may be difficult to distinguish from other forms of rhinitis not caused by an allergic reaction, such as polyps or a sinus condition. Allergic rhinitis often occurs together with asthma and can make asthma symptoms worse.

Allergic rhinitis, also known as hay fever, is the most common allergy type, afflicting 15 percent of Americans. People with allergic rhinitis may be allergic to pollen, ragweed, dust, mold, animal dander, or feathers. Allergies may be seasonal or may persist year-round.

People with allergy symptoms, such as the runny nose of allergic rhinitis, may at first suspect they have a cold—but the "cold" lingers on. It is important to see a doctor about any respiratory illness that lasts longer than a week or two.

Uy, William C. *Healing from Allergy (Hay Fever & Perennial Rhinitis) and Vasometer Rhinitis.* William C. Uy Book Marketing, 2000.

allergy   An inappropriate, abnormal, or exaggerated reaction of the immune system to certain substances, called allergens. In similar amounts and circumstances, these substances are harmless to nonallergic people. Overall, allergic diseases are among the major causes of illness and disability in the United States, affecting as many as 40 to 50 million Americans.

Among the most common allergens are animal danders, pollens, house dust, dust mites, molds, some drugs, and foods such as fish, eggs, milk, strawberries, tomatoes, and nuts. Insect bites, such as from mosquitoes, wasps, and bees, can also cause allergic reactions. In addition, substances such as feathers, wool, dyes, cosmetics, and perfumes sometimes act as allergens. In a susceptible person (or allergic person), one of these normally harmless substances is perceived as a threat and is attacked by the immune system.

Allergic people make a special type of antibody called immunoglobulin E (IgE), which is responsible for most allergic reactions. Allergy sufferers have 10 times as much IgE in their blood as nonallergic people. The reaction between allergens and IgE antibodies causes the release of substances such as histamine, which produce allergic symptoms in the skin, the nose, the eyes, the chest, and so on.

This allergic reaction can manifest itself as hay fever, asthma, eczema, hives, or other symptoms.

Doctors use skin tests to determine whether a patient has IgE antibodies in the skin that react to a specific allergen. The doctor will use diluted extracts from allergens such as dust mites, pollens, or molds commonly found in the local area. The extract of each kind of allergen is injected under the patient's skin or is applied to a tiny scratch or puncture made on the patient's arm or back.

Skin tests are also one way of measuring the level of IgE antibody in a patient. With a positive reaction, a small, raised, reddened area (called a wheal) with a surrounding flush (called a flare) will appear at the test site. The size of the wheal can give the physician an important diagnostic clue, but a positive reaction does not prove that a particular pollen is the cause of a patient's symptoms. Although such a reaction indicates that IgE antibody to a specific allergen is present in the skin, respiratory symptoms do not necessarily result.

Although skin testing is the most sensitive and least costly way to identify allergies in patients, some patients, such as those with widespread skin conditions like eczema, should not be tested using that method. Other diagnostic tests use a blood sample from the patient to detect levels of IgE antibody to a particular allergen. One such blood test is called the RAST (radioallergosorbent test), which can be performed when eczema is present or if a patient has taken medications that interfere with skin testing.

Treatment

Doctors are three general approaches to help people with allergies: advise them on ways to avoid the allergen as much as possible, prescribe medication to relieve symptoms, and give a series of allergy shots. Although there is no cure for allergies, one of these strategies or a combination of them can provide varying degrees of relief from allergy symptoms.

Avoidance Complete avoidance of allergenic pollen or mold means moving to a place where the offending substance does not grow and where it is not present in the air. However, even this extreme solution may offer only temporary relief since a person who is sensitive to a specific pollen or mold may

subsequently develop allergies to new allergens after repeated exposure. For example, people allergic to ragweed may leave their ragweed-ridden communities and relocate to areas where ragweed does not grow, only to develop allergies to other weeds or even to grasses or trees in their new surroundings. Because relocating is not a reliable solution, allergy specialists do not encourage this approach.

There are other ways to evade the offending pollen: remaining indoors in the morning, for example, when the outdoor pollen levels are highest. Sunny, windy days can be especially troublesome. If individuals with pollen allergy must work outdoors, they can wear face masks designed to filter pollen out of the air and keep it from reaching their nasal passages. As another approach, some people take their vacations at the height of the expected pollinating period and choose a location where such exposure would be minimal. The seashore, for example, may be an effective retreat for many with pollen allergies.

Mold allergens can be difficult to avoid, but some steps can be taken at least to reduce exposure to them. First, the allergy sufferer should avoid those hot spots mentioned earlier where molds tend to be concentrated. The lawn should be mowed and leaves should be raked up, but someone other than the allergic person should do these chores. If such work cannot be delegated, wearing a tightly fitting dust mask can greatly reduce exposure and resulting symptoms. Travel in the country, especially on dry, windy days or while crops are being harvested, should be avoided as should walks through tall vegetation. A summer cabin closed up all winter is probably full of molds and should be aired out and cleaned before a mold-sensitive person stays there.

Around the home, a dehumidifier will help dry out the basement. However, the water extracted from the air must be removed frequently to prevent mold growth in the machine.

Those with dust mite allergies should pay careful attention to dust proofing their bedrooms. The worst things to have in the bedroom are wall-to-wall carpets, venetian blinds, down-filled blankets, feather pillows, heating vents with forced hot air, dogs, cats, and closets full of clothing. Shades are preferred over venetian blinds because they do not trap dust. Curtains can be used if they are washed periodically in hot water to kill the dust mites. Most important, bedding should be encased in a zippered, plastic, airtight, and dust-proof cover.

Although shag carpets are the worst type for the dust mite-sensitive person, all carpets trap dust and make dust control impossible. In addition, vacuuming can contribute to the amount of dust unless the vacuum is equipped with a special high-efficiency particulate air (HEPA) filter. Wall-to-wall carpets should be replaced with washable throw rugs over hardwood, tile, or linoleum floors. Rugs on concrete floors encourage dust mite growth and should be avoided.

Reducing the amount of dust mites in a home may require new cleaning techniques as well as some changes in furnishings to eliminate dust collectors. Water is often the secret to effective dust removal. Washable items should be washed often using water hotter then 130 degrees Fahrenheit. Lower temperatures will not kill dust mites. If the water temperature must be set at a lower value, items can be washed at a commercial establishment that uses high wash temperatures. Dusting with a damp cloth or oiled mop should be done frequently.

The best way for a person allergic to pets, especially cats, to avoid allergic reactions is to find another home for the animal. Some suggestions, however, help lower the levels of cat allergens in the air: bathe the cat weekly and brush it more frequently (ideally, this should be done by someone other than the allergic person), remove carpets and soft furnishings, and use a vacuum cleaner with a high-efficiency filter and a room air cleaner (see section below). Wearing a face mask while house and cat cleaning and keeping the cat out of the bedroom are other methods that allow many people to live more happily with their pets.

Irritants such as chemicals can worsen airborne allergy symptoms and should be avoided as much as possible. For example, during periods of high pollen levels, people with pollen allergies should try to avoid unnecessary exposure to irritants such as insect sprays, tobacco smoke, air pollution, and fresh tar or paint.

Air conditioners and filters When possible, an allergic person should use air conditioners inside the home or in a car to help prevent pollen and mold allergens from entering. Various types of air-filtering devices made with fiberglass or electrically charged plates may help reduce allergens produced in the home. These can be added to the heating and cooling systems. In addition, portable devices that can be used in individual rooms are especially helpful in reducing animal allergens.

An allergy specialist can suggest which kind of filter is best for the home of a particular patient. Before buying a filtering device, the patient should rent one and use it in a closed room (the bedroom, for instance) for a month or two to see whether allergy symptoms diminish. The airflow should be sufficient to exchange the air in the room five or six times per hour; therefore, the size and efficiency of the filtering device should be determined in part by the size of the room.

Persons with allergies should be wary of exaggerated claims for appliances that cannot really clean the air. Very small air cleaners cannot remove dust and pollen—and no air purifier can prevent viral or bacterial diseases such as influenza, pneumonia, or tuberculosis. Buyers of electrostatic precipitators should compare the machine's ozone output with federal standards. Ozone can irritate the nose and airways of persons with allergies, especially those with asthma, and can increase the allergy symptoms. Other kinds of air filters, such as HEPA filters, do not release ozone into the air. HEPA filters, however, require adequate air flow to force air through them and must be changed periodically.

Medications For people who find they cannot adequately avoid airborne allergens, the symptoms can often be controlled with medications. Effective medications that can be prescribed by a physician include antihistamines and topical nasal steroids —either of which can be used alone or in combination. Many effective antihistamines and decongestants are also available without a prescription.

ANTIHISTAMINES As the name indicates, an antihistamine counters the effects of histamine, which is released by the mast cells in the body's tissues and contributes to allergy symptoms. For many years, antihistamines have proven useful in relieving sneezing and itching in the nose, throat, and eyes and in reducing nasal swelling and drainage.

Many people who take antihistamines experience some distressing side effects: drowsiness and loss of alertness and coordination. In children, such reactions can be misinterpreted as behavior problems. During the last few years, however, antihistamines that cause fewer of these side effects have become available by prescription. These nonsedating antihistamines are as effective as other antihistamines in preventing histamine-induced symptoms but do so without causing sleepiness. Some of these nonsedating antihistamines, however, can have serious side effects, particularly if they are taken with certain other drugs. A patient should always let the doctor know what other medications he/she is taking.

TOPICAL NASAL STEROIDS This medication should not be confused with anabolic steroids, which are sometimes used by athletes to enlarge muscle mass and can have serious side effects. Topical nasal steroids are anti-inflammatory drugs that stop the allergic reaction. In addition to other beneficial actions, they reduce the number of mast cells in the nose and reduce mucus secretion and nasal swelling. The combination of antihistamines and nasal steroids is a very effective way to treat allergic rhinitis, especially in people with moderate or severe allergic rhinitis. Although topical nasal steroids can have side effects, they are safe when used at recommended doses. Some of the newer agents are even safer than older ones.

CROMOLYN SODIUM Cromolyn sodium for allergic rhinitis is a nasal spray that in some people helps to prevent allergic reactions from starting. When administered as a nasal spray, it can safely inhibit the release of chemicals like histamine from the mast cell. It has few side effects when used as directed and significantly helps some patients with allergies.

DECONGESTANTS Sometimes reestablishing drainage of the nasal passages will help to relieve symptoms such as congestion, swelling, excess secretions, and discomfort in the sinus areas that can be caused by nasal allergies. (These sinus areas are hollow air spaces located within the bones of the skull surrounding the nose.) The doctor may recommend using oral or nasal decongestants to reduce congestion along with an antihistamine to control allergic symptoms. Over-the-counter and

prescription decongestant nose drops and sprays, however, should not be used for more than a few days. When used for longer periods, these drugs can lead to even more congestion and swelling of the nasal passages.

Immunotherapy Immunotherapy, or a series of allergy shots, is the only available treatment that has a chance of reducing the allergy symptoms over a longer period of time. Patients receive subcutaneous (under the skin) injections of increasing concentrations of the allergen(s) to which they are sensitive. These injections reduce the amount of IgE antibodies in the blood and cause the body to make a protective antibody called IgG. Many patients with allergic rhinitis will have a significant reduction in their hay fever symptoms and in their need for medication within 12 months of starting immunotherapy. Patients who benefit from immunotherapy may continue it for three years and then consider stopping. Although many patients are able to stop the injections with good, long-term results, some do get worse after immunotherapy is stopped. As better allergens for immunotherapy are produced, this technique will become an even more effective treatment.

Cutler, Ellen W. *Winning the War Against Immune Disorders and Allergies: A Drug Free Cure for Allergies.* Albany, N.Y.: Delmar Publishers, 1998.
Roberts, Angela M., and Matthew R. Walker, eds. *Allergic Mechanisms and Immunotherapeutic Strategies.* New York: Wiley, 1997.
"Something in the Air: Airborne Allergens," National Institute of Allergy and Infectious Diseases. Available online. URL: http://www.niaid.nih.gov/publications, allergens/title.htm. Updated 21 May 2001.

allograft Transplant tissue from one individual to another, as in bone marrow or organ transplants. Recipients of allografts take immunosuppressive drugs to prevent tissue rejection.

alopecia areata A disease in which the hair suddenly falls out, at times as quickly as within one or two days. It usually affects the scalp, often involving one side of the head more than the other, but hair loss can occur elsewhere on the body, including the falling out of eyebrows and eyelashes. Unlike mechanical damage to the hair, no stubble of regrowth can be found in the affected areas, so the scalp looks as if it is naturally hairless. Alopecia areata usually starts with one or more small, round, smooth patches. It occurs in males and females of all ages and races but most frequently during childhood. It is estimated that approximately 2 percent of the U.S. population, or more than 4.5 million people, will be affected at some point in their lives.

Scientists suspect it is an autoimmune disease, with the affected hair follicles mistakenly being attacked in groups by the person's own white blood cells, resulting in the disruption of normal hair formation. These affected follicles become very small, drastically slow down production, and grow no hair visible above the surface for months or years. Biopsies of affected skin show immune cells (lymphocytes) inside of the hair follicles where they are not normally present and with no known reason for their presence.

Some people develop only a few bare patches that regrow hair within a year. In others, extensive patchy loss occurs. In a few, all scalp hair is lost (referred to as alopecia totalis) or hair is lost from the entire scalp and body (referred to as alopecia universalis). No matter how widespread the hair loss, the hair follicles remain alive and are ready to resume normal hair production whenever they receive the appropriate signal. Spontaneous remission of the disease, along with hair regrowth, may occur even where there has been no treatment and even after many years or hair loss. It also can fall out again with no warning, even after it has grown back in. However, alopecia areata occurring at a young age or over a prolonged period often has a less satisfactory recovery.

Causes

The specific cause of alopecia areata is unknown, although a family history of alopecia is present in about 20 percent of all cases. Those who develop alopecia areata for the first time after age 30 are less likely to see it in another family member. Those who develop their first patch of alopecia areata before the age of 30 have a higher possibility that other family members will also have it.

It is not known what triggers the immune system to suppress the hair follicle nor whether the stimulus comes from outside the body like a virus or from inside. Recent research indicates that some persons have genetic markers that increase both their susceptibility to develop alopecia areata as well as the degree of disease severity. There is no known prevention.

Alopecia areata often occurs in families whose members have had asthma, hay fever, atopic eczema, or autoimmune diseases such as thyroid disease, early-onset diabetes, rheumatoid arthritis, lupus erythematosus, vitiligo, pernicious anemia, or Addison's disease.

Clinical Features

Roundish patches of hair loss with smooth hairless scalp in the affected areas, complete loss of all scalp hair, or complete loss of all body hair. Diagnosis is made with the finding of exclamation point hair in areas of hair loss. These hairs are short, broken-off hairs that are narrower closer to the scalp (thereby looking like an exclamation point). In some cases, a biopsy of the scalp is necessary for diagnosis. In some people, the nails develop a fine pitting that looks as if a pin had made rows of tiny dents. In a few, the nails are severely distorted into abnormal shapes. However, other than the hair and occasionally the nails, no other part of the body is affected.

Complications

Permanent hair loss can occur. Alopecia areata is not medically disabling; persons with alopecia areata are usually in excellent health. Emotionally, however, this disease can be challenging, especially for those with extensive hair loss. One of the purposes of the National Alopecia Areata Foundation is to reach out to individuals and families with alopecia areata and help them live full, productive lives.

Treatment

In about half the cases, hair will regrow within a year without any treatment. For those cases where the hair does not resume growth on its own, no fully effective treatments are available. As with many chronic disorders for which there is no proven treatment, a variety of remedies are promoted that, in fact, have no benefit. Those treatments that are used are most effective in milder cases. Current treatments do not stop the alopecia areata. Instead, they stimulate the follicle to produce hair again, and treatments need to be continued until the disease turns itself off.

The most common treatment where there is less than 50 percent of scalp hair loss is the injection of cortisone into the bare skin patches. The injections are usually given by a dermatologist who uses a tiny needle to give easily tolerated, multiple injections into the skin in and around the bare patches. The injections are repeated once a month. If new hair growth occurs, it is usually visible within four weeks. Treatment, however, does not prevent new patches from developing. There are few side effects from local cortisone injections. Occasionally, temporary depressions in the skin result from the local injections, but these "dells" usually fill in by themselves.

Another treatment is a 5 percent topical minoxidil solution applied twice daily, which may grow hair in alopecia areata. Scalp, eyebrows, and beard hair may also respond. If scalp hair regrows completely, treatment can be stopped.

Yet another treatment is the application of anthralin cream or ointment. Anthralin is a synthetic, tarlike substance that has been used widely for psoriasis. Anthralin is applied to the bare patches once daily and washed off after a short time, usually 30 to 60 minutes later. If new hair growth occurs, it is seen in eight to 12 weeks. Anthralin can be irritating to the skin and can cause temporary, brownish discoloration of the treated skin.

Where there is greater than 50 percent hair loss, cortisone pills are sometimes given. Cortisone taken internally is much stronger than local injections of cortisone into the skin. Healthy young adults often tolerate cortisone pills with few side effects. In general, however, cortisone pills are used in relatively few patients with alopecia areata due to health risks from prolonged use. Also, regrown hair is likely to fall out when the cortisone pills are stopped. Another method of treating extensive alopecia areata or alopecia totalis/universalis is known as topical immunotherapy. Chemicals such as diphencyprone (DPCP) or squaric acid dibutyl ester (SADBE) are applied to the scalp to produce

an allergic rash resembling poison oak or poison ivy. Approximately 40 percent of patients treated with topical immunotherapy will regrow scalp hair after six months of treatment. Those who do successfully regrow scalp hair still need to continue the treatment to maintain the hair regrowth, at least until the disease turns itself off. An itchy rash may be uncomfortable in very hot weather, especially under a wig. These treatments are not widely available in the United States, although they are used frequently in Canada and Europe. Clinical trials on these agents began in 2001 at select institutions in the United States.

A recent study in Scotland showed the effectiveness of aromatherapy essential oils (cedarwood, lavender, thyme, and rosemary oils) in some patients. In the study, 44 percent of the patients using the essential oils showed improvement compared with only 15 percent of patients in the control group. The researchers noted that they had found references from 100 years ago documenting the use of oils similar to those used in this study for hair loss.

For those patients where treatments are not very effective, especially for extensive alopecia areata (particularly alopecia totalis/alopecia universalis), wigs or hair transplantation are often used to hide the baldness.

Because of the stigma from hair loss and the usual young age of patients, professional counseling from a psychiatrist, psychologist, or social worker is sometimes recommended to develop the patient's self-confidence and positive self-image.

Hay, Isabelle C., Margaret Jamieson, and Anthony D. Ormerod. "Randomized Trial of Aromatherapy: Successful Treatment for Alopecia Areata." *Archives of Dermatology* 134, no. 11 (November 1998): 602–603.

"What You Should Know About Alopecia Areata and the National Alopecia Areata Foundation." San Rafael, Cal.: NAAF, 2001.

Wireman, Marni C., Jerry Shapiro, Nina McDonald, and Harvey Oui. "Predictive Model for Immunotherapy of Alopecia Areata With Diphencyprone." *Archives of Dermatology* 137, no. 8 (August 2001): 1,063–1,068.

alopecia areata research   A national registry for alopecia areata was established in 1991 by the National Institute of Arthritis and Musculoskeletal and Skin Diseases (NIAMS), a part of the National Institutes of Health (NIH). The registry is located at the University of Texas M.D. Anderson Cancer Center in Houston, with affiliated centers at the University of Colorado, the University of California San Francisco, the University of Minnesota and Columbia University.

Registry scientists will seek out and classify medical and family history data for patients with the three major forms of alopecia areata. Families with multiple affected members will be especially helpful to further research studies. The project will offer a future central information source where researchers can obtain statistical data associated with the disease. A website is currently being developed for the registry.

The registry will serve as a liaison between affected families and investigators interested in studying this disorder. Scientists hope the registry will be useful in locating the gene or genes associated with alopecia areata. It will also link patients with other researchers studying the cause or treatment of this disease.

alternative medical treatments Also referred to as complementary, natural, or environmental health care, alternative medical treatments comprise those health care and medical practices that are not currently an integral part of conventional medicine. A list of practices considered alternative would change continually as those proven safe and effective become accepted as mainstream health care treatments. For example, many doctors now treat patients with arthritis by suggesting that they take glucosamine sulfate. The National Center for Complementary and Alternative Medicine (NCCAM), a component of the National Institutes of Health (NIH), groups alternative practices and therapies into five major categories:

1. Alternative medical systems—Complete systems of theory and practices that have evolved independent of and often prior to conventional health care. Examples would be traditional oriental medicine (including acupuncture, herbal medicine, and oriental massage), Ayurveda, Native American, homeopathic, and naturopathic.

2. Mind-body interventions—Many mind-body interventions, such as cognitive-behavioral approaches, have been well documented and are now considered mainstream. Others, such as certain uses of hypnosis, music and art therapy, and prayer, are categorized as complementary and alternative.

3. Biological based therapies—These include herbal, special diet, and orthomolecular (varying concentrations of chemicals, such as magnesium and vitamins), many of which overlap with conventional medicine's use of dietary supplements. An example of a biological therapy is bee pollen used to treat autoimmune and inflammatory diseases.

4. Manipulative and body-based methods—These include chiropractors, some osteopaths, and massage therapists. FIBROMYALGIA patients, for example, have been known to benefit from massage and warm-water exercise that loosen muscles and alleviate pain.

5. Energy therapies—Energy therapies focus on either energy fields originating within the body (biofields) or those from other sources (electromagnetic fields). Examples include Reiki and therapeutic touch. Bioelectromagnetic-based therapies involve the unconventional use of electromagnetic fields to treat, for example, asthma or to manage pain.

The NCCAM's purpose is to explore complementary and alternative healing practices in the context of rigorous science. As part of its congressional mandate, NCCAM maintains an information clearinghouse, which was established in 1996. Available through its website (http://nccam.nih.gov/) are fact sheets, alerts and advisories, consensus reports, a complementary and alternative medicine database, NCCAM research, and clinical trials.

Many practitioners insist that natural medicine yields excellent results with autoimmune diseases. Newspapers, magazines, and websites are replete with anecdotal accounts of how various alternative treatments have alleviated—even cured—any number of autoimmune symptoms and disorders. Too often, people learn about alternative medical treatments through friends, family, and the tabloid press—none of which go into the medical research or potential hazards. Because alternative medicines and treatments invariably have their own side effects and can interact unfavorably with traditional drugs and treatments, it is critical to inform the patient's doctors about all alternative medications and treatments being taken or being considered.

Of particular interest or concern to autoimmune patients are the following popular alternative treatments:

- Echinacea—an herb that stimulates the immune system. American Indians used echinacea on cuts and wounds to prevent infection. Generally considered a safe herb, it should not be used at all by patients with lupus, multiple sclerosis, rheumatoid arthritis, or other autoimmune diseases.

- Cat's claw—a plant that grows in Peruvian rain forests. Its inner bark is used for treating a variety of ailments. Because it stimulates the immune system, it should not be taken by anyone with an autoimmune disease. Other immune-stimulating herbs to be avoided by those with autoimmune diseases are astragalus, ginseng, hydrastis (golden seal), larch, ligusticum (osha), lomatium, maitake, Oregon grape, reishi, and shiitake.

- Kava—a member of the pepper family and an herbal supplement. Products containing kava are sold in the United States for a variety of uses, including insomnia and short-term reduction of stress and anxiety. In March 2002, the U.S. Food and Drug Administration issued a consumer advisory that people with liver disease or liver problems or who are taking drugs that can affect the liver should talk to their health care practitioners before using kava after health authorities in five different countries linked kava to at least 25 cases of liver toxicity.

- Exercise—in a small study at Glasgow University in Scotland, researchers found that women with rheumatoid arthritis could walk 30 percent farther when they listened to music of their choice than when they walked in silence.

- Oils—including fish oils or omega-3 fatty acids in the diet is known to benefit the heart. However, University of Texas researchers have dis-

covered that when fed a combination of restricted diets and marine fish oil, autoimmune-prone mice lived 150 days longer (645 days versus 494 days). Likewise, according to *Arthritis Today,* "There is strong evidence that fish oil supplements with omega-3 fatty acids can ease rheumatoid arthritis (RA) symptoms, help prevent Raynaud's syndrome spasms, and possibly relieve some lupus symptoms." Doctors caution that researchers do not know the optimal dosage or if a combination of oils might work better than one alone. Flaxseed oil is believed by some to lower inflammation in rheumatoid arthritis. However, oils do thin the blood, so caution must be used when the patient is also taking blood-thinning drugs.

- Hot mineral spring baths—purported to help numerous functions, from improving circulation to unstuffing noses to aiding digestion. However, doctors caution that rheumatoid arthritis sufferers need to check with their doctors before soaking because the heat can aggravate the condition during flares.

- Tanning beds—at the 2002 Annual Meeting of the American Academy of Dermatology, light was shed on the fact that tanning beds, in combination with acitretin therapy, offer an effective and less costly alternative treatment to individuals who suffer from moderate to severe PSORIASIS.

- Vitamins—a Finnish study of more than 10,000 children showed that newborns who receive 2,000 IU of vitamin D daily during their first month appear to be less susceptible to Type 1 diabetes when they get older. The recommended intake of vitamin D for infants in the United States is 200 IU. Others caution that Northern Finland's limited amounts of sunlight may have a bearing on the results and that the finding may not apply everywhere.

A McGill University Health Centre (Montreal, Quebec) study assessed the use of alternative medicine therapies by patients with SYSTEMIC LUPUS ERYTHEMATOSUS (SLE) in three countries—Canada, United States, and United Kingdom. Among the 707 patients, 352 (49.8 percent) were found to use alternative therapies and at similar rates across all three countries. Users were younger and better educated than nonusers, exhibited poorer levels of satisfaction with traditional medical care, and had minimal to no objective evidence of worse disease. The study also determined that users of many alternative medical therapies accrue greater conventional medical costs compared with nonusers.

Draper, Kim. "Herbs to Avoid: For Lupus Patients," Lupus Den. Available online. URL: http://www.lupusden.com/article1005.html. Downloaded on 12 July 2002.

Goldberg, Burton. *Alternative Medicine Guide to Chronic Fatigue, Fibromyalgia and Environmental Illness.* Puyallup, Wash.: Future Medicine Publishing, 1998.

Horstman, Judith. "Medical Oils." *Arthritis Today* 13, no. 2 (July 1999): 56–58.

Moore, A. D., M. A. Petri, S. Manzi, D. A. Isenberg, et al. "The Use of Alternative Medical Therapies in Patients with Systemic Lupus Erythematosus. Trination Study Group." *Arthritis and Rheumatism* 43, no. 6 (June 2000): 1,410–1,418.

Skelly, Mark, et al. *Alternative Treatments for Fibromyalgia & Chronic Fatigue Syndrome: Insights from Practitioners and Patients.* Alameda, Calif.: Hunter House, 1999.

Vernarec, Emil. "Neonates, Vitamin D, and the Risk of Diabetes." *Complementary Therapies Update, RN.* 65, no. 3 (March 1, 2002): 23.

American Autoimmune Related Diseases Association (AARDA)   A 501(c)(3) tax exempt national voluntary health agency that sponsors physicians' conferences, research, legislative advocacy, and a national awareness campaign to bring a national focus to autoimmunity.

American trypanosomiasis   See CHAGAS' DISEASE.

anergy   A state of immune unresponsiveness in which the antigen-specific lymphocytes fail to react with the antigen but are not deleted.

ankylosing spondylitis (AS)   A form of chronic, painful, inflammatory arthritis that primarily affects the spine and the sacroiliac joints. The sacroiliac joints are located in the low back between the spine and the pelvis where the sacrum (the bone directly above the tailbone) meets the iliac bones (the bones on either side of the upper buttocks). Chronic inflammation in these areas causes pain and stiffness in and around the spine. Over time, as the diseases progresses, chronic spinal inflammation (spondylitis) can result in new bone growth that extends into the ligaments and tendons, leading to a complete growing together (fusion) of the vertebrae, a process called ankylosis. Ankylosis causes total loss of mobility of the spine, restricting the ability to move.

Ankylosing spondylitis is also a systemic rheumatic disease. Therefore, it can cause inflammation in other joints, tendons, and ligaments away from the spine, including the chest wall. It can also involve other organs, such as the eyes, heart, lungs, and kidneys.

Ankylosing spondylitis is two to three times more common in males than in females. In women, joints away from the spine are more frequently affected than in men. Ankylosing spondylitis affects all age groups, including children, but usually begins between ages 20 and 40.

When spondylitis begins before the age of 17, it is called juvenile ankylosing spondylitis (JAS). JAS and diseases related to it are uncommon but account for a significant proportion of all young people with arthritis. JAS may occur in one out of 1,000 children, and it occurs more commonly in boys than in girls. It usually begins in the preteen or teen years. JAS is usually a chronic disorder. It can last months or years with periods of remission (when the patient seems cured). It may persist into adulthood, and children with enthesitis may develop back problems as adults.

Causes

The tendency for developing ankylosing spondylitis is believed to be genetically inherited, and about 90 percent of patients with ankylosing spondylitis are born with the HLA-B27 gene. Blood tests have been developed to detect the HLA-B27 gene marker and have furthered the understanding of the relationship between HLA-B27 and ankylosing spondylitis. The HLA-B27 gene appears only to increase the tendency of developing ankylosing spondylitis, while some additional factor(s), perhaps environmental, are necessary for the disease to appear or become expressed. For example, while 7 to 8 percent of the United States population have the HLA-B27 gene, only 1 percent of the population actually has or will get the disease ankylosing spondylitis. In Northern Scandinavia (Lapland), 1.8 percent of the population have ankylosing spondylitis while 24 percent of the general population have the HLA-B27 gene. Even among HLA-B27-positive individuals, the risk of developing ankylosing spondylitis appears to be further related to heredity. In HLA-B27-positive individuals who have relatives with the disease, their risk of developing ankylosing spondylitis is 12 percent (six times greater than for those whose relatives do not have ankylosing spondylitis).

How inflammation occurs and persists in different organs in ankylosing spondylitis is a subject of active research. The initial inflammation may be a result of an activation of the body's immune system by a bacterial infection. Once activated, the body's immune system becomes unable to turn itself off even though the initial bacterial infection may have long subsided. Chronic tissue inflammation resulting from the continued activation of the body's own immune system in the absence of active infection is the hallmark of an autoimmune disease.

Clinical Features

The most common symptoms of ankylosing spondylitis are related to inflammation of the spine, joints, and other organs, which cause pain and stiffness in the low back, upper buttock area, neck, and the remainder of the spine. The onset of pain and stiffness is usually gradual, beginning with a dull ache deep in the buttocks or lower back, and progressively worsens over a period of at least three months. Occasionally, the onset is rapid and intense. The symptoms of pain and stiffness are often worse in the morning or after prolonged periods of inactivity. The pain and stiffness are often eased by motion, heat, and a warm shower in the morning. Because ankylosing spondylitis often affects patients in adolescence, the onset of low back pain is sometimes incorrectly attributed to athletic injuries in younger patients.

Patients who have chronic, severe inflammation of the spine can develop a complete bony fusion of the spine (ankylosis). Once fused, the pain in the spine disappears, but the patient has a complete loss of spine mobility. These fused spines are particularly brittle and vulnerable to breakage (fracture) when involved in trauma, such as motor vehicle accidents. A sudden onset of pain and mobility in the spinal area of these patients can indicate bone fracture. The lower neck (cervical spine) is the most common area for such fractures.

Chronic spondylitis and ankylosis cause forward curvature of the upper torso (thoracic spine), limiting breathing capacity. Spondylitis can also affect areas where ribs attach to the upper spine, further limiting lung capacity. Ankylosing spondylitis can cause inflammation and scarring of the lungs, causing coughing and shortness of breath, especially with exercise and infections. Therefore, breathing difficulty can be a serious complication of ankylosing spondylitis.

Patients with ankylosing spondylitis can also have arthritis in joints other than the spine. Patients may notice pain, stiffness, heat, swelling, warmth, and/or redness in joints such as the hips, knees, and ankles. Occasionally, the small joints of the toes can become inflamed, or "sausage" shaped. Inflammation can occur in the cartilage around the breast bone (costochondritis) as well as in the tendons where the muscles attach to the bone (tendinitis) and ligament attachments to bone. Some patients with this disease develop Achilles tendinitis, causing pain and stiffness in the back of the heel, especially when pushing off with the foot while walking up stairs.

The diagnosis of ankylosing spondylitis is based on evaluating the patient's symptoms, a physical examination, X-ray findings, and blood tests. Symptoms include pain and morning stiffness of the spine and sacral areas with or without accompanying inflammation in other joints, tendons, and organs. Early symptoms of ankylosing spondylitis can be very deceptive, as stiffness and pain in the low back can be seen in many other conditions. It can be particularly subtle in women, who tend to (though not always) have more mild spine involvement. Years can pass before the diagnosis of ankylosing spondylitis is even considered. In this condition, back pain and stiffness are worse in the morning and relieved by exercise; other causes of back pain are usually mechanical and improve with resting.

X rays are taken of the sacroiliac joints to note changes in tissues caused by inflammation. However, tissue changes do not always appear on X rays in the early stages of the disease. Because starting treatment early is critical to minimize years of uncontrolled inflammation and pain, experienced physicians will often diagnose the disease and start treatment even before X-ray findings are conclusive.

The examination can demonstrate signs of inflammation and decreased range of motion of joints. This can be particularly apparent in the spine. Flexibility of the low back and/or neck can be decreased. The sacroiliac joints of the upper buttocks may be tender. The expansion of the chest with full breathing can be limited because of rigidity of the chest wall. Severely affected persons can have a stooped posture. Inflammation of the eyes can be further evaluated with an ophthalmoscope.

Further clues to the diagnosis are suggested by X-ray abnormalities of the spine and the presence of the blood test genetic marker, the HLA-B27 gene. Other blood tests may provide evidence of inflammation in the body. For example, a blood test called the sedimentation rate is a nonspecific marker for inflammation throughout the body and is often elevated in conditions such as ankylosing spondylitis. Urinalysis is often done to look for accompanying abnormalities of the kidney as well as to exclude kidney conditions that may produce back pain that mimics ankylosing spondylitis.

Complications

Other areas of the body affected by ankylosing spondylitis include the eyes, heart, and kidneys. Patients with ankylosing spondylitis can develop inflammation of the iris, called "iritis." Iritis is characterized by redness and pain in the eye, especially when looking at bright lights. Recurrent attacks of iritis can affect either eye. In addition to the iris, the ciliary body and choroid of the eye can become inflamed, and this is referred to as uveitis. Iritis and uveitis can be serious complications of ankylosing spondylitis that can damage the eye and impair vision. They may require an ophthalmologist's urgent care.

Inflammation of the eye usually occurs in one eye at a time. The typical symptoms are redness, pain, and sensitivity to light. However, the degree of these symptoms can vary considerably. Inflammation of the eye requires prompt treatment by an ophthalmologist to prevent permanent eye damage.

The medical term *uveitis* refers to inflammation inside the eye. Iritis and iridocyclitis are two types of anterior uveitis, and the three terms are often used interchangeably. There are many types of uveitis, and different parts of the eye may be affected.

Iritis is associated with a variety of potential complications related to the eyes. These complications include scarring of the iris to the lens, scarring of the iris to more anteriorly located structures, cataract formation, and leakage from the blood vessels in the back of the eye. The scarring may lead to a secondary glaucoma, which can result in a permanent visual loss.

A rare complication of ankylosing spondylitis involves scarring of the heart's electric system, causing an abnormally slow heart rate. A small number of people with spondylitis will display signs of chronic inflammation in the base of the heart—around the aortic valve and origin of the aorta (i.e., the vessel that takes all blood from the heart to be distributed throughout the body). Years of chronic and silent inflammation at these sites can eventually lead to heart block and valve leakage, sometimes requiring surgical treatment. Although well recognized, these cardiac lesions are probably seen in fewer than 2 percent of all patients with spondylitis and nearly always in males. The lesions are readily detectable by the physician's examination and, when necessary, cardiac testing. A heart pacemaker may be necessary in these patients to maintain adequate heart rate and output. These patients can develop shortness of breath, dizziness, and heart failure.

Advanced spondylitis can lead to deposits of protein material called amyloid into the kidneys and result in kidney failure. Progressive kidney disease can lead to chronic fatigue and nausea. It can require removal of accumulated blood poisons by a filtering machine (dialysis).

Poor chest wall movement may result in decreased vital capacity. A few patients may develop scarring or fibrosis at the top of the lungs detected only by routine chest X ray (recommended every five years unless there is a special need).

Treatment

There is not yet a cure for ankylosing spondylitis, so treatment consists of medicines to alleviate the pain and stiffness, special daily exercises that incorporate stretching and strengthening, good posture habits, and a healthy diet. Medications decrease inflammation in the spine, other joints, and organs. Physical therapy and exercise help improve posture, spine mobility, and lung capacity. Plus they help reduce the stiffness. Treatment is typically most effective in the early stages of the disease before it causes irreversible damage.

Aspirin and other nonsteroidal anti-inflammatory drugs (NSAIDs) are the most commonly used medications; they decrease pain and stiffness of the spine and other joints. Commonly used NSAIDs include indomethacin (Indocin), tolmetin (Tolectin), sulindac (Clinoril), naproxen (Naprosyn), and diclofenac (Voltaren), and ibuprofen. Their common side effects include stomach upset, nausea, abdominal pain, diarrhea, and even bleeding ulcers. These medicines are frequently taken with food in order to minimize side effects. Each person responds differently to each of the many NSAIDs available, so a period of trial and error is sometimes required until the right medication and dosage is found.

In some patients with ankylosing spondylitis, inflammation of the spine and other joints may not respond to NSAIDs alone. In these patients, the addition of sulfasalazine (Azulfidine) may bring about long-term reduction of inflammation.

Oral or injectable corticosteroids (cortisone) are potent anti-inflammatory agents and can effectively control spondylitis and other inflammations in the body. Unfortunately, corticosteroids can have serious side effects when used on a long-term basis. These side effects include cataracts, thinning of the skin and bones, easy bruising, infections, diabetes, and destruction of large joints, such as the hips.

For persistent ankylosing spondylitis that is unresponsive to anti-inflammatory medications, agents that suppress body immunity are considered. Methotrexate (Rheumatrex) can be administered orally or by injection. Frequent blood tests are performed during methotrexate treatment because of its potential for toxicity to the liver, which can even lead to cirrhosis, and for toxicity to bone marrow, which can lead to severe anemia.

Physical therapy for ankylosing spondylitis includes instructions and exercises to maintain proper posture. This includes deep breathing for lung expansion and stretching exercises to improve spine and joint mobility. Because ankylosis of the spine tends to cause forward curvature, patients are instructed to maintain erect posture as much as possible and to perform back extension exercises. Patients are also advised to sleep on a firm mattress and avoid the use of a pillow in order to prevent spine curvature. Ankylosing spondylitis can involve the areas where the ribs attach to the upper spine as well as the vertebral joints, thus limiting lung breathing capacity. Patients are instructed to expand their chest maximally and frequently throughout each day to minimize this limitation.

Exercise programs are customized for the individual patient. Swimming is preferred, as it avoids jarring impact of the spine. Ankylosing spondylitis need not limit a patient's involvement in athletics. Patients can participate in carefully chosen aerobic sports when their disease is inactive. Aerobic exercise is generally encouraged as it promotes full expansion of the breathing muscles and opens the airways of the lungs.

Inflammation and diseases in other organs are treated separately. For example, inflammation of the iris of the eyes (iritis or uveitis) may require cortisone eye drops (Pred Forte) and high doses of cortisone by mouth. Additionally, atropine eye drops are often given to relax the muscles of the iris. Sometimes injections of cortisone into the affected eye are necessary when the inflammation is severe. Heart disease in patients with ankylosing spondylitis may require a pacemaker or medications for congestive heart failure.

Cigarette smoking is strongly discouraged in patients with ankylosing spondylitis, as it can accelerate lung scarring and seriously aggravate breathing difficulties. Occasionally, patients with severe lung disease relate to ankylosing spondylitis may require oxygen supplementation and medications to improve breathing.

Patients may need to modify their activities of daily living and adjust features of the workplace.

For example, workers can adjust chairs and desks for proper postures. Drivers can use wide rearview mirrors and prism glasses to compensate for the limited motion in the spine. However, with treatment, most people suffer only minor deformity of the spine and are able to lead a normal life.

Finally, patients who have severe disease of the hip joints and spine may require orthopedic surgery.

Shiel, William C., Jr. "Ankylosing Spondylitis." Focus On Arthritis. Available online. URL: http://www.focusonarthritis.com, last editorial review 21 April 2002.

antibody   A protein molecule compound (also called an immunoglobulin), produced by B cells, that controls the immune response to a specific and unique antigen. At first, an antibody is bound to a B cell. However, when it encounters its specific antigen, the antibody/antigen complex stimulates the B cell to produce copies of the antibody—all of which are designed to recognize the infecting antigen. Then the new group of antibodies bind to the infecting antigen, controlling or destroying the antigen.

antibody-dependent cell-mediated cytotoxicity (ADCC)   The process by which target cells coated with antibody are destroyed by specialized killer cells (NK cells, killer T cells and, macrophages). These killer cells carry antibody specific for the target cell, attached to their Fc receptors. The cells involved in the killing may be passive carriers of the antibody. ADCC is an immune response in which antibody, by coating the target cells, makes the targets vulnerable to attack by immune cells.

antigen   A substance that induces an immune response. The antigen can be foreign material from the environment or formed within the cells of one's own body, such as viruses or bacteria. Antigens on the body's own cells are called autoantigens. Antigens on all other cells are called foreign antigens. Usually, reactions of T cells and B cells are part of the specific immune response.

antigen-antibody complex   When the antibody binds to the antigen, this forms an antigen-antibody complex. This complex may make the antigen harmless or may trigger an inflammatory response.

antigen-presenting cell (APC)   Also called antigen-processing cell. A cell that displays an antigen with a major histocompatibility complex (MHC) molecule on the cell surface. In order for an antigen to be recognized by a T lymphocyte, it must be first processed and presented in a form the T cell can recognize. This is the function of APCs, also referred to as accessory cells. In the process, an APC engulfs an antigen. Enzymes in the APC break down the antigen into smaller fragments. These fragments are transported to the surface of the APC, bound with class II MHC molecules. A T cell receptor can now recognize the antigen linked with the MHC and thus binds to it. Examples of antigen-presenting cells include macrophages (large white blood cells that ingest antigens and other foreign substances) and dendritic cells (the principle APC involved in primary immune responses). The major function of dendritic cells is to take up antigen in tissues, migrate to lymphoid organs, and activate T cells and B cells.

antigen receptors   Receptors on white blood cells that bind an antigen molecule, stimulating an immune response.

antiglomerular basement membrane (anti-GBM) disease   A rare autoimmune kidney disorder characterized by the presence of antibodies directed against glomerular basement membrane (GBM), which is damaged in the reaction. The kidney itself may be the source of the antigen. An IgG autoantibody forms to the glomerular basement membrane (anti-GBM) and is capable of binding to the Goodpasture antigen, a component of the normal GBM. As a result, either focal or diffuse proliferative glomerular nephritis (GN) develops, usually with crescents. Linear deposits of IgG can be detected on the GBM, and anti-GBM antibodies can be detected in the circulation. Patients with Goodpasture's syndrome are most often young males under age 40. However, when the disease does not include the lung hemorrhage (anti-GBM disease), it strikes older people and males and females equally. The cause of anti-GBM disease is unknown. However, there is a genetic predisposition, and it does occasionally occur in identical twins. Patients with anti-GBM disease frequently show blood in the urine. In half to three-quarters of cases, the antibody also reacts with the alveolar basement membrane, causing pulmonary hemorrhage (referred to as Goodpasture's syndrome), which may be life threatening. Treatment with corticosteroids or plasmapheresis limits damage. The condition itself runs a definite course and is little modified by treatment.

antinuclear antibodies (ANA) A circulating group of autoantibodies that are produced by the body when the immune system mistakenly recognizes normal components of its own cell nucleus as foreign. Numerous of these antibodies have been detected in a variety of autoimmune diseases, including systemic lupus erythematosus (SLE), progressive systemic sclerosis, Sjögren's syndrome, scleroderma, polymyositis, rheumatoid arthritis, and dermatomyositis. Tests for ANA are used in the diagnosis and management of autoimmune diseases, especially SLE. Some ANAs have identified subgroups of patients within a disease and have prognostic and therapeutic significance. They are detected by looking at a blood sample for immunoglobulins that bind to nuclear antigens. Because certain drugs can provoke ANA and thus give a positive test result, persons being administered the test usually need to withhold these drugs, which include antibiotics, birth control pills, procainamide, some antihypertensive drugs, steroids, thiazide diuretics, and tranquilizers.

Aitcheson C. T., C. Peebles, F. Joslin, et al. "Characteristics of Antinuclear Antibodies in Rheumatoid Arthritis." *Arthritis and Rheumatism* 23 (2001): 528.

antiphospholipid syndrome (APS) Also referred to as antiphospholipid antibody syndrome, Hughes syndrome, and sticky blood, APS is a recently discovered immune disorder in which the body appears to recognize certain phospholipids (fatty molecules that are important components of a cell's membrane) as foreign substances and produces antibodies against them. During the late 1970s, it was recognized that blood-clotting disorders can be

linked with the appearance of certain antibodies in the blood. Then in 1983, British physician Graham Hughes provided the first detailed description of the antiphospholipid syndrome. In 1990, a journal estimated that 100,000 individuals in the United States have APS, with a cost to the U.S. Government of more than $100 million per year.

APS does not make the patient feel ill or stop the immune system from working to fight disease. People with APS may experience blood clots leading to heart attack, stroke, or loss of the fetus during pregnancy. It is not contagious and is rarely a terminal disease. Many people go throughout life without even knowing their body makes these antibodies.

For people with APS, though, there is a greater chance of certain problems. APS may occur in patients with lupus and related autoimmune diseases or as a primary syndrome in otherwise healthy individuals. Although lupus patients often have APS, people who have APS do not necessarily have lupus.

Antiphospholipid antibodies are present in the blood of about one-third of patients who have lupus. Approximately one-third of those with antibodies (10 to 15 percent of all lupus patients) have clinical signs of the syndrome. Antiphospholipid antibodies have also been identified in people who do not have an autoimmune disorder like lupus and who may not have any symptoms. These antibodies are found in about 2 percent of all women. Not all of these will have the disease.

The first thrombosis often occurs during the midteen years and is followed by recurring thromboses. Women may experience recurring miscarriage, usually during the second or third trimester, or their babies may have an unexpected low birth weight. People with APS may have a history of migraine headaches, memory loss, and fatigue going back several years.

The disease is diagnosed by carrying out two tests, one for lupus anticoagulant and the other for anticardiolipin antibodies. Higher levels of the antibody appear to correlate with an increased risk of unwanted blood clots. The levels of antibody can go up and down, and even disappear. Consequently, blood tests need to be repeated at least eight weeks from the initial positive tests and still be positive.

Causes

There is no known cause for the disease. However, APS may run in families, although not all members are necessarily affected. To what extent this happens is not exactly clear. APS, though, can be suspected where several members of a family have had a series of miscarriages or thromboses. A thrombosis is a blood clot that forms when it should not, such as in a deep vein of the leg (DVT) or in an artery. Antiphospholipid syndrome occurs two to five times more frequently in women than in men.

Clinical Features

In some patients, the only manifestation of the syndrome is recurrent miscarriage. In others, it is headaches or either speech or visual/neurological disturbance. The most dramatic sign that the disease is present is thrombosis, especially deep vein thrombosis (DVM), in the leg or arm. This may be recurrent or complicated by a lung clot (pulmonary embolus). "Internal" veins may also clot, affecting organs such as the eye, the kidney, the liver, and so on. Arteries can also clot, but major artery thrombosis is less common than DVM.

Another clinical feature common in patients with APS is blotchy skin. This blotchiness was described in Dr. Hughes's original clinical reports as "blue knees and purplish vein coloration on the back of the wrists."

In a small percentage of patients, according to Hughes, the platelet numbers are affected. Rarely, platelet counts may fall to dangerously low numbers. Thus, patients who have been diagnosed as having low platelet counts, thrombocytopenia, should be checked for APS.

In quite a few patients, headaches, frequently with migraine features like flashing lights or speech disturbances, are an important symptom. In many patients, the headaches predate the clotting problem by many years. For example, Hughes relates, a 25-year-old woman with recurrent miscarriages due to APS had a history of troublesome teenage migraines, possibly suggesting that the antibodies had been there for at least a decade before.

For reasons not completely understood, the brain appears particularly sensitive to the clotting effects of antiphospholipid antibodies. The brain has only a limited number of ways of complaining at any disturbances in its supply of blood. The patient may develop transient memory loss or a slight speech disturbance, suggestive of a ministroke. In others, the effect may be more insidious, with a gradually failing ability to put words, sentences, lists, and so on together.

Complications

Clots from the leg can dislodge and move to more dangerous places, such as the lung (pulmonary embolism). In APS, blood clots may affect any part of the body. In addition to stroke and heart attack, abnormalities of the heart valves, kidney disease, thrombocytopenia (a low level of platelets in the blood), and leg ulcers have been associated with the disorder. APS takes a particular toll during pregnancy, when the syndrome may cause miscarriage, stillbirth, retarded growth of the fetus, or preeclampsia (toxemia and high blood pressure). In such cases, the blood is unable to flow through the small and delicate blood vessels to the placenta and fetus. The placenta withers, and the fetus is spontaneously aborted (miscarried). In the general population, APS may account for 20 percent of deep vein thrombosis cases, one-third of strokes in people under age 50, and 5 to 15 percent of recurrent miscarriages.

Treatment

The optimal treatment of patients with antiphospholipid syndrome has not been defined. In some instances, patients need no treatment. Generally, APS is treated over the long term with anticlotting drugs such as warfarin (Coumadin), heparin, or low-dose (baby) aspirin. Severe, acute progression of antiphospholipid syndrome can be treated additionally with immunosuppressive agents (for example, steroids), hydroxychloroquine sulfate, and plasmapheresis.

One of the most common problems with APS is that of recurrent miscarriage. A promising treatment that helps prevent this is the use of low-dose aspirin in early pregnancy. This is sometimes combined with another drug called heparin, which is given by injection. Knowing that someone has APS means that the pregnancy can be monitored much more closely than usual, for example with ultrasound scans to watch for poor growth. The decision on treatment at a particular time (such as during pregnancy) depends upon the antibody levels and any previous medical problems.

APS can make someone more likely to get thrombosis. At specific times when thrombosis is already a risk, for example after major surgery, during prolonged illness or bed rest, during pregnancy, and for a short time after delivery, extra clot prevention may be needed. This might mean using some tight medical stockings or receiving heparin treatment. In more severe cases of thrombosis, it may mean long-term treatment with tablets to thin the blood.

Amengual, O., T. Atsumi, M. A. Khamashta, and G. R. Hughes. "Advances in Antiphospholipid (Hughes') Syndrome." *Annals of the Academy of Medicine* (Singapore) 27, no. 1 (January 1998): 61–66.

De Jong, A., V. Ziboh, and D. Robbins. "Antiphospholipid Antibodies and Platelets." *Current Rheumatology Reports* 2, no. 3 (June 2000): 238–245.

Greco, T. P., A. M. Conti-Kelly, and J. Ijdo. "Impact of the Antiphospholipid Syndrome: A Critical Coagulation Disorder in Women." *Medscape Womens Health* 2, no. 1 (January 1997): 7.

Gromnica-Ihle, E., and W. Schossler. "Antiphospholipid Syndrome." *International Archives of Allergy and Immunology* 123, no. 1 (September 2000): 67–76.

Hughes, G. R. V. "The Antiphospholipid Syndrome—Ten Years On." *The Lancet* (Symposium Supplement) 342 (1993): 341–344.

Hughes, Graham. "Hughes' Syndrome: A Patient's Guide to the Antiphospholipid Syndrome," OMNI: Organising Medical Networked Information. Available online. URL: http://www.infotech.demon.co.uk/HS.htm. Downloaded 12 July 2002.

Khamashta, M. A., A. E. Gharavi, and W. A. Wilson, eds. *7th International Symposium on Antiphospholipid Antibodies Lupus* 5 (1996): 343–558.

Khamashta, M. A., and G. R. Hughes. "Antiphospholipid Antibodies and Antiphospholipid Syndrome." *Current Opinions in Rheumatology* 7, no. 5 (September 1995): 389–394.

Khamashta, M. A., and C. Mackworth Young. "Antiphospholipid (Hughes') Syndrome—A Treatable Cause for Recurrent Pregnancy Loss." *British Medical Journal* 314 (1997): 244.

Wilson W. A., and A. E. Gharavi. "Hughes' Syndrome: Perspectives on Thrombosis and Antiphospholipid Antibody." *American Journal of Medicine* 101 (1996): 574–575.

antiphospholipid syndrome research Only recently were APS-related antibodies discovered and their significance understood. Therefore, the information available is somewhat limited, but research is ongoing. In April 2001, a new national registry and tissue repository was established by the National Institute of Arthritis and Musculoskeletal and Skin Diseases (NIAMS) and the National Center on Minority Health and Health Disparities (NCMHD). The coordinating center will reside at the University of North Carolina, Chapel Hill (UNC). Biomedical researchers at eight medical centers will collect and update clinical, demographic, and laboratory information from patients with APS and make it available to researchers and to medical practitioners concerned with the diagnosis and treatment of this syndrome. The availability of this information will permit better comparisons among clinical research projects and help rheumatologists, obstetricians, and other physicians resolve problems associated with the many manifestations of the syndrome. Registry scientists will collect data on patients with clinical signs of APS and on asymptomatic individuals who have antibodies but have not yet developed any clinical signs.

antitoxin An antibody formed in the bloodstream of an animal or human being in response to and capable of neutralizing (making inactive) the effects of a specific bacterial toxin or poison, such as those that cause diphtheria or tetanus. By introducing small amounts of a specific toxin into the healthy body, the production of antitoxin can be stimulated so that the body's defenses will have already been established if invaded by the bacteria or other organisms that produce the toxin. In 1890, the German physician von Behring and the Japanese physician Kitasoto were the first to demonstrate that animals immune to diphtheria have substances in their blood serum that neutralize the toxin produced by the diphtheria bacterium. Serum antitoxins were first prepared by immunizing horses with diphtheria toxin and were used in the treatment of diphtheria. Von Behring won the first Nobel prize for his discovery. Today, similar antitoxins are used to combat the toxins produced by tetanus and botulism. Antitoxins for use in human beings are produced in animals such as horses and cattle. The animal is injected with increasingly higher doses of the toxin, and its defense processes respond by producing antitoxin. Some of the animal's blood is then extracted and processed for use in human beings. An animal may be used to produce antitoxin for many years without apparent damage to itself. Antitoxins are usually administered by injection into a muscle. In a few instances, an antitoxin may cause an allergic reaction in the individual being given it.

apoptosis The process by which a cell actively commits suicide, also referred to as the programmed cell death due to genetic limitation of its life span. Apoptosis is essential in many aspects of normal development and is required for maintaining tissue homeostasis (equilibrium). For example, the removal by absorption of the tadpole tail at the time of the animal's metamorphosis into a frog occurs by apoptosis. The formation of the fingers and toes of the fetus requires the removal, by apoptosis, of the tissue between them. The sloughing off of the inner lining of the uterus (the endometrium) at the start of menstruation occurs by apoptosis.

Failure to regulate apoptosis properly can have catastrophic consequences. Apoptosis is a normal part of immune regulation. It is one of the ways the body protects itself against autoimmune disease. Cancer and many diseases (for example, AIDS, Alzheimer's disease, Parkinson's disease, heart attack, and stroke) are thought to arise from deregulation of apoptosis. Defects in the apoptotic machinery is associated with autoimmune diseases such as lupus erythematosus and rheumatoid arthritis.

Kimball, John W. *Biology,* 6th ed. New York: WCB/ McGraw-Hill, 1994.

Asians/Pacific Islander Americans (APIA) and autoimmune disease Asian American women experience RHEUMATOID ARTHRITIS at rates higher than the general population. Likewise, lupus is more common in women of Asian descent than in those of Caucasian European lineage. Young women in Southeast Asia, especially Japanese women, show a propensity for TAKAYASU'S ARTERITIS.

However, other autoimmune diseases are less likely to strike APIAs. DERMATITIS HERPETIFORMIS is rare in Asians. INSULIN-DEPENDENT DIABETES rarely occurs in Asian-Pacific Americans and their populations of origin. However, cases of nonautoimmune diabetes are increasing among several Asian/Pacific Islander Americans as well as in their populations of origin. The Japanese and other Asian peoples have very low incidence rates of MULTIPLE SCLEROSIS.

autoantibody An antibody, produced by B cells, that reacts against the body's own organs and tissues. Autoantibodies are the basis for recognizing autoimmune diseases. The most commonly accepted theory as to their development is that they are due to a combination of hereditary and environmental risk factors that cause a self antigen to be seen as foreign by B cells. As a result, antibodies are produced to destroy this self antigen.

autoantigen See ANTIGEN.

autograft A graft transferred from one part of a patient's body to another part of his or her body.

autoimmune disease The basic definition of an autoimmune disease is a disorder caused by an autoimmune response, i.e., an immune response directed against something in the body of the patient. The word *auto* is the Greek word for *self.* The immune system is a complicated network of cells and cell components that normally work to defend the body and eliminate infections caused by bacteria, viruses, and other invading microbes. If a person has an autoimmune disease, the immune system mistakenly attacks the self, targeting the cells, tissues, and organs of a person's own body. It has been described as an immune system that cannot be turned off. A collection of immune system cells and certain mediator molecules at a target site is broadly referred to as inflammation.

Nearly 100 different autoimmune diseases have been identified. They can each affect the body in different ways. For example, the autoimmune reaction is directed against the brain in multiple sclerosis and against the gut (intestines) in Crohn's disease. In other autoimmune diseases such as systemic lupus erythematosus (lupus), affected tissues and organs may vary among individuals with the same disease. One person with lupus may have affected skin and joints whereas another may have affected kidney and lungs. Ultimately, damage to certain tissues by the immune system may be permanent, as with destruction of insulin-producing cells of the pancreas in Type 1 diabetes mellitus. Some autoimmune diseases are mild; indeed, not all person's affected are even aware they have a disease. Other autoimmune diseases can be disabling, even life-threatening.

Most of the individual autoimmune diseases are rare. As a group, however, autoimmune diseases afflict millions of Americans. Most autoimmune diseases strike women far more often than men. In particular, they affect women of working age and during their childbearing years. Of the estimated 50 million Americans who suffer from autoimmune disease, 75 percent are women. These diseases now comprise the fifth leading cause of death among women aged 15 to 44. The reason for the sex-related difference is not known, but it may reflect the involvement of hormones in regulation of the immune response.

Some autoimmune diseases occur more frequently in certain minority populations. For example, lupus is more common in African-American and Hispanic women than in Caucasian women of European ancestry. Rheumatoid arthritis and scleroderma affect a higher percentage of residents in some Native-American communities than in the general U.S. population. Thus, the social, economic, and health impact from autoimmune diseases is far-reaching and extends not only to family but also to employers, coworkers, and friends.

Sometimes autoimmunity can be the initiating cause of the disease. In other cases, autoimmunity can contribute to, or exacerbate, a disease caused by something else.

The exact cause of autoimmune diseases is not known, but many theories exist. Among these is that because the surface markers of enemy antigens closely resemble those of healthy cells, the antibodies intended to target the antigens attack the healthy cells instead.

No autoimmune disease has ever been shown to be contagious or catching. Autoimmune diseases do not spread to other people like infections. They are not related to AIDS, nor are they a type of cancer, although they may occur in patients with cancer.

The genes people inherit contribute to their susceptibility for developing an autoimmune disease. Certain diseases such as psoriasis can occur among several members of the same family. This suggests that a specific gene or set of genes predisposes a family member to psoriasis. In addition, individual family members with autoimmune diseases may inherit and share a set of abnormal genes, although they may develop different autoimmune diseases. For example, one first cousin may have lupus, another may have dermatomyositis, and one of their mothers may have rheumatoid arthritis.

All the autoimmune diseases show evidence of genetic predisposition. No single gene by itself causes an autoimmune disease. Instead, a coalescence of several genes in certain individuals, in the aggregate, significantly heightens the overall possibility of developing an autoimmune disease. Some of these genes may be specific for a certain disease, but others predispose one to autoimmunity in general. That explains why a single patient may have more than one autoimmune disease or why autoimmune diseases are more common in some families than others.

Researchers also believed that for someone who is susceptible to an autoimmune disease, an outside or environmental trigger, such as stress or a virus, may lead to the development of an autoimmune disease in that person. Some autoimmune diseases are known not only to begin but to worsen with certain triggers such as viral infections. A well-known autoimmune disease, rheumatic fever, is associated with a preceding infection by a streptococcus. Sunlight not only acts as a trigger for lupus but can worsen the course of the disease. Sometimes components of the diet may influence the development of disease. For example, in autoimmune diseases of the thyroid, dietary iodine may be an important enhancing factor.

These environmental triggers act only in individuals with a genetic predisposition toward the disease and not in the population at large. If the trigger can be identified and the patient warned to avoid it, the autoimmune disease may never occur. So carriers of the genetic markers should be aware of the factors that can be avoided to help prevent or minimize the amount of damage from the autoimmune disease. Other less understood influences affecting the immune system and the course of autoimmune diseases include aging, chronic stress, hormones, and pregnancy.

The diagnosis of an autoimmune disease is based on an individual's symptoms, findings from a physical examination, and results from laboratory tests. Autoimmune diseases can be difficult to diagnose, particularly early in the course of the disease. Symptoms of many autoimmune diseases—such as fatigue, headaches, fever, rashes, and painful joints—are nonspecific. They also appear with other nonautoimmune diseases and conditions. Adding to the difficulty of making a diagnosis is that autoimmune diseases tend to flare up or go into remission periodically. Laboratory test results may help but are often inadequate to confirm a diagnosis.

If an individual has skeletal symptoms such as joint pain and a positive but nonspecific lab test, she or he may be diagnosed with the confusing name of early or undifferentiated connective tissue disease. In this case, a physician may want the patient to return frequently for follow-up. The early phase of disease may be a very frustrating time for both the patient and physician. On the other hand, symptoms may be short-lived, and inconclusive laboratory tests may amount to nothing of a serious nature. The average patient visits six different doctors over a period of five years before finally being diagnosed with an autoimmune disease. According to the American Autoimmune Related Diseases Association (AARDA), 65 percent of patients subsequently diagnosed with an autoimmune disease have been accused of being hypochondriacs in the earliest stages of their illnesses.

In some cases, a specific diagnosis can be made. A diagnosis shortly after onset of a patient's symptoms will allow for early aggressive medical therapy. For some diseases, patients will respond completely to treatments if the reason for their symptoms is discovered early in the course of their disease.

Although autoimmune diseases are chronic, the course they take is unpredictable. A doctor cannot foresee what will happen to the patient based on how the disease starts. Patients need to be monitored closely by their doctors so environmental factors or triggers that may worsen the disease can be discussed and avoided and so new medical therapy can be started as soon as possible. Frequent visits to a doctor are important initially in order for the physician to manage complex treatment regimens and watch for medication side effects.

Because autoimmune disease is somewhat of a mystery, the usual treatments give relief for the symptoms. The problem has been finding out how to turn off the immune response that has been the cause of the damage (an immune system that keeps attacking itself). Autoimmune diseases are often chronic, requiring lifelong care and monitoring, even when the person may look or feel well. Currently, few autoimmune diseases can be cured or made to disappear with treatment. However, many people with these diseases can live normal lives when they receive appropriate medical care.

Physicians most often help patients manage the consequences of inflammation caused by the autoimmune disease. For example, in people with Type 1 diabetes, physicians prescribe insulin to control blood sugar levels so that elevated blood sugar will not damage the kidneys, eyes, blood vessels, and nerves. However, the goal of scientific research is to prevent inflammation from causing destruction of the insulin-producing cells of the pancreas, which are necessary to control blood sugars.

On the other hand, in some diseases such as lupus or rheumatoid arthritis, medication can occasionally slow or stop the immune system's destruction of the kidneys or joints. Medications or therapies that slow or suppress the immune system response in an attempt to stop the inflammation involved in the autoimmune attack are called immunosuppressive medications. These drugs include corticosteroids (prednisone), methotrexate, cyclophosphamide, azathioprine, and cyclosporine. Unfortunately, these medications also suppress the ability of the immune system to fight infection and have other potentially serious side effects.

In some people, a limited number of immuno-suppressive medications may result in disease remission. Remission is the medical term used for the disappearance of a disease for a significant amount of time. Even if their disease goes into remission, patients are rarely able to discontinue medications. The possibility that the disease may restart when medication is discontinued must be balanced with the long-term side effects from the immunosuppressive medication.

A current goal in caring for patients with autoimmune diseases is to find treatments that produce remissions with fewer side effects. Much research is focused on developing therapies that target various steps in the immune response. New approaches such as therapeutic antibodies against specific T cell molecules may produce fewer long-term side effects than the chemotherapies that are now routinely used.

Ultimately, medical science is striving to design therapies that prevent autoimmune diseases. To this end, a significant amount of time and resources are spent studying the immune system and pathways of inflammation. Some researchers believe that one important outcome of the human genome project will be the identification of genes that contribute to an unusual autoimmune susceptibility. Individuals with the greatest risk will then be able to be forewarned. Others suggest that genes may not provide as many clues for autoimmune diseases as proteins, the product of those genes.

Cooke, Robert. "Women's Vulnerability." *Newsday* (13 March 2001), c6.

Goldsmith, Marsha F. "Are Autoimmunologists in Many Women's Future?" *Journal of the American Medical Association* 285, no. 11 (March 2001): 1,433–1,434.

Jarvis, Louise. "The Traitor Within." *Harper's Bazaar,* February 2001, 150, 156.

National Institutes of Health. *Understanding Autoimmune Diseases,* NIH Publication Number 98-4273, May 1998.

Rose, Noel R., and Ian R. MacKay, eds. *The Autoimmune Diseases,* 3rd ed. San Diego, Calif.: Academic Press, 1998.

autoimmune hemolytic anemia (AIHA) An autoimmune disorder that leads to the premature destruction of red blood cells by antibodies produced by the patient's own immune system. A normal red blood cell has a life span of approximately 120 days before the spleen removes it from circulation. Red blood cells are made in the bone marrow and released into circulation. In persons with autoimmune hemolytic anemia, the red blood cells are destroyed prematurely, and bone marrow production of new cells cannot make up for their loss. The severity of this disorder is determined by the length of time the red blood cell survives and by the capability of the bone marrow to continue red blood cell production.

Autoimmune hemolytic anemia is an uncommon disorder that occurs in persons who have formerly had a normal red blood cell count. The disorder usually occurs in conjunction with some other medical condition, very often another autoimmune disease. It may sometimes occur alone and without a triggering factor. It affects twice as many women as men, specifically women in their childbearing years. Several autoimmune blood diseases are related. Cold antibody hemolytic anemia (COLD AGGLUTININ DISEASE) most commonly affects elderly persons, and warm antibody hemolytic anemia can affect anyone at any age. Drug-induced hemolytic anemias are clinically indistinguishable from AIHA. For that reason, they are classified with this disorder, which is often referred to as idiopathic autoimmune hemolytic anemia. AIHA accounts for one-half of all immune hemolytic anemias.

Autoimmune hemolytic anemia has no known cause and thus no known way to prevent it. In many patients, the antibodies disappear or diminish to insignificant levels after a period varying from a few months to more than 10 years. It most often continues long-term in adults but is most often short-lived in children. Treatment to keep the patient in the best possible health until the autoantibody disappears begins with prednisone. If that does not improve the condition, removal of the spleen may be necessary. If neither of these treatments are effective, immunosuppressive therapy (Imuran, Cytoxin) is administered.

Hashimoto, C. "Autoimmune Hemolytic Anemia." *Allergy Immunology* 16, no. 3 (1998): 285–295.

Wheby, M. S., ed. *Anemia. Medical Clinics of North America.* Philadelphia: W. B. Saunders Co., 1992.

autoimmune inner ear disease (AIED) A syndrome of progressive sensory hearing loss, which may or may not be accompanied by dizziness, caused by antibodies attacking the inner ear. Tinnitus (noises such as ringing or roaring in the ear) or pressure may also occur. AIED is also seen in people with other autoimmune diseases. Autoimmune inner ear disease is rare, accounting for less than 1 percent of all cases of sensory hearing loss or dizziness. Because the disease has been recognized only since 1979 and is still being defined, the exact number of cases is unknown. Additionally, because it is new and uncommon, experts suspect that many cases go unrecognized. Unlike other hearing loss disorders, AIED may be reversed. Thus, researchers are actively investigating its causes and treatments in the hope that their findings may provide leads for understanding other forms of sensory hearing loss.

Autoimmune inner ear disease most commonly affects middle-aged women, which follows the pattern of many other autoimmune diseases. Reports show that 65 percent of AIED patients are female and 35 percent male. About 30 percent of the women have coexistent systemic autoimmune disease. The majority of AIED patients are young—in their 20s, 30s, and 40s.

Causes

Little is known for sure about exactly how AIED begins. However, several theories have been proposed about how damage done to the inner ear by either antibodies or immune cells can be compared with the effects of other autoimmune disorders. One theory is that damage to the inner ear causes cytokines to be released that provoke, after a delay, additional immune reactions. This theory might explain the attack/remission cycle of disorders such as Ménière's disease. In the cross-reactions theory, which has the most support, antibodies or rogue T cells cause accidental inner ear damage because the ear shares common antigens with a potentially harmful substance, virus, or bacteria that the body is fighting. Evidence also suggests that genetically controlled aspects of the immune system may increase or otherwise be associated with increased susceptibility to common hearing disorders such as Ménière's disease and AIED.

Clinical Features

Hearing loss involving the sensory nerves is usually bilateral (affecting both ears) and occurs rapidly over several weeks or months. This loss may fluctuate then stabilize at a certain level, or it may continue to progress. Occasionally, only one ear will be involved in the beginning, with the other ear developing hearing loss at a later time. About half of the patients will experience dizziness or vertigo. About half of the patients will also have symptoms of tinnitus and fullness in the ear (pressure), which may fluctuate in severity. Typically, patients are first treated with antibiotics for other suspected ear ailments; then when that treatment has no effect and hearing loss begins to appear also in the other ear, AIED will first be suspected.

Treatment

Steroids (prednisone or Decadron) are the initial treatment of choice and are effective in many cases. However, some patients are not able to tolerate the dosage or the length of time required for such therapy. Also, exact dosage and duration of therapy continue to be debated. In many cases, steroids are given in a high dose for a short time and then gradually lowered to a maintenance dose.

Barna, B. P., and G. B. Hughes. "Autoimmune Inner Ear Disease—A Real Entity?" *Clinics in Laboratory Medicine* 17, no. 3 (September 1997): 581–594.

Boulassel, M. R., N. Deggouj, J. P. Tomasi, and M. Gersdorff. "Inner Ear Autoantibodies and Their Targets in Patients with Autoimmune Inner Ear Diseases." *Acta Oto-Laryngologica* 121, no. 1 (January 2001): 28–34.

Campbell, K. C., and J. J. Clemens. "Sudden Hearing Loss and Autoimmune Disease." *Journal of the American Academy of Audiology* 11, no. 7 (July–August 2000): 361–367.

Hurley, Raymond M., and Janet P. Sells. "Autoimmune Inner Ear Disease (AIED): A Tutorial." *American Journal of Audiology* 6, no. 1 (March 1997).

Roland, J. T. "Autoimmune Inner Ear Disease." *Current Rheumatology Reports* 2, no. 2 (April 2000): 171–174.

autoimmune lymphoproliferative syndrome (ALPS) A recently recognized disease, first described in 1995, in which a genetic defect (mutation) in programmed cell death, or apoptosis, leads to the breakdown of lymphocyte homeostasis and normal immunologic tolerance. Some authors have referred to ALPS as Canale-Smith syndrome or lymphoproliferative syndrome with autoimmunity. Because patients with ALPS have defective apoptosis, their lymphocytes are not killed off in the normal fashion. This results in an expansion of lymphocytes and enlargement of tissues where lymphocytes normally reside: the lymph nodes and spleen. Moreover, lymphocytes that should be eliminated, because they recognize self, persist. These lymphocytes can cause autoimmune disease.

Patients with ALPS also have an increased risk of developing lymphoma, a cancer of the lymphoid tissues. The increased risk is 15 to 50 times greater than in normal individuals and usually occurs many years after the initial diagnosis of ALPS. Although the risk is significantly increased, the number of patients developing lymphoma is still rather small. In a study published by the investigators at the National Institutes of Health, 10 patients developed lymphoma among 130 patients with ALPS being followed.

Autoimmune lymphoproliferative syndrome is very rare. However, by studying patients with ALPS, scientists may learn more about how autoimmune disease occurs spontaneously and how autoimmune disease may predispose to lymphoma in a small percentage of patients.

Bleesing, J. J., S. E. Straus, and T. A. Fleisher. "Autoimmune Lymphoproliferative Syndrome. A Human Disorder of Abnormal Lymphocyte Survival." *Pediatric Clinics of North America* 47, no. 6 (December 2000): 1,291–1,310.

Chun, H. J., and M. J. Lenardo. "Autoimmune Lymphoproliferative Syndrome: Types I, II and Beyond." *Advances in Experimental Medicine and Biology* 490 (2001): 49–57.

Fleisher, T. A., J. M. Puck, W. Strober, J. K. Dale, M. J. Lenardo, R. M. Siegel, S. E. Straus, and J. J. Bleesing. "The Autoimmune Lymphoproliferative Syndrome. A Disorder of Human Lymphocyte Apoptosis." *Clinical Reviews in Allergy & Immunology* 20, no. 1 (February 2001): 109–120.

Jackson, Christine E., and Jennifer M. Puck. "Autoimmune Lymphoproliferative Syndrome: A Disorder of Apoptosis." *Current Opinions in Pediatrics* 11, no. 6 (December 1999): 521–527.

Straus, S. E., E. S. Jaffe, J. M. Puck, et al. "The development of Lymphomas in Families with Autoimmune Lymphoproliferative Syndrome with Germline Fas Mutations and Defective Lymphocyte Apoptosis." *Blood* 98, no. 1 (July 2001): 194–200.

autoimmunity A condition in which the cells and other components of the body's immune system mistakenly attack the person's own organs, tissues, and cells. One of the functions of the immune system is to protect the body by responding to invading microorganisms, such as viruses or bacteria, by producing antibodies or activated lymphocytes (types of white blood cells). In certain cases, immune cells make a mistake and attack the very host that they are meant to protect. This can lead to autoimmune disease. This term encompasses a broad category of related diseases in which the person's immune system attacks his or her own tissue.

bacteria The plural of *bacterium*, bacteria are single-cell microorganisms that lacks a nucleus and have a cell wall, or shell, composed of peptidoglycan, a protein-sugar molecule. Some bacteria, commonly called germs, are classified as pathogens because they cause disease, but most are harmless to people. Some even provide helpful services like producing antibiotics such as bacitracin, helping digest food in people's intestines, putting the tart taste into yogurt and the sour in sourdough bread, and helping to break down dead organic matter—the important function of biodegrading.

Bacteria are the largest class of creatures and therefore the most common organisms on Earth. They are found in the bodies of most living and nonliving things and in all environments, from deserts to oceans to mountaintops to glaciers. Most bacteria range in size from 0.5 to 1 micrometer in diameter and from 10 to 20 micrometers in length. To illustrate, hundreds of thousands of bacteria can fit into a space the size of the dot above the letter *i*. Yet colonies of bacteria containing millions of cells, such as those grown on a laboratory culture plate, can be viewed easily without a microscope.

Bacteria were discovered in the late 17th century, with the introduction of the microscope. Antoni van Leeuwenhoek, a Dutch microscope maker and the father of microbiology, was the first person to study bacteria systematically. However, not until the middle of the 19th century did researchers such as French chemist Louis Pasteur and German physician Robert Koch establish beyond a doubt that bacteria could cause disease.

Of the thousands of bacterial species on Earth, only a small fraction cause disease. Yet some of the most devastating diseases throughout history have been caused by bacteria—namely, plagues, cholera, and tuberculosis. Other diseases caused by bacteria include pneumonia, tonsilitis, meningitis, toxic shock syndrome, leprosy, typhoid fever, whooping cough, tetanus, diphtheria, legionnaires' disease, botulism, syphilis, and Lyme disease. Bacterial infections can aggravate psoriasis. In rheumatic fever, the individual produces antibodies to antigens of streptococcal bacteria that cross-react with heart tissue (i.e., autoantibodies). About 90 percent of hospitalized infections in developing countries are caused by bacteria.

Bacteria may infect certain organs or tissues that will later become targets of autoimmune disease in genetically predisposed individuals. Microorganisms may also affect different cell populations of the immune system, either stimulating or inhibiting their functions.

"Bacteria," Microsoft Encarta Online Encyclopedia 2002. Available online. URL: http://encarta.msm.com. Downloaded 13 July 2002.

Mattman, Lida H. *Cell Wall Deficient Forms: Stealth Pathogens,* 3rd ed. Boca Raton, Fla.: Lewis Publishers, Inc., 2001.

Nataro, James P., Martin J. Blaser, and S. Cunningham-Rundles, eds. *Persistent Bacterial Infections.* Washington, D.C.: American Society for Microbiology, 2000.

basophil A specific circulating white blood cell that stains readily with basic dyes, such as methylene blue. Basophils make up less than 1 percent of white blood cells. However, they are important in the body's immune response to inflammation because they release a stream of chemicals, including histamine, that dilate blood vessels when the immune response is triggered. These chemicals contribute to allergic symptoms.

Bechet's disease A common misspelling for BEHÇET'S DISEASE.

Behçet's disease   A rare and chronic autoimmune disorder that involves inflammation of blood vessels, called vasculitis, throughout the body. Common pronunciations include bay shetts, buh shetts, and buh setz. The disorder is named for Hulusi Behçet (1889–1948), a Turkish dermatologist and professor of dermatology in Istanbul. In 1937, he first described it as a triad syndrome due to its symptoms of recurring ulcers in the mouth that resemble but are more severe than canker sores, recurring genital ulcers, and eye inflammation. It is now known that in addition to those three primary symptoms, skin rashes, arthritis (swollen, painful, stiff joints), inflammation of the digestive tract, and meningitis may also occur. Behçet's disease is uncommon in the United States, affecting approximately 15,000 people. Although it does appear worldwide, it is most common in the eastern Mediterranean area and in Japan. In these regions, it appears most generally in young men and is the leading cause of blindness. In the United States, it affects more women, most generally in their 20s and 30s, although it can occur in children and older adults. Behçet's disease is not contagious and does not spread from one person to another.

Behçet's is a multisystem disease. It may involve all organs and affect the central nervous system, causing memory loss and impaired speech, balance, and movement. The effects of the disease may include blindness, stroke, swelling of the spinal cord, and intestinal complications.

Behçet's disease is a lifelong disorder characterized by a series of remissions (lack of disease activity) and active attacks, called flares. The length of time between active attacks is irregular; it may be as short a few days or as long as years. The disease is serious and painful, but it is not fatal. Most people with Behçet's can and do lead a normal life as long as they receive proper treatment.

Causes

The exact cause of Behçet's disease is unknown. Most of the symptoms are caused by inflammation of the blood vessels, particularly veins. Doctors think that an autoimmune reaction may cause blood vessels to become inflamed, but they do not know what triggers this reaction. Researchers think that two factors are probably important in its development. First, abnormalities of the immune system may make some people susceptible to the disease. Researchers suspect that this problem may be inherited through one or more specific genes. Second, something in the environment, possibly a bacterium or unknown virus, might trigger or activate the disease in susceptible people. Researchers have found that people who have frequent strep infections (caused by streptococcus bacteria) are more likely to develop Behçet's disease.

Clinical Features

Behçet's disease affects each person differently. Some people have only mild symptoms, such as skin sores or ulcers in the mouth or on the genitals. Others have more severe disease, such as meningitis or inflammation of the membranes that cover the brain and spinal cord. However, these more severe symptoms usually appear months or years after the first signs of Behçet's disease appear. Symptoms can last for a long time or can come and go in a few weeks. Typically, symptoms appear, disappear, and then reappear.

Mouth sores (aphthous ulcers) affect almost all patients with Behçet's disease. They are often the first symptom that a person notices and may occur long before any other symptoms appear. The sores usually have a red border with a white or yellow center, and several may appear at the same time, referred to as crops. They can be painful, especially when on the tongue, and make eating difficult. Mouth sores go away in 10 to 14 days but often come back. Small sores usually heal without scarring, but larger ones may scar.

Genital sores affect more that half of all people with Behçet's disease, appearing on the scrotum in men and vulva in women. These are not herpes related. The sores look similar to mouth sores and may be painful, but they do not recur as frequently as those in the mouth. After several outbreaks, they may cause scarring.

Inflammation of the middle part of the eye (the uvea), including the iris, occurs in more than half of all people with Behçet's disease. This symptom is more common among men than women and typically begins within two years of the first symptoms.

Arthritis, or inflammation of the joints, occur in more than half of all patients with Behçet's disease. Arthritis causes pain, swelling, and stiffness in the joints, especially the knees, ankles, wrists, and elbows. Arthritis that results from Behçet's disease usually lasts a few weeks and does not cause permanent damage to the joints. Behçet's disease causes various skin sores that look like red bumps on a black-and-blue mark. The sores are red, are raised, and typically appear on the legs and upper torso. Because these lesions are usually painless, they frequently are not paid serious attention by either patient or physician. In some people, sores or lesions may appear when the skin is scratched or pricked. Behçet's patients in the United States rarely have a skin reaction; however, more than half of the patients in Middle Eastern countries and Japan do have a reaction.

Behçet's disease affects the central nervous system in about 10 percent of all patients with the disease. It can cause meningoencephalitis—inflammation of the brain and the thin membrane that covers and protects it.

Only rarely does Behçet's disease cause inflammation and ulceration (sores) in the digestive tract and lead to stomach pain, diarrhea, constipation, and vomiting. These symptoms are very similar to symptoms of other diseases of the digestive tract, such as a peptic ulcer, ulcerative colitis, and especially Crohn's disease.

Diagnosing Behçet's disease is very difficult because no specific test confirms it, and some of its symptoms occur in other diseases such as lupus, Lyme disease, and Crohn's disease. Less than half of the patients initially thought to have Behçet's disease actually have it. Because several months or even years may pass before all the common symptoms appear, the diagnosis may not be made for a long time. Also, not all the symptoms are likely to appear at the same time. A patient may even visit several different kinds of doctors for the different symptoms before the diagnosis is finally made. The diagnosis relies on three or more of the major characteristic symptoms being present.

Complications

Eye inflammation can cause blurred vision and, rarely, pain and redness. Partial loss of vision or blindness can result if the eye frequently becomes inflamed. Meningitis can cause fever, a stiff neck, and headaches. If left untreated, a stroke can result. About 10 percent of patients with Behçet's disease have blood clots resulting from inflammation in the veins (thrombophlebitis), usually in the legs. Symptoms include pain and tenderness in the affected area, which may also be swollen and warm. A few patients may experience artery problems such as aneurysms (a stretching or expanding of a weakened blood vessel).

Treatment

Although no cure exists for Behçet's disease, most patients' symptoms can be controlled with medication to reduce inflammation and/or regulate the immune system, rest, and exercise. Treatment goals are to reduce discomfort and prevent serious complications such as disability from arthritis or blindness. The type of medicine and the length of treatment depend on the person's symptoms and their severity. In most cases, a combination of treatments is needed to relieve specific symptoms.

Topical medicine is applied directly on the sores to relieve pain and discomfort. For example, doctors prescribe rinses to treat mouth sores. Creams are used to treat skin and genital sores. The medicine usually contains corticosteroids, which reduce inflammation, or an anesthetic, which relieves pain.

Oral medicine is prescribed to reduce inflammation throughout the body, suppress the overactive immune system, and relieve symptoms. Prednisone is a corticosteroid prescribed to reduce pain and swelling throughout the body in people with severe joint pain and inflammation, skin sores, eye disease, or central nervous system symptoms. Immunosuppressive drugs (including corticosteroids) help control an overactive immune system in people with Behçet's disease, reduce inflammation throughout the body, and can lessen the number of flares. Doctors may use immunosuppressive drugs when a person has eye disease or central nervous system involvement.

Azathioprine is used to treat uveitis and central nervous system involvement in Behçet's disease. Chlorambucil is used to treat uveitis and meningoencephalitis. Cyclosporine is used to reduce uveitis and central nervous system involvement. Colchicine is sometimes used to treat eye inflammation and skin symptoms in patients with Behçet's disease. If these medicines do not reduce symptoms, doctors may use other drugs such as cyclophosphamide and methotrexate. Cyclophosphamide is similar to chlorambucil. Methotrexate can relieve Behçet's symptoms because it suppresses the immune system and reduces inflammation throughout the body.

Although rest is important during flares, moderate exercise such as swimming or walking carried out after the symptoms have improved or disappeared can help people with Behçet's disease keep their joints strong and flexible.

When treatment is effective, flares usually become less frequent after one or two years. Many patients eventually enter a period of remission. In some people, however, treatment does not relieve symptoms, and gradually more serious symptoms such as eye disease may occur. Serious symptoms may appear months or years after the first signs of Behçet's disease. A major "problem" for patients is the unpredictability of the disease and not knowing when another flare may occur.

Plotkin, Gary R., John J. Calabro, and J. Despond O'Duffy, eds. *Behçet's Disease: A Contemporary Synopsis.* Armonk, N.Y.: Futura Publishing Co., Inc., 1988.
"Questions and Answers About Behçet's disease," National Arthritis and Musculoskeletal and Skin Diseases Information Clearinghouse (NAMSIC), National Institutes of Health. Available online. URL: http://www.niams.nih.gov/du/topics/behcets/behcets.htm. Posted on January 1999.

Behçet's disease research   Researchers are exploring possible genetic, bacterial, and viral causes of Behçet's disease as well as improved drug treatment. They hope to identify genes that increase a person's chance of developing the disease. Studying these genes and how they work may lead to a new understanding of the disease and possibly new treatments.

Researchers are also investigating factors in the environment, such as a bacterium or virus, that could trigger Behçet's disease. They are particularly interested in whether streptococcus, the bacterium that causes strep throat, is associated with the dis-

ease. Many people with Behçet's disease have had several strep infections. In addition, researchers suspect that herpes virus type I, a virus that causes cold sores, may be associated with the disease.

Finally, researchers are identifying other medicines to treat Behçet's disease better. Thalidomide, for example, appears effective in treating severe mouth sores, but its use is experimental and very limited. Thalidomide is not used in women of childbearing age because it causes severe birth defects.

birth control   Because of the greater incidence of many autoimmune diseases in women, there has been much conjecture as to whether sex hormones, particularly estrogens, could be a factor in autoimmune diseases. Researchers do not completely agree about the effects of estrogen on SYSTEMIC LUPUS ERYTHEMATOSUS (SLE). Estrogen has been shown to exacerbate SLE in lab animals. However, experiments with human patients using estrogen-laden birth control pills were inconclusive. Limited data suggest oral contraceptives may be safe for some women with lupus. Similarly, there is a lack of clarity regarding the effects of estrogen on RHEUMATIC FEVER and no significant information on the effects of estrogen on other autoimmune diseases.

A small retrospective study looked at two groups of women who subsequently developed MULTIPLE SCLEROSIS. One group had taken birth control pills and one had not. The MS appeared to have developed later in the group using oral contraceptives. However, larger studies need to be done before any conclusions can be drawn.

A few reports have surfaced that autoimmune diseases such as INTERSTITIAL CYSTITIS (IC) have occurred following use of the birth control implant Norplant. It is believed, though, that the occurrence of autoimmune diseases among Norplant users is coincidental. Also, no proof exists that birth control devices will protect against autoimmune diseases.

Giesser, Barbara S. *Hormones in Multiple Sclerosis.* New York: The National Multiple Sclerosis Society, 1999.
"Hormones & Autoimmunity." *InFocus.* American Autoimmune Related Diseases Association. Available

online. URL: http://www.aarda.org/hormone_art2.
html. Downloaded 13 July 2002.

blindness   Little is known about the factors that
determine susceptibility of the visual system to
autoimmune diseases. The National Eye Institute's
research program is actively investigating the cause
of a number of autoimmune diseases, including
UVEITIS, a potentially blinding eye condition and
the third leading cause of blindness in the United
States. Other autoimmune diseases also may lead
to blindness:

- In the eastern Mediterranean countries and in
  eastern Asia, BEHÇET'S DISEASE is a leading cause
  of blindness. However, it is not a leading cause
  of blindness in the western world.

- CICATRICIAL PEMPHIGOID is a rare autoimmune
  blistering condition that causes blistering and
  scarring of moist tissue areas. In particular, the
  lining of the eyes and eyelids (conjunctiva) may
  be involved, which may lead to scarring and
  blindness.

- COGAN'S SYNDROME can lead to deafness or blindness.

- When uncontrolled or inadequately controlled,
  INSULIN-DEPENDENT DIABETES leads to blindness.
  Blindness is the only complication of diabetes
  that can be prevented.

- The initial symptom of MULTIPLE SCLEROSIS is
  often blurred or double vision, red-green color
  distortion, or even blindness in one eye.

- Inflammation of the eye occurs infrequently in
  POLYCHONDRITIS but can lead to blindness when
  it does.

- In a few cases of SARCOIDOSIS, cataracts, glaucoma, and blindness occur.

- SCLERITIS, which is inflammation of the outer
  layer of the eyeball, typically manifests with
  deep eye pain and redness. It is most commonly
  seen in older patients with systemic vascular or
  connective tissue disease such as rheumatoid
  arthritis. Scleritis can threaten vision and
  requires emergent ophthalmic evaluation.

- SJÖGREN'S SYNDROME is an autoimmune disease
  that causes the eye to become dry. If not treated,

dry eye can cause cloudiness or ulcerations of
the cornea, ultimately leading to blindness.

- If left untreated, SYMPATHETIC OPHTHALMIA can
  progress to complete blindness over a period of
  months or years.

- TEMPORAL ARTERITIS causes blindness if not
  treated adequately.

blood pressure   Blood pressure is the force of
blood against the walls of arteries. Blood pressure is
recorded as two numbers—the systolic pressure (as
the heart beats) over the diastolic pressure (as the
heart relaxes between beats). The measurement is
written with the systolic number above or before
the diastolic number. For example, a blood pressure measurement of 120/80 mm Hg (millimeters
of mercury) is expressed verbally as "120 over 80."
Normal blood pressure is less than 130 mm Hg systolic and less than 85 mm Hg diastolic. Optimal
blood pressure is less than 120 mm Hg systolic and
less than 80 mm Hg diastolic.

Blood pressure rises and falls during the day.
When blood pressure stays elevated over time, it is
called high blood pressure or hypertension. High
blood pressure increases one's chance (or risk) of
getting heart disease and/or kidney disease and of
having a stroke. It is especially dangerous because
it often has no warning signs or symptoms.

When blood pressure remains too low, inadequate amounts of blood are flowing to the heart,
brain, and other vital organs. Very low systolic
blood pressure (hypotension) can cause fainting.

A change in blood pressure—lower or higher
than usual for that person—is a symptom of several
autoimmune diseases. Low blood pressure can
occur with ADDISON'S DISEASE and HASHIMOTO'S THY-
ROIDITIS. High blood pressure can occur with
GRAVES' DISEASE, IDIOPATHIC PULMONARY FIBROSIS
(IPF), POLYARTERITIS NODOSA, and TAKAYASU'S
ARTERITIS. High blood pressure is also a complication of INSULIN-DEPENDENT DIABETES; those with diabetes are more likely to develop high blood
pressure than people without diabetes.

B lymphocyte (B cell)   White blood cells, which
develop in the bone marrow from pluripotent stem
cells. They may develop into plasma cells, which

produce immunoglobulins (antibodies). The antibody-producing cell of the immune system.

bone marrow   A soft, jellylike tissue found in the cavities of long bones (yellow marrow) and in the spaces between the tissue of spongy bone in the sternum (breastbone) and other flat and irregular bones (red marrow). Yellow marrow is mostly fat, stored energy. Red marrow produces white blood cells, which fight infection; red blood cells, which carry oxygen and nutrients to and remove waste products from organs and tissues throughout the body; and platelets, which enable blood clotting and healing. These cells are critical for life. Red marrow is present in all bones at birth. During the teens, it is gradually replaced in the long bones by yellow marrow. In adults, red marrow appears mainly in the spine, breastbone, ribs, collarbone, shoulder blades, pelvis (hipbones), and skull bones.

Immature hematopoietic cells, commonly called stem cells, within the red marrow are stimulated to form red blood cells by erythropoietin, a hormone produced in the kidney. The blood cells go through various stages in the red marrow before they are ready to be released into the circulation. Yellow marrow produces some white cells.

Sometimes bone marrow fails to produce the normal amount of blood cells, as in anemia or when the marrow has been displaced by tumor cells. At other times, it may overproduce only certain blood cells, as in polycythemia and leukemia. Symptoms of possible bone marrow dysfunction include easy bruising, lack of energy, bleeding problems, and recurring infections.

bone marrow transplant (BMT)   A surgical procedure used to transfer normal, healthy bone marrow to a patient who has malignant bone marrow or defective bone marrow resulting from chemotherapy or radiation treatment for cancer. The healthy bone marrow may come from three sources. First, it may be taken from the patient's own bone marrow prior to his or her chemotherapy or radiation treatment and stored for use after these treatments have caused the marrow's deterioration. This type of transplantation is called autologous. Second, it may be taken from an identical twin, yielding genetically identical bone marrow.

This type of transplantation is called syngeneic. Third, it may be taken from another person who is not genetically identical to the recipient but who has a similar enough tissue type to the patient for a successful graft. This type of transplantation is called allogeneic. Often, allogeneic transplantation is from a brother or sister. However, only 30 to 40 percent of patients have suitably matched siblings or parents. When no sibling or other relative with matching bone marrow is available, national and international bone marrow registries may yield unrelated donors with suitable matches. The odds of finding a marrow donor in the general population are typically one in 20,000. At any given time, an average of 3,000 patients are searching the National Marrow Donor Program (NMDP) Registry. As of 31 May 2001, the total number of volunteer potential donors was 4,389,410. Donated bone marrow must match the patient's tissue type. Donors are matched through special blood tests called human leukocyte-associated (HLA) tissue typing. Approximately 30 percent of allogeneic bone marrow transplants come from donors not related to the recipients.

Although the first successful bone marrow transplant did not take place until 1968, the discovery of human leukocyte antigens in 1958 was a major breakthrough because it allowed recipients to be matched with donors. Since then, the procedure has steadily advanced as research uncovered ways to improve transplant techniques. Donor registries have grown significantly, and drugs that prevent rejection and infection have improved. The Food and Drug Administration reviews new drugs used to prepare patients for bone marrow transplants and drugs that aid in recovery. The FDA also reviews so-called growth factors, genetically engineered substances that stimulate growth of the transplanted cells.

Patients need bone marrow transplants because they have dangerously low white blood cells, which are needed to fight infection. Bone marrow transplant patients are usually treated in centers specializing in the procedure, where they can stay in special nursing units in order to limit exposure to infections. Because of the risks involved, bone marrow transplantation is done only for potentially fatal blood and immune disorders.

In general, the procedure for obtaining bone marrow, which is also called *harvesting,* is similar for all three types of BMTs (autologous, syngeneic, and allogeneic). The donor is given either general anesthesia, which puts the person to sleep during the procedure, or local anesthesia, which causes loss of feeling in the area of the body where the bone marrow will be removed. Usually, several small cuts (not requiring stitches) are made in the skin over the pelvic bone or, in rare cases, the sternum. A large needle is inserted through the cuts and into the bone marrow to draw the marrow out of the bone. The process of obtaining the marrow takes about an hour.

The harvested bone marrow is then filtered to remove blood and bone fragments. Harvested bone marrow may be transported immediately or can be combined with a preservative and placed into a liquid nitrogen freezer to keep the stem cells alive until they are needed. This technique is known as cryopreservation. Marrow may be cryopreserved for many years.

Because only a small amount of bone marrow is removed, donating usually does not pose any significant problems for the donor. The most serious risk associated with donating bone marrow involves the use of anesthesia during the procedure.

Within a few weeks, the donor's body will have replaced the donated marrow. The area where the bone marrow was taken out may feel sore for a few days, and the donor may feel tired. The time required for a donor to recover varies. Some people are back to their usual routine within two or three days, while others may take up to three to four weeks to recover their strength.

After being treated with high-dose anticancer drugs and/or radiation, the patient receives the bone marrow through a central venous catheter, a flexible tube called an IV line, that is placed into a large vein in the neck or chest area. This part of the transplant is called the *rescue process.*

After entering the bloodstream, the transplanted cells travel to the bone marrow, where they begin to produce new white blood cells, red blood cells, and platelets in a process known as *engraftment.* Engraftment usually occurs within about two to four weeks after transplantation and is monitored by frequently checking blood counts. Complete recovery of immune function takes much longer, however—up to several months for autologous transplant recipients and one to two years for patients receiving allogeneic or syngeneic transplants. Doctors evaluate the results of various blood tests to confirm that new blood cells are being produced. Bone marrow aspiration (the removal of a small sample of bone marrow through a needle for examination under a microscope) can also help doctors determine how well the new marrow is working.

The major risk of a bone marrow transplant is an increased susceptibility to infection and bleeding as a result of any high-dose cancer treatment. Patients who undergo these procedures may experience short-term side effects such as nausea, vomiting, fatigue, loss of appetite, mouth sores, hair loss, and skin reactions. Additionally, patients receiving BMT may experience nausea and vomiting while receiving the transplant and also chills and fever during the first 24 hours after the transplant.

Potential long-term risks include infertility (the inability to produce children), cataracts (clouding of the lens of the eye, which causes loss of vision) and secondary (new) cancers. Complications in the liver, kidneys, lungs, and/or heart can also result.

With allogeneic BMT, a complication known as graft-versus-host disease (GVHD) sometimes develops. GVHD occurs when white blood cells from the donor marrow (the graft) identify the cells of the patient's body (the host) as foreign and attack it. GVHD can generally be treated with steroids or another immunosuppressive agent. Clinical trials are being conducted to find ways to prevent GVHD from occurring.

The immunosuppressive drug cyclosporine plays a major role in the success of an allogeneic transplant because it can help prevent GVHD and interstitial pneumonia, a lung infection caused by cytomegalovirus. For patients who have had this virus and then undergo a bone marrow transplant, a high chance exists that it will reactivate. Sometimes doctors also give patients growth factors, genetically engineered substances that stimulate a faster return of white cells. Examples are granulocyte-macrophage colony-stimulating factor (GM-CSF) and granulocyte colony-stimulating factor (G-CSF).

As for success rates of bone marrow transplants, experts generally agree there is no clear-cut answer. These rates depend on many factors, including the type and stage of disease, the condition of the patient at the time of the transplant, the donor, and the age of the patient. Success can range from 80 to 90 percent for children with inherited abnormalities of the immune system to as low as 10 percent for patients with aggressive, resistant diseases.

Diseases treatable by bone marrow transplant include acute lymphoblastic leukemia, acute myelogenous leukemia, chronic myelogenous leukemia, histiocytic disorders, Hodgkin's lymphoma, inherited erythrocyte abnormalities, inherited immune system disorders, inherited metabolism disorders, inherited platelet abnormalities, myelodysplastic disorder syndromes, non-Hodgkin's lymphoma, other leukemias, other malignancies, other nonmalignant diseases, plasma cell disorders, and severe aplastic anemia.

Meadows, Michelle. "Bone Marrow Transplants Come of Age." *FDA Consumer* 34, no. 4 (July/August 2000). Available online. URL: http://www.fda.gov/features/ 2000/400_bone.html. Posted August 2000.

breast-feeding with autoimmune disease

Mothers who have autoimmune diseases are sometimes told that because antibodies get into the milk, the mother should not breast-feed because she will cause illness in her baby. This is not true, according to Dr. Jack Newman. "The antibodies that make up the vast majority of the antibodies in the milk are of the type called secretory IgA. Autoimmune diseases are not caused by secretory IgA. Even if they were, secretory IgA is not absorbed by the baby. Therefore, mothers with autoimmune diseases may continue breast-feeding."

Studies have shown a possible association between breast-feeding and Type I diabetes. In Japan and Korea, where a high percentage of mothers nurse their infants, the disease is least prevalent. Where fewer mothers breast-feed—in Finland, Denmark, and the United States—the disease is far more common.

Cerrato, Paul L. "Does Milk Cause Juvenile Diabetes?" *RN,* 56 no. 1 (January 1993): 69.
Newman, Jack. "Breastfeeding: Illness in the Mother or Baby." Available online. URL: http://www.keepkids healthy.com/breastfeeding/guide/breastfeeding_illness.html. Posted January 2000.

bullous pemphigoid A relatively benign autoimmune disease characterized by formation of large blisters, which usually appear on the areas of the body that flex or move (called flexural surfaces), such as the inside of the elbow or back of the knee. About 15 to 30 percent of persons with bullous pemphigoid also develop blisters on mucous membranes such as the mouth, nose, or eyes. The disorder may occur in various forms, from no symptoms, to mild redness and irritation, to multiple blisters. Bullous pemphigoid typically occurs in middle-aged or elderly persons and rarely occurs in young people. However, children as young as several months of age have been reported with the condition. It tends to be chronic, with flare-ups after long remissions of five or six years.

Causes
Patients with bullous pemphigoid develop blisters as a consequence of autoantibodies directed against a normal protein in the skin. The cause is not known, and there is no known way to prevent this disorder.

Clinical Features
Multiple bullae, which is the name for the large blisters filled with clear fluid and greater than 1 cm in diameter, are usually located on the arms, legs, or trunk, although they may also occur in the mouth. These blisters may weep or crust over, may appear deep below the surface of the skin, or may erode the skin, forming ulcers or open sores. Also present will be itching, rashes, mouth sores, and bleeding gums. A skin lesion biopsy will show a blister beneath the outer skin layer and the inner skin layers and also immunoglobulin deposits.

Complications
Infection of the skin lesions is the most common complication.

Treatment
Treatment of patients with bullous pemphigoid focuses on relief of symptoms and prevention of infection. Corticosteroids are often the treatment of choice, given by mouth or by injection. Topical cor-

ticosteroids are sometimes used on early, localized lesions. Also for patients with localized disease, topical steroids or intralesional steroids may be tried initially. For patients with more severe or widespread disease, systemic corticosteroids such as prednisone are commonly used. Other anti-inflammatory drugs that have been reported successful in some patients with bullous pemphigoid include antibiotics (tetracycline or erythromycin), niacinamide, and dapsone. Some patients may require treatment with immunosuppressants such as azathioprine (Imuran), cyclophosphamide (Cytoxan), cyclosporine (Sandimmune or Neoral), methotrexate, chlorambucil (Leukeran), or mycophenolate mofetil (CellCept).

Up to 70 percent of patients with bullous pemphigoid will experience a remission within five years of initial diagnosis. Some patients may relapse. However, in general, the course for patients with bullous pemphigoid is not protracted.

Bullous pemphigoid lesions should heal without scarring unless secondary infection occurs.

Recently, researchers have identified the target antigens present in the skin that bind the autoantibodies associated with bullous pemphigoid. Circulating antibodies in patients with this disorder are specific for two distinct proteins found within the major cells of the epidermis, the keratinocytes. These two proteins are called BPAG1 (BP antigen1, the 230 kD BP antigen) and BPAG2 (BP antigen2, the 180 kD BP antigen).

These proteins are part of a complex of proteins that make up the hemidesmosome. Hemidesmosomes are critical for adhesion of the epidermis to the dermis. Investigators are trying to determine what parts of the target antigen are most important in turning on the immune response in patients with bullous pemphigoid and for normal epidermal-dermal adherence.

Canada and autoimmune diseases According to the Multiple Sclerosis Society of Canada, Canadians have one of the highest rates of MULTIPLE SCLEROSIS (MS) in the world. MS is the most common neurological disease affecting young adults in Canada. Every day, three more people in Canada are diagnosed with MS.

RHEUMATOID ARTHRITIS affects an estimated 293,000 Canadians, or one person in 100 statistically.

Estimates of the number of SYSTEMIC LUPUS ERYTHEMATOSUS (SLE) patients in Canada range from 15,000 (based on the number of patients followed in various University Hospital Lupus Clinics throughout the country) to 50,000 (based on the figures used by the Lupus Foundation of America, adjusted to the Canadian population). Other reports have stated the number to be between 20,000 and 25,000.

cancer Diseases in which abnormal cells divide and grow unchecked. Cancer can spread from its original site to other parts of the body (i.e., metastasize) and can also be fatal if not treated adequately.

cardiomyopathy A disease of the heart muscle. The heart loses its ability to pump blood and, in some instances, heart rhythm is disturbed, leading to irregular heartbeats, or arrhythmias. Usually, the exact cause of the muscle damage is never found. Cardiomyopathy differs from many other heart disorders in a couple of ways. First, it is fairly uncommon, affecting about 50,000 Americans annually. Second, unlike many other forms of heart disease that affect middle-aged and older persons, cardiomyopathy can, and often does, occur in the young. The condition tends to be progressive and sometimes worsens fairly quickly. The condition is a leading reason for heart transplantation.

The various types of cardiomyopathy fall into two major categories: ischemic and nonischemic cardiomyopathy. Ischemic cardiomyopathy typically refers to heart muscle damage that results from coronary artery disease, such as heart attack. Nonischemic cardiomyopathy includes several types, the main ones of which are dilated, hypertrophic, and restrictive. The name of each describes the nature of its muscle damage.

By far the most common type of nonischemic cardiomyopathy is the dilated (stretched) form. It occurs when disease-affected muscle fibers lead to enlargement, or dilation, of one or more chambers of the heart. This weakens the heart's pumping ability. The heart tries to cope with the pumping limitation by further enlarging and stretching—a process known as *compensation*. Dilated cardiomyopathy occurs most often in middle-aged people and more often in men than women.

In most cases, the disease is idiopathic—a specific cause for the damage is never identified. Some factors, though, have been linked to the disease's occurrence. For instance, alcohol has a direct suppressant effect on the heart. Dilated cardiomyopathy can be caused by chronic, excessive consumption of alcohol, particularly in combination with dietary deficiencies. Also, dilated cardiomyopathy occasionally occurs as a complication of pregnancy and childbirth.

Rarely, a virus may affect the heart of a normal person, sometimes causing no symptoms and sometimes causing mild or severe symptoms of the viral infection itself. This is called viral myocarditis and is commonly caused by a group of viruses called *Coxsackie B viruses*. The majority of people affected, though, do not have any permanent damage to their heart.

However a small proportion of people who develop such a myocarditis can develop dilated cardiomyopathy. This occurs because the virus severely damages the heart during the initial infection or because the virus triggers the body's own defense system (immune system) to attack and damage the heart. Researchers think that some cases of an idiopathic dilated cardiomyopathy may have resulted from a previous mild virus infection that produced no symptom at the time.

Treatment

Dilated cardiomyopathy is not currently curable, although some patients improve spontaneously. Treatment is usually with drugs. It is aimed at minimizing symptoms and preventing the development of complications and progression of the disease. A minority of patients deteriorate in spite of treatment and may require a heart transplant.

"Dilated Cardiomyopathy." Cardiomyopathy Association. Available online. URL: http://cardiomyopathy.org/docs/dilated_cardiomyopathy.pdf. Downloaded on 13 July 2002.

National Institutes of Health. *Facts About Cardiomyopathy.* NIH Publication Number: 97-3082, 1997.

cardiovascular disease (CVD) Cardiovascular disease (CVD) is defined as any serious, abnormal condition of the heart or blood vessels (arteries, veins). Cardiovascular disease includes coronary heart disease (CHD), stroke, peripheral vascular disease, congenital heart disease, endocarditis, and many other conditions, including autoimmune disorders such as rheumatic fever.

According to 1999 estimates, 61,800,000 Americans have one or more forms of cardiovascular disease. These diseases claimed 949,619 lives in 1998 (40.6 percent of all deaths). This number compares with 541,532 total cancer deaths, 97,835 accidental deaths, and 13,426 deaths from HIV (AIDS) in 1998. About one-sixth of all people killed by CVD are under age 65.

The American Heart Association statistics show that rheumatic fever and rheumatic heart disease killed 3,676 Americans in 1999, of which 1,042 (28.4 percent of total deaths from rheumatic

fever/rheumatic heart disease) were males and 2,634 (71.6 percent) females. Modern antibiotic therapy has sharply reduced mortality. In 1950, about 15,000 Americans died of these diseases. From 1989 to 1999, the death rate from rheumatic fever/rheumatic heart disease fell 34.6 percent. Actual deaths declined 26.4 percent. In 1999, the death rates per 100,000 for white males were 0.9, for African-American males were 0.8, for white females were 1.7, and for African-American fe males were 1.2.

ANTIPHOSPHOLIPID SYNDROME (APS) has been indicated as a causative factor in cardiovascular disease in women. Long-term complications in INSULIN-DEPENDENT DIABETES mellitus include accelerated cardiovascular disease.

The prevalence of preclinical cardiovascular disease was determined in women with SYSTEMIC LUPUS ERYTHEMATOSUS (SLE) and control subjects matched for traditional risk factors. When compared with control subjects, patients with SLE had a higher prevalence of carotid atherosclerosis (41 percent versus 9 percent) and left ventricular hypertrophy (32 percent versus 5 percent), supporting the possibility that chronic inflammation predisposes one to premature cardiovascular disease in SLE.

Roman M. J., J. E. Salmon, R. Sobel, M. D. Lockshin, L. Sammaritano, J. E. Schwartz, and R. B. Devereux. "Prevalence and Relation to Risk Factors of Carotid Atherosclerosis and Left Ventricular Hypertrophy in Systemic Lupus Erythematosus and Antiphospholipid Antibody Syndrome." *The American Journal of Cardiology* 87, no. 5 (March 1, 2001): 663–666, A11.

CD4 molecule A lymphocyte antigen molecule (protein) that plays a key role in the recognition of foreign antigens by helper T cells. Antibody-like molecules called T cell receptors, or TCRs, are found on the surface of helper T cells. It is the function of the TCRs to bind to any alien protein, including virus fragments that are presented on the surface of other cells that have ingested and digested these invaders. However, the bond between TCRs and the presented antigen fragments is weak. The recognition works only because of the CD4 molecules' ability to strengthen the union between helper T cells and their antigen-presenting partners. In addition, CD4 molecules trigger the increased metabolic activity and release from the T cell of stimulatory—helper—chemicals that follow this antigen binding.

CD8 molecule   Plays a role on cytotoxic T cells similar to that of CD4 on helper T cells. Cytotoxic T cells mediate transplantation rejection and killing of viral-infected or cancer cells.

celebrities with autoimmune diseases   Autoimmune diseases do not not leave the famous untouched. Several well-known athletes, authors, entertainers, and other public figures have had or are dealing with any number of autoimmune disorders.

ALOPECIA AREATA: Princess Caroline of Monaco, Al Pacino—actor.

AUTOIMMUNE INNER EAR DISEASE: Rush Limbaugh—radio talk show host.

CHRONIC FATIGUE SYNDROME: Michelle Akers—star of the United States women's national soccer team, Keith Jarrett—jazz pianist, Amy Peterson—Olympic speed skating medal winner.

CHURG-STRAUSS SYNDROME: Ben Watt—singer with Everything But The Girl.

GRAVES' DISEASE: George and Barbara Bush—former United States President and First Lady, Gail Devers—Olympic track gold medalist, Carla Overbeck—United States women's national soccer team captain.

HASHIMOTO'S THYROIDITIS: Linda Ronstadt—singer.

INSULIN-DEPENDENT DIABETES: Halle Berry—actress, Mary Tyler Moore—actress, Richard Mulligan—actor, Park Overall—actress, Anne Rice—author, Jackie Robinson—baseball player, Ron Santo—baseball player, Jason Johnson—baseball player.

MULTIPLE SCLEROSIS: Neil Cavuto—anchor on Fox News Channel, Michael Crichton—author of *ER* and *Jurassic Park,* Joan Didion—author and director, Donna Fargo—country singer, Lola Folana—singer, Annette Funicello—singer and former Mouseketeer, Roman Gabriel—Los Angeles Rams football player, Lena Horne—actress and singer, Barbara Jordan—former Congress-

woman, David "Squiggy" Lander—actor in the TV show *Laverne & Shirley,* Alan Osmond—one of the singing Osmond Brothers, Richard Pryor—comedian and actor, Madeline Rhue—actress, Joan Sweeney—children's author, Montel Williams—talk show host and actor.

MYASTHENIA GRAVIS: Mabel Fairbanks—the first African-American woman inducted into the U.S. Figure Skating Hall of Fame, Suzanne Rogers—actress (Maggie Horton on *Days of Our Lives*).

RHEUMATOID ARTHRITIS: James Coburn—actor, Susan Lamontagne—Broadway star, Auguste Renoir—French impressionist painter, Kathleen Turner—actress, Aida Turturro—actress (Janice Soprano in *The Sopranos*).

SCLERODERMA: Linda Chavez Rodriguez—activist.

SYSTEMIC LUPUS ERYTHEMATOSUS: Tim Raines—major league baseball player.

VITILIGO: Michael Jackson—singer.

celiac disease (also called nontropical sprue, celiac sprue, and gluten-sensitive enteropathy)   A digestive disease that damages the small intestine and interferes with absorption of nutrients from food. People who have celiac disease cannot tolerate a protein called gluten, which is found in wheat, rye, and barley. When people with celiac disease eat foods containing gluten, their immune system responds in the same way it would to an infection—by damaging the small intestine. Specifically, tiny fingerlike protrusions, called villi, on the lining of the small intestine are lost. Nutrients from food are absorbed into the bloodstream through these villi. Without villi, a person becomes malnourished—regardless of the quantity of food eaten. In addition to causing weight loss, this loss of vitamins and minerals can lead to anemia and skin problems.

Because the body's own immune system causes the damage, celiac disease is sometimes considered an autoimmune disorder. However, it is also classified as a disease of malabsorption because nutrients are not absorbed.

There is a genetic predisposition to celiac disease, meaning that it occurs more frequently in certain families. Sometimes the disease is triggered—or becomes active for the first time—after surgery, pregnancy, childbirth, viral infection, or severe emotional stress.

Celiac disease affects people differently. Some people develop symptoms as children, others as adults. One factor thought to play a role in when and how celiac disease appears is whether and how long a person was breast-fed—the longer one was breast-fed, the later the symptoms of celiac disease appear and the more atypical the symptoms. Other factors include the age at which one began eating foods containing gluten and how much gluten is eaten.

The proportion of people suffering from celiac disease varies widely among different countries. It is the most common genetic disease in Europe. In Italy, about one in 250 people and in Ireland about one in 300 people have celiac disease. It is rarely diagnosed in African, Chinese, and Japanese people.

An estimated one in 4,700 Americans have been diagnosed with celiac disease. Some researchers question how celiac disease could be so uncommon in the United States since it is hereditary in part and many Americans descend from European ethnic groups in whom the disease is common. A recent study in which random blood samples from the Red Cross were tested for celiac disease suggests that as many as one in every 250 Americans may have it. Celiac disease could be underdiagnosed in the United States for a number of reasons. First, celiac symptoms can be attributed to other problems. Additionally, many doctors are not knowledgeable about the disease. Finally, only a handful of U.S. laboratories are experienced and skilled in testing for celiac disease.

Clinical Features

Symptoms may or may not occur in the digestive system. For example, one person might have diarrhea and abdominal pain, while another person may have irritability or depression. In fact, irritability is one of the most common symptoms in children. Symptoms of celiac disease may include one or more of the following: recurring abdominal bloating and pain, chronic diarrhea, weight loss, pale and foul-smelling stool, unexplained anemia (low count of red blood cells), gas, bone pain, behavior changes, muscle cramps, fatigue, delayed growth, failure to thrive in infants, pain in the joints, seizures, tingling numbness in the legs (from nerve damage), pale sores inside the mouth (called aphthous ulcers), painful skin rash (called dermatitis herpetiformis), tooth discoloration or loss of enamel, and/or missed menstrual periods (often because of excessive weight loss).

Anemia, delayed growth, and weight loss are signs of malnutrition—not getting enough nutrients. Malnutrition is a serious problem for anyone but particularly for children because they need adequate nutrition to develop properly.

Some people with celiac disease may not have symptoms. The undamaged part of their small intestine is able to absorb enough nutrients to prevent symptoms. However, people without symptoms are still at risk for the complications of celiac disease.

Diagnosing celiac disease can be difficult because some of its symptoms are similar to those of other diseases. These include irritable bowel syndrome, Crohn's disease, ulcerative colitis, diverticulosis, intestinal infections, chronic fatigue syndrome, and depression.

Recently, researchers discovered that people with celiac disease have higher than normal levels of certain antibodies in their blood. Antibodies are produced by the immune system in response to substances that the body perceives to be threatening. To diagnose celiac disease, physicians test blood to measure levels of antibodies to these antigens. These antibodies are antigliadin, antiendomysium, and antireticulin.

If the tests and symptoms suggest celiac disease, the physician may remove a tiny piece of tissue from the small intestine to check for damage to the villi. This is done in a procedure called a biopsy. The physician eases a long, thin tube called an endoscope through the mouth and stomach into the small intestine and then takes a sample of tissue using instruments passed through the endoscope. Biopsy of the small intestine is the best way to diagnose celiac disease.

Screening for celiac disease involves testing asymptomatic people for the antibodies described above. Americans are not routinely screened for celiac disease. However, because celiac disease is hereditary, family members—particularly first-degree relatives—of people who have been diagnosed may need to be tested for the disease. About 10 percent of an affected person's first-degree relatives (parents, siblings, or children) will also have the disease. The longer a person goes undiagnosed and untreated, the greater the chance of developing malnutrition and other complications.

In Italy, where celiac disease is common, all children are screened by age six so that even asymptomatic disease is caught early. In addition, Italians of any age are tested for the disease as soon as they show symptoms. As a result of this vigilance, the time between when symptoms begin and the disease is diagnosed is usually only two to three weeks. In the United States, the time between the first symptoms and diagnosis averages about 10 years.

Treatment

The only treatment for celiac disease is to follow a gluten-free diet, to avoid all foods that contain gluten. For most people, following this diet will stop symptoms, heal existing intestinal damage, and prevent further damage. Improvements begin within days of starting the diet. The small intestine is usually completely healed—meaning the villi are intact and working—in three to six months. (Healing may take up to two years for older adults.)

The gluten-free diet is a lifetime requirement. Eating any gluten, no matter how small an amount, can damage the intestine. This is true for anyone with the disease, including people who do not have noticeable symptoms. Depending on a person's age at diagnosis, some problems, such as delayed growth and tooth discoloration, may not improve.

A small percentage of people with celiac disease do not improve on the gluten-free diet. These people often have severely damaged intestines that cannot heal even after they eliminate gluten from their diets. Because their intestines are not absorbing enough nutrients, they may need to receive intravenous nutritional supplements. Drug treatments are being evaluated for unresponsive celiac disease. These patients may need to be evaluated for complications of the disease.

If a person responds to the gluten-free diet, the physician will know for certain that the diagnosis of celiac disease is correct.

Complications

Damage to the small intestine and the resulting problems with nutrient absorption put a person with celiac disease at risk for several diseases and health problems. These include lymphoma and adenocarcinoma (types of cancer that can develop in the intestine) and osteoporosis. This is a condition in which the bones become weak, brittle, and prone to breaking. Poor calcium and vitamin D absorption is a contributing factor to osteoporosis. Miscarriage and congenital malformation of the baby, such as neural tube defects, are risks for untreated pregnant women with celiac disease because of malabsorption of nutrients.

Short stature results when childhood celiac disease prevents nutrient absorption during the years when nutrition is critical to a child's normal growth and development. Children who are diagnosed and treated before their growth stops may have a catch-up period.

Seizures, or convulsions, result from inadequate absorption of folic acid. Lack of folic acid causes calcium deposits, called calcifications, to form in the brain, which in turn cause seizures.

People with celiac disease tend to have other autoimmune diseases as well, including dermatitis herpetiformis, thyroid disease, systemic lupus erythematosus, Type 1 diabetes, liver disease, collagen vascular disease, rheumatoid arthritis, and Sjögren's syndrome. The connection between celiac disease and these diseases may be genetic.

Celiac Disease. NIH Publication No. 01-4269. National Institutes of Health, 1998 and updated September 2001.

Howdle, P. D. "Celiac Disease: Methods and Protocols." Gut 49, no. 4 (October 2001): 598C.

Korn, Danna. Kids with Celiac Disease: A Family Guide to Raising Happy, Healthy, Gluten-Free Children. Bethesda, Md.: Woodbine House, 2001.

Sollid, L. M., S. N. McAdam, O. Molberg, H. Quarsten, H. Arentz-Hansen, A. S. Louka, and K. E. Lundin. "Genes and Environment in Celiac Disease." Acta Odontologica Scandinavica 59, no. 3 (June 2001): 183–186.

cell The basic structural unit of the human body as well as of all animals and plants. An adult human body contains about 100 trillion cells, with most cells measuring only a few thousandths of a millimeter in diameter. Each cell is a small container of chemicals and water wrapped in a membrane. Each human being starts life as a single cell, a fertilized egg, which divides into more cells during the embryonic development. In the course of this duplication, cells begin to differentiate into muscle cells, skin cells, nerve cells, and so on. Most cells continue to divide and differentiate throughout a person's life. The nucleus, or control center, of each cell regulates the types and amount of molecules (proteins) made in the cell. See also ANTIGEN-PRESENTING CELL; B LYMPHOCYTE; ERYTHROCYTES/RED BLOOD CELLS; LEUKOCYTES; MAST CELL; MEMORY CELL; NATURAL KILLER CELLS; PLASMA CELLS; STEM CELLS; T-CYTOTOXIC CELL; T-HELPER CELL; T LYMPHOCYTES; T-SUPPRESSOR CELL.

cellular immunity (cell-mediated immunity)

Immune protection provided by the direct action of immune cells, such as graft rejection or destruction of infected cells. The cells identify certain foreign substances (antigens) as harmful to the body. For this reason, the body can acquire resistance to a particular foreign agent. These foreign agents are then attacked by sensitized T lymphocytes (T cells). White blood cells, plasma cells, B lymphocytes, and other specialized immune system cells act in concert with T lymphocytes to produce antibodies that attach to the antigen directing T cells to attack. Antibodies also stimulate the release of special chemical mediators in the blood (e.g., complement, interferon) that further enhance antigen destruction.

Chagas' disease

Also called American trypanosomiasis, Chagas' disease is an infection caused by the protozoan parasite *Trypanosoma cruzi*, which is found in South and Central America. An estimated 16 to 18 million people are infected with Chagas' disease; of those infected, 50,000 will die each year. It is named after the Brazilian physician Carlos Chagas (1879–1934). Chagas' disease is spread to humans through the feces of reduviid bugs (referred to as kissing bugs because of their tendency to lodge on victims' faces during sleep), which live in cracks and holes of substandard housing in Argentina, Belize, Bolivia, Brazil, Chile, Colombia, Costa Rica, Ecuador, El Salvador, French Guiana, Guatemala, Guyana, Honduras, Mexico, Nicaragua, Panama, Paraguay, Peru, Suriname, Uruguay, and Venezuela.

Insects become infected after biting an animal or person who already has Chagas' disease. They do this biting with a needlelike appendage through which they draw human blood. Infection is spread to humans when an infected bug deposits trypanosome-containing feces on a person's skin, usually while the person is sleeping at night. The person often accidentally rubs the feces into the bite wound, an open cut, the eyes, or mucous membranes, where the trypanosomes infect multiple cell types and reproduce. As the parasites increase in number, they rupture their host cells and spread the blood to different tissues, with the muscles of the heart their primary target.

Animals can become infected the same way, and they can also contract the disease by eating an infected bug. Infected mothers can also pass along infection to their baby during pregnancy, at delivery, or while breast-feeding. In some countries, the blood supply may not always be screened for Chagas' disease, and blood transfusions may carry a risk of infection.

Chagas' disease primarily affects low-income people living in rural areas, with many people getting the infection during childhood. The early stage of infection (acute Chagas' disease) is usually not severe, but sometimes it can cause death, particularly in infants. However, in about one-third of those who get the infection, chronic symptoms develop after 10 to 20 years. For these persons who develop chronic symptoms, the average life expectancy decreases by an average of nine years.

Clinical Features

Three stages of infection occur with Chagas' disease, and each stage has different symptoms. Some persons may be infected and never develop symptoms.

Acute stage Acute symptoms occur in only about 1 percent of cases. Symptoms may occur within a few days to weeks. Most people infected do not seek medical attention. The most recognized symptom of acute Chagas' infection is the Romaña's sign, or swelling of the eye on one side of the face, usually at the bite wound or where feces were rubbed into the eye. Other symptoms are usually not specific for Chagas' infection. These symptoms may include fatigue, fever, enlarged liver or spleen, and swollen lymph glands. Sometimes, a rash, loss of appetite, diarrhea, and vomiting occur. In infants and in very young children with acute Chagas' disease, swelling of the brain can develop, and this can cause death. In general, symptoms last for four to eight weeks and then they go away, even without treatment.

Indeterminate stage Eight to 10 weeks after infection, the indeterminate stage begins. During this stage, people do not have symptoms.

Chronic stage Most people do not have symptoms until the chronic stage of infection, 10 to 20 years after first being infected. At that time, people may develop the most serious symptoms of Chagas' disease. Cardiac problems, including an enlarged heart, altered heart rate or rhythm, heart failure, or cardiac arrest are symptoms of chronic disease. Not everyone will develop the chronic symptoms of Chagas' disease. Chronic Chagas' disease is believed to be due to an autoimmune response to the heart.

Complications

Chagas' disease can also lead to enlargement of parts of the digestive tract, which result in severe constipation or problems with swallowing. In persons who are immune compromised, including persons with HIV/AIDS, Chagas' disease can be severe.

Treatment

Medication for Chagas' disease is usually effective when given during the acute stage of infection. Once the disease has progressed to later stages, no medication has been proven to be effective. In the chronic stage, treatment involves managing symptoms associated with the disease. No vaccine is available.

Bastien, Joseph William. *The Kiss of Death: Chagas' Disease in the Americas.* Salt Lake City: University of Utah Press, 1998.

Chagas Disease Fact Sheet. Atlanta: Centers for Disease Control and Prevention. Available online. URL: http://www.cdc.gov/ncidod/dpd/parasites/chagasdisease/factsht_chagas_disease.htm. Downloaded on 13 July 2002.

Hagar, J. M., and S. H. Rahimtoola. "Chagas' Heart Disease." *Current Problems in Cardiology* 20 (1995): 825–824.

Herwaldt, B. L., and D. D. Juranek. "Laboratory-Acquired Malaria, Leishmaniasis, Trypanosomiasis, and Toxoplasmosis." *The American Journal of Tropical Medicine and Hygiene* 48 (1993): 313–323.

Kirchhoff, L. V. "American Trypanosomiasis (Chagas' Disease)." *Gastroenterology Clinics of North America* 25 (1996): 517–532.

Kirchhoff, L. V. "American Trypanosomiasis (Chagas' Disease)—A Tropical Disease Now in the United States." *The New England Journal of Medicine* 329 (1993): 639–644.

chemokines   A class of cytokines (proteins) that attract and activate leukocytes (white blood cells) to assist in destroying an invading microorganism. Chemokines stands for *chemo*tactic cyto*kines*. They act as chemical messengers between cells of the immune system and have been studied intently by immunologists since 1986. To date, more than 40 different chemokines have been isolated and characterized.

chemotaxis   The movement of additional white blood cells toward an area of inflammation in response to the release of chemical mediators by neutrophils and injured tissue. It recruits the cells to the tissue where they are needed to ingest the invading organism, antigens, or debris from the inflammation.

children of parents with autoimmune diseases According to a Swiss study of children with parents affected by multiple sclerosis (MS), the gender of the child significantly influences his or her coping behavior. Daughters cope better than sons, independently of the gender of the MS-affected parent. Only the daughter's coping is positively affected by age and disease variables. The study concluded that gender seems to be an important moderating factor in chronic parental disease, and it has complex effects on the coping capacity of children.

In a Danish study targeted to explore the potential relationship between parental autoimmune diseases and childhood cancer in offspring, the authors concluded that children of parents with autoimmune diseases are slightly more susceptible to childhood lymphoma and leukemia than children in general. Because of their findings, the researchers recommended that further studies be conducted to evaluate this association.

Children whose parents have VITILIGO are more likely to develop the condition. However, most children will not get vitiligo even if a parent has it, and most people with vitiligo do not have a family history of the disorder.

Steck, B., F. Amsler, L. Kappos, and D. Burgin. "Gender-Specific Differences in the Process of Coping in Families with a Parent Affected by a Chronic Somatic Disease (e.g., Multiple Sclerosis)." *Psychopathology* 34, no. 5 (September–October 2001): 236–244.

children with autoimmune diseases (school-age)

Several autoimmune diseases either especially target children of school age or present special problems for children who suffer from them. Autoimmune diseases that affect children include juvenile rheumatoid arthritis, Type 1 diabetes, chronic fatigue syndrome, systemic lupus erythematosus, multiple sclerosis, inflammatory bowel disease (Crohn's and ulcerative colitis), scleroderma, thyroiditis, immune-mediated thrombocytopenia, and hemolytic anemia.

Generally, the prognosis is better for children with CHRONIC FATIGUE SYNDROME (CFS) than it is for adults. Research suggests that CFS produces more long-term sickness absence than any other condition in schoolchildren. Children with CFS often require homeschooling or distance learning; those severely affected may need these on a long-term basis. The most severely affected by their illness may not be able to participate in any form of education.

According to the Arthritis Foundation, nearly three of every 1,000 children are living with a form of arthritis. The most common form of the disease among children is juvenile rheumatoid arthritis (JRA), which affects the entire body (see JUVENILE ARTHRITIS). Characterized by inflammation of the membrane lining the joint, JRA invades the synovium—the joint lining—and damages bone and cartilage by releasing enzymes that digest the bone and cartilage. JRA may affect growth during active

periods of the disease. Onset occurs between the ages of two to five and nine to 12. Girls are at a higher risk than boys.

Although SYSTEMIC LUPUS ERYTHEMATOSUS (SLE) is considered a "woman's disease," it regularly appears in prepubertal children. However, the precise numbers are not well documented. Because little is known about child-onset lupus, the University of Southern California in 1999 launched a five-year study, backed by a grant from the National Institutes of Health, in an attempt to pin down the genes responsible for SLE in children. According to Chaim Jacob, USC associate professor of medicine, the face of childhood lupus does not look exactly like the adult version—while the sex ratio of SLE in adults is nine females to one male, it is two to one in children. In addition, although lupus may be relatively rare in children, it comes on with a vengeance. "The symptoms are more severe in children. And while in adults it is usually a slow, chronic disease that can be quite benign, it generally appears in children as a major disease."

Hunt, Nigel. "How Can We Help Sufferers of Chronic Fatigue Syndrome?" *Pulse,* (March 2002): 47.
Oliwenstein, Lori. "Genes Examined for Clues $2.8 Million USC Study Targets Childhood Lupus." *USC Health Sciences Weekly* 5, no. 29 (October 15, 1999).

chronic fatigue syndrome (CFS)

A debilitating and complex disorder characterized by profound fatigue that is not improved by bed rest and that may be worsened by physical or mental activity. It is also known as myalgic encephalomyelitis, postviral fatigue syndrome, and chronic fatigue and immune dysfunction syndrome. Chronic fatigue syndrome seems to involve interactions between the immune and central nervous systems, interactions about which scientists know relatively little. Persons with chronic fatigue syndrome most often function at a substantially lower level of activity than they were capable of before the onset of illness. In addition to these key defining characteristics, patients report various nonspecific symptoms, including weakness, muscle pain, impaired memory and/or mental concentration, insomnia, and postexertional fatigue lasting more than 24 hours. In some cases, chronic fatigue syndrome can persist for years.

Sometimes referred to as a "mystery," chronic fatigue syndrome is not like the normal tired or depressed feelings experienced in everyday life. The early sign of this illness is a strong and noticeable fatigue that comes on suddenly and often comes and goes or never stops. People with chronic fatigue syndrome feel too tired to do normal activities or are easily exhausted with no apparent reason. Unlike the mind fog of a serious hangover, to which researchers have compared CFS, the profound weakness of chronic fatigue syndrome does not go away with a few good nights of sleep. Instead, it slyly steals the patient's energy and vigor over months and sometimes years.

Chronic fatigue syndrome was once stereotyped as a new yuppie flu because those who sought help for and caused scientific interest in chronic fatigue syndrome in the early 1980s were mainly well-educated, well-off women in their 30s and 40s. The modern stereotype arose. Similar illnesses, known by different names, however, date back at least to the late 1800s. Since then, doctors have seen the syndrome in people of all ages, races, and social and economic classes from several countries around the world.

Still, chronic fatigue syndrome is diagnosed two to four times more often in women than in men, possibly because of biological, psychological, and social influences. For example, CFS may have a sex difference similar to diseases such as systemic lupus erythematosus and multiple sclerosis, which affect more women than men. Women may be more likely than men to talk with their doctors about CFS-like symptoms. Some members of the medical community and the public do not know about or are skeptical of the syndrome.

One of the earliest attempts to estimate the prevalence of chronic fatigue syndrome was conducted by the Centers for Disease Control and Prevention (CDC) from 1989 to 1993. Physicians in four U.S. cities were asked to refer possible chronic fatigue syndrome patients for clinical evaluation by medical personnel participating in the study. The study estimated that between 4.0 and 8.7 per 100,000 persons 18 years of age or older have chronic fatigue syndrome and are under medical care. However, these projections were underestimates and could not be generalized to the U.S. population because the study did not randomly select its sites. A more recent study of the Seattle area has estimated that chronic fatigue syndrome affects between 75 and 265 people per 100,000. This estimate is similar to the prevalence observed in another CDC study conducted in San Francisco, which put the occurrence of CFS-like disease (not clinically diagnosed) at approximately 200 per 100,000 persons. A more recent study conducted by researchers at DePaul University estimates chronic fatigue syndrome at approximately 422 per 100,000 persons in the U.S. This means as many as 800,000 people nationwide suffer from the illness. Therefore, 90 percent of patients have not been diagnosed and are not receiving proper medical care for their illness.

Evidence indicates that chronic fatigue syndrome affects all racial and ethnic groups and both sexes. The Seattle study found that 59 percent of the chronic fatigue syndrome patients were women and 83 percent were Caucasian. This is an underrepresentation, since over 90 percent of the patients in the study were white. The CDC's San Francisco study found that CFS-like disease was most prevalent among women, among persons with household annual incomes of under $40,000, and among African Americans and was least common among Asians and Caucasians. Adolescents can have chronic fatigue syndrome, but few studies of adolescents have been published. A recently published CDC study documented that adolescents 12 to 18 years of age had CFS significantly less frequently than adults and did not identify chronic fatigue syndrome in children under 12 years of age. CFS-like illness has been reported in children under 12 by some investigators, although the symptom pattern varies somewhat from that seen in adults and adolescents. The illness in adolescents has many of the same characteristics as it has in adults. However, it is particularly important that the unique problems of chronically ill adolescents (e.g., family social and health interactions, education, and social interactions with peers) be considered as a part of their care. The CDC and the National Institutes of Health (NIH) are currently pursuing studies of CFS in children and adolescents.

No evidence supports the view that chronic fatigue syndrome is a contagious disease. Contagious diseases typically occur in well-defined clusters, otherwise known as outbreaks or epidemics. Although some earlier studies have been cited as evidence for chronic fatigue syndrome acting as a contagious illness, they did not rigorously document the occurrence of person-to-person transmission. In addition, none of these studies included patients with clinically evaluated fatigue that fit the chronic fatigue syndrome case definition. Therefore, these clusters of cases cannot be construed as outbreaks of chronic fatigue syndrome. The CDC worked with state health departments to investigate a number of reported outbreaks of fatiguing illness and has yet to confirm a cluster of chronic fatigue syndrome cases.

Carefully designed case-control studies involving rigorously classified CFS patients and controls have found no association between chronic fatigue syndrome and a large number of human disease agents. Finally, none of the behavioral characteristics typically associated with a contagious disease, such as intravenous drug use, exposure to animals, occupational or travel history, or sexual behavior, have been associated with chronic fatigue syndrome in case-control studies. Chronic fatigue syndrome is therefore unlikely to be a transmissible disease. Nevertheless, the lack of evidence for clustering of chronic fatigue syndrome, the absence of associations between specific behavioral characteristics and chronic fatigue syndrome, and the failure to detect evidence of infection more commonly in chronic fatigue syndrome patients than in controls do not rule out the possibility that infectious agents are involved in or reflect the development of this illness. For example, important questions remain to be answered concerning possible reactivation of latent viruses (such as human herpesviruses) and a possible role for infectious agents in some cases of chronic fatigue syndrome.

Causes

For many people, chronic fatigue syndrome begins after a bout with a cold, bronchitis, hepatitis, or an intestinal infection. For some, it follows a bout of infectious mononucleosis, or mono, which temporarily saps the energy of many teenagers and young adults. Often, people say that their illnesses started during a period of high stress. In others,

chronic fatigue syndrome develops more gradually, with no clear illness or other event starting it.

Although no one knows what causes chronic fatigue syndrome, for more than a century doctors have reported seeing illnesses similar to it. In the 1860s, Dr. George Beard named the syndrome neurasthenia because he thought it was a nervous disorder with weakness and fatigue. Since then, health experts have suggested other explanations for this baffling illness: iron-poor blood (anemia), low blood sugar (hypoglycemia), environmental allergy, or a body-wide yeast infection (candidiasis).

The cause or causes of chronic fatigue syndrome have not been identified, and no specific diagnostic tests are available. Moreover, because many illnesses have incapacitating fatigue as a symptom, other known and often treatable conditions must be excluded before a diagnosis of chronic fatigue syndrome is made.

While a single cause for chronic fatigue syndrome may yet be identified, another possibility is that CFS represents a common endpoint of disease resulting from multiple precipitating causes. None of the possible causes has been formally excluded, nor are the presently considered largely unrelated possible causes mutually exclusive.

Conditions that have been proposed to trigger the development of chronic fatigue syndrome include viral infection or other transient traumatic conditions, stress, and toxins.

Infectious agent   Due in part to its similarity to chronic mononucleosis, chronic fatigue syndrome was initially thought to be caused by a virus infection, most probably Epstein-Barr virus (EBV). It now seems clear that chronic fatigue syndrome cannot be caused exclusively by EBV or by any single recognized infectious disease agent. No firm association between infection with any known human pathogen and chronic fatigue syndrome has been established. The CDC's four-city surveillance study found no association between chronic fatigue syndrome and infection by a wide variety of human pathogens, including EBV, human retroviruses, human herpesvirus 6, enteroviruses, rubella, *Candida albicans*, and more recently bornaviruses and mycoplasma. When taken together, these studies suggest that among identified human pathogens, no causal relationship appears for chronic fatigue syndrome. However, the possibility remains that chronic fatigue syndrome may have multiple causes leading to a common endpoint, in which case some viruses or other infectious agents might have a contributory role for a subset of chronic fatigue syndrome cases.

Immunology   Some researchers have proposed that chronic fatigue syndrome may be caused by an immunologic dysfunction, for example inappropriate production of cytokines, such as interleukin-1, or altered capacity of certain immune functions. One thing is certain at this juncture: there are no immune disorders in chronic fatigue syndrome patients on the scale traditionally associated with disease. Some investigators have observed antiself antibodies and immune complexes in many chronic fatigue syndrome patients, both of which are hallmarks of autoimmune disease. However, no associated tissue damage typical of autoimmune disease has been described in patients with chronic fatigue syndrome. The opportunistic infections or increased risk for cancer observed in persons with immunodeficiency diseases or in immunosuppressed individuals is also not observed in chronic fatigue syndrome. Several investigators have reported lower numbers of natural killer cells or decreased natural killer cell activity among chronic fatigue syndrome patients compared with healthy controls, but others have found no differences between patients and controls.

T cell activation markers have also been reported to have differential expression in groups of chronic fatigue syndrome patients compared with controls. Again, though, not all investigators have consistently observed these differences. One intriguing hypothesis is that various triggering events, such as stress or a viral infection, may lead to the chronic expression of cytokines and then to chronic fatigue syndrome. Administration of some cytokines in therapeutic doses is known to cause fatigue, but no characteristic pattern of chronic cytokine secretion has ever been identified in chronic fatigue syndrome patients. In addition, some investigators have noted clinical improvement in patients with continued high levels of circulating cytokines. If a causal relationship exists between cytokines and chronic fatigue syndrome, it is likely to be complex. Finally, several studies have shown that chronic fatigue syndrome patients are more likely to have a history of allergies than are healthy controls. Allergy could be one predisposing factor for chronic fatigue syndrome. However, it cannot be the only one, because not all chronic fatigue syndrome patients have it.

Hypothalamic-pituitary-adrenal (HPA) axis   Multiple laboratory studies have suggested that the central nervous system may have an important role in chronic fatigue syndrome. Physical or emotional stress, which is commonly reported as a preonset condition in CFS patients, activates the hypothalamic-pituitary-adrenal axis, or HPA axis, leading to an increased release of cortisol and other hormones. Cortisol and corticotrophin-releasing hormone (CRH), which are also produced during the activation of the HPA axis, influence the immune system and many other body systems. They may also affect several aspects of behavior. Recent studies revealed that chronic fatigue syndrome patients often produce lower levels of cortisol than do healthy controls. Similar hormonal abnormalities have been observed by others in chronic fatigue syndrome patients and in persons with related disorders like fibromyalgia.

Cortisol suppresses inflammation and cellular immune activation. Reduced cortisol levels might relax constraints on inflammatory processes and immune cell activation. As with the immunologic data, the altered cortisol levels noted in chronic fatigue syndrome cases fall within the accepted range of normal, and only the average between cases and controls allows the distinction to be made. Therefore, cortisol levels cannot be used as a diagnostic marker for an individual with chronic fatigue syndrome. A placebo-controlled trial was conducted in which 70 chronic fatigue syndrome patients were randomized to receive either just enough hydrocortisone each day to restore their cortisol levels to normal or placebo pills for 12 weeks. It concluded that low levels of cortisol itself are not directly responsible for symptoms of chronic fatigue syndrome and that hormonal replacement is not an effective treatment. However, additional research into other aspects of neuroendocrine correlates of chronic fatigue syndrome is necessary to define this important, and largely unexplored, field fully.

Neurally mediated hypotension　Studies have been conducted to determine whether disturbances in the autonomic regulation of blood pressure and pulse (neurally mediated hypotension, or NMH) were common in chronic fatigue syndrome patients. Many CFS patients experience lightheadedness or worsened fatigue when they stand for prolonged periods or when in warm places, such as in a hot shower. These conditions are also known to trigger NMH. One study observed that 96 percent of adults with a clinical diagnosis of chronic fatigue syndrome developed hypotension during testing, compared with 29 percent of healthy controls. Testing also provoked characteristic chronic fatigue syndrome symptoms in the patients. A study (not placebo controlled) was conducted to determine whether medications effective for the treatment of NMH would benefit chronic fatigue syndrome patients. A subset of chronic fatigue syndrome patients reported a striking improvement in symptoms, but not all patients improved. A placebo-controlled trial of NMH medications for chronic fatigue syndrome patients is now in progress.

Nutritional deficiency　No published scientific evidence indicates that chronic fatigue syndrome is caused by a nutritional deficiency. Many patients do report intolerances for certain substances that may be found in foods or over-the-counter medications, such as alcohol or the artificial sweetener aspartame. Although evidence is currently lacking for nutritional defects in chronic fatigue syndrome patients, a balanced diet can be conducive to better health in general and would be expected to have beneficial effects in any chronic illness.

Clinical Features

A great deal of debate has surrounded the issue of how best to define chronic fatigue syndrome. In an effort to resolve these issues, an international panel of chronic fatigue syndrome research experts convened in 1994 to draft a definition of chronic fatigue syndrome that would be useful both to researchers studying the illness and to clinicians diagnosing it. In essence, in order to receive a diagnosis of chronic fatigue syndrome, a patient must satisfy two criteria. First, the patient must have severe chronic fatigue of six months or longer duration with other known medical conditions excluded by clinical diagnosis. Second, the patient must concurrently have four or more of the following symptoms: substantial impairment in short-term memory or concentration; sore throat; tender lymph nodes; muscle pain; multijoint pain without swelling or redness; headaches of a new type, pattern, or severity; unrefreshing sleep; and postexertional malaise lasting more than 24 hours. The symptoms must have persisted or recurred during six or more consecutive months of illness and must not have predated the fatigue.

In addition to the eight primary defining symptoms of chronic fatigue syndrome, a number of other symptoms have been reported by some CFS patients. The frequencies of occurrence of these symptoms vary from 20 percent to 50 percent among chronic fatigue syndrome patients. They include abdominal pain, alcohol intolerance, bloating, chest pain, chronic cough, diarrhea, dizziness, dry eyes or mouth, earaches, irregular heartbeat, jaw pain, morning stiffness, nausea, night sweats, psychological problems (depression, irritability, anxiety, panic attacks), shortness of breath, skin sensations, tingling sensations, and weight loss.

A number of illnesses have a similar spectrum of symptoms to chronic fatigue syndrome. These include fibromyalgia syndrome, myalgic encephalomyelitis, neurasthenia, multiple chemical sensitivities, and chronic mononucleosis. Although these illnesses may present with a primary symptom other than fatigue, chronic fatigue is commonly associated with all of them.

The clinical course of CFS varies considerably among persons who have the disorder. The actual percentage of patients who recover is unknown, and even the definition of what should be considered recovery is subject to debate. Some patients recover to the point that they can resume work and other activities but continue to experience various or periodic chronic fatigue syndrome symptoms. Some patients recover completely with time, and some grow progressively worse. Chronic fatigue syndrome often follows a cyclical course, alternating between periods of illness and relative well-being. The CDC continues to monitor the patients enrolled in the four-city surveillance study; recovery is defined by the patient and may not reflect complete symptom-free recovery. Approximately 50 percent of patients reported "recovery," and most recovered within the first five years after onset of illness. No characteristics were identified that made one patient more likely to recover than another. At illness onset, the most commonly reported chronic fatigue syndrome symptoms were sore throat, fever, muscle pain, and muscle weakness. As the illness progressed, muscle pain and forgetfulness increased and the reporting of depression decreased.

Treatment

Because no cause for chronic fatigue syndrome has been identified, the therapies for this disorder are directed at relief of symptoms. Each case is treated differently, but treatment is based on some combination of therapies.

Physical activity In general, physicians advise patients with chronic fatigue syndrome to pace themselves carefully and encourage them to avoid unusual physical or emotional stress. A regular, manageable daily routine helps avoid the push-crash phenomenon characterized by overexertion during periods of better health, followed by a relapse of symptoms perhaps initiated by the excessive activity.

Physical activities and therapy Nonpharmacological therapies sometimes used by chronic fatigue syndrome patients include acupuncture, aquatic therapy, chiropractic, cranial-sacral, light exercise, massage, self-hypnosis, stretching, tai chi, therapeutic touch, and yoga.

Psychotherapy and supportive counseling Certain psychotherapies, such as cognitive behavior therapy, have shown promise for facilitating patient coping and for alleviating some of the distress associated with chronic fatigue syndrome. In addition, any chronic illness can affect the patient's caregivers and family. In such instances, family therapy may foster good communication and reduce the adverse impact of chronic fatigue syndrome on the family. Learning how to manage fatigue may help the patient improve his or her level of functioning and quality of life despite one's symptoms. A rehabilitation medicine specialist can evaluate and teach how to plan activities to take advantage of times when one usually feels better.

Pharmacological therapy Pharmacological therapy is directed toward the relief of specific symptoms experienced by the individual patient. Patients with chronic fatigue syndrome appear particularly sensitive to drugs, especially those that affect the central nervous system. Thus, the usual treatment strategy is to begin with very low doses and to escalate the dosage gradually as necessary.

LOW-DOSE TRICYCLIC AGENTS Tricyclic agents are sometimes prescribed for chronic fatigue syndrome patients to improve sleep and to relieve mild, generalized pain. Examples include doxepin (Adapin, Sinequan), amitriptyline (Elavil, Etrafon, Limbitrol, Triavil), desipramine (Norpramin), and nortriptyline (Pamelor). Some adverse reactions include dry mouth, drowsiness, weight gain, and elevated heart rate.

ANTIDEPRESSANTS Antidepressants have been used to treat depression in chronic fatigue syndrome patients. However, nondepressed CFS patients receiving treatment with serotonin reuptake inhibitors have been found by some physicians to benefit from this treatment as well as or better than depressed patients. Examples of antidepressants used to treat chronic fatigue syndrome include serotonin reuptake inhibitors such as fluoxetine (Prozac), sertraline (Zoloft), and paroxetine (Paxil); venlafaxine (Effexor); trazodone (Desyrel); and bupropion (Wellbutrin). A number of mild adverse reactions, varying with the specific drug, may be experienced.

ANXIOLYTIC AGENTS Anxiolytic agents are used to treat panic disorder in chronic fatigue syndrome patients. Examples include alprazolam (Xanax), clonazepam (Klonopin), and lorazepam (Ativan). Common adverse reactions include sedation, amnesia, and withdrawal symptoms (insomnia, abdominal and muscle cramps, vomiting, sweating, tremors, and convulsions).

NONSTEROIDAL ANTI-INFLAMMATORY DRUGS These drugs may be used to relieve body aches and fever in chronic fatigue syndrome patients. Some are available as over-the-counter medications. Examples include naproxen (Aleve, Anaprox, Naprosen), ibuprofen (Advil, Bayer Select, Motrin, Nuprin), and piroxicam (Feldene). These medications are generally safe when used as directed but can cause a variety of adverse effects, including kidney damage, gastrointestinal bleeding, abdominal pain, nausea, and vomiting.

ANTIMICROBIALS An infectious cause for chronic fatigue syndrome has not been identified. Antimicrobial agents are not commonly prescribed for CFS unless the patient has been diagnosed with a concurrent infection. A controlled trial of the antiviral drug acyclovir found no benefit for the treatment of patients with chronic fatigue syndrome.

ANTIALLERGY THERAPY Some chronic fatigue syndrome patients have histories of allergy, and these symptoms may flare periodically. Nonsedating antihistamines may be helpful for CFS patients. Examples include astemizole (Hismanal) and loratadine (Claritin). Some of the more common adverse reactions associated with their use include drowsiness, fatigue, and headache. Sedating antihistamines can also be of benefit to patients at bedtime.

ANTIHYPOTENSIVE THERAPY Fludrocortisone (Florinef) has sometimes been prescribed for CFS patients who have had a positive tilt table test. Florinef is currently being tested in controlled studies for its efficacy in the treatment of CFS patients. Beta blockers such as atenolol (Tenormin) have also been prescribed for patients with a positive tilt table test. Increased salt and water intake is also recommended for these patients. Adverse reactions include elevated blood pressure and fluid retention.

Experimental drugs and treatments Several drugs and treatments are currently being tested. The following describes three of them.

AMPLIGEN This is a synthetic nucleic acid product that stimulates the production of interferons, a family of immune response modifiers that are also known to have antiviral activity. One report of a double-blinded, placebo-controlled study of chronic fatigue syndrome patients documented modest improvements in cognition and performance among Ampligen recipients compared with the placebo group. These preliminary results will need to be confirmed by further study. Ampligen is not approved by the Food and Drug Administration (FDA) for widespread use, and the administration of this drug in CFS patients is considered experimental. Although the recipients of Ampligen in this study tolerated the drug well, the adverse reactions of this material are still incompletely characterized, and some participants did experience reactions that might be attributable to Ampligen.

DEHYDROEPIANDROSTERONE (DHEA) This was reported in preliminary studies to improve symptoms in some patients. However, this finding has not been confirmed, and the use of DHEA in patients is regarded as experimental.

GAMMA GLOBULIN (GAMMAR) This is pooled human immune globulin. It contains antibody molecules directed against a broad range of common infectious agents. It is ordinarily used as a means for passively immunizing persons whose immune systems have been compromised or who have been exposed to an agent that might cause more serious disease in the absence of immune globulin. Its use with chronic fatigue syndrome patients is experimental and based on the unsubstantiated hypothesis that CFS is characterized by an underlying immune disorder. Serious adverse reactions are uncommon, although in rare instances gamma globulin may initiate anaphylactic shock.

Dietary supplements and herbal preparations A variety of dietary supplements and herbal preparations are claimed to have potential benefits for chronic fatigue syndrome patients. With few exceptions, the effectiveness of these remedies for treating CFS patients has not been evaluated in controlled trials. Contrary to common belief, the "natural" origin of a product does not ensure safety. Dietary supplements and herbal preparations can have potential side reactions, and some can interfere or interact with prescription medications.

VITAMINS, COENZYMES, MINERALS Preparations that have been claimed to have benefit for CFS patients include adenosine monophosphate; coenzyme Q-10; germanium; glutathione; iron; magnesium sulfate; melatonin; NADH; selenium; l-tryptophan; vitamins B_{12}, C, and A; and zinc. An early chronic fatigue syndrome study found reduced red blood cell magnesium sulfate in CFS patients, but two subsequent studies have found no difference between patients and healthy controls. The therapeutic value of all these preparations has not been validated.

HERBAL PREPARATIONS Plants are known sources of pharmacological materials. However, unrefined plant preparations contain variable levels of the active compound as well as many irrelevant, potentially harmful substances. Preparations that have been claimed to benefit chronic fatigue syndrome patients include astragalus, borage seed oil, bromelain, comfrey, echinacea, garlic, *Ginkgo biloba*, ginseng, primrose oil, quercetin, St. John's wort, and shiitake mushroom extract. Only primrose oil was evaluated in a controlled study, and the beneficial effects noted in chronic fatigue syndrome patients have not been independently confirmed. Some herbal preparations, notably comfrey and high-dose ginseng, have recognized harmful effects.

Because of the current debate among health care professionals and patients about appropriate strategies for management of chronic fatigue syndrome, Whiting et al. recently evaluated studies in order to assess the effectiveness of all interventions that have been evaluated for use in the treatment of management of CFS in adults or children. Studies were grouped into six different categories. In the behavioral category, graded exercise therapy and cognitive behavioral therapy showed positive results and also scored highly on the validity assessment. In the immunological category, both immunoglobulin and hydrocortisone showed some limited effects, but overall, the evidence was inconclusive. There was insufficient evidence about effectiveness in the other four categories (pharmacological, supplements, complementary/alternative, and other interventions).

Warning issued by the Centers for Disease Control Because the cause of chronic fatigue syndrome has not been identified and its effect on the body is not well understood, periodically new unvalidated beliefs about cures and causes of CFS are widely circulated. These may be based on one or more recent reports from the peer-reviewed scientific literature, or they may evolve from the anecdotal remarks of clinicians or scientists at medical meetings. In some cases the origin is obscure. Even work that is of sufficiently high caliber to be published in the scientific literature is not without limitations and design flaws. Additionally, all published work needs to be verified and expanded on by others before it can be applied with confidence in clinical situations. With regard to some stories that are currently circulating about chronic fatigue syndrome: there is evidence that CFS patients lose their fingerprints; there is no scientific evidence of any nutritional deficiency in CFS patients; and suicides of CFS patients have been reported, but the rate of occurrence has not been well studied. Additionally, regarding suicides, researchers do not know whether the rate is higher or lower than what would be expected in the general population. Addressing all of the information that circulates or emerges regarding CFS is not practical. One should simply be advised to be wary of information that points to sure cures or that alludes to pathological damage as a consequence of chronic fatigue syndrome. Specific questions should be discussed with the patient's physician, local or state health department, the Centers for Disease Control, or one of the national patient support organizations.

Chronic Fatigue Syndrome. Atlanta: Centers for Disease Control and Prevention. Available online. URL: http://www.cdc.gov/ncidod/diseases/cfs/info.htm. Downloaded on 15 July 2002.

Jason, L. A., J. A. Richman, A. W. Rademaker, K. M. Jordan, A. V. Plioplys, R. R. Taylor, W. McCready, C. F. Huang, and S. Plioplys. "A Community-Based Study of Chronic Fatigue Syndrome." *Archives of Internal Medicine* 159, no. 18 (1999): 2,129–2,137.

National Institute of Allergy and Infectious Diseases, National Institutes of Health. *Chronic Fatigue Syndrome Fact Sheet,* January 2001.

Patarca-Montero, Roberto. *Chronic Fatigue Syndrome: Critical Reviews and Clinical Advances.* Binghamton, N.Y.: Haworth Press, 2000.

Whiting, P., A. M. Bagnall, A. J. Sowden, J. E. Cornell, C. D. Mulrow, and G. Ramirez. "Interventions for the Treatment and Management of Chronic Fatigue Syndrome: A Systematic Review." *The Journal of the American Medical Association* 286, no. 11 (September 19, 2001): 1,360–1,368.

chronic inflammatory demyelinating polyneuropathy (CIDP) A rare autoimmune disorder, which is sometimes called chronic relapsing polyneuropathy, in which there is swelling of nerve roots and destruction of the covering (myelin sheath) over the nerves. (The myelin sheath is the fatty covering that acts as an insulator on fibers in the nerves.) This causes weakness, paralysis, and/or impairment in motor function, especially of the arms and legs. Sensory loss may also be present, causing numbness, tingling, and burning sensations. The motor and sensory impairments are usually found on both sides of the body. The severity of CIDP can vary from mild to severe. Although it can occur at any age and in both genders, CIDP is more common in young adults and in men more so than in women.

Symptoms include tingling or numbness (beginning in the toes and fingers), weakness of the arms and legs, aching pain in the muscles, loss of deep tendon reflexes (areflexia), fatigue, and abnormal sensations. CIDP is closely related to acute Guillain-Barré syndrome, and it is considered the chronic counterpart of the acute disease.

The course of CIDP varies widely among individuals. Some patients may follow a slow, steady pattern of symptoms, while other patients may have symptoms that flare and remit. The most severe symptoms usually occur after many months of symptoms that come and go. One characteristic that differentiates this disorder from other similar demyelinating diseases is that there is typically no preceding viral infection at least three to four months prior to the onset of the disorder, such as is the case in Guillain-Barré syndrome.

Treatment for CIDP includes corticosteroids such as prednisone, which may be prescribed alone or in combination with immunosuppressant drugs. Plasmapheresis (plasma exchange) and intravenous immunoglobulin (IVIg) therapy are thought to be effective. IVIg may even be used as a first-line therapy. Physiotherapy may improve muscle strength, function, and mobility and may minimize the development of contractures.

Churg-Strauss syndrome   Also known as allergic granulomatosis, Churg-Strauss syndrome is an autoimmune disorder accompanied by the formation of characteristic autoantibodies (ANCA), abnormal clustering of certain white blood cells (eosinophilia), inflammation of blood vessels (vasculitis), and development of inflammatory nodular lesions (granulomatosis). It was defined and differentiated in 1951 by Dr. Jacob Churg and Dr. Lotte Strauss. Other names used for Churg-Strauss syn-

drome include allergic angiitis and granulomatosis, eosinophilic granulomatous vasculitis, and Churg-Strauss vasculitis.

An allergic reaction or asthma may precede the syndrome's development by several years. Although Churg-Strauss syndrome patients may have a prior history of pulmonary disease, the syndrome tends, instead, to impair kidneys or other organs or to cause nerve damage in affected areas. Diagnosis is difficult because early symptoms mimic the common flu. Also, lung tissue infiltrations (short-term or persistent), fever, loss of appetite, and weight loss are often initial signs. Speedy diagnosis and treatment increase a patient's chances of resuming a normal life. Onset typically occurs from 15 to 70 years of age, and the disease affects both males and females. The exact cause is unknown. Corticosteroids are the treatment of choice for patients with hypersensitivity vasculitis who need specific therapy. Without appropriate treatment, serious organ damage may result.

cicatricial pemphigoid (CP)   A chronic autoimmune disease of the mucous membranes and/or skin (also known as mucous membrane pemphigoid [MMP] or benign pemphigoid) in which binding of anticonjunctival basement membrane antibodies results in inflammation. Lesions commonly appear on the lining of the mouth or conjunctiva (mucous membrane lining the inner surface of the eyelid and covering the front of the eyeball). Other less-frequent sites for lesions include the esophagus, trachea, and genitalia. The incidence is roughly one in 20,000 ophthalmic patients. Cicatricial pemphigoid is predominantly a disease of the elderly, most often occurring between 60 and 80 years of age; it is rarely seen in young adults or children. Most studies have shown a two-to-one female-to-male ratio.

Causes

Cicatricial pemphigoid is an autoimmune blistering disease associated with autoantibodies directed against basement membrane zone target antigens. Autoantibodies of the IgG subclass, particularly IgG4, are associated with CP; however, IgA antibodies have also been detected.

Clinical Features

Usually beginning as a chronic conjunctivitis and pain or the sensation of grittiness in the eye, the condition progresses to scarring of the membrane lining, inturning eyelashes, and possible blindness. Diminished tear production may lead to drying of the eyes and further trauma. Patients often present following cataract or other eye surgery. Ulcers and scars on the mouth's mucous membrane is common, with the gums most frequently affected, followed by the palate and cheek membrane, but any area within the mouth may blister. Nasal involvement may occur with bleeding following nose blowing, crusting, and discomfort. Other mucosal sites, such as the perianal area or the genitalia, may be involved. Scarring blisters or rashes on the skin are less common. Skin lesions occur in about 20 percent of patients and are usually brief in duration. When the lesions are present, they consist of small intact blisters or erosions, usually in the head and neck areas. Blisters frequently itch, and recurring lesions are frequently quite painful.

Complications

Recurring lesions will produce scarring, which can be dangerous on the mucosal surface. When the gums are involved, gingivitis can occur. Eye membranes are affected in about two-thirds of the cases of cicatricial pemphigoid. Many patients will experience severe visual loss due to ocular surface scarring, despite the most aggressive management. When the esophagus is involved, hoarseness or asphyxiation can follow. Scalp involvement may lead to loss of hair.

Treatment

Spontaneous remissions are rare, thus the organs involved require medical treatment. However, cicatricial pemphigoid frequently does not respond quickly to treatment, and some patients continue to develop blisters even with the closest of attention and treatment.

Surgery Surgery is sometimes used to remove ingrown eyelashes and prevent further risk of eye infection. Tsubota et al. reported the long-term outcome in patients with cicatricial ocular disorders treated with limbal allografts. Transfer of epithelial stem cells restored useful vision in these patients, including several with ocular cicatricial pemphigoid. A caution by Rico is that cicatricial pemphigoid patients frequently experience flares of disease activity after surgery.

Medication Treatment is with corticosteroids and immunosuppressive agents. Patients with mild localized disease may benefit from topical steroids such as triamcinolone (Kenalog in Orabase) or gel-based topical agents for mouth blisters and ointment-based topical steroids for skin lesions. Patients with more extensive disease may require treatment with systemic agents. Dapsone is used for patients with eye and mouth disease and is the first-line agent for patients with pure ocular cicatricial pemphigoid. Occasionally, patients respond to oral dapsone. Those that respond well do so quickly, but these patients have been reported to be in the minority. Patients with more severe cases may require high doses of prednisone. Patients with progressive scarring may require immunosuppressants such as azathioprine, cyclophosphamide, cyclosporin, or mycophenolate mofetil. The treatment of choice is oral cyclophosphamide (Cytoxan). About three-quarters of the patients treated with this regimen tolerate the drug. At the end of this period, most of these patients will have complete clinical remission. Azathioprine is an alternative for patients who cannot tolerate Cytoxan.

Wound care of erosions includes daily gentle cleaning or compresses, topical agents to promote wound healing, and biologic dressings. The ocular surface disease must be treated with lubrication therapy and perhaps antibiotics.

Chan, L. S., K. B. Yancey, and C. Hammerberg. "Immune-Mediated Subepithelial Blistering Diseases of Mucous Membranes." *Archives of Dermatology* 129 (1993): 448–455.

Rico, M. Joyce. "Cicatricial Pemphigoid," *eMedicine Journal* 2, no. 11 (July 13, 2001). Available online. URL: http://www.emedicine.com/DERMA/Topic79.htm. Downloaded on 15 July 2002.

Shimizu, H., T. Masunaga, and A. Ishiko. "Autoantibodies from Patients with Cicatricial Pemphigoid Target Different Sites in Epidermal Basement Membrane." *The Journal of Investigative Dermatology* 104 (1995): 370–373.

Tsubota, K., Y. Satake, and M. Kaido. "Treatment of Severe Ocular-Surface Disorders with Corneal Epithelial

Stem-Cell Transplantation." *The New England Journal of Medicine* 340 (1999): 1,697–1,703.
"What is Cicatricial Pemphigoid?" Albany, Calif.: The National Pemphigus Foundation, November 2001.

clinical studies/research   Research based mainly on observations of patients by medical personnel rather than on laboratory work.

The National Institute of Allergy and Infectious Diseases (NIAID) supports research studies on the function of the immune system in various diseases. A basic understanding of the human immune system is central to the understanding of the development of an autoimmune disease (disease pathogenesis). Scientists searching for ways to prevent and treat autoimmune diseases are studying disease pathogenesis and investigating new ways to modify the immune system.

Specifically, investigators supported by NIAID are focusing on five areas of research. First, they are studying the immune system during the progression of an autoimmune disease. They are analyzing the influence of genetics on autoimmune disease expression and progression. These investigators are researching the role of infectious agents in autoimmune diseases. They are also conducting studies of animal models of autoimmune diseases. Lastly, these researchers are investigating the effects of therapeutic intervention on the immune system in an autoimmune disease.

clonal deletion   A major mechanism of immune tolerance. A key mechanism through which the immune system eliminates potentially self-reactive lymphocytes. Via programmed cell death, immature lymphocytes are killed by binding to antigen. For T lymphocytes, this occurs in the thymus and ensures that mature T lymphocytes are self-tolerant. B lymphocytes may also undergo clonal deletion in the bone marrow. In this way, most cells bearing receptors that recognize self are deleted before they are capable of participating in immune responses.

clonal expansion   The selective proliferation of mature naive lymphocytes that encounter antigen. Only those lymphocytes bearing receptors specifi-

cally recognizing antigen are activated to proliferate and differentiate into effector cells.

clones   Exact copies. A group of genetically identical cells or organisms replicated from a single common ancestor. In the case of B cells, each B cell has a typical Ig. Therefore, all the cells that descend from one B cell (the clone) have the same Ig. Typically, a cancer is a clone of cells. Cell cloning is the process of producing a group of cells (clones), all genetically identical, from a single ancestral cell.

Cogan's syndrome   Defined as nonsyphilitic interstitial keratitis (an inflammation of the eye) and bilateral audiovestibular deficits (hearing problems and dizziness). Generally, a brief episode of inflammatory eye disease, tinnitus, and vertigo symptoms occur. The ocular symptoms typically regress within days, but any deafness is only rarely reversible. This condition is named after David Glendenning Cogan (1908–93), the American ophthalmologist who first described it in 1945. The syndrome features not only problems of the hearing and balance portions of the ear but also inflammation of the front of the eye (cornea) and often fever, fatigue, and weight loss. Joint and muscle pains can also be present. Less frequently, it can involve blood vessels elsewhere in the body and affect the skin, kidneys, nerves, or other organs. Cogan's syndrome can lead to deafness or blindness. It most often affects young adults, with the average age of onset at 29 years.

Cogan's syndrome is extremely rare, and its cause is not known. An autoimmune mechanism has long been suggested, but whether this process is mediated by cellular or humoral immunity has remained unclear. Some pathological and immunological findings such as lymphocytes, and plasma cell infiltration in the cochlea and in the cornea, presence of antibodies (IgG) against inner ear and cornea, as well as the beneficial effect of corticosteroids and immunosuppressants all support an autoimmune pathogenesis. Moreover, most of the patients exhibit variable, multiple organ involvement similar to other autoimmune diseases.

Treatment of Cogan's syndrome is directed toward stopping the inflammation of the blood vessels. Cortisone-related medications, such as prednisone, are often used. Some patients with severe disease can require immune suppression medications, such as cyclophosphamide (Cytoxan). Recent work has suggested that high-resolution MRI and antibodies to inner ear antigens may be helpful. Some reports indicate that the hearing loss may be reversible if the diagnosis is made within the first two weeks and high doses of corticosteroid therapy is begun promptly. See also AUTOIMMUNE INNER EAR DISEASE.

Allen, N. B., et al. "Use of Immunosuppressive Agents in the Treatment of Severe Ocular and Vascular Manifestations of Cogan's Syndrome." *The American Journal of Medicine* 88 (1990): 296–301.

Cogan, D. G. "Syndrome of Nonsyphilitic Interstitial Keratitis and Vestibuloauditory Symptoms." *Archives of Ophthalmology* 33 (1945): 144–149.

Garcia, Berrocal, J. R., et al. "Cogan's Syndrome: An Oculo-Audiovestibular Disease." *Postgraduate Medicine* 75 (1999): 262–264.

Helmchen, C., L. Jager, U. Buttner, M. Reiser, and T. Brandt. "Cogan's Syndrome: High Resolution MRI Indicators of Activity." *Journal of Vestibular Research: Equilibrium & Orientation* 8, no. 2 (1998): 155–167.

Helmchen, C., et al. "Cogan's Syndrome: Clinical Significance of Antibodies Against the Inner Ear and Cornea." *Acta Oto-Laryngologica* 119 (1999): 528–536.

Hughes, G. B., et al. "Autoimmune Reactivity in Cogan's Syndrome: A Preliminary Report." *Otolaryngology and Head and Neck Surgery* 91 (1983): 24–32.

Majoor, M. H. J. M. et al. "Corneal Autoimmunity in Cogan's Syndrome? Report of Two Cases." *The Annals of Otology, Rhinology, and Laryngology* 101 (1992): 679–684.

Miserocchi, Elisabetta. *Cogan's Syndrome.* Boston, Mass.: Harvard Medical School, 1996.

cold agglutinin disease   An autoimmune disease in which antibody directly agglutinates human red cells at low temperatures. Cold agglutinin diseases is an acquired AUTOIMMUNE HEMOLYTIC ANEMIA due to an IgM autoantibody usually directed against the I antigen on red blood cells. These IgM autoantibodies characteristically will not react with cells at 37 degrees Celsius or higher but only with those at lower temperatures. Because the blood temperature (even in the most peripheral parts of the body) rarely goes lower than 20 degrees Celsius, only antibodies active at higher temperatures than this will produce clinical effects. In the cooler parts of the body (fingers, nose, ears), agglutination of red blood cells by the IgM antibodies will transiently occur. Hemolysis results indirectly from attachment of IgM, which in the cooler parts of the circulation binds and fixes complement. When the red blood cells return to a cooler temperature, the IgM antibodies dissociate, leaving complement on the cells. Lysis, or destruction, of cells rarely occurs. Rather, C3b present on the red cells is recognized by Kupffer cells (which have receptors for C3b), and red blood cell formation follows.

Most cases of chronic cold agglutinin disease are of undetermined origin. Others occur in association with Waldenström's macroglobulinemia, a malignant lymphoproliferative disease in which a monoclonal IgM paraprotein is produced. Acute postinfectious cold agglutinin disease occurs following mycoplasmal pneumonia or, rarely, infectious mononucleosis; however, most cases of cold agglutinin disease are of undetermined etiology. In patients with cold agglutinin disease, open heart operations with hypothermia carry the risk of red cell agglutination resulting in complications such as hemolysis, myocardial infarction, renal insufficiency, and cerebral damage. Because of the limited number of cases reported, the optimal guidelines for detection and management of this condition remain controversial.

Lauchli, S., L. Widmer, and S. Lautenschlager. "Cold Agglutinin Disease—The Importance of Cutaneous Signs." *Dermatology* 202, no. 4 (2001): 356–368.

Rosenwasser, L. J., and B. Z. Joseph. "Immunohematologic Disorders." *The Journal of the American Medical Association* 268 (1992): 2,940–2,945.

complement   A term originally used to refer to the unstable heat factor in serum that causes immune cytolysis, the killing of antibody-coated cells, and now refers to the entire functionally related system of enzymes in normal serum. (See also COMPLEMENT SYSTEM.)

complement system   The complement system is made up of a series of about 25 proteins that work to "complement" the activity of antibodies in destroying bacteria, either by facilitating phagocytosis or by puncturing the bacterial cell membrane. Complement also helps to rid the body of antigen-antibody complexes. In carrying out these tasks, it induces an inflammatory response.

Complement proteins circulate in the blood in an inactive form. When the first of the complement substances is triggered—usually by antibody interlocked with an antigen—it sets in motion a ripple effect. As each component is activated in turn, it acts upon the next in a precise sequence of carefully regulated steps known as the *complement cascade*.

In the so-called classical pathway of complement activation, a series of proteins gives rise to a complex enzyme capable of cleaving a key protein, C3. In the alternative pathway—which can be triggered by suitable targets in the absence of antibody—C3 interacts with a different set of factors and enzymes. However, both pathways end in creation of a unit known as the membrane attack complex. When inserted in the wall of the target cell, the membrane attack complex constitutes a channel that allows fluids and molecules to flow in and out. The target cell rapidly swells and bursts.

Meanwhile, various fragments flung off during the course of the cascade can produce other consequences. One by-product causes mast cells and basophils to release their contents, producing the redness, warmth, and swelling of the inflammatory response. Another stimulates and attract neutrophils. Yet another, C3b, opsonizes or coats target cells so as to make them more palatable to phagocytes, which carry a special receptor for C3b.

The C3b fragment also appears to play a major role in the body's control of immune complexes. By opsonizing antigen-antibody complexes, C3b helps prevent the formation of large and insoluble (and thus potentially damaging) immune aggregates. Moreover, receptors for C3b are also present on red blood cells, which appear to use the receptors to pick up complement-coated immune complexes and deliver them to the Kupffer cells in the liver.

Schindler, Lydia, Donna Kerrigan, and Jeanne Kelly. *Understanding the Immune System. NCI Cancer Related Tutorials.* Bethesda, Md.: National Institutes of Health, National Cancer Institute. Available online: URL: http://newscenter.cancer.gov/sciencebehind/. Downloaded on 15 July 2002.

congenital heart block (CHB) Congenital heart block is characterized by an abnormal fetal heart rate due to interference with the transfer of electrical nerve impulses (conduction) that regulate the normal rhythmic pumping activity of the heart muscle (heart block). Most often, a delay occurs in the electrical conduction between the atria and the ventricles of the heart. The severity of such conduction abnormalities may vary among affected individuals.

Sometimes this condition occurs when other structural abnormalities occur in the heart. Other times it occurs in women with connective tissue autoimmune diseases, such as lupus. In many cases, there is no explanation for the condition.

The normal heart has four chambers. The two upper chambers are known as the atria, and the two lower chambers are known as the ventricles. In the mild form of heart block (first degree), the two upper chambers of the heart (atria) beat normally, but the contractions of the two lower chambers (ventricles) slightly lag behind. In the more severe forms (second degree), only a half to a quarter of the atrial beats are conducted to the ventricles. In complete heart block (third degree), the atria and ventricles beat independently. In most cases, infants with first or second degree experience no symptoms. However, infants with complete heart block may experience episodes of unconsciousness, breathlessness, and/or fatigue.

Complete congenital heart block (CCHB) is a rare disease of the newborn that carries significant morbidity and mortality. It generally occurs as a result of the presence of maternal autoantibodies that are transferred to the fetus and affect the fetal heart, or it may be associated with a congenital structural abnormality of the heart. Infants with complete congenital heart block are at risk for diminished cardiac output and the subsequent development of congestive heart failure. Many infants require the placement of a cardiac pacemaker. To date, congenital heart block is irreversible.

Klassen, Lisa Renee. "Complete Congenital Heart Block: A Review and Case Study." *Neonatal Network* 18, no. 3 (April 1999): 33–42.
Tseng, C., D. Friedman, and J. P. Buyon. "Spectrum of Cardiac Histopathology in Cases of Autoimmune-

Associated Congenital Heart Block (CHB) Obtained from the Research Registry for Neonatal Lupus." *Arthritis and Rheumatism* 40, Supp. (1997): S333.

corticosteroid In contrast to anabolic steroids (used by bodybuilders), corticosteroids are used in inflammatory conditions for their anti-inflammatory effects. They have a rapid onset of action and profoundly affect many parts of the immune system as well as most other body systems. Corticosteroids are a cornerstone of treating most types of vasculitis and are often used in combination with other immunosuppressive medications.

costimulation An event in the immune system involving the delivery of a second signal by an antigen-presenting cell. The second signal rescues the activated T cell from anergy (which is a state of immune unresponsiveness), allowing the T cell to produce the lymphokines necessary for the growth of additional T cells.

coxsackie myocarditis An infection of the heart muscle caused by coxsackie viruses, especially severe in newborns, who can be infected from their mothers. Infants with coxsackie myocarditis develop a fever within two weeks after birth and have trouble breathing. They may eat poorly, move very little, and sometimes develop cyanosis, a bluish color to the skin, lips, and nails caused by too little oxygen in the blood. Chest pain, increasing shortness of breath, irregularities of cardiac rhythm, and heart failure sometimes develop. Some patients wind up with long-term heart failure if the heart muscle is significantly affected. These cases may be due to an autoimmune response to the heart.

The coxsackie viruses are part of the enterovirus family of viruses (including ECHO, polio, and hepatitis A viruses) that live in the human digestive tract. The viruses can spread from person to person, usually on unwashed hands and surfaces contaminated by tiny amounts of feces, where they can live for several days. They can even survive freezing temperatures outdoors. In tropical parts of the world, the viruses actively infect humans year-round. However, in cooler climates, outbreaks of coxsackie virus most often occur in the summer and fall.

Coxsackie myocarditis can be fatal, especially in newborns. Even older children with coxsackie myocarditis may need special care in a hospital. However, these complications are rare.

"Viral Infections in Childhood: Coxsackie." Health on the Net Foundation. Available online. URL: http://www.hon.ch/Dossier/MotherChild/child_virus/virus_coxsackie.html. Posted 2001; last modified 25 June 2002.

C-reactive protein An acute-phase protein produced by the liver that circulates in increased amounts during acute inflammation and after tissue damage. Its major importance is its interaction with the complement system, which is one of the body's defense mechanisms against foreign bodies.

CREST syndrome An acronym for a collection of symptoms that occur to some degree in all people with systemic sclerosis—*c*alcinosis, *R*aynaud's phenomenon, *e*sophageal dysfunction, *s*clerodactyly, and *t*elangiectasia. It is a variant of the two groups of scleroderma, localized and systemic. It is characterized by calcium deposits, usually in the fingers; loss of muscle control of the esophagus, which can cause difficulty swallowing; a tapering deformity of the bones of the fingers; and small red spots on the skin of the fingers, face, or inside of the mouth. CREST is a relatively stable and slow-moving form of scleroderma and has a much more favorable prognosis than other forms. Because of the predominance of CREST symptoms in people with limited systemic sclerosis, some people use the term CREST syndrome when referring to that form of the disease. There is no evidence that the basic process differs from the usual scleroderma. However, the tempo of CREST seems to be different in that visceral involvement comes slower and later in the course of the disease.

Crohn's disease A chronic form of inflammatory bowel disease (IBD), the general name for diseases that cause inflammation in the intestines. Crohn's disease can be difficult to diagnose because its symptoms are similar to other intestinal disorders such as irritable bowel syndrome and to another type of IBD called ulcerative colitis. Ulcerative colitis causes inflammation and ulcers in the top layer of the lining of the large intestine. Crohn's disease afflicts more than 500,000 Americans, most of them under age 30. It affects men and women equally and seems to run in some families. About 20 percent of people with Crohn's disease have a blood relative with some form of IBD, most often a brother or sister and sometimes a parent or child. Crohn's disease (named for U.S. gastroenterologist Burrill B. Crohn, 1884–1983) may also be called ileitis or enteritis.

Most often Crohn's disease causes inflammation in the small intestine, marked by patchy areas of full-thickness inflammation. It usually occurs in the lower part of the small intestine, called the ileum, but it can affect any part of the digestive tract, from the mouth to the anus. The inflammation extends deep into the lining of the affected organ. The inflammation can cause pain and can make the intestines empty frequently, resulting in diarrhea.

Causes

Theories about what causes Crohn's disease abound, but none has been proven. The most popular theory is that the body's immune system reacts to a virus or a bacterium by causing ongoing inflammation in the intestine. People with Crohn's disease tend to have abnormalities of the immune system, but doctors do not know whether these abnormalities are a cause or result of the disease. Crohn's disease is not caused by emotional distress.

Clinical Features

The most common symptoms of Crohn's disease are abdominal pain, often in the lower right area, and severe and persistent diarrhea. Rectal bleeding, weight loss, fatigue, and fever may also occur. Bleeding may be serious and persistent, leading to anemia. Children with Crohn's disease may suffer delayed development and stunted growth.

A thorough physical exam and a series of tests may be required to diagnose Crohn's disease. Blood tests may be done to check for anemia, which could indicate bleeding in the intestines. Blood tests may also uncover a high white blood cell count, which is a sign of inflammation somewhere in the body. By testing a stool sample, the doctor can tell if there is bleeding or infection in the intestines.

The doctor may do an upper gastrointestinal (GI) series to look at the small intestine. For this test, the patient drinks barium, a chalky solution that coats the lining of the small intestine, before X rays are taken. The barium shows up white on X-ray film, revealing inflammation or other abnormalities in the intestine.

The doctor may also do a colonoscopy. For this test, the doctor inserts an endoscope—a long, flexible, lighted tube linked to a computer and TV monitor—into the anus to see the inside of the large intestine. The doctor will be able to see any inflammation or bleeding. During the exam, the doctor may do a biopsy, which involves taking a sample of tissue from the lining of the intestine to view with a microscope.

If these tests show Crohn's disease, more X rays of both the upper and lower digestive tract may be necessary to see how much is affected by the disease.

Complications

The most common complication is blockage of the intestine. Blockage occurs because the disease tends to thicken the intestinal wall with swelling and scar tissue, narrowing the passage. Crohn's disease may also cause sores, or ulcers, that tunnel through the affected area into surrounding tissues such as the bladder, vagina, or skin. The areas around the anus and rectum are often involved. The tunnels, called fistulas, are a common complication and often become infected. Sometimes fistulas can be treated with medicine, but in some cases, they may require surgery.

Nutritional complications are common in Crohn's disease. Deficiencies of proteins, calories, and vitamins are well documented. These deficiencies may be caused by inadequate dietary intake, intestinal loss of protein, or poor absorption (malabsorption).

Other complications associated with Crohn's disease include arthritis, skin problems, inflammation in the eyes or mouth, kidney stones, gallstones, or other diseases of the liver and biliary system. Some of these problems resolve during treatment for disease in the digestive system, but some must be treated separately.

Treatment

Treatment for Crohn's disease depends on the location and severity of disease, complications, and response to previous treatment. The goals of treatment are to control inflammation, correct nutritional deficiencies, and relieve symptoms like abdominal pain, diarrhea, and rectal bleeding. Treatment may include drugs, nutrition supplements, surgery, or a combination of these options. At this time, treatment can help control the disease, but there is no cure.

Some people have long periods of remission, sometimes years, when they are free of symptoms. However, the disease usually recurs at various times over a person's lifetime. This changing pattern of the disease means one cannot always tell when a treatment has helped. Predicting when a remission may occur or when symptoms will return is not possible. Someone with Crohn's disease may need medical care for a long time, with regular doctor visits to monitor the condition.

Drug therapy Most people are first treated with drugs containing mesalamine, a substance that helps control inflammation. Sulfasalazine is the most commonly used of these drugs. Patients who do not benefit from it or who cannot tolerate it may be put on other mesalamine-containing drugs, generally known as 5-ASA agents, such as Asacol, Dipentum, or Pentasa. Possible side effects of mesalamine preparations include nausea, vomiting, heartburn, diarrhea, and headache.

Some patients take corticosteroids to control inflammation. These drugs are the most effective for active Crohn's disease, but they can cause serious side effects, including greater susceptibility to infection. In October 2001, the Food and Drug Administration approved Entocort EC, saying the capsule promises fewer side effects than other steroids, such as prednisone, that are used to treat Crohn's. Entocort EC capsules are formulated to release the medication, known chemically as budesonide, once they reach the intestine. That means less of the steroidal drug is absorbed into the body than other Crohn's treatments allow.

Drugs that suppress the immune system are also used to treat Crohn's disease. Most commonly prescribed are 6-mercaptopurine and a related drug, azathioprine. Immunosuppressive agents work by blocking the immune reaction that contributes to inflammation. These drugs may cause side effects like nausea, vomiting, and diarrhea and may lower a person's resistance to infection. When patients are treated with a combination of corticosteroids and immunosuppressive drugs, the dose of corticosteroids can eventually be lowered. Some studies suggest that immunosuppressive drugs may enhance the effectiveness of corticosteroids.

The U.S. Food and Drug Administration has approved the drug infliximab (Remicade) for the treatment of moderate-to-severe Crohn's disease that does not respond to standard therapies (mesalamine substances, corticosteroids, immunosuppressive agents) and for the treatment of open, draining fistulas. Infliximab, the first treatment approved specifically for Crohn's disease, is an anti–tumor necrosis factor (TNF) substance. TNF is a protein produced by the immune system that may cause the inflammation associated with Crohn's disease. Anti-TNF removes TNF from the bloodstream before it reaches the intestines, thereby preventing inflammation. Investigators will continue to study patients taking infliximab to determine its long-term safety and efficacy.

Antibiotics are used to treat bacterial overgrowth in the small intestine caused by stricture, fistulas, or prior surgery. For this common problem, the doctor may prescribe one or more of the following antibiotics: ampicillin, sulfonamide, cephalosporin, tetracycline, or metronidazole.

Antibiotics are often paired with an anti-inflammatory drug. In a recent finding, patients with Crohn's of the small intestine who were treated with both drugs had a 33 percent remission rate, compared with 38 percent of those who took the anti-inflammatory and a placebo. The combination group also reported more diarrhea, dizziness, and taste disturbance. However, in those with Crohn's of the small intestine *and* the colon who took both drugs, the remission rate was 53 percent.

Diarrhea and crampy, abdominal pain are often relieved when the inflammation subsides, but additional medication may also be necessary. Several antidiarrheal agents could be used, including diphenoxylate, loperamide, and codeine. Patients who are dehydrated because of diarrhea will be treated with fluids and electrolytes.

Nutrition supplementation Nutritional supplements may be recommended, especially for children whose growth has been slowed. Special high-calorie liquid formulas are sometimes used for this purpose. A small number of patients may need periods of feeding by vein. This can help patients who need extra nutrition temporarily, those whose intestines need to rest, or those whose intestines cannot absorb enough nutrition from food.

Surgery Surgery to remove part of the intestine can help Crohn's disease but cannot cure it. The inflammation tends to return to the area of intestine next to that which has been removed. About half of all Crohn's patients at some point require surgery, either to relieve symptoms that do not respond to medical therapy or to correct complications such as blockage, perforation, abscess, or bleeding in the intestine.

Some people who have Crohn's disease in the large intestine need to have their entire colon removed in an operation called colectomy. A small opening is made in the front of the abdominal wall, and the tip of the ileum is brought to the skin's surface. This opening, called a stoma, is where waste exits the body. The stoma is about the size of a quarter and is usually located in the right lower part of the abdomen near the beltline. A pouch is worn over the opening to collect waste, and the patient empties the pouch as needed. The majority of colectomy patients go on to live normal, active lives. Sometimes only the diseased section of intestine is removed and no stoma is needed. In this operation, the intestine is cut above and below the diseased area and reconnected. Crohn's disease often recurs after surgery.

People with Crohn's disease may feel well and be free of symptoms for substantial spans of time when their disease is not active. Despite the need to take medication for long periods of time and occasional hospitalizations, most people with Crohn's disease are able to hold jobs, raise families, and function successfully at home and in society.

Crohn's Disease. NIH Publication No. 98-3410, December 1998. The National Institute of Diabetes and Digestive and Kidney Disease of the National Institutes of Health.

Gomez, Joan. *Positive Options for Crohn's Disease: Self-Help and Treatment.* Alameda, Calif.: Hunter House, 2000.

Greenbloom, S. L., A. H. Steinhart, and G. R. Greenberg. "Combination Ciprofloxacin and Metronidazole for Active Crohn's Disease." *Canadian Journal of Gastroenterology* (Canada) 12, no. 1 (January–February 1998): 53–56.

Trachter, Amy B., and Henry Wodnicki. *Coping with Crohn's Disease: Manage Your Physical Symptoms and Overcome the Emotional Challenges.* Oakland, Calif.: New Harbinger Publications, 2001.

Crohn's disease research Researchers continue to look for more effective treatments. Examples of investigational treatments include:

Anti-TNF Research has shown that cells affected by Crohn's disease contain a cytokine, a protein produced by the immune system, called tumor necrosis factor (TNF). TNF may be responsible for the inflammation of Crohn's disease. Anti-TNF is a substance that finds TNF in the bloodstream, binds to it, and removes it before it can reach the intestines and cause inflammation. In studies, anti-TNF seems particularly helpful in closing fistulas.

Interleukin 10 Interleukin 10 (IL-10) is a cytokine that suppresses inflammation. Researchers are now studying the effectiveness of synthetic IL-10 in treating Crohn's disease.

Antibiotics Antibiotics are now used to treat the bacterial infections that often accompany Crohn's disease. However, some research suggests that they might also be useful as a primary treatment for active Crohn's disease.

Methotrexate and cyclosporine These are immunosuppressive drugs that may be useful in treating Crohn's disease. One potential benefit of methotrexate and cyclosporine is that they appear to work faster than traditional immunosuppressive drugs.

Zinc Free radicals—molecules produced during fat metabolism, stress, and infection, among other things—may contribute to inflammation in Crohn's disease. Free radicals sometimes cause cell damage when they interact with other molecules in the body. The mineral zinc removes free radicals from the bloodstream. Studies are under way to determine whether zinc supplementation might reduce inflammation.

cross-reaction   The reaction of one antigen with antibodies that were generated against another different but similar antigen.

cryoglobulinemia   A medical condition caused by proteins (antibodies or immunoglobulins) called cryoglobulins being present in the blood. Cryoglobulins are abnormal proteins that by definition have the unusual property of clumping together in the laboratory when chilled and redissolving at normal body temperatures. The name literally means "cold antibody in the blood."

Cryoglobulins produce no symptoms in most people. In others, however, they cause cryoglobulinemia. This can manifest as conditions throughout the body, including problems resulting from abnormal thickness/viscosity of the blood (such as stroke or blood clots in the eyes leading to blindness) and inflammation of blood vessels, referred to as vasculitis. Vasculitis of arteries can result in blockage of arteries, leading to damage to the organ(s) supplied by the affected blood vessels, such as in the skin, kidneys, or elsewhere. Cryoglobulinemia is marked by skin rashes, joint and muscle aches, kidney disease, or neuropathy.

When the cryoglobulin proteins are a mixture of various antibody types, and have not formed because of any identifiable underlying disease, the condition is referred to as ESSENTIAL MIXED CRYOGLOBULINEMIA.

cytokines   Powerful nonantibody proteins secreted by inflammatory cells. Cytokines include lymphokines produced by lymphocytes (white blood cells) and monokines produced by monocytes and macrophages. They provide signals to regulate immunological aspects of cell growth, and they function during inflammation and immune response.

cytotoxic   Toxic (destructive) to cells.

cytotoxic T cells   See T CYTOTOXIC CELL.

cytotoxicity   See ANTIBODY-DEPENDENT CELL-MEDIATED CYTOTOXICITY.

death Autoimmune diseases constitute one of the 10 leading causes of all deaths among U.S. women age 65 and younger, according to a study published by researchers from the Department of Community Medicine at the University of Connecticut Health Center's School of Medicine.

The study, published in the September 2000 issue of the *American Journal of Public Health,* was the first to show mortality rates from autoimmune diseases among women of various age groups. Apart from accidents, homicides, and suicides, the study showed that autoimmune diseases are

- the seventh leading cause of death by disease among females aged one to 14,
- the fifth leading cause of death by disease among females aged 15 to 44, and
- the seventh leading cause of death by disease among females aged 45 to 65.

In that study, multiple sclerosis and rheumatic fever were the two leading autoimmune diseases based on the underlying cause of death among women below age 65. However, Type 1 diabetes deaths were included for women only younger than 35 years of age. Systemic lupus erythematosus was the underlying cause of death for more women between ages 25 and 44 than any other autoimmune disease. Type 1 diabetes, though counted for only ages 25 to 34, was second.

Connecticut Women's Health. Hartford: Connecticut Department of Public Health, 2001.

demyelinating neuropathies Inflammatory diseases of the nerves that destroy normal, healthy myelin (demyelination). Myelin is a fatty layer, or sheath, that surrounds and electrically insulates nerves, speeding the transmission of impulses along the nerve cells. Demyelination short-circuits that process, causing loss of sensation and coordination in various areas of the body. (See also CHRONIC INFLAMMATORY DEMYELINATING POLYNEUROPATHY, GUILLAIN-BARRÉ SYNDROME.)

denial of autoimmune diseases The first response to a diagnosis of any chronic disease is usually denial. In fact, a person commonly experiences a variety of emotional responses upon learning he or she has an autoimmune disease. Typically, newly diagnosed patients feel the "anger, denial, bargaining, depression, and acceptance" cycle identified by E. Kubler-Ross as a response to coping with a significant loss and major life changes. The patient may feel isolated from others and experience fear of the unknown future. The challenge at this initial phase of the illness is to move through the feelings of anger, denial, and sadness to reach an "accommodation" with the disease. This term is increasingly used to replace "acceptance." True acceptance of a serious chronic and potentially disabling disease probably never occurs.

Holland, Nancy J. *Psychosocial Aspects.* Washington, D.C.: The National Women's Health Information Center, The Office On Women's Health, U.S. Department of Health and Human Services, 1996.
Ladd, Virginia. "Coping With Autoimmunity," *InFocus,* American Autoimmune Related Diseases Association. Available online. URL: http://www.aarda.org/coping_art.html. Posted 2001.

depression When diagnosed with an autoimmune disease, the patient usually goes through a period of depression, usually between the DENIAL and anger stages.

Although depressive feelings are an expected consequence of the diagnostic phase, prolonged depression is cause for concern. Symptoms of significant depression include ongoing and pervasive sadness; loss of interest in—or enjoyment of—important activities and relationships; feelings of hopelessness and despair, sometimes including suicidal feelings or thoughts; and changes in sleep and eating patterns. It is important to recognize that relief from depression is readily available. Counseling and/or antidepressant medication are very successful in relieving symptoms of depression. Seeking help for this problem demonstrates an understanding of its significance, not personal weakness or deficiency.

Holland, Nancy J. *Psychosocial Aspects.* Washington, D.C.: The National Women's Health Information Center, The Office On Women's Health, U.S. Department of Health and Human Services, 1996.

dermatitis herpetiformis (DH) A chronic, severe, intensely itchy, blistering skin disease. Dermatitis herpetiformis is related to CELIAC DISEASE in that both are autoimmune disorders caused by gluten intolerance, but they are separate diseases. The rash usually appears in a symmetrical pattern of small clusters of red and itchy bumps. It most often occurs on the elbows, knees, back, scalp, and buttocks. In rare occasions, the lesions occur within the mouth. Although people with dermatitis herpetiformis do not usually have digestive symptoms, they sometimes experience the same chronic diarrhea as do people with celiac disease.

Originally called Duhring's disease, dermatitis herpetiformis usually first appears in the teens, 20s, or 30s. In the U.S., the presence of diagnosed cases is estimated to be about one in 10,000 with a male/female ratio of two to one. It occurs more commonly in Caucasians and rarely in African Americans and Asians. Although its severity may vary, it persists indefinitely and is a lifelong condition, with spontaneous remission over a 25-year period occurring in only 10 percent to 15 percent of patients.

Causes

Dermatitis herpetiformis is triggered by an allergy to gluten, a protein found in wheat and some other grains. Unlike other allergies, which are made by the body's IgE system and treatable with pills and injections of the antigen, dermatitis herpetiformis is an allergy of the IgA system. IgA is an antibody produced in the mucous membranes of the intestines, and the usual allergy treatments are useless. The rash is caused when gluten in the diet combines with IgA, and the IgA-gluten-antibody complex enters the bloodstream and circulates. The IgA or the complex settles in the skin, causing the intense reaction labeled dermatitis herpetiformis. Gluten proteins from ingested wheat and other grains find their way to the afflicted skin and trigger an immune attack.

Clinical Features

Before the lesions appear, the area usually has a burning feeling, followed by discolorations and then small bumps called papules and small water blisters called vesicles. These lesions tend to occur in groups much like the lesions of herpes, thus the term herpetiformis, meaning "like herpes." Because of the intense itching, the lesions are often scratched; these scratched areas will then develop crusts. Most DH patients can usually predict the location of a new lesion as much as eight to 12 hours before the actual onset because of the symptoms of localized burning and itching. Though the blisters tend to come out in crops, all stages can be seen at any one time. The blisters may take from seven to 10 days to lose their itching and burning sensations and then begin to crust. They are rarely inflamed and do not contain pus.

Dermatitis herpetiformis is diagnosed by a skin biopsy. This involves removing a tiny piece of skin near the rash and testing it for the IgA antibody.

Treatment

Dermatitis herpetiformis is treated with a gluten-free diet and medication, such as dapsone or sulfapyridine, to control the rash. Drug treatment may last several years or be lifelong as the severity of the disease builds and subsides.

Complete elimination of gluten is healing. However, significant improvement takes months, and a gluten-free diet is very difficult because tiny amounts of gluten are in almost all restaurants and prepared foods. It is worth the effort, however, because a gluten-free diet reduces the necessary dapsone dosage and its associated complications, provides an improvement in gastrointestinal symptoms, and attacks the cause rather than the symptoms of the disease. Cutting down on wheat and gluten may reduce the amount of medication needed but will not cure the disease.

In one study to determine the effectiveness of the gluten-free diet for dermatitis herpetiformis, 20 patients strictly adhered to a gluten-free diet. In 10 of them, the drug therapy could be completely discontinued; in six, the dosage could be reduced by at least 75 percent. In each case, however, adherence to the diet for at least five months was needed before any reduction of medication could be instituted. In a second follow-up study, however, one patient had no response until 14 months. The study also found that a reintroduction of gluten into the diet of four patients resulted in the production of symptoms and signs of DH in from one to three weeks. Even after one year of treatment with the gluten-free diet, the skin of the dermatitis herpetiformis patients still contained IgA.

Dapsone will improve dermatitis herpetiformis quickly. Because of its potential side effects, therapy is typically started with a small dosage. Usually, the patient's symptoms of itching and burning will subside within a few hours after taking the first pill. The dosage of dapsone is then adjusted upward to maintain adequate suppression of symptoms. Minor fluctuations in dermatitis herpetiformis severity do occur and are thought to be related to gluten intake. The on and off response of the dermatitis herpetiformis lesions to dapsone is dramatic. Itching and general symptoms are relieved within 48 to 72 hours after starting dapsone; lesions recur within 24 to 48 hours after discontinuation of dapsone therapy.

Because dapsone has potential side effects and may have adverse effects, weekly or biweekly blood tests are taken for the first three months. The two side effects of dapsone, if expressed at all, are anemia and allergic reactions. In anemia, a condition exists in which the old red blood cells disintegrate earlier than they normally would

without the influence of the drug. Allergic reactions, known as the *dapsone syndrome,* may develop days, months, or years later. Common symptoms include fever, swollen glands, rash, and abdominal pain.

Alternative treatments of sulfapyridine or tetracycline are available if dapsone cannot be used. However, they are not as effective.

Egan, C. A., E. P. Smith, T. B. Taylor, L. J. Meyer, W. S. Samowitz, and J. J. Zone. "Linear IgA Bullous Dermatosis Responsive to a Gluten-Free Diet." *The American Journal of Gastroenterology* 96, no. 6 (June 2001): 1,927–1,929.

Porter, W. M., S. A. Dawe, and C. B. Bunker. "Dermatitis Herpetiformis and Cutaneous T-Cell Lymphoma." *Clinical and Experimental Dermatology* 26, no. 3 (May 2001): 305–306.

dermatomyositis One of a group of acquired muscle diseases called inflammatory myopathies. The disease, which has a somewhat short and relatively severe onset, affects both children and adults. However, it most commonly occurs in adults 50 to 60 years old or in children from five to 15 years old. Females are affected twice as often as males. Overall, dermatomyositis is rare, having an incidence rate of five out of 1 million people. Dermatomyositis is characterized by a rash accompanying or, more often, preceding muscle weakness. The rash is described as patchy, bluish purple discolorations on the face, neck, shoulders, upper chest, elbows, knees, knuckles, and back. Some patients may also develop hardened bumps of calcium deposits under the skin. The most common symptom is muscle weakness, usually affecting those muscles that are closest to the trunk of the body (proximal). The muscle weakness may appear suddenly or gradually over weeks or months. Eventually, patients have difficulty rising from a sitting position, climbing stairs, lifting objects, or reaching overhead. In some cases, distal muscles (those not close to the trunk of the body) may be affected later in the course of the disease. Trouble with swallowing (dysphagia), painful joints, lung disease, and inflammation of the heart may occur. Occasionally, the muscles ache and are tender to touch. Patients may also feel fatigue and discomfort and have weight loss or a low-grade fever.

Causes

The precise cause of dermatomyositis is unknown. However, genetic factors, viral infection of the muscles involved in body movement, and autoimmune reaction are all suspected to contribute.

Treatment

Treatment for dermatomyositis generally begins with a steroid drug called prednisone. As muscle strength improves, the medication is slowly tapered to a maintenance level. For patients in whom prednisone is not effective, immunosuppressants such as azathioprine and methotrexate may be prescribed. Recently, a drug called intravenous immunoglobulin (IVIg) was claimed to be effective and safe in the treatment of the disease. Physical therapy is usually recommended to preserve muscle function and avoid muscle atrophy. Most cases of dermatomyositis respond to therapy. The disease is usually more severe and resistant to therapy in patients with cardiac or pulmonary problems.

Euwer, R. L., and R. D. Sontheimer. "Amyopathic Dermatomyositis: A Review." *The Journal of Investigative Dermatology* 100, Supp. (1993): 1,245–1,275.

Rockerbie, N. R., T. Y. Woo, J. P. Callen, et al. "Cutaneous Changes of Dermatomyositis Precede Muscle Weakness." *The Journal of the American Academy of Dermatology* 20 (1998): 629–632.

diagnosis of autoimmune diseases The diagnosis of an autoimmune disease is based on a review of the individual's symptoms; findings from a detailed physical examination; review of the patient's and family's medical history; analysis of results from laboratory tests such as blood, biopsy, X ray, vision, or hearing; and the ruling out of other diseases. Autoimmune diseases can be difficult to diagnose, particularly early in the course of the disease. Symptoms of many autoimmune diseases—such as fatigue—are nonspecific and can result from a myriad of diseases and conditions. Additionally, a variety of symptoms frequently accompany autoimmune diseases, thus confusing the diagnosis process. Sometimes the symptoms of one disease overlap with those of another. Laboratory test results may help but are often inadequate to confirm a diagnosis.

If an individual has sufficient symptoms of an autoimmune disease (e.g., joint pain) plus a positive but nonspecific lab test, the physician will likely request the patient to return frequently for follow-up. The early phase of disease may be a very frustrating time for both the patient and physician. On the other hand, symptoms may be short-lived, and inconclusive laboratory tests may amount to nothing of a serious nature.

For some autoimmune diseases, such as autoimmune inner ear disease, there are no specific tests. So a common approach is to look for other evidence of autoimmune involvement.

In some cases, a specific diagnosis can be made. A diagnosis shortly after onset of a patient's symptoms will allow for early aggressive medical therapy. For some diseases, patients will respond completely to treatments if the reason for their symptoms is discovered early in the course of their disease.

diet/nutrition Recent findings have emphasized the importance of nutritional factors in autoimmune diseases. Changes in diet have been linked to autoimmune disorders as a specific pathogenetic mechanism and also for the malnutrition conditions frequently documented in autoimmune patients. Although the precise function of different nutrients is not completely known, trace elements and vitamins are certainly important for the control of inflammation and of susceptibility in infections, even if their role is not clear. More research is necessary to clarify the link between the dietary component and autoimmune diseases. However, studies in SYSTEMIC LUPUS ERYTHEMATOSUS and RHEUMATOID ARTHRITIS have demonstrated that good nutrition can help diminish the severity of these disorders and help treatment with no side effects. In some autoimmune diseases, though, researchers believe that elements of the diet may be detrimental, such as in autoimmune diseases of the thyroid, where dietary iodine may be an important enhancing factor. Other autoimmune diseases are also affected by diet and nutrition.

CELIAC DISEASE—The only treatment for celiac disease is to follow a gluten-free diet, which means avoiding all foods that contain wheat (including spelt, triticale, and kamut), rye, barley, and possibly oats—that is, most grains, pasta, and cereals and many processed foods. Despite these restrictions, people with celiac disease can eat a well-balanced diet with a variety of foods, including bread and pasta. For example, instead of wheat flour, people can use potato, rice, soy, or bean flour. Alternatively, they can buy gluten-free bread, pasta, and other products from special food companies. A related, but separate, autoimmune disease, DERMATITIS HERPETIFORMIS is also treated with a gluten-free diet.

CHRONIC FATIGUE SYNDROME—According to the American Academy of Family Physicians, "Eat a well-balanced diet that's low in fat but high in fiber and complex carbohydrates. Avoid eating too many simple sugars such as candy and sweets. Eat more fruits and vegetables. They're good sources of energy and vitamins and minerals."

INSULIN-DEPENDENT DIABETES—In addition to taking insulin, diabetes patients must closely monitor their diet for successful disease management, adjusting it when necessary to optimize glucose control. A diabetes diet is a well-balanced meal plan that controls the types and amounts of food eaten.

INTERSTITIAL CYSTITIS (IC)—Some types of IC respond well to changes in the diet. No scientific evidence proves that diet affects IC, but many IC patients believe that eliminating certain foods from their diet helps treatment. Others say that specific foods cause flare-ups. Many physicians also see evidence of certain foods helping or hurting their IC patients.

MÉNIÈRE'S DISEASE—Some physicians recommend a change of diet to help control Ménière's symptoms. Eliminating caffeine, alcohol, and salt may relieve the frequency and intensity of attacks in some people. Restricting salt intake helps large numbers of Ménière's patients, but there is no scientific explanation for why a low-sodium diet works.

SYSTEMIC LUPUS ERYTHEMATOSUS (SLE)—It appears that substantial dietary intake of alfalfa seeds or sprouts may produce lupus and lupuslike symptoms in humans, monkeys, and mice. A non-protein amino acid, L-canavanine, naturally present in alfalfa seeds and sprouts, is thought to be responsible for the autoimmune effects. It has been suggested that patients with autoimmune disease such as SLE avoid large amounts of alfalfa seeds and sprouts.

"Chronic Fatigue Syndrome: How to Help Yourself." *American Family Physician* 65, no. 6 (March 2002): 1,095.

Danieli, M. G., and M. Candela. "Diet and Autoimmunity." *Recenti Progressi in Medicina* 81, no. 7–8 (July–August 1990): 532–538.

"Interstitial Cystitis Diet Tips." Available online. URL: http://www.elmiron100.com/diet.html. Downloaded on 15 July 2002.

Malinow, M. R., E. J. Bardana, B. Pirofsky, S. Craig, and P. McLaughlin. "Systemic Lupus Erythematosus-Like Syndrome in Monkeys Fed Alfalfa Sprouts: Role of a Nonprotein Amino Acid." *Science* 216 (1982): 415–417.

Montanaro, A., and E. J. Bardana. "Dietary Amino Acid-Induced Systemic Lupus Erythematosus." *Rheumatic Diseases Clinics of North America* 17 (1991): 323–332.

Prete, P. E. "Effects of L-Canavanine on Immune Function in Normal and Autoimmune Mice: Disordered B-Cell Function by a Dietary Amino Acid in the Immunoregulation of Autoimmune Disease." *Canadian Journal of Physiology and Pharmacology* 63 (1985): 843–854.

Rall, Laura C., and Ronenn Roubenoff. "Nutrition and Connective Tissue Health." *Nutrition Today* 35, no. 4 (July 2000): 142.

disability/disability benefits Autoimmune diseases cause varying degrees of disability and affect all patients differently. In many cases, though, the disability is sufficient to curtail or prohibit the patient from his or her normal work. When taken as a whole, autoimmune diseases represent the fourth-largest cause of disability among women in the United States.

Social Security pays disability benefits under two programs: the Social Security Disability Insurance Program and the Supplemental Security Income (SSI) Program. Medical requirements for disability payments under both programs are the same. Eligibility for Social Security disability is based on prior work history, and SSI payments are made on the basis of financial need.

discoid lupus A benign, distinctive disk-shaped rash that is chronic. It affects only the skin and not the internal organs. Females outnumber males with this condition three to one. Discoid lupus is neither cancerous nor contagious. The initial lesion is a small or moderate-sized, coin-shaped red patch that arises spontaneously or after mild injury or exposure to sunlight. The disease spreads to other areas. However, it may be confined to the exposed areas of the body, such as the face, scalp, ears, chest, and arms. The inflammation occurring on the skin may cause destruction of hair follicles and glands and thinning of the skin, with loss of normal color. These lesions may cause permanent scarring and loss of hair. The disease usually comes and goes. Discoid lupus will rarely go away and not come back.

Lupus is named after a characteristic butterfly-shaped rash on the nose and cheeks that in ancient times was thought to make the person look like a wolf (*lupus* in Latin). The disease has many forms, including discoid, systemic, and drug induced. Discoid lupus is confined to the skin and can be relatively mild. However, in some cases, the disease can proceed to the more serious system form where antibodies attack healthy tissues and organs throughout the body. Several common medications can also induce a temporary syndrome that resembles lupus.

The cause of the disease is an autoimmunity. Researchers believe that changes in the skin may be caused by an autoimmune reaction of the immune system, skin injury, or an inherited factor because it tends to run in families. However, there is no clearly defined predisposition to the disease.

Treatments for discoid lupus are directed at symptom control. They include avoiding Sun exposure, antimalarial medications (hydroxychloroquine/Plaquinil and others), local cortisone injections, dapsone, and immune suppression medications.

Cortisone ointment applied to the skin in the affected areas will often improve the lesions and slow down their progression. Cortisone injections into the lesions usually are more effective than the ointment form of cortisone. Plaquenil will often improve the condition, but patients on Plaquenil need eye exams once a year to prevent damage to the retina of the eye, plus periodic blood work. Patients whose condition is sensitive to sunlight need to wear a sunscreen of SPF 15 or higher daily and a hat while outdoors. At present, the disease has no known cure. (See also SYSTEMIC LUPUS ERYTHEMATOSUS.)

disease A condition or impairment that interferes with the performance of the vital functions and having a specific history, clinical signs, symptoms, and laboratory findings. It may be caused by environmental factors, infections, genetic factors, or to a combinations of these.

DNA (deoxyribonucleic acid) A double-stranded molecule that encodes (stores) genetic information about the cell growth, division, and function of most living organisms. It plays a central role in the determination of hereditary characteristics by controlling protein synthesis in cells. DNA is a nucleic acid composed of two chains of nucleotides. When the cell divides, its DNA also replicates in such a way that each of the two daughter molecules are identical to the parent molecule.

Dressler's syndrome This is also called post-MI pericarditis, postcardiac injury syndrome, and postcardiotomy pericarditis. It is an uncommon disorder that may occur following a heart attack, heart surgery, stab wounds to the heart, or blunt chest trauma. It is characterized by pleurisy (inflammation of the outer lining of the lungs) and fever, which may occur within days to several weeks after a heart attack. This complication is thought to be autoimmune, with the body's immune system producing antibodies that attack the damaged areas of heart muscle. Dressler's syndrome may be life threatening if untreated. Recurrences are common even with adequate treatment. It occurs in approximately four out of 100,000 people.

Causes

Dressler's syndrome is caused by an inflammatory response in the pericardial sac (the outer covering membrane of the heart) or necrotic (dead or severely damaged) tissue in the heart muscle. Pain occurs when the inflamed pericardium rubs on the heart.

Clinical Features

Symptoms include chest pain that may come and go. It is either tight and crushing or sharp and stabbing pain radiating to the neck, shoulder, back or abdomen. The chest pain possibly increases when breathing. The patient will feel pain relief when upright, standing, or sitting. He or she will experience difficulty breathing, dry cough, anxiety, fatigue, fever, and general malaise. The diagnosis is confirmed by detecting specific antibodies in the blood.

Complications

If untreated, the condition can lead to a compression of the heart caused by blood or fluid accumulation in the sac around the heart (pericardium), heart failure, or an accumulation of fluid in the lungs.

Treatment

The goals of treatment are to improve heart function and reduce symptoms. Aspirin or nonsteroidal anti-inflammatory medications (NSAIDS) will usually relieve the inflammation of the pericardium. In more severe cases, oral corticosteroids may be needed. Other medications may include analgesics to relieve pain and diuretics to remove excess fluid.

driving   Operating a motor vehicle may at times be dangerous for autoimmune patients. This is sometimes due to medication being taken, at other times it is because of the disease itself.

CHRONIC FATIGUE SYNDROME—Many autoimmune diseases cause patients to be tired, but CFS patients are particularly likely to be exhausted to the point where they give up driving.

INSULIN-DEPENDENT DIABETES—Progressive diabetic hypoglycemia leads to neuroglycopenia, which impairs driving. Research suggests that persons with Type 1 diabetes may not judge correctly when their blood glucose level is too low to permit safe driving and may consider driving with a low blood glucose level even when they are aware of the low level. Health care professionals should counsel their patients about the risk of driving with hypoglycemia and the importance of measuring blood glucose level before driving.

MULTIPLE SCLEROSIS (MS)—MS patients who experience cognitive difficulties have impaired driving skills, according to a recent study. Based on two computerized driving tests, MS patients with cognitive difficulties had a slower response time than the other MS patients. Additionally, 29 percent of these subjects tested as high risk for getting into an accident.

MYASTHENIA GRAVIS—A person's legs may become so weak that while driving, he or she will find it difficult to lift their foot from accelerator to brake.

eating disorders INSULIN-DEPENDENT DIABETES mellitus (IDDM) and eating disorders are relatively common among young women in North America. In a Canadian study, 29 percent of young women with IDDM had highly or moderately disordered eating behavior at the beginning of the study, which persisted over four years in 18 percent and improved in 11 percent. Of those with normal eating behavior at the beginning, 15 percent had disordered eating four to five years later. Among their weight loss practices was the intentional omission or underuse of insulin to control weight. Those with disordered eating behavior had a higher risk of retinopathy (damage to the retina, which can lead to blindness).

It has been suggested that the emphasis placed on weight and eating habits for young diabetics adds fuel to the "diet fire" lit under so many adolescents and teenagers in today's image-conscious culture. As the diabetics learn that drastically decreasing food intake can diminish their diabetic symptoms for the short term or that misusing their insulin can contribute to weight loss, some begin to use these tactics beyond what is safe. In some cases, they may even be praised for keeping their weight under control by family and friends, who are not aware of the extent of the methods being used.

Rydall, Anne C., et al. "Disordered Eating Behavior and Microvascular Complications in Young Women with Insulin-Dependent Diabetes Mellitus." *The New England Journal of Medicine* 336 (1997): 1,849–1,854.

economic cost of autoimmune diseases In industrialized societies, autoimmune diseases are serious medical problems because of their chronic and disabling effects. For example, the end stage renal failure caused by Type 1 INSULIN-DEPENDENT DIABETES mellitus (IDDM) costs the U.S. Medicare program over $2 billion per year for renal dialysis. Similarly, providing medical care to children with IDDM costs the Australian government $1.5 million per year. Therapy for autoimmune diseases continues to advance, thus increasing the demand for clinical laboratory testing that can help diagnose and monitor treatments and progress. Overall, autoimmune conditions cost an estimated $87 billion a year in healthcare expenditures in the United States, according to a 1999 report.

- The estimated economic costs of asthma in the United States in 1996 were $14 billion. The largest single indirect cost in 1990 was $1 billion for decreased productivity due to loss of school days. Despite the widespread assumption that asthma is a mild illness, 43 percent of the cost was due to emergency room use, hospitalization, and death. According to the National Institute of Environmental Health Sciences, ALLERGIC ASTHMA itself costs an estimated $6.2 billion per year.

- Economic costs for CROHN'S DISEASE and ULCERATIVE COLITIS are estimated at between $1.8 and $2.6 billion per year.

- According to a 1996 NIH-sponsored study, insulin-dependent diabetes mellitus (IDDM) patients on intensive therapy who maintain near-normal blood sugar for life are predicted to gain on average an extra five years of life, eight years of sight, six years free from kidney disease, and six years free from amputations and nerve damage, compared with patients on standard therapy. Intensive treatment costs about $4,500 per patient each year, and standard treatment costs $1,700 per patient annually.

- The economic costs of INTERSTITIAL CYSTITIS (IC) can be profound. The average annual medical cost per IC patient in year 2000 dollars is approximately $5,870. This leads to an estimated annual cost in the U.S. of $258 million. Research has estimated that one in four female IC patients are less likely to be employed full-time compared with a healthy female population. Total lost incomes would amount to $472.2 million.

- MULTIPLE SCLEROSIS (MS) is a lifelong chronic disease diagnosed primarily in young adults who have a virtually normal life expectancy. Consequently, the economic, social, and medical costs associated with the disease are significant. The National Multiple Sclerosis Society estimates that direct and indirect costs associated with MS exceed $9 billion annually.

- According to "Psoriasis Causes as Much Disability as Other Major Medical Diseases," an article published in the September 1999 *Journal of the American Academy of Dermatology,* PSORIASIS costs the nation between $2 billion and $3 billion each year.

- The direct medical costs of RHEUMATOID ARTHRITIS (RA) approach $5 billion annually, with nearly 70 percent of these costs attributable to hospitalizations and home nursing care. Rheumatoid arthritis patients make more than 9 million physician visits and account for over 250,000 hospitalizations annually. The direct cost to patients is considerable, even for those with insurance.

In a review of RA costs published in 2000, total average medical costs per patient were reported to range from $5,720 to $5,822. Medication constituted between 8 percent and 24 percent of total medical costs, physician visits between 8 percent and 21 percent, and in-patient stays between 17 percent and 88 percent. The average number of days absent from work due to a person's RA was reported to range from 2.7 to 30 days per year.

Lost productivity costs due to rheumatoid arthritis approach $20 billion annually. Rheumatoid arthritis patients lose, on average, 50 percent of potential earnings, with approximately 50 percent of patients unable to work within 10 years of onset. The lifetime indirect costs of rheumatoid arthritis are similar to those for stroke or coronary artery disease. Increased absenteeism, disability, and early retirement all contribute to the loss of personal income resulting from rheumatoid arthritis.

In April 2002, the Canadian Rheumatology Association (CRA) called for the provinces to cover the costs of biologic response modifiers in the treatment of RA. Their statement addressed the economic considerations of biologic therapies, which cost approximately $12,000 to $17,000 per year. Because these medications can prevent the direct cost of joint damage, including frequent hospitalizations and joint replacement surgery, as well as indirect costs, such as disability and premature death, the CRA's research found the use of biologics justified in appropriate patients.

Most of the 300,000 Canadians with RA develop the disease between the ages of 25 and 50. Half of them will be disabled within 10 years of diagnosis, so the long-term cost of not treating patients who require biologics will be immense. The CRA estimated that approximately 15,000 Canadians would be realistic candidates for this treatment. Without these drugs, the CRA said, millions of dollars will be spent down the road caring for these patients who otherwise could lead productive lives if they received the treatment they need now.

- Because SYSTEMIC LUPUS ERYTHEMATOSUS affects multiple organ systems, it can be an expensive disease to manage. Treatment requires the participation of many different medical specialists and expensive specialized testing and procedures. The average annual cost of medical treatment for a lupus patient is between $6,000 and $10,000. However, for some people with lupus, medical costs may exceed several thousand dollars every month. Lupus can be financially devastating for many families.

Lupus patients often must take many medications to control symptoms or health effects of the disease. A survey of Lupus Foundation of America (LFA) members revealed that four of 10 people with lupus take six or more medications at a time.

Medications for seriously ill lupus patients easily can exceed $1,000 per month.

About one in five lupus sufferers is disabled and receives disability payments. Often people are disabled by lupus at a very young age. LFA statistics reveal that more than one in four lupus patients receives his or her medical care through Medicare or Medicaid. When combined with the cost of Social Security disability benefits and lost wage tax revenue, the LFA estimates the economic impact of lupus on the federal treasury is several billion dollars annually.

Fink, David B. "Interstitial Cystitis: A Family Physician's Perspective." *Osteopathic Family Physician News* 2, no. 2. (February 2002): 1, 10–13. The American College of Osteopathic Family Physicians.

Pincus, T. "The Underestimated Long Term Medical and Economic Consequences of Rheumatoid Arthritis." *Drugs* 50, Supp. (1995): 1–14.

Stone, C. E. "The Lifetime Economic Costs of Rheumatoid Arthritis." *The Journal of Rheumatology* 11 (1984): 819–827.

Yelin, E. "The Costs of Rheumatoid Arthritis: Absolute, Incremental, and Marginal Estimates." *The Journal of Rheumatology* 23, Supp. (1996): 47–51.

education about autoimmune diseases All but a few autoimmune diseases are relatively unknown by the general public and even by many in the medical profession. Because of this, educating physicians, nurses, patients, and families of patients is critical—with knowledge comes better understanding, more effective treatment, and improved disease management. The National Institutes of Health (NIH) supports a variety of educational programs aimed at improving disease management and quality of life for patients with chronic illness, their families, and their caregivers. To support the recruitment and development of health care professionals who treat patients with chronic illnesses, the NIH supports training programs in this area. Among recent educational activities cosponsored by NIH Institutes, Centers and Offices:

- Infectious Etiologies of Chronic Diseases
- Discovery of Human Response Genes
- Linking Environmental Agents and Autoimmune Diseases

- New Immunotherapies for Autoimmune Diseases
- Workshop on Accelerated Atherosclerosis in Systemic Lupus Erythematosus
- Neuropsychiatric Manifestations of Systemic Lupus Erythematosus
- Gene Therapy Approaches for Diabetes and Its Complications

Also heavily involved in the education and public awareness of autoimmune diseases is the nonprofit AMERICAN AUTOIMMUNE RELATED DISEASES ASSOCIATION (AARDA). One of the purposes of the John Hopkins Autoimmune Disease Research Center is to enhance education about the autoimmune diseases among medical students, graduate students, residents, and postdoctoral fellows while encouraging the inclusion of, and greater attention to, the autoimmune diseases in the medical curriculum. The Center arranges training opportunities for fellows wishing to emphasize research on the autoimmune disease in their career development. A goal of the Center is to assist in recruiting and supporting junior faculty interested in autoimmunity aimed at sparking fresh insights into the pathogenesis of autoimmune disease, seeking novel treatments, and developing strategies to prevent these diseases among those at risk. Another goal is to serve as a clearinghouse for reliable information about autoimmune diseases to the wider professional and lay public, fostering collaboration with the American Autoimmune Related Disease Association and the World Health Organization to disseminate accurate, up-to-date information.

emergency medical identification Cards, bracelets, or necklaces that have written messages on them. These are used by people with diabetes or other serious medical problems to alert paramedics or other emergency care providers in case of a medical emergency. (See Appendix IV—Medical Alert Jewelry.)

employment/work One of the concerns employers have when hiring or retaining employees who have any chronic condition is the amount of work time that might be lost. According to a 2001 report, days when workers have to cut back on activities because of health problems are more common than days when workers are totally unable to work. The research team led by Ronald Kessler, Ph.D., of Harvard Medical School, believe that because previous research on workplace costs of specific illnesses has largely ignored cutback days, it has substantially underestimated productivity loss due to illness. In the findings, 4.3 percent of the 2,000 adult employees were affected by autoimmune diseases, and these employees averaged 3.2 days of impairment (either lost or cutback) out of 30 days.

Some autoimmune patients are unable to work at all because of the debilitating pain, fatigue, or loss of function. However, others continue to work, although accommodations often are needed. For example, individuals with CHRONIC FATIGUE SYNDROME (CFS) may need to reduce their activity levels in order to avoid overstimulation. Jobs with intense physical requirements, eight-hour days, and multiple or complicated steps may not be feasible. Researchers have found that jobs for CFS individuals that are home based, part-time, job sharing, or with flextime are more viable. Appropriate jobs could be those that allow extra time to complete activities, minimize distractions, establish a routine for daily activities that will minimize the stress on fragile cognitive capacities, and permit schedule relaxation to reduce confusion and improve attention. Because individuals with CFS are often chemically sensitive, the environment in which they work must be relatively chemical free of odors and scents.

Similarly, SYSTEMIC LUPUS ERYTHEMATOSUS, sufferers who work in offices may be affected by any fluorescent lights, causing them to tire quickly. Under the Americans with Disabilities Act (ADA), the employer may be obligated to protect an affected lupus employee from such lighting. Passed by Congress in 1990, the ADA bans discrimination against people with disabilities in many areas, including hiring and employment. At the same time, it protects employers from having to make changes that are unreasonable or expensive. The ADA applies to companies employing 15 or more people. Many of the terms in the law, such as

"unreasonable," are being decided by the courts in test cases.

Also helpful to workers with chronic autoimmune diseases is the Family and Medical Leave Act (FMLA) of 1993. It allows qualified employees of companies with 50 or more workers to take up to three months unpaid medical leave per year if they are unable to work because of a serious health condition. This can be done intermittently or by working fewer hours per day, all with employer approval. Such working arrangements are especially helpful when the employee has an autoimmune disease that periodically flares up.

"Arthritis on the Job," iVillage. Available online. URL: http://www.ivillagehealth.com. Posted 30 July 1999.
"Chronic Conditions Cause Work Impairment." *Business & Health* 19, no. 6 (June 2001): 19.
Harley, Debra A. "Recognizing and Understanding Chronic Fatigue Syndrome: Implications for Rehabilitation Counselors." *The Journal of Rehabilitation* 67, no. 2 (April 2001): 22.
Kessler, Ronald, Paul Greenberg, Kristin Mickelson, Laurie Meneades, and Philip Wang. "The Effects of Chronic Medical Conditions on Work Loss and Work Cutback." *Journal of Occupational and Environmental Medicine* 4, no. 3 (March 2001): 218–225.

endocrine autoimmunity   Endocrine autoimmunity deals with autoimmune disorders that affect specific endocrine glands. Hashimoto's thyroiditis (low thyroid function) and Graves' disease (overactive thyroid function) are among the most commonly occurring endocrine autoimmune diseases. The general features of endocrine autoimmune disorders are similar to those for all autoimmunity. Treatment for endocrine autoimmunity usually consists of hormone replacement or agents to suppress overactive glands. The current advances related to endocrine autoimmunity involve improved hormone preparations for therapy and greater awareness leading to earlier detection and treatment.

Luborsky, Judy. "Endocrine Autoimmunity." *InFocus.* American Autoimmune Related Diseases Association, Inc., 1998.
Weetman, Anthony P. *Endocrine Autoimmunity and Associated Conditions.* Dordrecht, The Netherlands: Kluwer Academic Publishers, 1998.

endometriosis The name *endometriosis* comes from the word "endometrium," the tissue that lines the inner walls of the uterus. During normal menstrual cycles, uterine endometrial tissue debris and blood are shed in the process of menstruation. When this tissue moves outside its usual location, it is known as endometriosis—a problem that affects as many as 5 million American women or one in seven of childbearing age. Endometriosis strikes when the endometrium implants on the ovaries, fallopian tubes, pelvic ligaments, abdominal organs, old scars, and, in rare cases, other parts of the body.

When this occurs, the misplaced tissue continues to respond to the menstrual cycle as if it were still in the uterus. So at the end of every monthly cycle, when hormones cause the uterus to shed its endometrial lining, endometrial tissue growing outside the uterus will break apart and bleed. However, unlike menstrual fluid from the uterus, which is discharged from the body during menstruation, blood from the misplaced tissue cannot escape. Instead, it causes the formation of slowly growing, blood-filled cysts, which have been known to grow to the size of a grapefruit. These endometrial tissue sites may develop into what are called lesions, implants, nodules, or growths. Tissues surrounding the area of endometriosis may become inflamed or swollen. The inflammation may produce scar tissue around the area of endometriosis. Scarring may also form tough fibrous adhesions between pelvic and abdominal structures. The adhesions can cause pain in the pelvic area, irregular and heavy menstrual bleeding, painful menstruation, painful intercourse, and infertility.

Physicians use stages to describe the severity of endometriosis. Endometrial implants that are small and not widespread are considered minimal or mild endometriosis. Moderate endometriosis means that larger implants or more extensive scar tissue is present. Severe endometriosis is used to describe large implants and extensive scar tissue.

Causes

The cause of endometriosis is still unknown. One theory is that during menstruation, some of the menstrual tissue backs up through the fallopian tubes into the abdomen, where it implants and grows. Another theory suggests that endometriosis may be a genetic process or that certain families may have predisposing factors to endometriosis. In the latter view, endometriosis is seen as the tissue development process gone awry. Others have proposed that it is a disease influenced by delayed childbearing. Because the hormones made by the placenta during pregnancy prevent ovulation, the progress of endometriosis is slowed or stopped during pregnancy and the total number of lifetime cycles is reduced for a woman who had multiple pregnancies.

Whatever the cause of endometriosis, its progression is influenced by various stimulating factors such as hormones or growth factors. In this regard, the National Institute of Child Health and Human Development investigators are studying the role of the immune system in activating cells that may secrete factors that, in turn, stimulate endometriosis.

In fact, a large body of evidence accumulated over the last two decades indicates that endometriosis is, in large part, an autoimmune disease. Many of the diseases that are found more frequently in women with endometriosis and their immediate families are also autoimmune.

The Endometriosis Association's research registry tracks health problems that are reported by women with endometriosis and their families. This tracking shows higher rates of immune-related problems and diseases than are found in the general population. These range from allergies and chemical sensitivities to severe autoimmune disorders such as lupus.

Research suggests that endometriosis is associated with abnormal polyclonal B cell activation, a classic characteristic of autoimmune disease. This contention is further supported in that immunoglobulin levels (particularly IgG) are elevated in patients with endometriosis.

Researchers think that a healthy immune system prevents normal body cells from implanting in unusual sites. With a weakened immune system, the stray endometrial cells are not captured by the body's natural defenses and are able to implant themselves.

Some studies suggest that cytokines (substances produced by cells in the immune system) may influence the ability of endometrial growths to spread and flourish where they do not belong. A fairly recent realization is that environmental pollutants like dioxin also have profound immunological impacts. Although the precise impact of environmental pollutants on humans is unknown, endometriosis may be the first human disease definitely linked to hormonal and immunological disruption due to pollutants.

Clinical Features

Most commonly, the symptoms of endometriosis start years after menstrual periods begin. Over the years, the symptoms tend to increase gradually as the endometriosis areas increase in size. After menopause, the abnormal implants shrink away and the symptoms subside.

The most common symptom is pain, especially excessive menstrual cramps (dysmenorrhea), which may be felt in the abdomen or lower back, or pain during or after sexual activity (dyspareunia). Infertility occurs in about 30 percent to 40 percent of women with endometriosis. Rarely, the irritation caused by endometrial implants may progress into infection or abscesses causing pain independent of the menstrual cycle. Endometrial patches may also be tender to touch or pressure. Intestinal pain may also result from endometrial patches on the walls of the colon or intestine.

The amount of pain is not always related to the severity of the disease. Some women with severe endometriosis have no pain, while others with just a few small growths have incapacitating pain.

A diagnosis of endometriosis begins with a gynecologist evaluating the patient's medical history. A complete physical exam, including a pelvic examination, is also necessary. However, a diagnosis of endometriosis is complete only when proven by a laparoscopy, a minor surgical procedure in which a laparoscope (a tube with a light in it) is inserted into a small incision in the abdomen. The laparascope is moved around the abdomen, which has been distended with carbon dioxide gas to make the organs easier to see. The surgeon can then check the condition of the abdominal organs and see the endometrial implants. The laparoscopy will show the locations, extent, and size of the growths and will help with decisions about treatment.

Complications

Severe endometriosis with extensive scarring and organ damage may affect fertility. It is considered one of the three major causes of female infertility. However, unsuspected or mild endometriosis is a common finding among infertile women and how this type of endometriosis affects fertility is still not clear. While the pregnancy rates for patients with endometriosis remain lower than those of the general population, most patients with endometriosis do not experience fertility problems.

Endometrial cancer is very rarely associated with endometriosis, occurring in less than 1 percent of women who have the disease. When it does occur, it is usually found in more advanced patches of endometriosis in older women and the long-term outlook in these unusual cases is reasonably good.

Treatment

While the treatment for endometriosis has varied over the years, doctors now agree that if the symptoms are mild, no further treatment other than medication for pain may be needed. For those patients with mild or minimal endometriosis who wish to become pregnant, doctors are advising that, depending on the age of the patient and the amount of pain associated with the disease, the best course of action is to have a trial period of unprotected intercourse for six months to one year. If pregnancy does not occur within that time, then further treatment may be needed.

For patients not seeking a pregnancy where treatment specific for the management of endometriosis is required and a definitive diagnosis of endometriosis by laparoscopy has been made, a physician may suggest hormone suppression treatment. Because this therapy shuts off ovulation, women being treated for endometriosis will not get pregnant during such therapy, although some may elect to become pregnant shortly after therapy is stopped. Hormone treatment is most effective when the implants are small. The doctor may prescribe a weak synthetic male hormone called danazol, a synthetic progestin alone, or a combination of estrogen and progestin such as oral contraceptives.

Danazol has become a more common treatment choice than either progestin or the birth control pill. Disease symptoms are improved for 80 percent to 90 percent of the patients taking danazol, and the size and the extent of implants are also reduced. Although side effects with danazol treatment are not uncommon (e.g., acne, hot flashes, or fluid retention), most of them are relatively mild and stop when treatment is stopped. Overall, pregnancy rates following this therapy depend on the severity of the disease. However, some recent studies have shown that with mild-to-minimal endometriosis, danazol alone does not improve pregnancy rates.

Another type of hormone treatment is a synthetic pituitary hormone blocker called gonadotropin-releasing hormone agonist, or GnRH agonist. This treatment stops ovarian hormone production by blocking pituitary gland hormones that normally stimulate ovarian cycles.

These hormones are currently being tested using different methods of administration. One such treatment involves a drug that is administered as a nasal spray twice daily for six months. It works by suppressing production of estrogen, which controls the growth of the endometrial tissue. Other treatments being developed in this category include daily or monthly hormone injections. One concern is the loss of bone mineral that occurs with this type of hormone therapy. This may limit the duration and frequency of this type of treatment.

Although pregnancy rates for women with fertility problems resulting from endometriosis are fairly good with no therapy and with only a trial waiting period, some women may need more aggressive treatment. Those women who are older and who feel the need to become pregnant more quickly or those women who have severe physical changes due to the disease may consider surgical treatment. Also, women who are not interested in pregnancy but who have severe, debilitating pain may also consider surgery.

Conservative surgery attempts to remove the diseased tissue without risking damage to healthy surrounding tissue. This surgery is called laparotomy and is performed in a hospital under anesthesia. Pregnancy rates are highest during the first year after surgery, as recurrences of endometriosis are fairly common.

Some patients may need more radical surgery to correct the damage caused by untreated endometriosis. Hysterectomy and removal of the ovaries may be the only treatments possible if the ovaries are badly damaged. In some cases, hysterectomy alone without the removal of the ovaries may be reasonable.

New surgical treatments are being developed that further utilize the laparoscope instead of full abdominal surgery. During routine laparoscopy, the surgeon can cauterize small areas of endometriosis. Other evolving techniques include using a laser during laparoscopy to vaporize abnormal tissue. This involves a shorter recovery time. Laparoscopy treatment is possible, however, only if the surgeon can see pelvic structures clearly through the laparoscope. These newer techniques should be performed by surgeons specializing in such delicate procedures. Although these techniques are promising, more study is needed to determine if they yield results comparable to conventional surgical management.

Corwin, Elizabeth J. "Endometriosis: Pathophysiology, Diagnosis, and Treatment." *The Nurse Practitioner* 22, no. 10 (October 1997): 35–38, 40–42, 45–46, passim; quiz 56–57.

DuBrow, Andrea. "Endometriosis Update from the National Women's Health Network." *Network News* 24, no. 5 (September–October 1999): 1, 6.

National Institutes of Health: National Institute of Child Health and Human Development. *Facts About Endometriosis.* NIH Publication Number 91–2413. Last modified September 18, 2001.

environment and autoimmune diseases While attempting to solve the mystery of how autoimmune diseases begin and develop, scientists have been exploring what role, if any, environmental factors might play in the process. To date, they still have not reached a consensus. A 1998 National Institute of Environmental Health Sciences (NIEHS) workshop, Linking Environmental Agents and Autoimmune Disease, highlighted the need for solid data linking exposure to a specific environmental agent with a specific autoimmune disease. Researchers stressed that the field of autoimmune study as it relates to environmental exposures is in its infancy, noting that they are not yet at a point where they can say that there are known environmental causes of autoimmune diseases. *Potential* environmental links are under consideration, but the necessary combination of a theoretical framework and experimental and human data needed to fully support them does not exist. Heimer explained the situation as follows:

> Identifying specific environmental risk factors for autoimmune diseases is highly speculative. What data exist from epidemiologic studies are often contradictory or show weak effects of individual risk factors. In fact, most candidates for environmental links to autoimmune disease come primarily from a few well-known large-scale chemical or drug exposures that produced autoimmune syndromes. For example, in 1981, 35,000 people in Spain developed acute "toxic oil syndrome" after ingesting contaminated rapeseed oil. Their initial symptoms, including fever, fatigue, and joint and muscle pain, were similar to symptoms seen in autoimmune diseases. In most cases, patients were eventually categorized as having a "lupus-like" or "scleroderma-like" disorder. (Systemic scleroderma is an autoimmune disease that manifests through a thickening of the skin.) A similar syndrome was caused in the United States in 1989 by contaminants in the dietary supplement L-tryptophan. A large number of medicinal drugs, approximately 40 of which are still in use today, have also produced lupus-like syndromes in some patients. Most prominent among the more than 70 drugs that have caused lupus-like syndromes are procainamide, a cardiac antiarrhythmic medicine, and hydralazine, an antihypertensive drug.
>
> Occupational exposure to vinyl chloride also has been linked to a lupus-like syndrome, and silica dust is known to induce scleroderma. But because these syndromes differ in some respects from the spontaneous diseases and because they generally resolve when the chemical or drug exposure is ended, researchers wonder whether these syndromes provide real insight into the etiology of the spontaneous or idiopathic diseases.

The NIEHS workshop concluded that in most cases a definitive role for environmental agents, chemical, physical, or infectious, in the initiation or exacerbation of autoimmune disease is not strong, and that hypothesis-generating feasibility studies are needed to move the field forward. As a result, the NIEHS, in collaboration with other NIH institutes, has initiated several programs aimed at developing the preliminary data needed to link exposures to environmental agents to the initiation or progression of specific autoimmune diseases.

Ermann, Joerg, and C. Garrison Fathman. "Autoimmune Diseases: Genes, Bugs and Failed Regulation." *Nature Immunology* 2, no. 9: 759–761.

Heimer, Hakon. "Outer Causes of Inner Conflicts: Environment and Autoimmunity." *Environmental Health Perspectives* 107, no. 10 (October 1999): A504–509.

Heindel, Jerrold J. "The Environment and Autoimmune Disease." *Environmental Health Perspectives* 107, no. 5 (May 1999). Available online. URL: http:.//ehpnet1.niehs.nih.gov/docs/1999/107-5/extram-speaking.html. Last updated on 19 April 1999.

enzyme A protein, produced by living cells, that promotes the chemical processes of life without itself being permanently altered.

eosinophil A white blood cell that contains granules filled with chemicals damaging to parasites and enzymes that decrease inflammatory reactions. Eosinophils are believed to destroy parasitic worms and to play a major role in allergic reactions. They release some of the major chemical mediators that cause bronchoconstriction in asthma.

epitope A unique shape or marker carried on an antigen's surface, which triggers a corresponding antibody response.

erythrocytes/red blood cells The erythrocytes make up the largest population of blood cells, numbering from 4.5 million to 6 million per cubic millimeter of blood. They carry out the exchange of oxygen and carbon dioxide between the lungs and the body tissues. To combine with oxygen effectively, the erythrocytes must contain a normal amount of the red protein pigment hemoglobin, the amount of which in turn depends on the iron level in the body. A deficiency of iron and therefore of hemoglobin leads to anemia and poor oxygenation of the body tissues. Erythrocytes are constantly developing from stem cells.

essential mixed cryoglobulinemia A rare autoimmune disorder that may involve the blood and various other tissues and organs. The major symptoms include unusual response to cold, skin abnormalities, blood disorders, and generalized weakness. There may also be joint pain, inflamed blood vessels, and kidney problems.

Causes
The exact cause of essential mixed cryoglobulinemia is not known, but it is considered to be an autoimmune disorder. In this condition, the immune system appears to be triggered by cold temperatures. Cryoglobulins are abnormal proteins in the blood that become apparent when the blood is cooled. These cryoglobulins can affect many different bodily systems, causing pain and dysfunction. When the cryoglobulin proteins are a mixture of various antibody types, and forming for unknown reasons, the condition is referred to as essential mixed cryoglobulinemia. A link between CRYOGLOBULINEMIA and hepatitis B infection is possible.

Clinical Features
Essential mixed cryoglobulinemia is characterized by joint pains and swelling (arthritis), enlargement of the spleen, skin vasculitis with purplish patches, and nerve and kidney disease. This can lead to recurrent pain in the abdomen, heart attack, and bleeding in the lungs. Weight loss can occur as well as poor appetite.

Complications
Kidney damage can be serious. Recent reports state that permanent failure of the kidney occurs in approximately 10 percent of patients. Death can occur, usually from serious heart disease, infection, or brain hemorrhage.

Treatment
Essential mixed cryoglobulinemia is treated with combinations of medications that reduce inflammation and suppress the immune system. Medications used include nonsteroid antiinflammatory drugs (ibuprofen, aspirin), cortisone preparations (prednisone, prednisolone), cyclophosphamide (Cytoxan), chlorambucil (Leukeran), and azathioprine (Imuran). Plasmapheresis, a procedure whereby the blood's serum is replaced with saline (salt water), is also performed for severe symptoms. Recent studies have demonstrated some benefit when using interferon alpha for those patients with evidence of hepatitis C virus, particularly those with mild disease or in those with remission of manifestations after immune suppression treatment.

Shiel Jr., William C. "Essential Mixed Cryoglobulinemia," MedicineNet.com. Available online. URL: http://www.medicinenet.com. Downloaded on 16 July 2002.

Evans' syndrome A rare autoimmune disorder in which the body makes antibodies that destroy the red blood cells, platelets, and white blood cells. It was first mentioned in 1951 by American physician Robert S. Evans (1882–1971) and associates who described a group of patients with "primary thrombocytopenic purpura" and "acquired hemolytic anemia." Although these patients had varying symptoms, there was a strong suggestion of a common autoimmune mechanism. Other similar reports followed until 1980, when Pui, Williams, and Wang published the first significant report describing Evans' syndrome in childhood. Their criteria for diagnosis included both thrombocytopenia and autoimmune hemolytic anemia with no other known underlying cause for the disease. Evans' syndrome patients may be affected by low levels of all three types of blood cells at one time or may have problems with only one or two of them.

Causes
The specific cause for Evans' syndrome is unknown. Researchers have speculated that for every case, the cause may be different. No genetic links have been identified.

Clinical Features
The course of Evans' syndrome varies by case. The patient may be symptomatic of whatever blood levels are down. If the red blood cells are down, the problems complained of may be weakness, fatigue, shortness of breath, and the usual things associated with anemia. With low platelets, the patient may be susceptible to bleeding and major bruising from minor bumps and cuts. A bump on the head could

cause severe brain hemorrhage and death. With low white blood cells, the patient has increased susceptibility to infections and difficulty in fighting these infections. The patient may have problems with one, two, or all three of these blood lines at one time.

Complications

Patients with Evans' syndrome are reported to have a greater tendency to develop other autoimmune disorders such as lupus and rheumatoid arthritis. They have a tendency to develop various malignancies.

Treatment

Treatment of Evans' syndrome varies and so far has been unsatisfactory, with no "magic bullets" identified as a cure. Steroids are frequently used to help suppress the immune system or to decrease the production of the "bad antibodies." Intravenous immune globulin or IVIg is often tried as is chemotherapy when responses to other treatments are not satisfactory. Splenectomy has frequently been done, but the benefits of this are usually short-lived. In a recent study, the beneficial effects from splenectomy had lasted an average of one month. Closely monitoring the patients' complete blood count is crucial to the patients' treatment. Blood transfusions are done in crisis situations to help stabilize the patient. However, this is not a long-lasting solution because these cells are usually destroyed very quickly by the body. The prognosis with Evans' syndrome is guarded. Some patients have episodes of major blood cell destruction followed by long remissions, while others have chronic problems with no remissions.

Pegels, J. G. et al. "The Evans Syndrome: Characterization of the Responsible Autoantibodies." *British Journal of Haematology* 51 (1982): 445–450.

Pui, C. H., et al. "Evans' Syndrome in Childhood." *The Journal of Pediatrics* 97 (1980): 754–758.

What Is Evans Syndrome? Port Orange, Fla.: Evans Syndrome Support and Research Group, Legal Nurse Associates. Available online. URL: http://legalnursesassociates.com/evans.htm. Downloaded on 16 July 2002.

exercise   In some autoimmune diseases, exercise is an important component of disease manage-ment. In INSULIN-DEPENDENT DIABETES mellitus, for example, exercise makes the insulin more efficient.

Exercise is a commonly recommended treatment for ANKYLOSING SPONDYLITIS (AS). In one study, researchers concluded that unsupervised recreational exercise improves pain and stiffness and that back exercise improves pain and function in patients with AS. However, these effects differ with the duration of AS. Health status is improved when patients perform recreational exercise at least 30 minutes per day and back exercises at least five days per week. In a Dutch study of patients with AS, a three-week course of combined spa-exercise therapy, in addition to drug treatment and weekly group physical therapy alone, provided beneficial effects. The researchers concluded that these beneficial effects may last for at least 40 weeks.

Most patients with SYSTEMIC LUPUS ERYTHEMATOSUS can use exercise to increase aerobic capacity of cells and improve immune function. However, clearing any exercise program with one's doctor is very important. Generally, aerobic exercise is best for lupus patients; isometric exercises should be pursued with caution and only with medical approval. Also, exercise is usually not recommended during flares, when feeling fatigued, or if muscles ache.

Because lupus causes joint pain and inflammation, muscle pain, and fatigue, the very thought of exercising can be a challenge. In addition, because lupus is a disease that requires a large amount of rest, exercise is not always considered to be so important. Although rest is important in managing fatigue, too much rest can be harmful to muscles, bones, joints, and overall fitness. Keeping fit through an exercise program planned for the specific individual can help that person feel better, both mentally and physically. Many types of exercises are appropriate for lupus patients, such as swimming and walking. Regular exercise will

- increase muscle strength,
- help prevent joints from getting stiff,
- help prevent osteoporosis,
- help keep weight under control,

- improve cardiovascular health, and
- help reduce stress.

Similarly, although bed rest is considered therapy for many RHEUMATOID ARTHRITIS (RA) patients, it is recommended only until inflammation subsides. After that, the acute inflammatory response becomes more chronic from the downward spiraling of the patient's physical condition. RA patients die 10 to 15 years earlier than nonafflicted individuals, but the research shows a predictably higher mortality rate in RA patients who are inactive. Thus, exercise and physical activity is an important part of the treatment of rheumatoid arthritis. Daily exercise can reduce joint pain and stiffness and also increase flexibility, muscle strength, and endurance—generally helping to promote a better and longer life. It is important, however, that individual needs are assessed before developing an exercise program. RA patients are divided into four classifications based on their physical abilities and handicaps. Different types of exercise should be implemented according to the level of the patient. In one study, a short-term intensive exercise program in active RA was found to be more effective in improving muscle strength than a conservative exercise program and did not have deleterious effects on disease activity.

In a Canadian study, 59 women with FIBROMYALGIA, evaluated over a three-year period, most frequently identified physical exercise as the most helpful treatment.

Individuals with MULTIPLE SCLEROSIS (MS) have long been advised to avoid participation in exercise in order to minimize the risk of exacerbation and symptoms of fatigue. There is, however, increasing interest in how acute and chronic exercise affect physiological and psychological functioning in MS.

According to the Chronic Syndrome Support Association (CSSA), stretching and gentle aerobic exercise are essential for many autoimmune conditions. However, some experts caution against implementing an exercise program for those with CHRONIC FATIGUE SYNDROME (CFS). According to the American Academy of Family Physicians, modest exercise reduces fatigue and improves functioning and fitness in up to 75 percent of people with CFS. "It's important to exercise within your limits. Begin with as little as five minutes of light to moderate exercise a day. Then slowly increase how long and how hard you exercise. Always stop exercising before you feel overly tired. Try different forms of physical activity, such as walking, swimming, pool exercises, stationary exercise machines, stretching, T'ai chi, and yoga."

The CSSA suggests that the optimum time of day for exercise is approximately five hours before bedtime, although any time of day may be beneficial. Stretching can and should be done several times a day—simple things like shoulder rotation can be done in almost any setting. The CSSA cautions that some traditional repetitive regimens should not be performed because they can exacerbate pain. Those people who cannot tolerate aerobic exercise may respond better to a program of simple basic stretches. Many people with severe pain have found that water therapy in a heated pool provides some relief.

Most importantly, the CSSA cautions, people with autoimmune diseases need to listen to their bodies and not push too hard. A general rule of thumb is "always stop exercising while you still could do a little more." The old adage "no pain, no gain" does *not* apply to autoimmune conditions.

Writing in *IDEA Health & Fitness Source* magazine, Rosemary Lindle, Ph.D. emphasized the need to assess each person individually, "A growing body of evidence suggests that while the immune system is enhanced by moderate exercise, intense long-duration exercise (overtraining) may impair immune function. Although certainly not conclusive, many studies indicate that further research on the link between overtraining and autoimmunity is warranted. Since overtraining has been shown to have such a deleterious effect on the immune system, it seems entirely plausible that overtraining could trigger an autoimmune response in genetically predisposed individuals."

"Chronic Fatigue Syndrome: How to Help Yourself." American Family Physician 65, no. 6 (March 2002): 1,095.
Lindle, Rosemary. "Autoimmune Disease and Overtraining." *IDEA Health & Fitness Source* 18, no. 9 (October 2000): 30–36.

Lovett, Kate. *Exercise and Disease Prevention.* Vanderbilt University. Available online. URL: http://www.vanderbilt.edu/AnS/psychology/health_psychology/exercise.htm. Downloaded 16 July 2002.

LUPUS: A Patient Care Guide for Nurses and Other Health Professionals. National Institute of Arthritis and Musculoskeletal and Skin Diseases, National Institutes of Health.

Pinelli, L., A. Pietrobelli, F. Tomasselli, A. Verrotti, M. Catino, and F. Chiarelli. "Nutrition and Exercise in Children with Diabetes." *Diabetes, Nutrition & Metabolism* 12, no. 2 (April 1999): 102–107.

Poyhia, R., D. Da Costa, and M. A. Fitzcharles. "Pain and Pain Relief in Fibromyalgia Patients Followed for Three Years." *Arthritis and Rheumatism* 45, no. 4 (August 2001): 355–361.

Sutherland, G., and M. B. Andersen. "Exercise and Multiple Sclerosis: Physiological, Psychological, and Quality of Life Issues." *The Journal of Sports Medicine and Physical Fitness* 41, no. 4 (December 2001): 421–432.

Uhrin, Z., S. Kuzis, and M. M. Ward. "Exercise and Changes in Health Status in Patients with Ankylosing Spondylitis." *Archives of Internal Medicine* 160, no. 19 (October 2000): 2,969–2,975.

van den Ende, C. H., F. C. Breedveld, S. le Cessie, B. A. Dijkmans, A. W. de Mug, and J. M. Hazes. "Effect of Intensive Exercise on Patients with Active Rheumatoid Arthritis: A Randomized Clinical Trial." *Annals of the Rheumatic Diseases* 59, no. 8 (August 2000): 615–621.

van Tubergen, A., R. Landewe, D. van der Heijde, A. Hidding, N. Wolter, M. Asscher, A. Falkenbach, E. Genth, and S. van der Linden. "Combined Spa-Exercise Therapy Is Effective in Patients with Ankylosing Spondylitis: A Randomized Controlled Trial." *Arthritis and Rheumatism* 45, no. 5 (October 2001): 430–438.

experimental allergic encephalomyelitis (EAE)
This is also called experimental autoimmune encephalomyelitic. It is a disease of the central nervous system that can be induced in laboratory animals. This disease serves as an animal model for MULTIPLE SCLEROSIS (MS). Animal models of human diseases are diseases of nonhuman species that closely resemble their human counterparts and are studied with a view to understanding and treating the human form better. EAE is not multiple sclerosis, nor is it a single disease in a single species, but its different forms resemble the various forms and stages of MS very closely in a number of ways. Like multiple sclerosis, EAE is a demyelinating disease—it destroys the myelin, the fatty sheath that protects and surrounds nerve fibers. EAE can be induced in rats, mice, guinea pigs, rabbits, and monkeys. It has both relapsing-remitting and progressive-relapsing forms.

Much of the current knowledge about the pathology and immunology of MS has been gained from studies of animals with EAE. Information derived from microscopic and biochemical examination of the brain, blood, and spinal cord of animals with EAE includes identifying sites in the central nervous system that are more likely to develop MS lesions—damaged areas—also known as plaques, finding out which immune cells are involved in the formation of plaques and how they interact, and developing experimental treatments or manipulations that can stop or reverse the demyelinating process.

It has been possible to promote remyelination—the growth of new myelin—in animals with EAE using a protein normally found in the brain. Ongoing studies of EAE in the laboratory will continue to be an important early step in the development of new therapies for multiple sclerosis.

"Experimental Allergic Encephalomyelitis," *The MS Information Sourcebook,* New York: The National Multiple Sclerosis Society, 2001.

eye diseases A number of autoimmune diseases exist in which the eye or various parts of the eye may be attacked by white blood cells. Often the autoimmune disease is systemic, with a variety of organs throughout the body system being attacked. Examples of such diseases include rheumatoid arthritis, systemic lupus erythematosus, polyarteritis nodosa, scleroderma, relapsing polychondritis, and inflammatory bowel disease (ulcerative colitis and Crohn's disease). All these can affect the eye, causing corneal ulcers, sclerosis, uveitis, or other inflammation. The eye may be affected as a target of immune inflammatory attack in any of these diseases. The eye may, however, in certain instances be the specific and only target affected by certain autoimmune diseases. Some such diseases include ocular cicatricial pemphigoid, Mooren's corneal ulcer, and various forms of uveitis. Any autoimmune disease affecting the eye will require systemic (e.g., oral as opposed to local, topical, or ocular) therapy. The components of the immune system reside not in the eye but, rather, are systemic and, therefore, regulation of those components will require systemic therapy.

Ekong, A. S., C. S. Foster, and M. R. Roque. "Eye Involvement in Autoimmune Blistering Diseases." *Clinics in Dermatology* 19, no. 6 (November–December 2001): 742–749.

Q&A on Uveitis and Immunology. Boston, Mass.: The Massachusetts Eye and Ear Infirmary. Available online. URL: http://www.meei.harvard.adulshared/ophtho/uveit.html. Downloaded on 16 July 2002.

family, the impact of autoimmune diseases
Diagnosis of an autoimmune disease will have a profound impact on the entire family. The American Autoimmune Related Diseases Association (AARDA) cautions that initially one must "give yourself and your family time to adjust. Nobody adjusts overnight to something that may significantly impact on the rest of his or her life." In some cases, the patient must deal with the disintegration of a marriage or family support network due to the added stresses of a chronic illness. Within the family, changes in primary relationships usually occur as a result of the illness. Assistance may be necessary for everyday activities or to fulfill one's role as a spouse, parent, worker, and friend. Patterns of giving and taking may need to be adjusted.

The fact that a preponderance of autoimmune patients are young women exacerbates the impact of these diseases on family. When a wife and mother faces disability, the family structure can be threatened. When the husband has the autoimmune disease, his customary role and responsibility as primary financial provider and involved father may be disrupted. Conflict can arise when the chronically ill husband feels tension and frustration because he cannot function in every capacity that he once did. Children, in particular, may feel frightened or upset by a parent's illness.

In a 1993 study of the families of RHEUMATOID ARTHRITIS (RA) sufferers, for most children the effect of living with a parent suffering from a painful, chronic illness was not detrimental, but a minority suffered verbal and physical abuse. The disease had wide-ranging effects on sexual and working relationships. However, marriage to a partner with RA did not result in a threat to the relationship for the majority.

In a later study, researchers found that depression for both RA patients and their partners were slightly elevated and that 35.7 percent of patients and 23.3 percent of well partners had scores high enough for possible clinical depression. Interestingly, there was no significant difference between the patients' level of distress and that of the partners.

Another autoimmune disease with great impact on the family is MULTIPLE SCLEROSIS (MS). In a Danish study, more than half of the patients (56.4 percent) were dependent on help from close relatives, most frequently spouses. The need for help, the risk of divorce, loss of contact with relatives, difficulty in going out, the need for structural changes in the home, and the need for a pension became greater with increasing physical handicap.

A British study in 2000 assessed the effects of MS on the patients' ability to fulfill their chosen family and social roles and examined the impact of the disease on their relatives. The standards of living of 37 percent of patients and their families had declined as a direct result of the disease. Most family caregivers reported symptoms that clearly related to anxiety and symptoms of depression. The occurrence of these symptoms was associated with disease severity. The professional career of 57 percent of relatives was also adversely affected by the patient's illness.

However, the family is affected not only when a parent has a chronic illness. Autoimmune diseases in children impact the family as well. As May wrote, "In families the whole is greater than the sum of the parts. All family members are interconnected, interdependent and exist in a fragile balance. What happens to one affects all the others. Having a child with a chronic illness or disability creates permanent change in family dynamics.

Often roles become stratified, communication may break down and personal needs can go unmet."

In a study of the impact of childhood chronic illness within a family context, the mothers of asthmatic children reported a greater number of internalizing behavior problems in their children, perceived their own social support as less adequate, and reported a greater number of stressful events than mothers of healthy children of the same age and sex. Regression analyses demonstrated that family functioning, maternal social support, and chronic illness were significantly related to the psychological adjustment of the child.

Several studies have examined family functioning where a child has Type 1 or INSULIN-DEPENDENT DIABETES mellitus (IDDM). Faulkner and Clark found that parental life satisfaction was most affected by the burden the child's diabetes placed on the family. The event having the most impact on parental quality of life was the frequency of telling others about the child's diabetes. The greatest worry was that the child would develop complications from diabetes. Parents of elementary school-age children experienced significantly greater life satisfaction than parents of adolescents. Married parents had higher life satisfaction than those who were divorced. Metabolic control was associated with the life satisfaction of parents.

An Australian study examined the initial impact and subsequent adjustment to the diagnosis of IDDM. Children between one and 14 years of age and their families were assessed several weeks after diagnosis and again a year later using standardized measures of child behavior, parental mental health, and family functioning. Their findings suggest that most children and their parents exhibit satisfactory individual adjustment after a period of initial stress but family functioning is affected in complex ways.

Beneton, C., and L. Rumbach. "Social and Economic Impact of Multiple Sclerosis." *La Revue du Practicien* 49, no. 17 (November 1999): 1,890–1,893.

"Dealing with Chronic Illness—A Family Concern." *The Menninger Letter,* 3, no. 6 (June 1995): 4.

Faulkner, M. S., and F. S. Clark. "Quality of Life for Parents of Children and Adolescents with Type 1 Diabetes." *The Diabetes Educator* 24, no. 6 (November–December 1998): 721–727.

Hakim, E. A., A. M. Bakheit, T. N. Bryant, M. W. Roberts, S. A. McIntosh-Michaelis, A. J. Spackman, J. P. Martin, and D. L. McLellan. "The Social Impact of Multiple Sclerosis—A Study of 305 Patients and Their Relatives." *Disability and Rehabilitation* 22, no. 6 (April 2000): 288–293.

Hamlett, K. W., D. S. Pellegrini, and K. S. Katz. "Childhood Chronic Illness as a Family Stressor." *Journal of Pediatric Psychology* 1 (February 1992): 33–47.

le Gallez, P. "Rheumatoid Arthritis: Effects on the Family." *Nursing Standard* 7, no. 39 (June 1993): 30–34.

May, J. "Rebalancing and Mobile: The Impact of Chronic Illness/Disability on the Family." *The Journal of Rheumatology Supplement* 33 (April 1992): 2–5.

Northam, E., P. Anderson, R. Adler, G. Werther, and G. Warne. "Psychosocial and Family Functioning in Children with Insulin-Dependent Diabetes at Diagnosis and One Year Later." *Journal of Pediatric Psychology* 21, no. 5 (October 1996): 699–717.

Schwartz, L., and G. H. Kraft. "The Role of Spouse Responses to Disability and Family Environment in Multiple Sclerosis." *American Journal of Physical Medicine & Rehabilitation* 78, no. 6 (November–December 1999): 525–532.

Stenager, E., E. N. Stenager, L. Knudsen, and K. Jensen. "Multiple Sclerosis: The Impact on Family and Social Life." *Acta Psychiatrica Belgica* 94, no. 3 (May–June 1994): 165–174.

Walsh, J. D., E. B. Blanchard, J. M. Kremer, and C. G. Blanchard. "The Psychosocial Effects of Rheumatoid Arthritis on the Patient and the Well Partner." *Behaviour Research and Therapy* 37, no. 3 (March 1999): 259–271.

fatigue Fatigue is an overwhelming continual sense of exhaustion and the inability to perform mental and physical activities at normal levels. Complaints of being fatigued are common in today's time-pressured culture. Reports have stated that as many as 20 percent of adults claim to be fatigued most of the time and that 15 million doctor visits per year in the United States are motivated by the feeling of fatigue. For some people, fatigue is equated to being sleepy during nonsleep hours, general malaise, or physical weakness—most often from lifestyle factors such as lack of sleep, excessive activity, or overwork. For others, fatigue is more debilitating and more chronic—likely to stem from a disease or other serious medical condition.

Fatigue accompanies many of the autoimmune diseases. Learning how to pace their activity levels can help patients maintain control of their illnesses. This means listening to their bodies and stopping before feeling tired in order to sustain relatively normal and consistent energy levels. According to the American Autoimmune Related Diseases Association, patients often feel guilty if they slow their pace and therefore rest only when they are not feeling well or are very tired. This forced rest period can last a few days and patients then try to "catch up" and accomplish all they were unable to do during the time they were resting.

Among the autoimmune diseases where fatigue is a prominent symptom are Addison's disease, celiac disease, chronic fatigue syndrome, fibromyalgia, Graves' disease, Hashimoto's thyroiditis, inflammatory bowel disease, insulin-dependent (Type 1) diabetes, Sjögren's syndrome, and systemic lupus erythematosus (SLE).

Ladd, Virginia. "Coping With Autoimmunity." *In Focus.* American Autoimmune Related Diseases Association, Inc. Available online. URL: http://aarda.org/coping _art.html. Posted 2001.

fertility   The condition, quality, or degree of being capable of contributing to reproduction; in women, the ability to conceive. Although autoimmune diseases generally do not impair fertility of patients, important exceptions exist. The role antibodies play in infertility is unclear, and studies often contradict each other. Still, many physicians will check the immune system for antiphospholipid antibodies (APA).

Individuals with a history of repeated pregnancy loss are among those at high risk for developing antiphospholipid antibodies. Detection of APA is helpful in identifying individuals at risk for recurrent pregnancy loss and thrombosis as well as in selecting appropriate treatment. APA have been reported to identify women experiencing infertility associated with endometriosis, premature ovarian failure, failure to conceive after in vitro fertilization or embryo transfer procedures, and unexplained fertility.

The presence of thyroid antibodies may directly result in infertility or pregnancy loss. Moreover, if these antibodies have damaged the thyroid and a low thyroid hormone level is present, fertility may be hampered. Some women who have fertility problems actually have undiagnosed underlying autoimmune thyroid problems.

Researchers have also determined that women destined to develop RHEUMATOID ARTHRITIS may have reduced fertility that would have occurred prior to the onset of arthritis.

Sterility and fertility rates for women with SYSTEMIC LUPUS ERYTHEMATOSUS are comparable to control groups without disease, but fertility may be decreased during FLAREs. This may be the result of hormonal changes caused by lupus or from side effects of medications used to treat lupus.

Because of the high incidence of autoantibodies they found in patients with primary infertility, Cubillos et al. suggest the possibility of a direct involvement of these antibodies in reproductive failure. They conclude, therefore, that patients with a history of reproductive failure should be immunologically evaluated and treated before undergoing assisted fertilization techniques.

Antispermatozoal antibodies in semen affect male fertility by reducing the capacity of the spermatozoa to penetrate cervical mucus. Several ANTIGENs of the human sperm cell can stimulate production of autoantibodies in certain individuals. This occurs in a number of spontaneous cases and leads to a condition of immunological infertility. It also occurs in a majority of men who have had a vasectomy. Many recent developments allow for the detection of the antibody, the study of its significance, and the treatment of this autoimmune disease.

(See also ANTIPHOSPHOLIPID SYNDROME, SPERM [TESTICULAR] AUTOIMMUNITY.)

Cubillos, J., A. Lucena, C. Lucena, J. C. Mendoza, H. Ruiz, A. Arango, G. Quiroga, J. Ferro, and E. Lucena. "Incidence of Autoantibodies in the Infertile Population." *Early Pregnancy.* 3, no. 2 (June 1997): 119–124.

Jager, S., and J. Kremer. "Immunological Aspects of Male Infertility." *Annales de Biologie Clinique* 45, no. 3 (1987): 340–345.

Shomon, Mary J. "Fertility and Thyroid Disease: Frequently Asked Questions About How to Overcome Thyroid-Related Infertility and Get Pregnant When You Have Thyroid Disease." Available online. URL: http://www.Thyroid-Info.com. Downloaded 16 July 2002.

Shulman, S. "Sperm Antigens and Autoantibodies: Effects on Fertility." *American Journal of Reproductive*

Immunology and Microbiology: AJRIM 10, no. 3 (March 1986): 82–89.

fibromyalgia Fibromyalgia is a chronic disorder characterized by widespread pain in the muscles and tissues surrounding the joints, fatigue, and multiple tender points (tenderness that occurs in precise, localized areas, particularly in the neck, spine, shoulders, and hips). People with this syndrome may also experience sleep disturbances, morning stiffness, irritable bowel syndrome, anxiety, and other symptoms. Fibromyalgia is also often accompanied by depression. Other names for this disorder have been fibromyitis, fibromyositis, fibrositis, and tension myalgia.

According to the American College of Rheumatology, fibromyalgia affects 3 to 6 million Americans. It primarily occurs in women of childbearing age, but children, the elderly, and men can also be affected. Nine in 10 fibromyalgia patients are female. In the United States, 3 to 6 million people may be afflicted with its symptoms, and an estimated 15 percent to 20 percent of patients (90 percent of them women) seen in rheumatology practice have fibromyalgia.

Fibromyalgia has only recently gained recognition as a distinct clinical entity with the establishment of diagnostic criteria in 1990. This common and perplexing disorder, which superficially resembles other disorders such as rheumatoid arthritis, has often been dismissed as an imaginary or psychiatric problem or a form of malingering. Patients commonly complain of widespread pain and tenderness, fatigue, and exhaustion after minimal effort. Often they feel unrested after sleep, and sleep laboratory tests are usually normal. A diagnosis can be confirmed by a characteristic pattern of specific points on the body that are exquisitely tender to palpitation. Fibromyalgia has not been identified as an autoimmune disorder itself. However, it is well known that fibromyalgia often accompanies other endocrine and rheumatic autoimmune disorders.

Causes
Although the cause of fibromyalgia is unknown, researchers have several theories about causes or triggers of the disorder. Some scientists believe that the syndrome may be caused by an injury or trauma. This injury may affect the central nervous system. Fibromyalgia may be associated with changes in muscle metabolism, such as decreased blood flow, causing fatigue and decreased strength. Others believe the syndrome may be triggered by an infectious agent such as a virus in susceptible people, but no such agent has been identified. Researchers have found pain-processing abnormalities in the spines and brain stems of those with fibromyalgia.

In 1999, researchers found antipolymer antibodies in approximately one-half of all patients who were diagnosed with fibromyalgia and in more than 60 percent of the fibromyalgia patients with severe fibromyalgia symptoms. Patients with diseases frequently confused with fibromyalgia, including rheumatoid arthritis, systemic lupus erythematosus, and systemic sclerosis/scleroderma, had a much lower incidence of these antibodies than did the fibromyalgia patients. It is possible, the researchers pointed out, that antipolymer antibodies are associated with one of the several different causes of fibromyalgia, perhaps the cause that tends to produce the most severe symptoms. The published data indicate that this may be the case, although more research is needed. In addition to serving as a marker for fibromyalgia, these antibodies may also be directly involved in initiating or promoting fibromyalgia.

Clinical Features
Fibromyalgia is difficult to diagnose because many of the symptoms mimic those of other disorders. The physician reviews the patient's medical history and makes a diagnosis of fibromyalgia based on a history of chronic widespread pain that persists for more than three months. The American College of Rheumatology (ACR) has developed criteria for fibromyalgia that physicians can use in diagnosing the disorder. According to ACR criteria, a person is considered to have fibromyalgia if he or she has widespread pain in combination with tenderness in at least 11 of 18 specific tender point sites. Fibromyalgia is characterized by the constant presence of widespread pain so severe that it is often incapacitating. It is also characterized by the total absence of any definable pathophysiological or

laboratory abnormality, even under that most intense scrutiny.

Treatment

Treatment of fibromyalgia requires a comprehensive approach, with the physician, physical therapist, and patient all playing active roles in its management. Studies have shown that aerobic exercise, such as swimming and walking, improves muscle fitness and reduces muscle pain and tenderness. In a 2001 study, fibromyalgia patients found exercise to be more effective in easing their symptoms than medication or alternative treatments. The researchers, led by Dr. Reino Poyhia of Helsinki University Central Hospital in Finland, also discovered that fibromyalgia patients' symptoms tended to get better with time.

In a recent study, fibromyalgia patients who meditated for up to 45 minutes six days a week felt less depressed, slept better, and were less likely than nonmeditators to report that their condition was adversely affecting their lives. The theory for this result is that meditation may help reduce pain by lowering levels of the stress hormone cortisol. In some cases, meditation can increase tolerance without changing pain intensity. The benefits of meditation lasted all day.

Heat and massage may also give short-term relief. Antidepressant medications may help elevate mood, improve quality of sleep, and relax muscles. Patients with fibromyalgia may benefit from a combination of exercise, medication, physical therapy, and relaxation.

Poyhia, R., D. Da Costa, and M. A. Fitzcharles. "Pain and Pain Relief in Fibromyalgia Patients Followed for Three Years." *Arthritis and Rheumatism* 45, no. 4 (August 2001): 355–361.

Sephton, Sandra E. "Effects of a Meditation Program on Disease Symptoms in Women with Fibromyalgia." Presented at American Psychosomatic Society Annual Meeting, held March 7–10, 2001 in Monterey, Calif.

Wilson, Russell B. et al. "Anti-Polymer Antibody Reactivity in a Subset of Patients with Fibromyalgia Correlates with Severity." *Journal of Rheumatology* 26, no. 2 (February 1999): 402–407.

fibromyalgia research The National Institute of Arthritis and Musculoskeletal and Skin Diseases (NIAMS) is sponsoring research that will increase understanding of the specific abnormalities that cause and accompany fibromyalgia with the hope of developing better ways to diagnose, treat, and prevent this disorder.

Recent NIAMS studies show that abnormally low levels of the hormone cortisol may be associated with fibromyalgia. At Brigham and Women's Hospital in Boston, Massachusetts, and at the University of Michigan Medical Center in Ann Arbor, researchers are studying regulation of the function of the adrenal gland (which makes cortisol) in fibromyalgia. People whose bodies make inadequate amounts of cortisol experience many of the same symptoms as people with fibromyalgia. It is hoped that these studies will increase understanding about fibromyalgia and may suggest new ways to treat the disorder.

NIAMS research studies are looking at different aspects of the disorder. At the University of Alabama in Birmingham, researchers are concentrating on how specific brain structures are involved in the painful symptoms of fibromyalgia. At George Washington University in Washington, D.C., scientists are investigating the causes of a post–Lyme disease syndrome as a model for fibromyalgia. Some patients develop a fibromyalgia-like condition following Lyme disease, an infectious disorder associated with arthritis and other symptoms.

NIAMS-supported research on fibromyalgia also includes several projects at the Institute's Multipurpose Arthritis and Musculoskeletal Diseases Centers. Researchers at these centers are studying individuals who do not seek medical care but who meet the criteria for fibromyalgia. (Potential subjects are located through advertisements in local newspapers asking for volunteers with widespread pain or aching.) Other studies at the centers are attempting to uncover better ways to manage the pain associated with the disorder through behavioral interventions such as relaxation training.

In March 1998, NIAMS and several other NIH institutes and offices issued a Request for Proposals to promote research studies of fibromyalgia. As a result of this request, NIAMS and its partners recently funded 15 new fibromyalgia projects totaling more than $3.6 million.

flare In autoimmune diseases, a period of active immune reaction initiated by some trigger, such as stress, surgery, drugs, or even exposure to sunlight.

fungi Members of a class of relatively primitive vegetable organisms. Fungi include mushrooms, yeasts, rusts, molds, and smuts.

gamma globulin A group of proteins found in blood plasma that contains immunoglobulins or antibodies produced by that individual. These antibodies are produced as a protective reaction of the body's immune system to the invasion of disease-producing organisms. It can be extracted from the blood of a person who is immune to a certain infection and injected into another person who has been exposed to the disease. These extracts can provide quick but temporary immunity to infectious diseases such as hepatitis, rubeola (measles), poliomyelitis, tetanus, or yellow fever. The gamma globulin used for such purposes is extracted from blood plasma from a large, diverse adult population. The resulting mixture is thus likely to contain a wide variety of antibodies, because it includes the combined gamma globulin of all the donors. Gamma globulin is also administered to people who cannot produce enough antibodies and to some patients who have low blood platelet counts because of autoimmune diseases. Also known as immune serum globulin and immune globulin.

gene The functional and physical unit of heredity passed from parent to offspring. A gene is part of a deoxyribonucleic acid (DNA) molecule. Humans have between 50,000 and 100,000 genes. Genes carry instructions that allow the cells to produce specific proteins (the building blocks of bodies) such as enzymes. The body buries genes deep in the heart of every cell, the nucleus, and organizes them in the chromosomes that hold the DNA. Only certain genes in a cell are active at any given moment. As cells mature, many genes become permanently inactive. The pattern of active and inactive genes in a cell and the resulting protein composition determine what kind of cell it is and what it can and cannot do. Genes determine obvious traits, such as hair and eye color, as well as more subtle characteristics, such as the ability of the blood to carry oxygen. Complex traits, such as physical strength, may be shaped by the interaction of a number of different genes along with environmental influences. When the DNA is damaged, it no longer makes all the needed proteins and disease results. The word *gene* was derived from De Vries' term *pangen*, itself a derivative of the word *pangenesis*, which Darwin (1868) had coined.

gene therapy An evolving technique used to treat, cure, or ultimately prevent disease by changing the expression of a person's genes. Gene therapy is in its infancy. Current gene therapy is primarily experimental, with most human clinical trials in only the research stages. The medical procedure involves either replacing, manipulating, or supplementing nonfunctional genes with healthy genes.

To reverse disease caused by genetic damage, researchers isolate normal DNA and package it into a vector, a molecular delivery truck usually made from a disabled virus. Doctors then infect a target cell—usually from a tissue affected by the illness, such as liver or lung cells—with the vector. The vector unloads its DNA cargo, which then begins producing the missing protein and restores the cell to normal.

French researchers reported dramatic results in treating a disease called severe combined immune deficiency (SCID), the disorder suffered by David Vetter, a boy who lived all 12 years of his life inside a sealed plastic bubble, which protected him from infections. In SCID, a broken gene eliminates the production of an enzyme essential for the development of a normal immune system. Scientists isolated the normal copy of the gene and packaged it into a vector. In the laboratory, they then used the vector to transport the gene into the patient's own bone marrow cells. Bone marrow cells create the immune system. The treated bone marrow cells are then given back to the patient in a germ-free isolation room, where they reconstitute a normal, functioning immune system, freeing the patient from the need to remain in isolation. Researchers are also investigating the use of gene therapy for such diverse conditions as hemophilia, Parkinson's disease, diabetes, a hereditary form of dangerously high cholesterol, and AIDS.

One of the goals of gene therapy is to supply cells with healthy copies of missing or altered genes. Instead of giving a patient a drug, doctors attempt to correct the problem by altering the genetic makeup of some of the patient's cells. Examples of diseases that could be treated this way include cystic fibrosis and hemophilia.

Gene therapy is also being studied as a way to change how a cell functions. Examples include stimulating immune system cells to attack cancer cells and introducing resistance to human immunodeficiency virus (HIV), the virus that causes acquired immunodeficiency syndrome (AIDS).

In general, a gene cannot be directly inserted into a person's cell. It must be delivered to the cell using a carrier known as a vector. The most common types of vectors used in gene therapy are viruses. Scientists use viruses because they have a unique ability to enter a cell's DNA. Viruses used as vectors in gene therapy are genetically disabled; they are unable to reproduce themselves.

Most gene therapy clinical trials rely on mouse retroviruses to deliver the desired gene. Other viruses used as vectors include adenoviruses, adeno-associated viruses, poxviruses, and the herpes virus.

In most gene therapy clinical trials, cells from the patient's blood or bone marrow are removed and grown in the laboratory. The cells are exposed to the virus that is carrying the desired gene. The virus enters the cells, and the desired gene becomes part of the cells' DNA. The cells grow in the laboratory and are then returned to the patient by injection into a vein. This type of gene therapy is called

ex vivo, which means "outside the body." The gene is transferred into the patient's cells while the cells are outside the patient's body.

In other studies, vectors or liposomes (fatty particles) are used to deliver the desired gene to cells in the patient's body. This form of gene therapy is called in vivo, because the gene is transferred to cells inside the patient's body.

Gene therapy can be targeted to somatic (body) or germ (egg and sperm) cells. In somatic gene therapy, the recipient's genome is changed, but the change is not passed along to the next generation. In germline gene therapy, the parents' egg and sperm cells are changed with the goal of passing on the changes to their offspring. Germline gene therapy is not being actively investigated, at least in larger animals and humans, although a lot of discussion is being conducted about its value and desirability.

Many people falsely assume that germline gene therapy is already being done with regularity. News reports of parents selecting a genetically tested egg for implantation or choosing the sex of their unborn child may lead the public to think that gene therapy is occurring. Actually, in these cases, genetic information is being used for selection. No cells are altered or changed.

Many factors have prevented researchers from developing successful gene therapy techniques. The first hurdle is the gene delivery tool or vectors (gene carriers), which deliver therapeutic genes to the patients' cells. Currently, the most common vectors are viruses. Viruses have evolved a way of delivering their genes to human cells in a pathogenic manner. Scientists have tried to take advantage of the virus's biology and manipulate its genome to remove the disease-causing genes and insert therapeutic genes. Viruses, while effective, introduce other problems to the body—toxicity, immune and inflammatory responses, and gene control and targeting issues. Some alternatives to viruses that have been considered are complexes of DNA with lipids and proteins.

Researchers are also experimenting with introducing a 47th (artificial human) chromosome to the body. It would exist autonomously alongside the standard 46 chromosomes—not affecting their workings or causing any mutations. It would be a large vector capable of carrying substantial amounts of genetic code. Scientists anticipate that because of its construction and autonomy, the body's immune systems would not attack it.

Another hurdle is understanding gene function. Of the estimated 100,000 genes, scientists know the function of only a very few. Attempting gene therapy without knowing how everything works could address only some of the genes implicated in particular diseases. Likewise, genes may have more than one function.

For example, consider that sickle cell anemia is caused by an error in the gene that tells the body how to make hemoglobin. Sickle cell anemia is prevalent among African Americans. Children who inherit two copies (one from each of their parents) of the gene for sickle-cell anemia will have the disease. Children who inherit only one copy will not. The error in the hemoglobin gene results from a genetic mutation that occurred many thousands of years ago in people in parts of Africa, the Mediterranean basin, the Middle East, and India. A deadly form of malaria was very common at that time, and malaria epidemics caused the death of great numbers of people. Studies show that in areas where malaria was a problem, children who inherited one sickle hemoglobin gene—and who, therefore, carried the sickle cell trait—had a survival advantage. Unlike the children who had normal hemoglobin genes, they survived the malaria epidemics; they grew up, had their own children, and passed on the gene for sickle hemoglobin.

Once the human genome sequence is complete, the next step in genome research will be functional genomics—understanding what the function of each gene is.

A third hurdle is multigene disorders. Most genetic disorders involve more than one gene. In only a handful of genetic diseases, like Huntington's disease, inheriting one particular gene means that the individual has a 100 percent chance of developing the disorder.

Most diseases involve the interaction of several genes and the environment. Many people who develop cancer not only inherit the disease gene for their disorder, they may also have not inherited particular tumor-suppressor genes. Diet, exercise,

smoking, and other environmental factors may have also contributed to their disease.

Studies of identical twins show that individuals with the same genetic makeup do not develop the same diseases and disorders. This is irrefutable evidence of the role environment plays in gene expression.

The high costs associated with developing gene therapy technology and regulations associated with human experimentation are also hurdles for researchers in this field.

Gene Therapy, Germantown, Md.: U.S. Department of Energy Office of Science, Office of Biological and Environmental Research, Human Genome Program. Last modified June 2002.

National Cancer Institute. *Questions and Answers About Gene Therapy,* Fact Sheet 7.18, June 2000.

Thompson, Larry. *Fundamentals of Gene Therapy,* Rockville, Md.: FDA/Office of Public Affairs, August 2000.

genetic   Having to do with reproduction; determined by genes. Inherited; having to do with information that is passed from parents to offspring through genes in sperm and egg cells.

genetic engineering   More formally known as recombinant DNA technology, genetic engineering allows scientists to pluck genes (segments of DNA) from one type of organism and combine them with genes of a second organism. In this way, relatively simple organisms such as bacteria or yeast, or even mammalian cells in culture and mammals such as goats and sheep, can be induced to make quantities of human proteins, including hormones such as insulin as well as lymphokines and monokines. Microorganisms can also be made to manufacture proteins from infectious agents such as the hepatitis virus or the AIDS virus for use in vaccines.

Genes can be packaged for delivery in a variety of ways: inserted into the genetic material of such carriers as the familiar vaccinia virus or inactivated retroviruses, grafted onto a protein carrier that magnifies the immune response (an adjuvant), or tucked into fat globules known as liposomes.

Schindler, Lydia, Donna Kerrigan, and Jeanne Kelly. *Understanding Gene Testing,* Bethesda, Md.: National Cancer Institute, National Institutes of Health, 1997.

genetic marker A segment of DNA with an identifiable physical location on a chromosome and whose inheritance can be followed. A marker can be a gene, or it can be some section of DNA with no known function. Because DNA segments that lie near each other on a chromosome tend to be inherited together, markers are often used as indirect ways of tracking the inheritance pattern of a gene that has not yet been identified, but whose approximate location is known.

genetics The branch of biology that deals with heredity and the transmission of inherited characteristics.

genotype The genetic identity of an individual that does not show as outward characteristics.

globulin Any of the group of plasma proteins that are widely distributed throughout the plant and animal kingdoms. Globulins make up 38 percent of all plasma proteins. The term globulin is used in classifying an otherwise diverse group of proteins that are soluble in water or dilute salt solutions. Among the most important are the immunoglobulins (Ig), the antibodies of the immune system. They are classified into five types based upon structure: IgA, IgD, IgE, IgG, and IgM. IgG is the most common and forms about 70 percent of the immunoglobins in the blood. Other globulins are involved in the transport of a variety of substances, including lipids, hormones, and inorganic ions.

glucocorticoid A compound that belongs to the family of compounds called corticosteroids (steroids). Glucocorticoids affect metabolism and have anti-inflammatory and immunosuppressive effects. They may be naturally produced (hormones) or synthetic (drugs).

Goodpasture's syndrome Goodpasture's syndrome is a rare autoimmune disease that can affect the lungs and kidneys. It can cause people to cough up blood or feel a burning sensation when urinating. However, the first signs of this disease may be vague, like fatigue, nausea, dyspnea (difficult breathing), or pallor. These signs are followed by kidney involvement, represented first with small amounts of blood in the urine, protein excretion in the urine, and other clinical and laboratory findings. In 1918, U.S. pathologist Ernest William Goodpasture (1886–1960) reported the association of pulmonary hemorrhage and glomerulonephritis, which has subsequently been termed Goodpasture's syndrome.

Causes

No one knows why in Goodpasture's syndrome the immune system makes antibodies that end up attacking the lungs and kidneys. A combination of factors has been implicated, and among these is the presence of an inherited component.

Clinical Features

To diagnose Goodpasture's syndrome, doctors can now use a blood test. However, a kidney biopsy may be necessary to check for the presence of the harmful antibody.

Complications

Goodpasture's syndrome may last only a few weeks or as long as two years. Bleeding in the lungs can be very serious in some cases. However, Goodpasture's syndrome does not usually lead to permanent lung damage. Damage to the kidneys, however, may be long lasting. If the kidneys fail, kidney transplantation or dialysis therapy to remove waste products and extra fluid from the blood may become necessary.

Treatment

Goodpasture's syndrome is treated with immunosuppressive drugs given by mouth to keep the immune system from making antibodies. Corticosteroids may be given intravenously to control bleeding in the lungs. A process called plasmapheresis may be helpful and necessary to filter the harmful antibodies from the blood; this is usually done in combination with the steroid treatment. (See also ANTIGLOMERULAR BASEMENT MEMBRANE [ANTI-GBM] DISEASE.)

National Institutes of Health. *Goodpasture Syndrome,* NIH Publication No. 01-4558, 1998.

graft   Material, especially living tissue or an organ, surgically attached to or implanted in a part of the body to repair a defect or replace a damaged part. An allograft is a graft of material from another individual of the same species. A xenograft is a graft of material from another individual of another species.

graft rejection   A consequence of organ or tissue transplantation caused by an immune response that damages or destroys the transplanted organ/tissue. The immune response protects the body from potentially harmful substances (antigens) such as microorganisms, toxins, and cancer cells. The immune system distinguishes self from foreign and reacts against substances it recognizes as foreign. The presence of foreign blood or tissue in the body triggers an immune response that results in blood transfusion reactions and transplant rejection.

Blood and tissue contain identifying proteins on the surface that aid in distinguishing self from foreign tissues. These proteins can act as antigens that trigger the immune response, and antibodies are formed against foreign antigens. Tissue is typed according to the antigens it contains.

No two people (except identical twins) have identical tissue antigens. Therefore, organ and tissue transplantation almost always causes an immune response against the foreign tissue (rejection), which results in destruction of the transplant. Tissue typing ensures that the organ or tissue is as similar as possible to the tissues of the receiving person. This is performed because greater antigen difference causes more rapid and severe rejection.

A few exceptions occur. Corneal transplants are rarely rejected because they have no blood supply, so lymphocytes and antibodies do not reach the cornea to cause rejection. Identical twins have identical tissue antigens, so transplantation between identical twins almost never causes rejection. (See also GRAFT-VERSUS-HOST DISEASE [GHVD].)

graft-versus-host disease (GVHD)   A life-threatening condition that occurs following bone marrow transplants in which the donor's immune cells, in the transplanted marrow, make antibodies against the host's tissues.

Bone marrow transplants are done when a person has certain types of leukemia or the bone marrow has been invaded by other types of malignancy. In the transplant, bone marrow is destroyed by drugs, radiation, or both and is replaced with compatible marrow from a donor. While marrow destruction kills the cancer, it also suppresses the person's immune system, thus allowing the new donor marrow to implant without being destroyed by the recipient's immune system.

Graft-versus-host disease occurs when the new donor marrow makes antibodies against the host (person who received the marrow) and tries to destroy the host as if it were a disease or foreign material.

Varying degrees of graft-versus-host disease are viewed as an expected complication of bone marrow transplantation since tissue typing can find close but not perfect tissue matches between donor and recipient. Only identical twins have identical tissue types.

granulocytes   White blood cells filled with granules containing potent chemicals that allow the cells to digest microorganisms or to produce inflammatory reactions. The granulocytes form in the bone marrow and account for about 70 percent of all white blood cells. Neutrophils, eosinophils, and basophils are examples of granulocytes. Neutrophils constitute the vast majority of granulocytes. They travel about by amoeboid movement. They can surround and destroy bacteria and other foreign particles. The eosinophils, ordinarily about 2 percent of the granulocyte count, increase in number in the presence of allergic disorders and parasitic infestations. The basophils account for about 1 percent of the granulocytes. They release chemicals such as histamine and play a role in the inflammatory response to infection.

Graves' disease   A glandular autoimmune disease affecting the thyroid gland; Graves' disease is the most common cause of hyperthyroidism in the United States. In Graves' disease, the autoantibodies (immunoglobulins) bind to the thyroid gland to induce an increase in the production of thyroid hormone. Thyroid hormone plays a major role in metabolism (the regulation of the body's ability to utilize fuel). Similar antibodies may also attack the tissues in the eye muscles and in the skin on the front of the lower leg. Graves' disease is not curable, but it is a completely treatable disease. A good example is Olympic track and field gold medalist Gail Devers, who struggled with the symptoms of Graves' disease for two years before discovering what was wrong with her. After treatment, she went on to win her gold medal.

Although both men and women can have Graves' disease, it is much more prevalent in women between the ages of 20 and 30. However, it also occurs in children, adolescents, and the elderly. The prevalence of total patients in the United States and Europe approaches 3,000,000, with 37,000 new patients per year in the United States.

Causes

Any of several factors may contribute to the development of Graves' disease. There is a genetic predisposition to autoimmune disorders. Infections and stress play a part. Graves' disease may have its onset after an external stressor. In other instances, it may follow a viral infection or pregnancy. Many times, the exact cause of Graves' disease is simply not known. It is not contagious, although it has been known to occur coincidentally between husbands and wives. One example occurred when First Lady Barbara Bush developed Graves' disease with exophthalmos (eye protrusion). Her husband, President George Bush, also has Graves' disease. The Graves' gene in DNA has not yet been identified.

Clinical Features

Mild forms of the disease can include symptoms such as nervousness, heat intolerance, diarrhea, sweating, insomnia, and weight loss with increased appetite. More serious complications may include irregular heartbeat, tachycardia (increased heartbeat), tremor and atrial fibrillation, extreme sensitivity to light, swelling in the legs and eyes, and clubbing of the fingers. The eyes may have a bulging appearance or a surprised expression. In rare extreme situations, there may be cardiovascular collapse and shock or coma.

Complications

In most instances, Graves' disease responds well to treatment and, after the initial period of hyperthyroidism, is relatively easy to manage. In a very few cases, patients do not respond well to treatment. However, the occurrence of complications is most often due to improper or no treatment. The more serious complications of Graves' disease include weakened heart muscle leading to heart failure, osteoporosis, or possible severe emotional disorders.

Treatment

Treatment selection depends on age, degree of illness, and personal preferences of physicians and patients.

Drugs Thionamides (methimazole or PTU), antithyroid drugs that inhibit production or conversion of the active thyroid hormone.

Radioactive iodine Destroys part or all of the thyroid gland and renders it incapable of overproducing thyroid hormone.

Surgery Subtotal thyroidectomy, in which a surgeon removes most of the thyroid gland and renders it incapable of overproducing thyroid hormone.

In a few cases, the treatments must be repeated. In all cases, lifetime follow-up laboratory studies must be done, and in almost all cases, lifetime replacement thyroid hormone must be taken.

Moore, Elaine A., Lisa Moore, and Kelly R. Hale. *Graves' Disease: A Practical Guide.* Jefferson, N.C.: McFarland & Company, Inc., Publishers, 2001.

Rapoport, Basil, and Sandra M. McLachlan, eds. *Graves' Disease: Pathogenesis and Treatment.* Dordrecht, The Netherlands: Kluwer Academic Publishers, 2000.

Guillain-Barré syndrome (GBS) A disorder in which the body's immune system attacks part of the peripheral nervous system—those nerves outside the brain and spinal cord. Also called acute inflammatory demyelinating polyneuropathy and Landry's ascending paralysis. The first symptoms of this disorder include varying degrees of weakness or tingling sensations in the legs. In many instances, the weakness and abnormal sensations spread to the arms and upper body. These symptoms can increase in intensity until certain muscles cannot be used at all, and when severe, the patient is almost totally paralyzed. In these cases, the disorder is life threatening—potentially interfering with breathing and, at times, with blood pressure or heart rate—and is considered a medical emergency. Such a patient is often put on a respirator to assist with breathing and is watched closely for problems such as an abnormal heartbeat, infections, blood clots, and high or low blood pressure. Most patients, however, recover from even the most severe cases of Guillain-Barré syndrome, although some continue to have a certain degree of weakness.

Guillain-Barré syndrome can affect anybody regardless of ethnic background. It can strike at any age, and both sexes are equally prone to the disorder. The syndrome is rare, however, afflicting only about one person in 100,000. Usually Guillain-Barré occurs a few days or weeks after the patient has had symptoms of a respiratory or gastrointestinal viral infection. Occasionally, surgery or vaccinations will trigger the syndrome. The disorder can develop over the course of hours or days, or it may take up to three to four weeks. Most people reach the stage of greatest weakness within the first two weeks after symptoms appear, and by the third week of the illness, 90 percent of all patients are at their weakest.

Causes

No one yet knows why Guillain-Barré strikes some people and not others. Nor does anyone know exactly what sets the disease in motion.

What scientists do know is that the body's immune system starts to destroy the myelin sheath that surrounds the axons of many peripheral nerves or even the axons themselves (axons are long, thin extensions of the nerve cells; they carry nerve signals). The myelin sheath surrounding the axon speeds up the transmission of nerve signals and allows the transmission of signals over long distances.

In diseases in which the peripheral nerves' myelin sheaths are injured or degraded, the nerves cannot transmit signals efficiently. That is why the muscles begin to lose their ability to respond to the brain's commands, commands that must be carried through the nerve network. The brain also receives fewer sensory signals from the rest of the body, resulting in an inability to feel textures, heat, pain, and other sensations. Alternately, the brain may receive inappropriate signals that result in tingling, "crawling skin," or painful sensations. Because the signals to and from the arms and legs must travel the longest distances, they are most vulnerable to interruption. Therefore, muscle weakness and tingling sensations usually first appear in the hands and feet and progress upward.

When Guillain-Barré is preceded by a viral or bacterial infection, it is possible that the virus has changed the nature of cells in the nervous system so that the immune system treats them as foreign cells. It is also possible that the virus makes the immune system itself less discriminating about what cells it recognizes as its own, allowing some of the immune cells, such as certain kinds of lymphocytes and macrophages, to attack the myelin. Sensitized T lymphocytes cooperate with B lymphocytes to produce antibodies against components of the myelin sheath and may contribute to destruction of the myelin. The cause and course of Guillain-Barré syndrome is an active area of neurological investigation, incorporating the cooperative efforts of neurological scientists, immunologists, and virologists.

Clinical Features

Guillain-Barré is called a syndrome rather than a disease because it is not clear that a specific disease-causing agent is involved. The signs and symptoms of the syndrome can be quite varied, so doctors may, on rare occasions, find it difficult to diagnose Guillain-Barré in its earliest stages.

Several disorders have symptoms similar to those found in Guillain-Barré, so doctors must examine and question patients carefully before making a diagnosis. Collectively, the signs and symptoms form a certain pattern that helps doctors differentiate Guillain-Barré from other disorders. For example, physicians will note whether the symptoms appear on both sides of the body (most common in Guillain-Barré) and the quickness with which the symptoms appear (in other disorders, muscle weakness may progress over months rather than days or weeks). In Guillain-Barré, reflexes such as knee jerks are usually lost. Because the signals traveling along the nerve are slower, a nerve conduction velocity (NCV) test can give a doctor clues to aid the diagnosis. In Guillain-Barré patients, the cerebrospinal fluid that bathes the spinal cord and brain contains more protein than usual. Therefore, a physician may decide to perform a spinal tap, a procedure in which the doctor inserts a needle into the patient's lower back to draw cerebrospinal fluid from the spinal column.

Complications

Guillain-Barré syndrome patients face not only physical difficulties but emotionally painful periods as well. It is often extremely difficult for patients to adjust to sudden paralysis and dependence on others for help with routine daily activities. Patients sometimes need psychological counseling to help them adapt.

Treatment

No cure is known for Guillain-Barré syndrome. However, some therapies lessen the severity of the illness and accelerate the recovery in most patients. There are also a number of ways to treat the complications of the disease.

Currently, plasmapheresis and high-dose immunoglobulin therapy are used. Both of them are equally effective, but immunoglobulin is easier to administer. Plasmapheresis is a method by which whole blood is removed from the body and processed so that the red and white blood cells are separated from the plasma, or liquid portion of the blood. The blood cells are then returned to the patient without the plasma, which the body quickly replaces. Scientists still do not know exactly why plasmapheresis works, but the technique seems to reduce the severity and duration of the Guillain-Barré episode. This may be because the plasma portion of the blood contains elements of the immune system that may be toxic to the myelin.

In high-dose immunoglobulin therapy, doctors give intravenous injections of the proteins that, in small quantities, the immune system naturally uses to attack invading organisms. Investigators have found that giving high doses of these immunoglobulins, derived from a pool of thousands of normal donors, to Guillain-Barré patients can lessen the immune attack on the nervous system. Investigators do not know why or how this works, although several hypotheses have been proposed.

The use of steroid hormones has also been tried as a way to reduce the severity of Guillain-Barré. However, controlled clinical trials have demonstrated that this treatment not only is not effective but may even have a deleterious effect on the patient.

The most critical part of the treatment for this syndrome consists of keeping the patient's body functioning during recovery of the nervous system. This can sometimes require placing the patient on a respirator, a heart monitor, or other machines that assist body function. The need for this sophisticated machinery is one reason why Guillain-Barré syndrome patients are usually treated in hospitals, often in an intensive care ward. In the hospital, doctors can also look for and treat the many problems that can afflict any paralyzed patient—complications such as pneumonia or bed sores. Often, even before recovery begins, caregivers may be instructed to move the patient's limbs manually to help keep the muscles flexible and strong. Later, as the patient begins to recover limb control, physical therapy begins.

Guillain-Barré syndrome can be a devastating disorder because of its sudden and unexpected onset. In addition, recovery is not necessarily quick. Patients usually reach the point of greatest weakness or paralysis days or weeks after the first symptoms occur. Symptoms then stabilize at this level for a period of days, weeks, or, sometimes, months. The recovery period may be as little as a few weeks or as long as a few years. About 30 percent of those with Guillain-Barré still have a residual weakness after three years. About 3 percent may suffer a relapse of muscle weakness and tingling sensations many years after the initial attack. Although most people recover, this can take months, and some may have long-term disabilities of varying degrees. Less than 5 percent die.

National Institute of Neurological Disorders and Stroke, National Institutes of Health. *Guillain-Barré Syndrome Fact Sheet,* July 2001.

Wilcox, Dorris R. *No Time for Tears: Transforming Tragedy into Triumph.* Mt. Pleasant, S.C.: Corinthian Books, 2000.

Hashimoto's thyroiditis Also referred to as autoimmune thyroiditis and chronic lymphocytic thyroiditis—a chronic inflammatory glandular autoimmune disease. It is named after the Japanese physician, Hakaru Hashimoto, who first described it in 1912. An autoimmune reaction to proteins in the thyroid is the underlying cause of Hashimoto's thyroiditis. The thyroid helps set the rate of metabolism—the rate at which the body uses energy. Hashimoto's prevents the gland from producing enough thyroid hormones for the body to work correctly. There is evidence of a genetic predisposition in the development of Hashimoto's thyroiditis. It is not uncommon for persons with autoimmune thyroid disease to have other coinciding autoimmune disorders.

The disease process can eventually destroy the thyroid, resulting in hypothyroidism. Usually, though, the person has an enlarged thyroid gland with normal or mildly abnormal thyroid function tests. Persons with Hashimoto's thyroiditis have autoantibodies against several different proteins in their thyroid gland. A family history of thyroid disease is not unusual. Hashimoto's thyroiditis is the most common cause of hypothyroidism (underactive thyroid); another thyroid-related autoimmune disease is GRAVES' DISEASE.

Men and women of any age can develop this disease. However, it is most common in women between the ages of 30 or 50, where the ratio of female to male is 50 to one.

Causes

Hashimoto's thyroiditis is caused by abnormal blood antibodies and white blood cells attacking and damaging thyroid cells. The end result of this autoimmune destruction is hypothyroidism caused by the complete absence of thyroid cells. However, in many patients, sufficient thyroid reserve remains to prevent hypothyroidism.

Clinical Features

Some patients with Hashimoto's thyroiditis may have no symptoms. However, the common symptoms are fatigue, depression, sensitivity to cold, weight gain, muscle weakness, coarsening of the skin, dry or brittle hair, constipation, muscle cramps, increased menstrual flow, and goiter (enlargement of the thyroid gland). Classically, Hashimoto's thyroiditis begins with a painless, gradual enlargement of the thyroid gland and is often discovered by the patient when she or he finds a fullness in the neck or a new lump while self-examining because of a vague discomfort in the neck. It is also frequently found by the physician during the course of an examination for some other complaint. In some instances, the thyroid gland may enlarge rapidly. Rarely, pain is persistent and unresponsive to medical treatment and requires medical therapy or surgery. The goiter of Hashimoto's thyroiditis may remain unchanged for decades, but usually it gradually increases in size.

The diagnosis of Hashimoto's thyroiditis is confirmed by finding high levels of antibodies in the blood. These work against the patient's own thyroid proteins. The diagnosis can be firmly established by doing a thyroid biopsy. A needle is inserted into the thyroid gland, and some cells are removed and smeared onto a glass slide. The pathologist will see many blood lymphocytes in the smear that indicate the nature of the inflammatory reaction in the thyroid gland.

Complications

Approximately 25 percent of patients with Hashimoto's thyroiditis may develop pernicious anemia, diabetes, adrenal insufficiency, or other autoimmune diseases. If left untreated, Hashimoto's thyroiditis can cause further complications, including changes in menstrual cycles, prevention of ovulation, and an increased risk of miscarriage. In addition, a British study reported in November 2000 that pregnant women with hypothyroidism have a 3.8 percent risk for second-trimester miscarriage as opposed to women with normal thyroid function who have a 0.9 percent rate. In an earlier study, the same researchers documented an association between undetected subclinical thyroidism during pregnancy and lower I.Q. in offspring. Women with untreated thyroid deficiency during pregnancy are four times more likely to have children with lower I.Q. scores.

Treatment

Treatment of Hashimoto's thyroiditis is to take thyroid hormone replacement (thyroxine) as soon as the diagnosis is made, even if thyroid function is, at that time, normal. Thyroid hormone is given for three reasons. First, it shrinks the goiter by suppressing production of thyroid-stimulating hormone (TSH) by the pituitary gland. It secondly anticipates the development of thyroid failure and the resulting low levels of thyroid hormone because the disease may progress with time. Finally, it seems to have an effect on blood lymphocytes that cause the damage and destruction in the thyroid gland. The goiter itself may remain for several years before disappearing, although it will shrink over a period of six to 18 months in most patients. When the gland has shrunk, it is not functioning and the patient would be hypothyroid if treatment were not given. Therefore, thyroxine treatment for Hashimoto's thyroiditis must be taken for life.

It is also important to know that too much thyroid replacement hormone can mimic the symptoms of hyperthyroidism. This is a condition where the thyroid gland produces more hormones than normal. These symptoms include insomnia, irritability, weight loss without dieting, heat sensitivity, increased perspiration, thinning of the skin, fine or brittle hair, muscular weakness, eye changes, lighter menstrual flow, rapid heartbeat, and hand tremors.

Generally, the progression to hypothyroidism has been considered an irreversible process due to thyroid cell damage and loss of thyroidal iodine stores. However, it is now clear that up to one-fourth of patients who are hypothyroid may spontaneously return to normal function over the course of several years. This sequence may reflect the initial effect of high titers of thyroid-stimulation-blocking antibodies that fall with time and allow thyroid function to return.

heat shock proteins A family of proteins that cells produce in response to stress from heat, injury, germs, or toxins. Also called stress proteins. They act as molecular chaperones, binding to other proteins and ferrying them to and from various compartments of the cell. A few years ago, immunologists noticed that heat shock proteins are particularly abundant in bacteria and are responsible for flagging the T cells and triggering cytotoxic T cells (CTLs) to attack infected or cancer cells and destroy them. Massachusetts Institute of Technology researchers found that heat shock proteins from the tuberculosis bacterium could elicit powerful immune responses and could be used as an immune system booster. Their continued research with mice showed that the heat shock proteins can function as vehicles to deliver viral proteins to a critical immune system and elicit a CTL response. When injected with a vaccine containing heat shock proteins, mice lacking healthy immune systems were able to mount cellular responses despite their compromised immune systems. If this vaccine behaves the same way in humans, the findings will have profound implications for developing safe vaccines to immunize similarly immunocompromised humans such as AIDS patients. Heat shock proteins have been related to a number of autoimmune diseases such as Type I diabetes and rheumatoid arthritis.

Kumar, Seema. "Protein May Play Key Role for Patients With Damaged Immune Systems." *MIT Tech Talk* 44, no. 18 (January 2000): 1, 12.
Qian, Huang, Joan F. L. Richmond, Kimiko Suzue, Herman N. Eisen, and Richard A. Young. "In Vivo Cytotoxic T Lymphocyte Elicitation by Mycobacterial Heat Shock Protein 70 Fusion Proteins Maps to a Discrete Domain and Is CD4+ T Cell Independent." *Journal of Experimental Medicine* 191 (2000): 403–408.

helper T cells   See T HELPER CELL.

hemoglobin   The predominant protein in the red blood cells (erythrocytes). It contains iron and carries oxygen from the lungs to the tissues.

hemolytic anemia   See AUTOIMMUNE HEMOLYTIC ANEMIA.

hepatitis (autoimmune)   A chronic inflammatory disease in which the body's immune system attacks liver cells. This causes the liver to become inflamed (hepatitis). About 70 percent of those with autoimmune hepatitis are women, most between the ages of 15 and 40. The disease is usually quite serious and, if not treated, gets worse over time. It can lead to cirrhosis (scarring and hardening) of the liver and eventually liver failure. It has been identified by a number of different names, including autoimmune chronic active hepatitis (CAH), idiopathic chronic active hepatitis, and lupoid hepatitis.

Autoimmune hepatitis is classified as either type I or II. Type I is the most common form in North America. It occurs at any age and is more common among women than men. About half of those with type I have other autoimmune disorders, such as thyroidosis, Graves' disease, Sjögren's syndrome, autoimmune anemia, and ulcerative colitis. Although the term *lupoid* hepatitis was originally used to describe this disease, patients with SYSTEMIC LUPUS ERYTHEMATOSUS do not have an increased incidence of autoimmune hepatitis and the two diseases are distinct entities. Type II autoimmune hepatitis is less common, typically affecting girls ages two to 14, although adults can have it too.

Causes
Cellular immune reactions may be a cause of chronic active hepatitis. A variety of circulating autoantibodies can be found in the blood of patients with chronic active hepatitis.

Clinical Features
Fatigue is the most common symptom of autoimmune hepatitis. Other symptoms include enlarged liver, jaundice, itching, skin rashes, joint pain, or abdominal discomfort. People in advanced stages of the disease are more likely to have symptoms such as fluid in the abdomen (ascites) or mental confusion. Women may stop having menstrual periods.

Symptoms of autoimmune hepatitis range from mild to severe. Because severe viral hepatitis or hepatitis caused by a drug—for example, certain antibiotics—have the same symptoms, tests may be needed for an exact diagnosis.

Blood tests   A routine blood test for liver enzymes can help reveal a pattern typical of hepatitis. However, further tests, especially for autoantibodies, are needed to diagnose autoimmune hepatitis. Antibodies are proteins made by the immune system to fight off bacteria and viruses. In autoimmune hepatitis, the immune system makes antinuclear antibodies (ANA), antibodies to smooth muscle cells (SMA), or liver and kidney microsomes (anti-LKM). The pattern and level of these antibodies help define the type of autoimmune hepatitis (type I or type II).

Blood tests also help distinguish autoimmune hepatitis from viral hepatitis (such as hepatitis B or C) or a metabolic disease (such as Wilson's disease).

Liver biopsy   A small sample of liver tissue, examined under a microscope, can help the doctor accurately diagnose autoimmune hepatitis and tell how serious it is.

Complications
When treatment is not administered promptly or when it is not effective, there may be complication of cirrhosis, liver cell failure, or hepatocellular carcinoma.

In addition, both prednisone and azathioprine have side effects. Because high doses of prednisone are needed to control autoimmune hepatitis, managing side effects is very important. However, most side effects appear only after a long period of time. Some possible side effects of prednisone are weight gain, anxiety and confusion, thinning of the bones (osteoporosis), thinning of the hair and skin, diabetes, high blood pressure, and cataracts.

Azathioprine can lower the white blood cell count and sometimes causes nausea and poor appetite. Rare side effects are allergic reaction, liver damage, and pancreatitis (inflammation of the pancreas gland with severe stomach pain).

Treatment

Treatment works best when autoimmune hepatitis is diagnosed early. With proper treatment, autoimmune hepatitis can usually be controlled. In fact, recent studies show that sustained response to treatment not only stops the disease from getting worse, but it may actually reverse some of the damage.

The primary treatment is medicine to suppress (slow down) an overactive immune system.

Both types of autoimmune hepatitis are treated with daily doses of a corticosteroid called prednisone. Doctors will usually start a patient on a high dose (20 to 60 mg per day) and lower the dose as the disease is controlled. The goal is to find the lowest possible dose that will control the disease.

Another medicine, azathioprine (Imuran) is also used to treat autoimmune hepatitis. Like prednisone, azathioprine suppresses the immune system but in a different way. It helps lower the dose of prednisone needed, thereby reducing prednisone's side effects. Azathioprine may be prescribed in addition to prednisone once the disease is under control.

Most people will need to take prednisone, with or without azathioprine, for years. Some people take it for life. Corticosteroids may slow down the disease, but everyone is different. In about one out of every three people, treatment can eventually be stopped. Continued monitoring of each patient's condition is important because the disease may return and be even more severe, especially during the first few months after stopping treatment.

People who do not respond to standard immune therapy or who have severe side effects may benefit from other immunosuppressive agents like cyclosporine or tacrolimus. People who progress to end stage liver disease (liver failure) may need a liver transplant. Transplantation is a promising alternative, with a one-year survival rate of 90 percent and a five-year survival rate of 70 to 80 percent.

In about seven out of 10 people, the disease goes into remission, with a lessening of severity of symptoms, within two years of starting treatment. A portion of persons with a remission will see the disease return within three years, so treatment may be necessary on and off for years, if not for life.

Autoimmune Hepatitis, NIH Publication No. 01-4761, Bethesda, Md.: National Digestive Diseases Information Clearinghouse (NDDIC), National Institutes of Health, September 2001.

Krawitt, E. L. "Autoimmune Hepatitis." *The New England Journal of Medicine.* 334 (1996): 897–903.

herbal medicines The American Autoimmune Related Diseases Association has cautioned that autoimmune disease patients need to be aware that some alternative treatments, such as natural supplements and herbals, may trigger an autoimmune response and worsen the patient's condition. It is in the patient's best interest to confer with his or her physician or professional to determine whether the compound or treatment being considered will help, harm, or, at least, do no harm.

herpes gestationis (HG) A rare autoimmune skin disease of pregnancy. Despite its name, this disease has no relationship to the herpes virus infection but rather was named based on the clinical feature of herpetiform blisters. In Europe, herpes gestationis is known as pemphigoid gestationis. In the United States, it occurs in one out of 50,000 pregnancies. It usually begins in the second or third trimester or immediately postpartum.

Causes

It is caused by the production of antibodies that bind the patient's own basement membrane zone, which separates the top layer of the skin (epidermis) from the underlying dermis. These antibodies elicit an immune reaction that causes separation of the epidermis and therefore blistering of the skin.

Clinical Features

Intensely itchy, herpes gestationis is characterized by bulbous lesions (blisters) and tends to recur in successive pregnancies. It may begin at any time between nine weeks' gestation and one week postpartum, with the average onset being 21 weeks' gestation. Usually, it lasts several weeks, but it may persist for many months after delivery. In a high proportion of patients, the eruption begins around the umbilicus and then spreads over the abdomen to the thighs. The extremities, palms, and soles can be markedly affected. The condition usually disappears in the weeks and months following delivery but may reappear with menses or with subsequent use of oral contraceptives. The diagnosis is confirmed by using immunofluorescence techniques to detect deposition of IgG antibodies at the basement membrane zone between the epidermis and underlying dermis. The disorder may be associated with other autoimmune diseases such as GRAVES' DISEASE and VITILIGO.

Complications

Herpes gestationis can have severe complications. The mother can develop necrosis (breakdown and death) of affected skin as well as kidney damage, which is diagnosed when blood and protein are found in the urine. Infants can be born with this rash, but it usually clears up within a few weeks of birth without treatment.

Treatment

Treatment includes oral or topical corticosteroids (prednisone).

Chen, S. H., K. Chopra, T. Y. Evans, S. S. Raimer, M. L. Levy, and S. K. Tyring. "Herpes Gestationis in a Mother and Child." *Journal of the American Academy of Dermatology* 40, no. 5, Pt. 2 (May 1999): 847–849.

Hispanics/Latinos and autoimmune diseases
Some autoimmune diseases occur more frequently in the Hispanic/Latino community; others occur noticeably less frequently.

- ALLERGIC ASTHMA morbidity and mortality have been increasing in the United States for the past 15 years and are particularly high among poor African-American and Hispanic/Latino inner-city residents, especially children. Low socioeconomic status, exposure to cockroach allergens and pollutants, lack of access to medical care, and lack of self-management skills all contribute to increased morbidity from asthma.

- INSULIN-DEPENDENT DIABETES mellitus (IDDM) has a lower incidence in Hispanics/Latinos and other cultural groups than in Caucasians. Interestingly, Hispanic Americans are almost twice as likely to have the nonimmune Type 2 (adult-onset) diabetes as non-Hispanic Caucasians of similar age.

- MULTIPLE SCLEROSIS—In June 2000, the Consortium of Multiple Sclerosis Centers/North American Research Committee on MS released demographic information showing 14,420 (89.0 percent) non-Hispanic whites with MS, while only 300 Hispanics/Latinos (1.9 percent) had the disease.

- SYSTEMIC LUPUS ERYTHEMATOSUS—Anyone can get lupus, but it is more common in Hispanic/Latino women, as well as in other minority groups. Hispanics/Latinos tend to develop lupus at a younger age and have more symptoms at diagnosis (including kidney problems). They also tend to have more severe disease than whites. For example, Hispanic/Latino patients have more heart problems. Researchers do not understand why some people seem to have more problems with lupus than others. (See also AFRICAN AMERICANS WITH AUTOIMMUNE DISEASE.)

Serrano-Rios, M., A. Goday, and T. Martinez Larrad. "Migrant Populations and the Incidence of Type 1 Diabetes Mellitus: An Overview of the Literature with a Focus on the Spanish-Heritage Countries in Latin America." *Diabetes/Metabolism Research and Reviews* 15, no. 2 (March–April 1999): 113–132.

histocompatibility testing A method of matching the self antigens (HLA) on the tissues of a transplant donor with those of the recipient. The closer the match, the better the chance that the transplant will take.

HIV Human immunodeficiency virus, a retrovirus that causes acquired immune-deficiency syndrome (AIDS). HIV is spread most commonly by having unprotected sex with an infected partner. The virus can enter the body through the lining of the vagina, vulva, penis, rectum, or mouth during sex.

HIV is also spread through contact with infected blood. Before donated blood was screened for evidence of HIV infection and before heat-treating techniques to destroy HIV in blood products were introduced, HIV was transmitted through transfusions of contaminated blood or blood components. Today, because of blood screening and heat treatment, the risk of getting HIV from such transfusions is extremely small.

HIV is frequently spread among injection drug users by the sharing of needles or syringes contaminated with very small quantities of blood from someone infected with the virus. It is rare, however, for a patient to give HIV to a health care worker or vice versa by accidental sticks with contaminated needles or other medical instruments.

Women can transmit HIV to their babies during pregnancy or birth. Approximately one-quarter to one-third of all untreated pregnant women infected with HIV will pass the infection to their babies. HIV can also be spread to babies through the breast milk of mothers infected with the virus. If the mother takes the drug AZT during pregnancy, she can significantly reduce the chances that her baby will get be infected with HIV. If health care providers treat mothers with AZT and deliver their babies by cesarean section, the chances of the baby being infected can be reduced to a rate of 1 percent.

A study sponsored by the National Institute of Allergy and Infectious Diseases (NIAID) in Uganda found a highly effective and safe drug regimen for preventing transmission of HIV from an infected mother to her newborn that is more affordable and practical than any other examined to date. Interim results from the study show that a single oral dose of the antiretroviral drug nevirapine (NVP) given to an HIV-infected woman in labor and another to her baby within three days of birth reduces the transmission rate by half compared with a similar short course of AZT.

Although researchers have found HIV in the saliva of infected people, there is no evidence that the virus is spread by contact with saliva. Laboratory studies reveal that saliva has natural properties that limit the power of HIV to infect. Research studies of people infected with HIV have found no evidence that the virus is spread to others through saliva by kissing. No one knows, however, whether so-called deep kissing, involving the exchange of large amounts of saliva, or oral intercourse increase the risk of infection. Scientists have also found no evidence that HIV is spread through sweat, tears, urine, or feces.

Studies of families of HIV-infected people have clearly shown that HIV is not spread through casual contact such as the sharing of food utensils, towels and bedding, swimming pools, telephones, or toilet seats. HIV is not spread by biting insects such as mosquitoes or bedbugs.

HIV can infect anyone who practices risky behaviors such as sharing drug needles or syringes, having sexual contact with an infected person without using a condom, or having sexual contact with someone whose HIV status is unknown.

Having a sexually transmitted disease such as syphilis, genital herpes, chlamydial infection, gonorrhea, or bacterial vaginosis appears to make people more susceptible to getting HIV infection during sex with infected partners. Many people do not have any symptoms when they first become infected with HIV. Some people, however, have a flu-like illness within a month or two after exposure to the virus. This illness may include fever, headache, tiredness, and enlarged lymph nodes (glands of the immune system easily felt in the neck and groin). These symptoms usually disappear within a week to a month and are often mistaken for those of another viral infection. During this period, people are very infectious, and HIV is present in large quantities in genital fluids.

More persistent or severe symptoms may not surface for a decade or more after HIV first enters the body in adults or within two years in children born with HIV infection. This period of asymptomatic infection is highly individual. Some people may begin to have symptoms within a few months, while others may be symptom free for more than 10 years.

Even during the asymptomatic period, the virus is actively multiplying, infecting, and killing cells of the immune system. HIV's effect is seen most obviously in a decline in the blood levels of CD4+ T cells (also called T4 cells)—the immune system's key infection fighters. At the beginning of its life in the human body, the virus disables or destroys these cells without causing symptoms.

As the immune system deteriorates, a variety of complications start to take over. For many people, their first sign of infection is large lymph nodes or swollen glands that may be enlarged for more than three months. Other symptoms often experienced months to years before the onset of AIDS include lack of energy, weight loss, frequent fevers and sweats, persistent or frequent yeast infections (oral or vaginal), persistent skin rashes or flaky skin, pelvic inflammatory disease in women that does not respond to treatment, and short-term memory loss. Some people develop frequent and severe herpes infections that cause mouth, genital, or anal sores or a painful nerve disease called shingles. Children may grow slowly or be sick a lot.

Because no vaccine for HIV is available, the only way to prevent infection by the virus is to avoid behaviors that put a person at risk of infection, such as sharing needles and having unprotected sex.

Many people infected with HIV have no symptoms. Therefore, there is no way of knowing with certainty whether a sexual partner is infected unless he or she has repeatedly tested negative for the virus and has not engaged in any risky behavior.

People should either abstain from having sex or use male latex condoms or female polyurethane condoms, which may offer partial protection, during oral, anal, or vaginal sex. Only water-based lubricants should be used with male latex condoms.

Although some laboratory evidence shows that spermicides can kill HIV, researchers have not found that these products can prevent a person from getting HIV.

The risk of HIV transmission from a pregnant woman to her baby is significantly reduced if she takes AZT during pregnancy, labor, and delivery and her baby takes it for the first six weeks of life.

National Institute of Allergy and Infectious Diseases, National Institutes of Health. *HIV Infection and AIDS: An Overview,* May 2001.

HMOs/managed care   The health maintenance organization (HMO) is the most common form of managed care, which began making serious inroads in health care in the early 1970s. It is the opposite of fee for service, where patients or their insurers pay health providers for each medical service rendered. The individual enrolling in an HMO pays the same monthly premium regardless of the amount of services received. Managed care is a method of providing health care coverage to patients at reduced costs to employers and others.

Under the managed care system, both the patient and the doctor are managed through rules imposed by the managed care company. These rules generally limit the patient's choice of both doctors and other health care providers such as labs, X-ray facilities, hospitals, and visiting nurse service. The managed care company also dictates to varying degrees the treatment choices a participating doctor may make. The original intent of this system was to emphasize preventive care in order to keep costs down, thereby making the HMO profitable. However, studies have indicated that costs have been held down not by preventive care but by restricting hospitalization and other expensive treatment avenues.

The current trend toward HMOs and other managed care forms is a growing concern of autoimmune patients, their families, and caregivers. Although the possibility of controlling costs is of great interest and hope, the overriding concern is whether patients with such chronic disorders, and frequently being treated for multiple chronic disorders, will receive inadequate care or be excluded from the more costly emerging treatments. Little is known about the numbers of autoimmune patients under age 65 who are enrolled in managed care programs. However, horror stories have proliferated, especially on disease-specific Internet websites. As in most areas, all forms of the media tend to repeat most frequently the bad news.

According to Lubeck, studies comparing the quality of care in HMOs and fee-for-service settings for RHEUMATOID ARTHRITIS (RA) have found few differences in outcomes, although reduced costs have been attributed to lower hospitalization rates in patients with RA. The Stanford University researchers reviewed 10 studies of direct costs of RA. In 1996 dollars, direct costs ranged from $2,299 (U.S.) per person per year in Canada to $13,549 in a U.S. study focusing on patients who had been hospitalized only. In managed care settings, costs of medications were proportionately higher than in fee-for-service settings. The researchers concluded that in studies of the direct costs of RA, the components of costs have remained relatively stable over time. However, they cautioned that this may change with the development and growing use of new RA medications including cyclooxygenase 2 inhibitors, interleukins, cytokines, treatments that inhibit tumor necrosis factor, and combination therapies. They added that the effectiveness of managed care in controlling direct costs needs to be evaluated in more targeted studies.

Studies do show, though, that physicians are more dissatisfied now than they were in the past and that this change correlates both over time and cross-sectionally with shifts in managed care penetration. In a 1997 national survey, physicians reported that over the previous three years, 38 percent had experienced a decline in their ability to make decisions they think are right for their patients, and 41 percent reported a decrease in the amount of time spent with patients. Overall, physicians reported feeling greater pressures on their clinical autonomy.

Another area of concern is in research. Sullivan and Furst wrote, "The emergence of managed care contracts and payer limitations in the United States could hinder the development of innovative, curative therapies."

Collins, Karen Scott, Cathy Schoen, and David R. Sandman. *The Commonwealth Fund Survey of Physician Experiences With Managed Care.* New York: Commonwealth Fund, 1997.

Grabois, Ellen. "What Every Person with a Disability Should Know about Managed Care Plans." Houston, Tex.: The Center for Research on Women with Disabilities, Baylor College of Medicine, Baylor University, 1999.

Lubeck, D. P. "A Review of the Direct Costs of Rheumatoid Arthritis: Managed Care Versus Fee-For-Service Settings." *Pharmaeconomics* 19, no. 8 (2001): 811–818.

"Managed Care Insurance." Cystic Fibrosis Foundation. Available online. URL: http://www.cff.org/living_with _cf/managed_care_insurance.cfm. Downloaded on 17 July 2002.

President's Advisory Commission on Consumer Protection and Quality in the Health Care Industry. "Quality First: Better Health Care for All Americans." chap. 2 in *Improving Health Care Quality in an Industry in Transition.* March 1998. Silver Spring, Md.: Agency for Healthcare Research and Quality Publications Clearinghouse.

Sullivan, K. M., and D. E. Furst. "The Evolving Role of Blood and Marrow Transplantation for the Treatment of Autoimmune Diseases." *The Journal of Rheumatology* 48, Supp. (1997): 1–4.

home health care   Home care, provided through both private and governmental agencies, is an integral part of the health care system and plays an important role in reducing overall health costs. In autoimmune disease treatment, for example, home care can provide an alternative to hospitals for people who need regular intravenous medications for pain management and chronic diseases such as RHEUMATOID ARTHRITIS and CROHN'S DISEASE. Home care saves payers or patients about $1,000 a day compared with an inpatient setting, according to studies. The Multiple Sclerosis Society of Canada says home care is frequently an essential component of daily life for people with MULTIPLE SCLEROSIS and one that enables them to remain in their home environment longer.

hospitalization   The average length of stay for U.S. hospital inpatients for all causes was 5.0 days and the average hospitalization rate was 116 per 1,000 population in 1999, according to a Centers for Disease Control and Prevention (CDC) report released in 2001. Precise hospitalization incidence is not known for most autoimmune diseases, basically because no single hospital or university has enough patients with any one autoimmune disease to support effective evaluation of causes or treatments.

In Connecticut, hospitalizations are used to estimate the prevalence of the most severe cases of autoimmune disease. For the five years between 1993 and 1997, over 2,300 women were hospitalized for a select number of autoimmune diseases. Rates of hospital discharges per 100,000 women per year were as follows: rheumatoid arthritis—9,334; lupus erythematosus—3,575; Crohn's disease—3,434; multiple sclerosis—3,212; ulcerative colitis—1,692; fibromyalgia—1,632; Graves' disease—955; scleroderma—805; Hashimoto's thyroiditis—775; and Sjögren's syndrome—564.

Although hospitalization is sometimes needed during treatment of autoimmune diseases, it is not always to be expected. The likelihood can range from rarely to absolutely. In many cases, hospitalization is needed only during times of disease flare-ups or adverse drug reactions or for treatment of another disease impacting the primary autoimmune disease (called a comorbid disease). Examples of the varying needs for autoimmune-related hospitalization include the following.

- ALLERGIC ASTHMA—In 1985, according to one study, annual hospitalizations for asthma totaled 463,500 admissions (median length of stay was 5.0 days), of which 34.6 percent were for persons under 18 years of age. At Children's Memorial Hospital in Chicago—the fourth largest children's hospital in the United States—asthma is the number one diagnosis for hospitalizations. This hospital has also noticed a marked increase in the number of admissions to the intensive care unit over the past few years. At Maine Medical Center from 1989 to 1992, admissions for children with a primary diagnosis of asthma increased by 33 percent.

- GUILLAIN-BARRÉ SYNDROME (GBS)—When writing in the March 2000 issue of *RN*, Treesa L. Worsham said, "Once GBS is suspected, hospitalization is a must. The patient's condition can rapidly deteriorate into paralysis that affects the respiratory muscles, necessitating intubation and mechanical ventilation. Depending on the severity of the patient's symptoms (not all will experience paralysis), he may be admitted to a medical or neurology floor or to an ICU."

- INSULIN-DEPENDENT DIABETES mellitus (IDDM)— Most children who develop diabetes are hospitalized for a few days to regulate their insulin and diet and to learn about the disease. The length of the initial hospitalization depends on the child's age, the availability of self-care training in the community, and the degree of glucose elevation.

There are approximately four hospital admissions per 100,000 children per year for diabetic ketoacidosis (DKA) in the United States. Current home-monitoring techniques allow most diabetic care to occur in an outpatient setting. However, DKA remains the most common cause of hospital admission for children with diabetes. One study reported that after an initial diagnosis of diabetes in children ages eight to 13 years, 25 percent were rehospitalized within 2.5 years, with DKA the most common reason.

- MYASTHENIA GRAVIS (MG)—When the muscle weakness is severe and involves the breathing muscles, hospitalization is usually necessary. These attacks seldom last longer than a few weeks.

- PSORIASIS—Although hospital treatment for psoriasis is usually reserved for patients with potentially life-threatening disease variants, some physicians consider it even for severe cases not requiring emergency care. At the University of Miami hospital, where in-patient psoriasis treatment is used for certain cases, length of stay at the hospital averages nine to 10 days for patients admitted for erythrodermic or pustular psoriasis and is typically six days for patients with severe psoriasis vulgaris.

- RHEUMATOID ARTHRITIS (RA)—Although the majority of RA patients are managed by the rheumatologist and primary care provider on an outpatient basis, hospitalization due to severity of illness or for procedures such as joint replacement does occur. From a survey conducted by the Centers for Disease Control and Prevention (CDC) about the impact of arthritis and rheumatic diseases on the U.S. health care system, data showed that in 1997, 744,000 people with arthritis and other rheumatic diseases accounted for 30,914,000 discharges from short-stay hospitalizations. They consumed 4 million days of care.

- SYSTEMIC LUPUS ERYTHEMATOSUS (SLE)—Although some people with lupus have severe recurrent attacks and are frequently hospitalized, most people with lupus rarely require hospitalization. Many lupus patients never have to be hospitalized, especially if they are careful and follow their physicians' instructions.

Lupus patients can experience life-threatening episodes of kidney inflammation known as flares, which can require expensive intensive-care hospitalization. Lupus accounts for more than 100,000 hospital admissions in the U.S. each year, averaging 10 days and about $20,000 per visit.

Cardiovascular and cerebrovascular diseases are important comorbid conditions in patients with SLE. In one population-based hospitalization study, women ages 18 to 44 with SLE had a substantially increased risk of hospitalization due to acute myocardial infarctions and cerebrovascular accidents compared with age-matched control subjects. Women of all ages with SLE had increased risk of hospitalizations due to congestive heart failure.

Connecticut Department of Public Health. *Connecticut Women's Health,* 2001.

Guttman, Cheryl. "In-Patient Therapy Plays Uncommon but Valuable Role in Psoriasis Care: Hospitalization Deserves Place in Armamentarium for Psoriasis Vulgaris." *Dermatology Times* 21, no. 12 (December 2000): 35.

National Institutes of Health: National Heart, Lung, and Blood Institute. *National Asthma Education and Prevention Program Task Force on the Cost Effectiveness, Quality of Care, and Financing of Asthma Care,* NIH Publication No. 55-807, 1996.

Human Genome Project An international research effort to chart and characterize the human genome—the entire package of genetic instructions for a human being. That entails laying out—in order—the 3 billion DNA letters (or base pairs) of the full human genetic code.

Begun in 1990, the U.S. Human Genome Project is a 13-year effort coordinated by the U.S. Department of Energy and the National Institutes of Health. The project was originally planned to last 15 years. However, effective resource and technological advances have accelerated the expected completion date to 2003. Project goals are to:

- identify all the approximate 30,000 genes in human DNA,

- determine the sequences of the 3 billion chemical base pairs that make up human DNA,

- store this information in databases,

- improve tools for data analysis,

- transfer related technologies to the private sector, and

- address the ethical, legal, and social issues (ELSI) that may arise from the project.

Several types of genome maps have already been completed. A working draft of the entire human genome sequence was announced in June 2000, with analyses published in February 2001. An important feature of this project is the federal government's long-standing dedication to the transfer of technology to the private sector. By licensing technologies to private companies and awarding grants for innovative research, the project is catalyzing the multibillion-dollar U.S. biotechnology industry and fostering the development of new medical applications.

A great profusion of discoveries about the genetic basis of a long list of diseases has already resulted from the Human Genome Project. Initially, these discoveries related to relatively rare conditions. Increasingly, though, the same powerful approaches are uncovering hereditary factors in diabetes and other common illnesses.

These revelations hold promise for transforming medical practice. In the years ahead, learning about individual susceptibilities to common disorders such as cancer and heart disease may be possible, allowing the design of programs of effective, individualized preventive medicine focused on life style changes, diet, and medical surveillance to keep people healthy.

The same discoveries ushered in by the Human Genome Project will enable scientists to predict who will respond most effectively to a particular drug therapy and who may suffer a side effect and ought to avoid that particular drug. In addition, these advances will lead to the next generation of designer drugs, targeted to each individual and engineered in a much more precise way than today's drugs.

As a part of the Human Genome Project, 16 research institutions in the United States, Great Britain, Germany, France, Japan, and China are currently generating a high-quality, accurate sequence of the human genetic code for scientists everywhere to use as a no-cost resource without restrictions. The project is being done in two stages: the working draft and the finished sequence.

The government agencies funding the Human Genome Project in the U.S. are the National Human Genome Research Institute (NHGRI), a part of the National Institutes of Health (NIH), and the Department of Energy (DOE). Most of the Human Genome Project sequencing occurs at four laboratories in the U.S. and one in Great Britain.

The three U.S. labs funded by the NHGRI are at Baylor College of Medicine in Houston, Washington University School of Medicine in St. Louis, and Whitehead Institute outside Boston. The DOE sponsors the Joint Genome Institute in Walnut Creek, California. The Wellcome Trust funds the Sanger Centre located outside London.

The Human Genome Project international consortium includes two laboratories at the University of Washington in Seattle and labs at Stanford University in Palo Alto, California; Genome Therapeutics Corp. in Waltham, Massachusetts; Genoscope in Evry, France, the RIKEN Institute and Keio University School of Medicine in Japan, the Max-Planck Institute for Molecular Biology, the Institute of Molecular Biotechnology, and the Gesellschaft fuer Biotechnologische in Germany; and the Beijing Human Genome Center in China.

All participants in the Human Genome Project have agreed to adhere to specific procedures, including maintaining quality standards and making daily deposits of sequence information into the public databases including GenBank, the European Bioinformatics Institute, and the DNA Database of Japan. Scientists by the thousands, located worldwide, tap into GenBank every day to search for data to advance their medical research.

human leukocyte antigens (HLA)   A pattern of cell surface proteins that identifies the cell to the immune system as "self" or "nonself." Any human Class I or Class II protein in markers of self used in histocompatibility (cell-mediated immunological similarity or compatibility) testing. Some HLA types also correlate with certain autoimmune diseases. These are important in presenting antigens to immune effector cells.

humoral immunity (antibody-mediated immunity)   Immune protection provided by soluble factors such as antibodies, which circulate in the body's fluids or *humors*, primarily serum and lymph.

idiopathic Unknown cause, from the Greek *idio*, meaning "peculiar" or "unusual," and from *pathy*, meaning "illness."

idiopathic autoimmune hemolytic anemia See AUTOIMMUNE HEMOLYTIC ANEMIA.

idiopathic pulmonary fibrosis (IPF) A disease of inflammation that results in scarring, or fibrosis, of the lungs. In time, this fibrosis can thicken and build up to the point where the lungs are unable to provide oxygen to the tissues of the body. Whatever the trigger is for IPF, it appears to set off a series of events in which the inflammation and immune activity in the lungs—and, eventually, the fibrosis processes, too—become uncontrollable. In a few cases, heredity appears to play a part, possibly making some individuals more likely than others to get IPF. In studies of patients with IPF, the average survival rate has been found to be four to six years after diagnosis. Those who develop IPF at a young age seem to survive longer.

The exact number of people who develop IPF each year is not known. It is known, however, that equal numbers of men and women get the illness and that most cases of IPF are diagnosed when the patients are between the ages of 40 and 70. Nearly 75 percent of people with IPF have smoked cigarettes.

Causes

Although a number of separate diseases can initiate pulmonary fibrosis, many times the cause is unknown. When this is so, the condition is called idiopathic (of unknown origin) pulmonary fibrosis. In IPF, careful examination of the patient's environmental and occupational history gives no clues to the cause.

Currently, researchers believe that IPF may result from either an autoimmune disorder or the aftereffects of an infection, most likely a virus. Other theories as to what may cause IPF include allergic or environmental exposure (including tobacco smoke). These theories are still being researched. Bacteria and other microorganisms are not thought to be the cause of IPF.

There is also a familial form of the disease, known as familial idiopathic pulmonary fibrosis. Additional research is being done to determine whether there is a genetic tendency to develop the disease as well as to determine other causes of IPF.

Clinical Features

Early symptoms of IPF are usually similar to those of other lung diseases. Very often, for example, patients suffer from a dry cough and dyspnea (shortness of breath). As the disease progresses, dyspnea becomes the major problem. Day-to-day activities such as climbing stairs, walking short distances, dressing, and even talking on the phone and eating become more difficult and sometimes nearly impossible. Enlargement (clubbing) of the fingertips may develop. The patient may also become less able to fight infection. In advanced stages of the illness, the patient may need oxygen all the time.

Although the course of IPF varies greatly from person to person, the disease usually develops slowly, sometimes over years. The early stages are marked by alveolitis, an inflammation of the air sacs called alveoli, in the lungs. The job of the air sacs is to allow the transfer of oxygen from the lungs into the blood and the elimination of carbon dioxide from the lungs and out of the body.

As IPF progresses, the alveoli become damaged and scarred, thus stiffening the lungs. The stiffening makes breathing difficult and brings on a feeling of breathlessness (dyspnea), especially during activities that require extra effort.

In addition, scarring of the alveoli reduces the ability of the lungs to transfer oxygen. The resulting lack of oxygen in the blood (hypoxemia) may cause increases in the pressure inside the blood vessels of the lungs, a situation known as pulmonary hypertension. The high blood pressure in the lungs then puts a strain on the right ventricle, the lower right side of the heart, which pumps the oxygen-poor blood into the lungs.

Complications

IPF can lead to death. Often the immediate cause is respiratory failure due to hypoxemia, right-side heart failure, a heart attack, blood clot (embolism) in the lungs, stroke, or lung infection brought on by the disease.

Treatment

The best chance of slowing the progress of IPF is by treatment as soon as possible. Most IPF patients require treatment throughout life, usually under the guidance of a lung specialist. Some major medical centers and large teaching hospitals do research on the disease and provide consultation and treatment to patients.

Treatment for IPF may vary a great deal. It depends on many things, including the age of the patient and stage of the disease. The aim of treatment is to reduce the inflammation of the alveoli and stop the abnormal process that ends in fibrosis. Once scar tissue has formed in the lung, it cannot be returned to normal.

Drugs are the primary way that IPF is treated. They are usually prescribed for at least three to six months to allow time to determine if a particular treatment is effective. Commonly used drugs are prednisone and cytoxan. Oxygen administration and, in special cases, transplantation of the lung are other choices.

Prednisone A corticosteroid, prednisone is the most common drug given to patients with IPF. About 25 to 35 percent of all patients respond favorably to this medicine. No one knows exactly how corticosteroids work or why some patients do well on prednisone while others do not. Patients take prednisone by mouth every morning, starting with a high dose for the first four to eight weeks. As they improve, they gradually take smaller amounts. Changes in mood are one of the more common side effects of prednisone. Most patients, however, can handle the mood changes—anxiety, depression, or sleeplessness—once they know what is causing the problem. A less common side effect is a rise in blood-sugar levels.

Cytoxan Cyclophosphamide, also referred to as cytoxan, may be taken together with prednisone or instead of it. Like prednisone, cytoxan is swallowed each day. One of the more serious side effects of cyclophosphamide is leukopenia, a condition in which the number of white blood cells drops to a dangerously low level. Leukopenia can be controlled by regularly checking the blood count and adjusting the dose of cytoxan if necessary.

Other medicines Azathioprine, penicillamine, chlorambucil, vincristine sulfate, and colchicine have been used in a few patients with IPF. Their effectiveness in treating IPF, however, has not been adequately tested.

Oxygen In addition to treatment with medicine, some patients may need oxygen, especially when blood oxygen becomes low. This treatment helps resupply the blood with oxygen. As a result, breathlessness is reduced, the patient can be more active, and the severity of pulmonary hypertension decreases.

Many IPF patients, particularly those in the early stages of the disease, respond to drug treatment and can continue to go about most of their normal activities, including working. Some patients with advanced IPF need to carry oxygen with them.

Exercise A daily walk or regular use of a stationary bicycle or treadmill can improve muscle strength and breathing ability and also increase overall strength. Supplemental oxygen is used when needed; sometimes it is the only way a patient is able to do a reasonable amount of activity.

Lung transplantation Lung transplantation, either of both lungs or only one, is an alternative to drug treatment for patients in the severe, final stages of IPF. It is most often performed in patients under 60 years of age who do not respond to any form of treatment. The one-year survival rate is approximately 60 percent.

National Heart, Lung, and Blood Institute, National Institutes of Health. *Facts About Idiopathic Pulmonary Fibrosis,* NIH Publication No. 93-2997, 1993.

idiopathic thrombocytopenic purpura (ITP)

Also called immune thrombocytopenic purpura. A disorder of the blood. *Thrombocytopenic* refers to a decrease in blood platelets. *Purpura* refers to the purplish looking areas of the skin and mucous membranes (such as the lining of the mouth) where bleeding has occurred as a result of decreased platelets.

Acute (temporary) thrombocytopenic purpura is most commonly seen in young children. Boys and girls are equally affected. Symptoms often, but do not necessarily, follow a viral infection. About 85 percent of children recover within one year and the problem does not return.

Thrombocytopenic purpura is considered chronic when it has lasted more than six months. Chronic ITP is an autoimmune disease of primarily young to middle-age adults, although the onset of illness may be at any age, which is at least twice as common in females as in males. It is relatively insidious in its onset and is not associated with preceding viral infection. ITP resolves spontaneously only on rare occasions. ITP is a common disorder. In fact, it may be the most common of all the autoimmune diseases in which the cell targeted by the immune system for auto-reaction has been clearly identified.

In ITP, autoantibodies are directed against platelets. Platelets are minute, disk-shaped components of the blood that are needed for prevention and control of bleeding. Platelets are formed in the bone marrow and are released into the blood. Platelets have a limited life span before they are replaced by new platelets. In ITP, the platelets are prematurely destroyed. This destruction results in a low blood platelet count (thrombocytopenia) that may produce bruising or excessive bleeding.

Causes

Some cases of ITP are caused by drugs, and others are associated with infection, pregnancy, or immune disorders such as systemic lupus erythematosus. About half of all cases are classified as idiopathic, meaning the cause is unknown.

Clinical Features

The main symptom is bleeding, which can include bruising (ecchymosis) and tiny red dots on the skin or mucous membranes (petechiae). In some instances, bleeding from the nose, gums, or digestive or urinary tracts may also occur. Rarely, bleeding within the brain occurs.

A careful review of medications the patient is taking is important because some drugs can be associated with thrombocytopenia. A complete blood count will be done. A low platelet count will establish thrombocytopenia as the cause of purpura. Often the next procedure is a bone marrow examination to verify that there are adequate platelet-forming cells (megakaryocytes) in the marrow and to rule out other diseases such as metastatic cancer (cancer that has spread to the bone marrow) and leukemia (cancer of the blood cells themselves). Another blood sample may be drawn to check for other conditions sometimes associated with thrombocytopenia such as lupus and infection.

Treatment

The treatment of idiopathic thrombocytopenic purpura is determined by the severity of the symptoms. In some cases, no therapy is needed. In most cases, drugs that alter the immune system's attack on the platelets are prescribed. These include corticosteroids (prednisone) and/or intravenous infusions of immune globulin. Another treatment that usually results in an increased number of platelets is removal of the spleen, the organ that destroys antibody-coated platelets. Other drugs such as vincristine, azathioprine (Imuran), danazol, cyclophosphamide, and cyclosporine are prescribed for patients only in the severe case where other treatments have not shown benefits since these drugs have potentially harmful side effects.

Except in certain situations, (e.g., internal bleeding and preparation for surgery), platelet transfusions are usually not beneficial and, therefore, are seldom performed. Because all therapies can have risks, it is important that overtreatment (treatment based solely on platelet counts and not on symptoms) be avoided. In some instances, lifestyle adjustments may be helpful for prevention of bleeding due to injury. These would include use of protective gear such as helmets and avoidance of contact sports in symptomatic patients or when platelet counts are less than 50,000. Otherwise, patients can usually carry on normal activities, but final decisions about activity are made in consultation with the patient's hematologist.

Karpatkin, S. "Autoimmune (Idiopathic) Thrombocytopenic Purpura." *Lancet* 349 (1997): 1,531.

McMillan, R., and P. A. Imbach. "Immune Thrombocytopenic Purpura." In *Thrombosis and Hemorrhage,* 2nd ed., edited by J. L. Loscalzo and A. I. Schafer. Philadelphia: Williams & Wilkins, 1998.

National Heart, Lung, and Blood Institute, National Institutes of Health. *Immune Thrombocytopenic Purpura (ITP),* NIH Publication No. 90-2114, September 1990.

idiotype   The unique and characteristic parts of an antibody's variable region, which can themselves serve as antigens. A set of one or more antigenic determinants (idiotopes) on an antibody that make that antibody unique. It is associated with the amino acids of immunoglobulin light and heavy chains.

IgA   See IMMUNOGLOBULINS.

IgA nephropathy   Primary IgA nephropathy is an autoimmune kidney disease caused by deposits of the protein immunoglobulin A (IgA) inside the glomeruli (filters) within the kidney. These glomeruli (the singular form is *glomerulus*) normally filter wastes and excess water from the blood and send them to the bladder as urine. The IgA protein prevents this filtering process, leading to blood and protein in the urine and swelling in the hands and feet. This chronic kidney disease may progress over a period of 10 to 20 years. If this disorder leads to end-stage renal disease, the patient must go on dialysis or receive a kidney transplant.

IgA nephropathy usually occurs in adolescents or young adults between the ages of 15 and 35. Males are affected two or three times more often than females. It occurs significantly more often in Native Americans than in any other ethnic group tested. It is more prevalent in Caucasians than in African Americans, and it is one of the leading causes of acute nephritis in young people in the United States, Europe, and Japan. One study of young men in the military showed an annual occurrence of 94 cases of IgA nephropathy out of 100,000 male inductees.

The IgA protein is a normal part of the body's system to protect against disease (the immune system). What causes IgA deposits in the glomeruli is not known. However, because IgA nephropathy may run in families, genetic factors probably contribute to the disease.

Kidney disease usually cannot be cured. Once the tiny filtering units are damaged, they cannot be repaired. Treatment focuses on slowing the progression of the disease and preventing complications. One complication is high blood pressure, which further damages glomeruli.

Some patients may benefit from limiting protein in their diet to reduce the buildup of waste in the blood. Patients with IgA nephropathy often have high cholesterol. Reducing cholesterol—through diet, medication, or both—appears to help slow the progression of IgA nephropathy.

National Institute of Diabetes and Digestive and Kidney Diseases (NIDDK), The National Institutes of Health. *IgA Nephropathy,* NIH Publication No. 01-4571, 1998, updated 2001.

IgD   See IMMUNOGLOBULINS.

IgE   See IMMUNOGLOBULINS.

IgG   See IMMUNOGLOBULINS.

IgM   See IMMUNOGLOBULINS.

immune   Protected from or resistant to a disease or infection because of the development of antibodies or CELLULAR IMMUNITY.

immune complex   A cluster of interlocking antigens and antibodies, formed when antibodies attach to the antigens in order to destroy them. These complexes circulate in the blood and may eventually attach to the walls of blood vessels, producing an inflammatory response at that point.

immune response The reactions of the immune system to foreign substances so that they are neutralized or eliminated, thereby preventing the diseases or injuries these foreign substances (antigens) might cause.

immune system The body's natural defense system, which protects it from infection, foreign substances, and organisms that could lead to illness. This protection may result from the formation of specialized white blood cells or the production of antibodies.

immunity Protection from diseases, especially infectious diseases. *Acquired immunity* is immunity that results from either exposure to an antigen or from the passive injection or IMMUNOGLOBULINS. (See also ACTIVE IMMUNITY, INNATE IMMUNITY.)

immunodeficiency The lack of an adequate or normal immune response. Immunodeficiency can be *primary*—intrinsic, not due to another illness or agent; *secondary*—due to another illness or agent, e.g., human immunodeficiency virus, cancer, or chemotherapy; or *combined*—deficiencies of both killer T lymphocytes and antibodies.

immunodeficiency diseases A group of serious but little known disorders in which immune system malfunction causes increased susceptibility to infection, autoimmune diseases, and malignancy. This is a group of more than 70 different diseases, many of which are inherited. Together they affect approximately 500,000 individuals in the United States. Of these, between 5,000 and 10,000 people, many of whom are children, are severely affected by serious, recurrent, and often life-threatening infections.

Primary immunodeficiency diseases are caused by intrinsic defects in the cells of the immune system and are often caused by inherited genetic defects. This is in contrast to *secondary* immunodeficiency diseases such as acquired immunodeficiency syndrome caused by infection with human immunodeficiency virus.

immunoglobulins A family of large protein molecules, also known as antibodies, that are found in the blood serum and in tissue fluids. They are produced by specific white cells (B lymphocytes) of the immune system and released into the circulation in response to the presence of an antigen. This antigen may be a protein on the surface of an infectious agent such as a bacteria or it may be a foreign chemical substance. Normal plasma cells manufacture immunoglobulins to match exactly and specifically the invading antigen.

Immunoglobulin is abbreviated as Ig. The structure of an Ig molecule consists of two heavy chains joined by bonds to two light chains. Five major types (classes) of Ig have been identified in human serum. Each class of Ig has a unique type of heavy chain that is defined by use of a Greek letter: gamma, mu, alpha, epsilon, or delta. The abbreviated name for the five classes of Ig are as follows:

1. IgG for Ig gamma—(immunoglobulin G). The most abundant class of antibodies found in blood serum and active against bacteria, fungi, viruses, and foreign particles. Immunoglobulin G antibodies trigger action of the complement system.
2. IgM for Ig mu—(immunoglobulin M). The class of antibodies found in circulating body fluids and the first antibodies to appear in response to an initial exposure to an antigen.
3. IgA for Ig alpha—(immunoglobulin A). The class of antibodies produced primarily against ingested antigens, found in body secretions such as saliva, sweat, or tears. Its function is to prevent viruses and bacteria from invading the body through epithelial surfaces (the epidermis of the skin and the surface layer of mucous and serous membranes). Its presence in colostrum and breast milk helps prevent infection in breast-feeding infants.
4. IgE for Ig epsilon—(immunoglobulin E). The class of antibodies produced in the lungs, skin, and mucous membranes and responsible for allergic reactions. Approximately one-half of patients with allergies have increased IgE levels.
5. IgD for Ig delta—(immunoglobulin D). The class of antibodies found only on the surface of B cells and possibly functioning as antigen receptors to initiate differentiation of B cells into plasma cells.

immunologist A person who specializes in researching and/or treating the functions and disorders of the immune system. Immunologists work with problems related to allergies, autoimmune disorders, immunodeficiency disorders, and transplant surgery.

immunology The study of the components of the immune system, their function, and their disorders.

immunosuppressive agents Drugs that slow or halt immune system activity. Immunosuppressive agents may be given to prevent the body from mounting an immune response after an organ transplant and thus reject the transplant or for treating a disease that is caused by the immune system.

immunotherapy The concept of using the immune system to treat disease, for example, developing a vaccine against cancer. Immunotherapy may also refer to the therapy of diseases caused by the immune system, allergies for example.

incidence How often a disease occurs; the number of new cases of a disease among a certain group of people for a certain period of time.

inclusion body myositis (IBM) This is also called inflammatory myopathy. It is an inflammatory muscle disease characterized by slow and relentlessly progressive but painless muscle weakness and atrophy of the muscles. The disorder is very similar to another inflammatory myopathy called polymyositis. In fact, IBM is often diagnosed in cases of polymyositis that are unresponsive to therapy. However, IBM has its own distinctive features. The onset of muscle weakness in IBM is generally gradual (over months or years). Also, IBM, which occurs more frequently in men than women, affects both the proximal (closest to the center of the body) and distal (farthest from the center of the body) muscles. There may be weakness of the wrist and finger muscles and atrophy of the quadriceps muscles in the legs. Atrophy or shrinking of the forearms is also characteristic. Difficulty swallow-

ing (dysphagia) occurs in approximately half of IBM cases. Symptoms of the disease usually begin after the age of 50, although the disease can occur in any age group. Falling and tripping are usually the first noticeable symptoms of IBM. For some patients, the disorder begins with weakness in the hands causing difficulty with gripping, pinching, and buttoning.

Causes

IBM is considered a sporadic disease—that is, there is no evidence that the disease is inherited and researchers do not yet know what causes it. Because of the inflammation associated with the disease, some doctors think IBM is a form of autoimmune disorder. Others speculate that the inflammation is secondary to a different problem in the muscles. For example, some researchers believe that the primary problem in IBM is an age-related inability of the muscle to deal with destructive free radicals and an abnormal accumulation of a number of proteins within the muscle fiber.

Very rarely, IBM with inflammation in the muscle biopsy can be present in families (familial IBM). Whether this form is inherited or whether some people have genes that make them susceptible to whatever causes the sporadic form is not yet clear.

Clinical Features

Symptoms of IBM may occur one at a time or appear simultaneously. Together, they can lead to difficulty grasping objects, rising from a sitting position, walking long distances, or going up stairs. Weakness of the quadriceps muscles can cause sudden falling, and lower-leg weakness can cause difficulty holding the foot up (*footdrop*), which can lead to tripping. If the esophageal muscles weaken, choking may become a problem when ingesting some types of food or liquids.

When viewed under the microscope, the muscle cells of persons with IBM contain vacuoles (typically, rounded empty spaces). Within the vacuoles are usually abnormal clumps of several proteins, one of which is amyloid. These characteristic protein clumps, which are called *inclusion bodies*, give this disorder its name. In addition, signs of inflammation in the form of invading immune cells are frequently seen in the muscle tissue. However, the amount varies and lack of them does not rule out a diagnosis of IBM.

The definitive way to diagnose IBM is with a muscle biopsy. Electromyography and blood enzyme levels, including creatine kinase, are not diagnostic.

Treatment

No standard course of treatment exists for IBM. The disease is unresponsive to corticosteroids and other immunosuppressive drugs. Some evidence suggests that intravenous immunoglobulin may have a slight, but transient, beneficial effect in a small number of cases. Physical therapy may be helpful in maintaining mobility. IBM is generally resistant to all therapies, and its rate of progression also appears to be unaffected by the presently available treatments.

Those with the disorder may eventually find that a cane, walker, or wheelchair is helpful for traversing long distances, but the disease does not seem to affect life expectancy. Sometimes, people with IBM will remain ambulatory for several years. Occasionally, dysphagia symptoms can be severe enough that a nonsurgical expansion of the throat muscles (called *dilation*) or a surgical division of specific throat muscles (called a *cricopharyngeal myotomy*) may be needed.

MDA Fact Sheet: Frequently Asked Questions About Inclusion Body Myositis, The Muscular Dystrophy Association. Available online. URL: http://mdausa.org/research/ibmfaq.html. Downloaded on 17 July 2002.

infants and preschool children with autoimmune diseases Although autoimmune diseases most often target adults and especially young adult women, most of these diseases can and do attack people of all ages, including infants and very young children, if only rarely. However, several autoimmune diseases appear frequently in infants or preschool children, and they present special problems for these age groups.

- ALLERGIC ASTHMA—Asthma can be difficult to diagnose in infants and children under age six and usually requires a specialist to be sure it is asthma. Common signs of childhood asthma include recurring coughing spells, wheezing (noisy breathing), shortness of breath, complaints of soreness (or "hurting") in the chest, and tiring more quickly than playmates of the same age. Exposure to high levels of house dust mites and tobacco smoke can increase the risk of asthma in infants.

- CELIAC DISEASE—During the first year of life, an infant may reveal celiac disease with intermittent vomiting, diarrhea, growth delay, and failure to thrive. The incidence of this early classic presentation in infants has decreased. However, to prevent significant growth problems in infants, confirmation of celiac disease is important.

- CHAGAS' DISEASE—In infants and in very young children with acute Chagas' disease, swelling of the brain can develop in acute Chagas' disease, and this can cause death.

- CONGENITAL HEART BLOCK (CHB)—CHB is a relatively uncommon yet life-threatening condition seen in fetuses, newborns, and older children. Although once thought to occur in approximately one in 20,000 live births, University of Alberta researchers say it appears to be at least twice as common—due, in most part, to improved methods of fetal diagnosis. In patients born to mothers with autoimmune diseases such as lupus erythematosus, the incidence is significantly higher at approximately five out of every 100 babies born. Approximately 60 percent of infants and children with CHB go on to require artificial pacemaker implantation. However, despite cardiac pacing, approximately 30 percent of these children die in the first year of life. A significant number of these patients, despite successful implantation of a cardiac pacemaker and survival beyond age one year, develop severe heart failure requiring, in many cases, heart transplants.

- INSULIN-DEPENDENT DIABETES mellitus (IDDM)—IDDM in infants is rare, but it is more common in preschool children, especially boys. Young children have special problems when dealing with diabetes. Because most children under age four do not recognize the symptoms of impending low blood sugar, caregivers must be especially vigilant for external symptoms such as pallor, sweatiness or unusual behavior. Also, for young children, getting the balance between insulin and food intake is difficult. The growth hormone in their bodies affects the way insulin works, and predicting exactly when and how much a young child will eat can be difficult. Nights also present a challenge for the toddler who eats at 5 P.M., goes to bed at 7 P.M., and wakes at 7 A.M., which is a long time without food. For this reason, low blood sugar occurs most commonly at night.

Florida announced in early 2002 that it would become the first state to offer screening to determine an infant's lifetime probability of developing IDDM. Funded by a $10 million grant from the American Diabetes Association, the program was scheduled to launch within the year. The parents of at-risk children will be offered the opportunity to have the child monitored for antibodies throughout his or her life.

In Washington, scientists at Seattle's Pacific Northwest Research Institute began in 2002 testing the blood samples of 32,000 Washington newborns to see if they carry a genetic marker for juvenile diabetes. The intent is to determine how well detection of certain versions of the gene called HLA DQ predicts diabetes. Early detection is critical because as much as 90 percent of the insulin-producing cells have been destroyed by the time a child shows symptoms of diabetes.

- JUVENILE ARTHRITIS—Symptoms of rheumatoid arthritis in infants are chronic irritability and crying when handled with no other reason apparent. Systemic onset juvenile rheumatoid arthritis (SoJRA) accounts for 10 to 20 percent of all juvenile rheumatoid arthritis, affecting males and females equally and occurring most frequently under the age of five years.

Collins, Jane. "Diabetic Dilemmas," *The Times* (London), 23 April 2002.

Hypponen, E., E. Laara, et al. "Intake of Vitamin D and Risk of Type 1 Diabetes: A Birth-Cohort Study." *Lancet* 358, no. 9,292 (2001): 1,500–1,503.

Jones Jr., H. R. "Guillain-Barré Syndrome: Perspectives With Infants and Children." *Seminars in Pediatric Neurology* 7, no. 2 (June 2000): 91–102.

King, Warren. "Goal: To Develop Test for Infants to Predict Diabetes," *Seattle Times*, 18 March 2002.

Pruessner, Harold T. "Detecting Celiac Disease in Your Patients." *American Family Physicians* 57, no. 5 (March 1, 1998): 1,023–1,039.

Robb, Michael. "Researchers Break Through Heart Block." *ExpressNews*, University of Alberta. Available online. URL: http://www.expressnews.ualberta.ca/expressnews/. Posted May 17, 2001.

Schneider, R., and R. M. Laxer. "Systemic Onset Juvenile Rheumatoid Arthritis." *Bailliere's Clinical Rheumatology* 12, no. 2 (May 1998): 245–271.

Tsao, C. Y., J. R. Mendell, W. D. Lo, M. Luquette, and R. Rennebohm. "Myasthenia Gravis and Associated Autoimmune Diseases in Children." *Journal of Child Neurology* 15, no. 11 (November 2000): 767–769.

infections The relationship between infections and autoimmune diseases has long been studied and conjectured. Increasing evidence suggests that some autoimmune disorders may be caused by certain chronic bacterial and viral infections. For example, RHEUMATIC FEVER always follows repeated strep throat infections during childhood. Other autoimmune diseases are worsened when infections are present in the body. Plus, many persons with autoimmune disorders are at a higher risk of infections. To complicate this fact, many of the medications used to treat autoimmune disorders suppress the immune system—to keep the immune system from attacking the body—and in the process reduce the body's ability to fight off infections.

In a study of 860,648 death certificates of public school teachers during an 11-year period, University of Connecticut researchers discovered that the mortality rate from autoimmune diseases for those teachers was twice the rate for people in other professional occupations. The finding also showed that the death rate from the diseases for high school teachers was 12 percent higher than for elementary school teachers. Because so many teachers work in old, poorly ventilated buildings and because teachers in high schools are exposed to many more students on a daily basis, several interpreters of the study have suggested that infections may have been an important component in the high incidence rate among teachers.

There are several possibilities for how infections may directly or indirectly lead to autoimmune diseases.

- A person's immune system may not be functioning properly in some area. So when an infection invades the body, the immune system may not react appropriately. After the infection runs its course, the immune system continues to malfunction. Under the influence of that infection, the malfunction develops into autoimmunity.

- In incidences similar to the development of multiple sclerosis, a viral infection creates a clone of lymphocytes that are capable of cross-reacting with self-tissue. According to Bone, "Because there is no immune dysregulation, no damaging cross-reaction occurs and these cells persist as memory cells after the virus has gone. They are then reactivated by exposure to the same virus, or one that is antigenically similar. If this event coincides with a state of immune dysregulation, autoimmune disease may develop."

Double-blind clinical studies sponsored by the National Institutes of Health indicate that some antibiotics are effective in treating RHEUMATOID ARTHRITIS. Although not proven in large, double-blind trials, anecdotal reports have claimed successful antibiotic treatment for CROHN'S DISEASE, GRAVES' DISEASE, HASHIMOTO'S THYROIDITIS, and SJÖGREN'S DISEASE.

Infection as a cause of autoimmune disease is difficult to prove. Studies have implicated involvement of multiple species of microorganisms with each autoimmune disease, and these microorganisms vary from region to region and from person to person.

Bone, Kerry. "Treating Autoimmune Disease—A Phytotherapeutic Perspective: Part 2." *The British Journal of Phytotherapy* 4, no. 2 (Winter 1995): 72–88.

Walsh, S. J., and L. M. DeChello. "Excess Autoimmune Disease Mortality Among School Teachers." *The Journal of Rheumatology* 28, no. 7 (July 2001): 1,537–1,545.

inflammation Part of the body's immunological defensive response against physical or chemical injury, allergy, or infection. It is characterized by redness, swelling, heat, and pain in the affected tissue and sometimes by loss of function.

inflammatory Characterized or caused by inflammation.

innate immunity Natural immunity that is present in a person from birth and is the first line of defense against most infectious agents. (See also NATURAL IMMUNITY.)

insulin-dependent diabetes (Type 1) Diabetes is a group of conditions in which glucose (sugar) levels are abnormally high. Diabetes occurs when the pancreas stops making enough insulin, which is necessary for the proper metabolism of digested foods.

About 14 million people in the United States have some form of diabetes, although only half are diagnosed. The three main types of diabetes are insulin dependent, also known as Type 1 diabetes; noninsulin dependent, also called Type 2 diabetes; and gestational diabetes, which occurs during pregnancy.

Insulin-dependent diabetes mellitus (IDDM) most often develops in children and young adults. Sometimes people over age 40 get IDDM, but it usually begins at younger ages. For this reason, IDDM used to be known as juvenile diabetes. IDDM is one of the most common chronic disorders in U.S. children. Each year, from 11,000 to 12,000 children are diagnosed with IDDM. Among the more than 7 million people in the United States who are being treated for diabetes, about 5 percent to 10 percent have IDDM.

Causes

When people eat, foods containing proteins, fats, and carbohydrates are broken down into simpler, easily absorbed chemicals. One of these is a form of simple sugar called glucose. Glucose circulates in the bloodstream where it is available for body cells to use. The body relies on glucose as a source of fuel for important organs such as the brain.

The pancreas, a large gland located behind the stomach, produces the hormone insulin. In people without diabetes, the pancreas makes the correct amount of insulin needed to allow glucose to enter body cells. In people with diabetes, however, not enough insulin is produced. As a result, glucose builds up in blood, overflows into the urine, and passes out of the body unused. Thus, the body loses an important source of fuel—even though the blood contains large amounts of glucose.

Insulin also allows the body to store excess glucose as fat, proteins as muscle protein, and important enzymes that control metabolism. A severe deficiency of insulin causes excess breakdown of stored fats and proteins.

In people with IDDM, the pancreas produces too little or no insulin at all. The pancreas is not able to produce insulin because the body's immune system has destroyed the insulin-producing cells.

Scientists do not know why the body's immune system attacks and destroys insulin-producing cells. A combination of factors may be involved, including exposure to common viruses or other substances early in life as well as an inherited risk for IDDM.

Researchers can now test family members of people with IDDM to identify those at increased risk for diabetes. Scientists hope to find a way to prevent the disease through a study called the Diabetes Prevention Trial-Type 1.

Clinical Features

The early symptoms of IDDM can be gradual or sudden. They include frequent urination (particularly at night), increased thirst, unexplained weight loss (in spite of increased appetite), and extreme tiredness. These symptoms are caused by the build up of sugar in the blood and its loss in the urine.

To eliminate sugar in the urine, the kidney borrows water from the body. The loss of this extra sugar and water in the urine results in dehydration, which causes increased thirst. In addition to causing high blood glucose, the lack of insulin causes the body to break down stored fats and proteins. As fats are broken down, the body can convert these fats into waste products called ketones. If ketone production is excessive, abnormal amounts of ketones in the blood can spill into the urine. If blood ketone levels rise too high, a life-threatening condition called ketoacidosis can develop, which requires immediate medical attention. Symptoms of ketoacidosis include abdominal pain, vomiting, rapid breathing, extreme tiredness, and drowsiness.

Diabetes often goes undetected because testing is done in the afternoon, researchers discovered through the Diabetes Prevention Trial-Type 1 Program. Blood glucose levels peak in the morning, then drop in the afternoon. Thus, people with symptoms of diabetes need to have a fasting blood glucose test repeated on a different day, with at least one of the tests performed in the morning.

Complications

Diabetes can cause damage to both large and small blood vessels, resulting in complications affecting the kidneys, eyes, nerves, heart, and gums. Maintaining blood sugar levels as close as possible to normal prevents or slows the development of many of these complications.

Diabetic kidney disease, called diabetic nephropathy, can be a life-threatening complication of IDDM in about 40 percent of people who have had diabetes for 20 or more years. The kidneys are vital to good health because they serve as a filtering system to clean waste products from the blood. Diabetic nephropathy develops when the small blood vessels that filter these wastes are damaged. Sometimes this damage causes the kidneys to stop working. This condition is called kidney failure or end-stage renal disease. People with kidney failure must either have their blood cleaned by a dialysis machine or have a kidney transplant.

High blood pressure (hypertension) also increases a person's chance of developing kidney disease. People with diabetes are more likely to develop high blood pressure than people without diabetes. Therefore, keeping blood pressure under control is especially important for someone with IDDM.

An early sign of kidney disease is albumin or protein in the urine. Intensive therapy can prevent the development and slow the progression of early diabetic kidney disease. A type of medication called an ACE inhibitor can help protect the kidneys from damage.

Diabetes can affect the small blood vessels in the back of the eye, a condition called diabetic retinopathy. Retinopathy means disease of the retina, the tissue at the back of the eye that is sensitive to light. Diabetes eventually causes changes in the tiny vessels that supply the retina with blood. These small changes are called background retinopathy. Most people who have had diabetes for a number of years have background retinopathy, which usually does not affect sight. Over time, the blood vessels may rupture or leak fluid. In a minority of patients, most often those with higher blood sugar, retinopathy becomes more severe and new blood vessels may grow on the retina. These vessels may bleed into the clear gel, or vitreous, that fills the eye or detach the retina from its normal position because of bleeding or scar formation. Laser treatment, as well as surgical procedures performed by eye doctors who specialize in diabetic problems, can often help preserve useful vision even in cases of advanced retinopathy.

Nerve disease caused by diabetes is called diabetic neuropathy. There are three types of nerve disease: peripheral, autonomic, and mononeuropathy. Peripheral neuropathy affects the hands, feet, legs, toes, or fingers. A person's feet, legs, and fingertips may lose feeling, burn, or become painful. To relieve the pain, doctors prescribe painkilling drugs and sometimes antidepressant drugs. Scientists are studying other substances to help relieve pain associated with diabetic peripheral neuropathy.

Another type of nerve disease that may occur after several years of diabetes is called autonomic neuropathy. Autonomic neuropathy affects the internal organs such as the heart, stomach, sexual organs, and urinary tract. It can cause digestive problems and lead to incontinence (a loss of ability to control urine or bowel movements) and sexual impotence. A doctor can help diagnose problems associated with internal organs and may prescribe medication to help relieve pain and other problems associated with autonomic neuropathy. Mononeuropathy is a form of nerve disease that affects specific nerves, most often in the torso, leg, or head. Mononeuropathy may cause pain in the lower back, chest, abdomen, or the front of one thigh. Sometimes, this nerve disease can cause aching in the eye, an inability to focus the eye, or double vision.

Mononeuropathy may also cause facial paralysis, a condition called Bell's palsy, or problems with hearing. Mononeuropathies occur most often in older people and can be quite painful. Usually the symptoms improve in weeks or months without causing long-term damage.

As with high blood pressure, heart disease is more common in people with diabetes than in people without diabetes. People with diabetes tend to have more fat and cholesterol in their arteries—the large blood vessels that keep the heart beating and the blood flowing. When too much fat and cholesterol build up in the arteries, the arteries and heart must work harder. Over time, this extra work can lead to a heart attack.

People with diabetes are also at greater risk for stroke and other forms of large blood vessel disease. A stroke is the result of damage to the blood vessels that circulate blood in the brain. Blockage of major blood vessels in the feet, legs, or arms is called peripheral vascular disease. Peripheral vascular disease causes poor circulation and can contribute to foot and leg ulcers.

People with diabetes, especially those with poor control of their blood sugar, are at risk for developing infections of the gums and bone that hold the teeth in place. Like all infections, gum infections can cause blood sugar to rise and make diabetes harder to control.

Periodontal disease starts as gingivitis, which causes sore, bleeding gums. If not stopped, gingivitis can lead to serious periodontal disease that can damage the bones that holds the teeth in their sockets. Without treatment, teeth may loosen and fall out.

Good blood sugar control lowers the risk of gum disease. People with good control have no more gum disease than people without diabetes. Good blood sugar control, daily brushing and flossing, and regular dental checkups are the best defense against gum problems.

Before the 1950s, most pregnant women with diabetes had little chance of having a normal baby. Since the 1960s, major advances in diabetes treatment have taken place in Europe and North America. Today, with careful planning, most women with diabetes can become pregnant and deliver healthy babies with the help of their doctors.

Treatment

Diabetes requires constant attention and daily care to keep blood sugar levels in balance. Injecting insulin, following a diet, exercising, and testing blood sugar are some of the day-to-day requirements. To feel good and stay healthy, a person with IDDM must follow a daily management routine. For this reason, diabetes is often referred to as a 24-hour disease. The federal government has issued treatment recommendations based on a 10-year study recently completed, called the Diabetes Control and Complications Trial (DCCT). The DCCT proved that lowering blood sugar levels delayed or prevented diabetes complications by 50 to 80 percent.

The DCCT compared two approaches to managing IDDM: intensive and standard treatment. People in the intensive-treatment group learned how to adjust their insulin according to food intake and exercise. They injected insulin three to four times a day or used an insulin pump and tested their blood sugar at least four times a day and once a week at 3 A.M. They also followed a diet and exercise plan and met once a month with a health care team composed of a physician, nurse educator, dietitian, and mental health professional.

People in the standard treatment group followed a plan that was not as strict. They took one or two insulin injections a day, tested sugar levels once or twice a day, and met with the doctor or nurse every three months.

At the end of the DCCT, volunteers on intensive treatment had lower rates of kidney, eye, and nerve damage than volunteers in the standard treatment group. The study showed that efforts to improve control of blood sugar made a major difference. In fact, the study found that any long-term lowering of blood sugar levels will reduce the risk of complications, even in people with poor control of their diabetes and early complications of diabetes. For this reason, people with IDDM are encouraged to do the best they can to keep their blood sugar levels as close to the normal range as possible.

However, intensive treatment does increase the risk of low blood sugar episodes, or hypoglycemia. Therefore, it is not recommended for everyone, particularly older adults, children under age 13, people with heart problems or advanced complications, and people with a history of frequent severe hypoglycemia. (See also INSULIN-DEPENDENT DIABETES: RESEARCH.)

National Diabetes Information Clearinghouse (NDIC), National Institute of Diabetes and Digestive and Kidney Diseases (NIDDK), National Institutes of Health. *Insulin Dependent Diabetes,* NIH Publication No. 94-2098, 1994.

insulin-dependent diabetes research   The Diabetes Control and Complications Trial (DCCT) was one of many recent research programs supported by the federal government and by nongovernment organizations to improve the health and well-being of people with diabetes and to find ways to prevent and cure the disorder. A 10-year follow-up to the DCCT, the Epidemiology of Diabetes Intervention and Complications Study, is focusing on the development of macrovascular and renal complications in DCCT volunteers.

The National Institute of Diabetes and Digestive and Kidney Diseases (NIDDK) conducts basic and clinical research in its own laboratories and supports research at centers and hospitals throughout the United States. Other institutes of the National Institutes of Health support studies on diabetic eye, heart, vascular, and nerve disease; pregnancy and diabetes; dental complications; and the immunological aspects of diabetes. This research has led to improved treatments for the complications of diabetes and ways to prevent complications from occurring.

Researchers are searching diligently for the causes of all forms of diabetes and ways to delay or prevent the disorder. Much progress has been made. Scientists have identified antibodies in the blood that make a person susceptible to IDDM, making it possible to screen relatives of people with diabetes and determine their risk for developing the disease.

A new NIDDK clinical trial, the Diabetes Prevention Trial-Type 1 (DPT-1), began in 1994. It is identifying relatives at risk for developing IDDM and treating them with low doses of insulin or with oral insulin-like agents in the hope of preventing IDDM. Similar research is being conducted at other medical centers throughout the world. These studies are based on encouraging results in laboratory animals with IDDM and on pilot studies in relatives of people with IDDM.

Many recent advances have improved treatment for people with diabetes:

• Genetically engineered insulin. Because it is identical to insulin produced by the human body, genetically engineered insulin is less apt to cause skin and other allergic reactions. Supplies of genetically engineered insulin are readily available.

• Self-monitoring of blood glucose. By testing their own blood sugar, patients enable doctors to offer them much better treatment than was available before 1980 when testing urine for glucose was the only way of estimating diabetes control.

• Hemoglobin A1c testing. By using only one blood test, doctors can now monitor average blood sugar control over a period of two to three months. This test tells how well the patient is doing and whether any changes are needed in the management routine.

• Insulin pumps, insulin pens, and other aids for administering insulin. Insulin pumps, including implantable pumps now under development, can supply insulin in a more natural pattern, similar to the way the pancreas in a person without diabetes makes insulin. Other injection aids make giving insulin easier and more convenient than in the past, even in young children and people who are visually impaired.

Other improvements in diabetes management being developed include insulin in the form of nasal sprays, patches, or pills and devices to test blood sugar levels without having to prick a finger to get a blood sample. Perhaps one of the most important advances has been the development of an entirely new approach to diabetes management in which IDDM patients take responsibility for much of their own care.

Transplantation of the pancreas or of the insulin-producing islets of the pancreas offer a hope for a cure for IDDM. Many people with IDDM have had successful pancreas transplants, and a few have had islet transplants. Unfortunately, pancreas and islet transplants cannot be offered to everyone with diabetes as yet. The body's immune system rejects foreign or transplanted tissue, and people who have transplants must take powerful drugs to prevent rejection. These drugs are costly and may cause serious health problems. Therefore, pancreas or islet transplants are usually given only to people who have had or require a kidney transplant because of advanced complications and are already taking drugs to prevent rejection.

Researchers are working to develop less harmful drugs and better methods of transplanting pancreatic tissue to prevent rejection by the body. Examples include encapsulating the islet cells in a semipermeable membrane that offers protection from immune attack, implanting the cells in the thymus gland to induce tolerance by the immune system, and using bioengineering techniques to create artificial islet cells that secrete insulin in response to increased sugar levels in the blood.

In 2001, CuraGen Corp. of New Haven, Connecticut, and Bayer AG announced approval from the Federal Trade Commission and that they have selected 12 targets for drug screening. The companies intend to use the targets to identify new therapies for the treatment of obesity and diabetes. CuraGen genomics technologies help scientists determine how genes and proteins function. Bayer is identifying chemicals that might interact with the drug targets and that could be developed into novel treatments.

insurance   Health insurance is crucial for autoimmune patients but can be difficult to obtain after the diagnosis is made. This causes women (usually) or their spouses to limit job mobility for fear of losing current insurance. In some cases, this problem is alleviated because of COBRA. The federal COBRA (Consolidated Omnibus Reconciliation Act) law requires continuation of group coverage for 18 months when the employee stops working or reduces work hours. Additionally, family coverage can be extended to 29 months if the covered employee was disabled at the time of employment stoppage or curtailment. However, the patient must take over the costs of the coverage, and the law applies only to businesses that have 20 or more employees. It does not cover employees who work for small companies of fewer than 20 employees, the federal government, or certain other organizations.

In cases of private (nongroup) insurance, diagnosis of autoimmune diseases such as diabetes or Addison's disease could lead to increased premiums or loss of health insurance benefits. For persons with chronic autoimmune illnesses, potentially high health care expenditures often make obtaining adequate insurance coverage impossible. Health insurance that excludes pharmaceutical benefits for chronic autoimmune illnesses represents inadequate and inappropriate coverage according to the National Institutes of Health (NIH). The NIH also found that insurance carriers vary dramatically in their policy coverage of durable medical equipment (DME) even though several types of equipment (e.g., spacers and home nebulizers) may be critical to the care of persons with asthma (and other autoimmune diseases).

Life insurance can also be a problem for people with autoimmune conditions that are chronic but not terminal. Multiple sclerosis (MS) is one example—though incurable, the majority of sufferers now live a normal life span, with life expectancy reduced by only a few years compared with the general population. Yet MS patients applying for life insurance have discovered that many insurance companies are taking their information about MS from old and misleading data. Compounding this is the fact that MS is an individual condition, with each person experiencing different symptoms and varying degrees of severity. However, insurance companies tend to calculate their approvals and rates on the worst-case scenarios. Autoimmune patients with lifelong but not life-threatening cases therefore must sometimes fight for coverage and then pay higher rates than other people of the same gender and age.

Miller, Deborah M. *Psychosocial Issues for Women With Autoimmune Disease.* The National Women's Health Information Center. Available online. URL: http://www.4woman.gov/owh/autoimm/miller.htm. Downloaded on 17 July 2002.
National Institutes of Health: National Heart, Lung, and Blood Institute. *National Asthma Education and Prevention Program Task Force on the Cost Effectiveness, Quality of Care, and Financing of Asthma Care,* NIH Publication No. 55-807, September 1996.

interferons   A group of glycoproteins that are produced by different body cells in response to various stimuli, such as viral infections, bacteria, parasites, or other antigens. They prevent viral replication in newly infected cells and, in some cases, increase the activity of natural killer cells, which form part of the body's innate immune system.

interleukins   A major group of lymphokines and monokines, which are produced by T lymphocytes and macrophages (a type of white blood cell) in the presence of antigens or mitogens. They cause the T lymphocytes to activate and proliferate. *Interleukin-1* (leukocyte-activating factor, IL-1) is a protein factor produced by macrophages (a type of white blood cell) that plays an important role in activating T lymphocytes and B lymphocytes when antigens or mitogens are present. *Interleukin-2* (IL-2) is a protein factor produced by T lymphocytes that have been activated by an antigen. Interleukin-2 stimulates other T lymphocytes to activate and differentiate regardless of what specific antigen is involved. Interleukin-1 and interleukin-2 are both known to be involved in achieving T-cell-mediated immunity. *Interleukin-3* (IL-3) is a protein factor produced by T lymphocytes that have been activated by a mitogen. Interleukin-3 stimulates bone marrow stem cells and mast cells.

interstitial cystitis (IC)   A chronic pelvic pain disorder resulting in recurring discomfort or pain in the bladder and the surrounding pelvic region. The symptoms of IC vary from case to case and even in the same individual. People may experience mild discomfort, pressure, tenderness, or intense pain in the bladder and surrounding pelvic area. Symptoms may include an urgent need to urinate, frequent need to urinate, or a combination of these symptoms. Pain may change in intensity as the bladder fills with urine or as it empties. Women's symptoms often get worse during menstruation.

In IC, the bladder wall may be irritated and become scarred or stiff. Glomerulations (pinpoint bleeding caused by recurrent irritation) may appear on the bladder wall. Some people with IC find that their bladders cannot hold much urine, which increases the frequency of urination. Frequency, however, is not always specifically related to bladder size; many people with severe frequency have normal bladder capacity. People with severe cases of IC may urinate as many as 60 times a day.

Also, people with IC often experience pain during sexual intercourse. IC is far more common in women than in men. Of the more than 700,000 Americans estimated to have IC, 90 percent are women.

Because IC varies so much in symptoms and severity, most researchers believe that it is not one but several diseases. In the past, cases were mainly categorized as ulcerative IC or nonulcerative IC, based on whether ulcers had formed on the bladder wall. However, many researchers and clinicians have questioned the usefulness of this classification because the vast majority of cases do not involve ulcers and their presence or absence does not influence treatment options as much as other factors do.

Factors that influence treatment options include whether bladder capacity under anesthesia is great or small and whether mast cells are present in the tissue of the bladder wall, which may be a sign of an allergic or autoimmune reaction. In some cases, the success or failure of a treatment helps characterize the type of IC. For example, some cases respond to changes in diet while others do not.

Causes

Some of the symptoms of IC resemble those of bacterial infection, but medical tests reveal no organisms in the urine of patients with IC. Furthermore, patients with IC do not respond to antibiotic therapy. Researchers are working to understand the causes of IC and to find effective treatments.

One theory being studied is that IC is an autoimmune response following a bladder infection. Another theory is that a bacterium may be present in bladder cells but not detectable through routine urine tests. Some scientists have suggested that certain substances in urine may be irritating to people with IC, but no substance unique to people with IC has as yet been isolated. Researchers are beginning to explore the possibility that heredity may play a part in some forms of IC. In a few cases, IC has

affected a mother and a daughter or two sisters, but it does not commonly run in families. No gene has yet been implicated as a cause.

Clinical Features

Because symptoms are similar to those of other disorders of the urinary system and because there is no definitive test to identify IC, doctors must rule out other conditions before considering a diagnosis of IC. Among these disorders are urinary tract or vaginal infections, bladder cancer, bladder inflammation or infection caused by radiation to the pelvic area, eosinophilic and tuberculous cystitis, kidney stones, endometriosis, neurological disorders, sexually transmitted diseases, low-count bacteria in the urine, and in men, chronic bacterial and nonbacterial prostatitis.

The diagnosis of IC in the general population is based on:

- presence of urgency, frequency, or pelvic/bladder pain,
- cystoscopic evidence (under anesthesia) of bladder wall inflammation, including glomerulations or Hunner's ulcers present in 90 percent of patients with IC, and
- absence of other diseases that could cause the symptoms.

Diagnostic tests that help identify other conditions include urinalysis, urine culture, cystoscopy, biopsy of the bladder wall, urine cytology, and in men, laboratory examination of prostate secretions. The most important test to confirm IC is a cystoscopy under anesthesia.

Treatment

Scientists have not yet found a cure for IC nor can they predict who will respond best to which treatment. Symptoms may disappear without explanation or coincide with an event such as a change in diet or treatment. Even when symptoms disappear, they may return after days, weeks, months, or years. Scientists do not know why.

Because the causes of IC are unknown, treatments are aimed at relieving symptoms. Most people are helped for variable periods by one or a combination of treatments. As researchers learn more about IC, the list of potential treatments will change. The following describes the presently available treatment options.

Bladder distension Because many patients have noted an improvement in symptoms after a bladder distension done to diagnose IC, the procedure is often thought of as one of the first treatment attempts. Researchers are not sure why distension helps, but some believe that it may increase capacity and interfere with pain signals transmitted by nerves in the bladder. Symptoms may temporarily worsen 24 to 48 hours after distension but should return to predistension levels or improve after two to four weeks.

Bladder instillation During a bladder instillation, also called a bladder wash or bath, the bladder is filled with a solution that is held for varying periods of time, averaging 10 to 15 minutes, before being emptied.

The only drug approved by the U.S. Food and Drug Administration (FDA) for bladder instillation is dimethyl sulfoxide (DMSO, RIMSO-50). DMSO treatment involves guiding a narrow tube called a catheter up the urethra into the bladder. A measured amount of DMSO is passed through the catheter into the bladder, where it is retained for about 15 minutes before being expelled. Treatments are given every week or two for six to eight weeks and repeated as needed. Most people who respond to DMSO notice improvement three or four weeks after the first six- to eight-week cycle of treatments. Highly motivated patients who are willing to catheterize themselves may, after consultation with their doctor, be able to have DMSO treatments at home. Self-administration is less expensive and more convenient than going to the doctor's office.

Doctors think DMSO works in several ways. Because it passes into the bladder wall, it may reach tissue more effectively to reduce inflammation and block pain. It may also prevent muscle contractions that cause pain, frequency, and urgency.

A bothersome but relatively insignificant side effect of DMSO treatments is a garliclike taste and odor on the breath and skin that may last up to 72 hours after treatment. Long-term treatment has caused cataracts in animal studies, but this side effect has not appeared in humans. Blood tests,

including a complete blood count and kidney and liver function tests, need to be done about every six months.

A variety of other drugs, not yet approved by the FDA, have been used experimentally for bladder washes. In 1997, researchers from William Beaumont Hospital in Royal Oak, Michigan, reported promising results from a bladder wash containing Bacillus Calmette-Guérin (BCG), a vaccine traditionally used to immunize against tuberculosis. This preparation is undergoing continuing clinical trials to determine how long the effect lasts in a larger sample of patients.

Oral drugs Pentosan polysulfate sodium (Elmiron), the first oral drug developed for IC, was approved by the FDA in 1996. In clinical trials, Elmiron improved symptoms in 38 percent of patients treated. Doctors do not know exactly how it works, but one theory is that it may repair defects that might have developed in the lining of the bladder.

The FDA-recommended dosage of Elmiron is 100 mg, three times a day. Patients may not feel relief from IC pain for the first two to four months. A decrease in urinary frequency may take up to six months.

Elmiron's side effects are limited primarily to minor gastrointestinal discomfort. A small minority of patients experienced some hair loss, but hair grew back when they stopped taking the drug. Researchers have found no negative interactions between Elmiron and other medications, but it may affect liver function.

Some patients have experienced improvement in their urinary symptoms by taking antidepressants or antihistamines. Antidepressants help reduce pain and may also help patients deal with the psychological stress that accompanies living with chronic pain. In patients with severe pain, narcotic analgesics such as Tylenol with codeine or longer acting narcotics may be necessary.

Transcutaneous electrical nerve stimulation With transcutaneous electrical nerve stimulation (TENS), mild electrical pulses enter the body for minutes to hours two or more times a day either through wires placed onto the lower back or just above the pubic area, between the navel and the pubic hair, or through special devices inserted into the vagina in women or into the rectum in men. Although scientists do not know exactly how TENS works, it has been suggested that the electrical pulses may increase blood flow to the bladder, strengthen pelvic muscles that help control the bladder, or trigger the release of substances that block pain.

TENS is relatively inexpensive and allows the patient to take an active part in treatment. Within some guidelines, the patient decides when, how long, and at what intensity TENS will be used. It has been most helpful in relieving pain and decreasing frequency in patients with Hunner's ulcers. Smokers do not respond as well as non-smokers. If TENS is going to help, improvement is usually apparent in three to four months.

Diet No scientific evidence links diet to IC. However, many doctors and patients find that alcohol, tomatoes, spices, chocolate, caffeinated and citrus beverages, and high-acid foods may contribute to bladder irritation and inflammation. Some patients also note that their symptoms worsen after eating or drinking products containing artificial sweeteners.

Smoking Many patients feel that smoking makes their symptoms worse. Because smoking is the major known cause of bladder cancer, one of the best things smokers can do for their bladder is to quit.

Exercise Many patients feel that gentle stretching exercises help relieve IC symptoms.

Bladder training People who have found adequate relief from pain may be able to reduce frequency by using bladder-training techniques. Methods vary, but basically patients decide to void (that is, empty their bladder) at designated times and use relaxation techniques and distractions to keep to the schedule. Gradually, patients try to lengthen the time between scheduled voids. A diary that records voiding times is usually helpful in keeping track of progress.

Surgery Many approaches and techniques are used, each of which has its own advantages and complications. Surgery is considered only if all available treatments have failed and the pain is disabling. Most doctors are reluctant to operate because the outcome is unpredictable—some people still have symptoms after surgery.

Two procedures—fulguration and resection of ulcers—can be done with instruments inserted through the urethra. Fulguration involves burning Hunner's ulcers with electricity or a laser. When the area heals, the dead tissue and the ulcers fall off, leaving new, healthy tissue behind. Resection involves cutting around and removing the ulcers. Both treatments are done under anesthesia and use special instruments inserted into the bladder through a cystoscope.

Another surgical treatment is augmentation, which makes the bladder larger. In most procedures, scarred, ulcerated, and inflamed sections of the patient's bladder are removed, leaving only the base of the bladder and healthy tissue. A piece of the patient's bowel (large intestine) is then removed, reshaped, and attached to what remains of the bladder. After the incisions heal, the patient may void less frequently. The effect on pain varies greatly; IC can sometimes recur on the segment of bowel used to enlarge the bladder.

Even in carefully selected patients—those with small, contracted bladders—pain, frequency, and urgency may remain or return after surgery. The patient may have additional problems with infections in the new bladder and difficulty absorbing nutrients from the shortened intestine. Some patients are incontinent, while others cannot void at all and must insert a catheter into the urethra to empty the bladder.

Bladder removal, called a cystectomy, is another surgical option. Once the bladder has been removed, different methods can be used to reroute urine. In most cases, ureters are attached to a piece of bowel that opens onto the skin of the abdomen; this procedure is called a urostomy, and the opening is called a stoma. Urine empties through the stoma into a bag outside the body. Some urologists are using a second technique that also requires a stoma but allows urine to be stored in a pouch inside the abdomen. At intervals throughout the day, the patient puts a catheter into the stoma and empties the pouch. Patients with either type of urostomy must be very careful to keep the area in and around the stoma clean to prevent infection. Serious potential complications may include kidney infection and small bowel obstruction.

A third method to reroute urine involves making a new bladder from a piece of the patient's bowel and attaching it to the urethra. After healing, the patient may be able to empty the newly formed bladder by voiding at scheduled times or by inserting a catheter into the urethra. Few surgeons have the special training and expertise needed to perform this procedure. Even after total bladder removal, some patients still experience variable IC symptoms in the form of phantom pain.

A surgical variation of TENS, called saccral nerve root stimulation, involves permanent implantation of electrodes and a unit emitting continuous electrical pulses. Studies of this experimental procedure are now under way.

Brody, J. "Interstitial Cystitis: Help for a Puzzling Illness," *New York Times*, 25 January 1995.

Hanno, P. "Interstitial Cystitis and Related Diseases." In *Campbell's Urology*, 7th ed., edited by P. C. Walsh, A. B. Retik, E. D. Vaughan, and A. J. Wein. Philadelphia, Pa.: W. B. Saunders Company, 1998.

National Kidney and Urologic Diseases Information Clearinghouse (NKUDIC), National Institute of Diabetes and Digestive and Kidney Diseases (NIDDK), National Institutes of Health. *Interstitial Cystitis*, NIH Publication No. 99-3220, August 1999.

Sant, G., ed. *Interstitial Cystitis*. Philadelphia, Pa.: Lippincott-Raven, 1997.

Wein, A., and P. Hanno, eds. "Interstitial Cystitis: An Update of the Current Information." *Urology* 49, no. 5A, Supp. (1997).

juvenile arthritis Arthritis means *joint inflammation* and refers to a group of diseases that cause pain, swelling, stiffness, and loss of motion in the joints. The word *arthritis* is often used as a more general term to refer to the more than 100 rheumatic diseases that may affect the joints but can also cause pain, swelling, and stiffness in other supporting structures of the body such as muscles, tendons, ligaments, and bones. Some rheumatic diseases can affect other parts of the body, including various internal organs. Children can develop almost all types of arthritis that affect adults, but the most common type of arthritis that affects children is juvenile rheumatoid arthritis.

Juvenile rheumatoid arthritis (JRA) is a rheumatic autoimmune disease characterized by chronic inflammation of the synovial tissue found in joints and stiffness for more than six weeks in a child of 16 years of age or less. Inflammation causes redness, swelling, warmth, and soreness in the joints, although many children with JRA do not complain of joint pain. Any joint can be affected, and inflammation may limit the mobility of affected joints.

Juvenile rheumatoid arthritis affects between 65,000 to 70,000 children in the United States and comprises about 10 percent of all incidences of juvenile chronic arthritis (JCA). The disease may develop at any age during childhood, and girls are more often affected than boys. JRA has been described as a childhood rheumatic illness that has many characteristics of adult onset autoimmune diseases, such as rheumatoid arthritis and lupus.

Doctors classify three kinds of JRA by the number of joints involved, the symptoms, and the presence or absence of certain antibodies in the blood. (Antibodies are special proteins made by the immune system.) These classifications help the doctor determine how the disease will progress.

- Pauciarticular (paw-see-are-tick-you-lar): *Pauciarticular* means that four or fewer joints are affected. Pauciarticular is the most common form of JRA; about half of all children with JRA have this type. Pauciarticular disease typically affects large joints, such as the knees. Girls under age eight are most likely to develop this type of JRA.Some children have special proteins in the blood called antinuclear antibodies (ANAs). Eye disease affects about 20 percent to 30 percent of children with pauciarticular JRA. Up to 80 percent of those with eye disease also test positive for ANA, and the disease tends to develop at a particularly early age in these children. Regular examinations by an ophthalmologist (a doctor who specializes in eye diseases) are necessary to prevent serious eye problems such as iritis (inflammation of the iris) or uveitis (inflammation of the inner eye, or uvea). Many children with pauciarticular disease outgrow arthritis by adulthood, although eye problems can continue and joint symptoms may recur in some people.

- Polyarticular: About 30 percent of all children with JRA have polyarticular disease. In polyarticular disease, five or more joints are affected. The small joints, such as those in the hands and feet, are most commonly involved, but the disease may also affect large joints. Polyarticular JRA is often symmetrical, that is, it affects the same joint on both sides of the body. Some children with polyarticular disease have a special kind of antibody in their blood called IgM rheumatoid factor (RF). These children often have a more severe form of the disease, which doctors consider to be the same as adult rheumatoid arthritis.

- Systemic: Besides joint swelling, the systemic form of JRA is characterized by fever and a light pink rash, and it may also affect internal organs such as the heart, liver, spleen, and lymph nodes. Doctors sometimes call it Still's disease. Almost all children with this type of JRA test negative for both RF and ANA. The systemic form affects 20 percent of all children with JRA. A small percentage of these children develop arthritis in many joints and can have severe arthritis that continues into adulthood.

The main difference between juvenile and adult rheumatoid arthritis is that many people with JRA outgrow the illness, while adults usually have lifelong symptoms. Studies estimate that by adulthood, JRA symptoms disappear in more than half of all affected children. Additionally, unlike rheumatoid arthritis in an adult, JRA may affect bone development as well as the child's growth.

Another difference between JRA and adult rheumatoid arthritis is the percentage of people who are positive for IgM rheumatoid factor (RF). About 70 percent to 80 percent of all adults with rheumatoid arthritis are positive for RF, but fewer than half of all children with rheumatoid arthritis are RF positive. The presence of RF indicates an increased chance that JRA will continue into adulthood.

Causes

JRA is an autoimmune disorder, which means that the body mistakenly identifies some of its own cells and tissues as foreign. The immune system, which normally helps to fight off harmful, foreign substances such as bacteria or viruses, begins to attack healthy cells and tissues. The result is inflammation marked by redness, heat, pain, and swelling. Doctors do not know why the immune system goes awry in children who develop JRA. Scientists suspect that it is a two-step process. First, something in the children's genetic makeup gives them a tendency to develop JRA; and then an environmental factor, such as a virus, triggers the development of JRA.

Clinical Features

The most common symptom of all types of JRA is persistent joint swelling, pain, and stiffness that typically is worse in the morning or after a nap. The pain may limit movement of the affected joint, although many children, especially younger ones, will not complain of pain. JRA commonly affects the knees and joints in the hands and feet. One of the earliest signs of JRA may be limping in the morning because of an affected knee. Besides joint symptoms, children with systemic JRA have a high fever and a light pink rash. The rash and fever may appear and disappear very quickly. Systemic JRA may also cause the lymph nodes located in the neck and other parts of the body to swell. In some cases (less than half), internal organs, including the heart and very rarely the lungs, may be involved.

Eye inflammation is a potentially severe complication that sometimes occurs in children with pauciarticular JRA. Eye diseases such as iritis and uveitis are often not present until some time after a child first develops JRA.

Typically, there are periods when the symptoms of JRA are better or disappear (remissions) and times when symptoms are worse (flares). JRA is different in each child—some may have just one or two flares and never have symptoms again, while others experience many flares or even have symptoms that never go away.

Some children with JRA may look different because they have growth problems. Depending on the severity of the disease and the joints involved, growth in affected joints may be too fast or too slow, causing one leg or arm to be longer than the other. Overall growth may also be slowed. Doctors are exploring the use of growth hormones to treat this problem. JRA may also cause joints to grow unevenly or to one side.

Children with JRA may also look different because of medication. Corticosteroids, a type of medication sometimes used to treat JRA, can result in weight gain and a round face. When the doctor stops giving the medication, these side effects may disappear.

Doctors usually suspect JRA, along with several other possible conditions, when they see children with persistent joint pain or swelling, unexplained skin rashes and fever, or swelling of lymph nodes or inflammation of internal organs. A diagnosis of JRA is also considered in children with an unexplained limp or excessive clumsiness.

No one test can be used to diagnose JRA. A doctor diagnoses JRA by carefully examining the patient and considering the patient's medical history and the results of laboratory tests that help rule out other conditions.

Symptoms One important consideration in diagnosing JRA is the length of time that symptoms have been present. Joint swelling or pain must last for at least six weeks for the doctor to consider a diagnosis of JRA. Because this factor is so important, keeping a record of when the symptoms first appeared and when they are worse or better is useful.

Laboratory tests Laboratory tests, usually blood tests, cannot by themselves provide the doctor with a clear diagnosis. However, these tests can be used to help rule out other conditions and to help classify the type of JRA that a patient has. Blood may be taken to test for RF or ANA and to determine the erythrocyte sedimentation rate (ESR).

ANA is found in the blood more often than RF, and both are found in only a small portion of JRA patients. The RF test helps the doctor tell the difference among the three types of JRA.

ESR is a test that measures how quickly red blood cells fall to the bottom of a test tube. Some people with rheumatic disease have an elevated ESR or "sed rate" (cells fall quickly to the bottom of the test tube), showing that there is inflammation in the body. Not all children with active joint inflammation have an elevated ESR.

X rays X rays are needed if the doctor suspects injury to the bone or unusual bone development. Early in the disease, some X rays can show cartilage damage. In general, X rays are more useful later in the disease when bones may be affected.

Other diseases Because there are many causes of joint pain and swelling, the doctor must rule out other conditions before diagnosing JRA. These include physical injury, bacterial infection, Lyme disease, inflammatory bowel disease, lupus, dermatomyositis, and some forms of cancer. The doctor may use additional laboratory tests to help rule out these and other possible conditions.

Complications
The complications associated with JRA include loss of vision or decreased vision and total joint destruction of the major weight-bearing joints.

Treatment
The main goals of treatment are to preserve a high level of physical and social functioning and maintain a good quality of life. To achieve these goals, doctors recommend treatments to reduce swelling; maintain full movement in the affected joints; relieve pain; and identify, treat, and prevent complications. Most children with JRA need medication and physical therapy to reach these goals.

Several types of medication are available to treat JRA.

Nonsteroidal anti-inflammatory drugs (NSAIDs) Aspirin, ibuprofen (Motrin, Advil, Nuprin), and naproxen or naproxen sodium (Naprosyn, Aleve) are examples of NSAIDs. They are often the first type of medication used. Most doctors do not treat children with aspirin because of the possibility that it will cause bleeding problems, stomach upset, liver problems, or Reye's syndrome. For some children, though, aspirin in the correct dose (measured by blood test) can control JRA symptoms effectively with few serious side effects.

If the doctor prefers not to use aspirin, other NSAIDs are available. For example, in addition to those mentioned above, diclofenac and tolmetin are available with a doctor's prescription. Studies show that these medications are as effective as aspirin but with fewer side effects. An upset stomach is the most common complaint.

Disease-modifying antirheumatic drugs (DMARDs) If NSAIDs do not relieve symptoms of JRA, the doctor is likely to prescribe this type of medication. DMARDs slow the progression of JRA. However, because they take weeks or months to relieve symptoms, they are often taken with an NSAID. Various types of DMARDs are available. In the past, doctors prescribed hydroxychloroquine, oral and injectable gold, sulfasalazine, and d-penicillamine; however, doctors are now much more likely to use methotrexate for children with JRA.

Methotrexate Researchers have learned that this type of DMARD is safe and effective for some children with rheumatoid arthritis whose symptoms are not relieved by other medications. Because only small doses of methotrexate are needed to relieve arthritis symptoms, potentially dangerous side effects rarely occur. The most serious complication is liver damage, but it can be avoided with regular blood screening tests and doctor follow-ups. Careful monitoring for side effects is important for people taking methotrexate. When side effects are noticed early, the doctor can reduce the dose and eliminate side effects.

Corticosteroids   In children with very severe JRA, stronger medicines may be needed to stop serious symptoms such as inflammation of the sac around the heart (pericarditis). Corticosteroids like prednisone may be added to the treatment plan to control severe symptoms. This medication can be given either intravenously (directly into the vein) or by mouth. Corticosteroids can interfere with a child's normal growth and can cause other side effects, such as a round face, weakened bones, and increased susceptibility to infections. Once the medication controls severe symptoms, the doctor may reduce the dose gradually and eventually stop it completely. Because it can be dangerous to stop taking corticosteroids suddenly, the patient must carefully follow the doctor's instructions about how to take or reduce the dose.

In addition to medications, physical therapy is an important part of a child's treatment plan. Exercise can help to maintain muscle tone and to preserve and recover the range of motion of the joints. A physical therapist can design an appropriate exercise program for a person with JRA. The physical therapist may also recommend using splints and other devices to keep joints growing evenly.

Although pain sometimes limits physical activity, exercise is important to reduce the symptoms of JRA and maintain function and range of motion of the joints. Most children with JRA can take part fully in physical activities and sports when their symptoms are under control. During a disease flare, however, the doctor may advise limiting certain activities depending on the joints involved. Once the flare is over, a child can start regular activities again. Swimming is particularly useful because it uses many joints and muscles without putting weight onto the joints.

Adams, B. S. "Juvenile Arthritis. More Common than you Think." *Michigan Medicine* 160, no. 3 (May–June 2001): 53–54.

National Institute of Arthritis and Musculoskeletal and Skin Diseases (NIAMS), National Institutes of Health. *Questions and Answers About Juvenile Rheumatoid Arthritis,* 2001.

Peacock, Judith. *Juvenile Arthritis (Perspectives on Disease and Illness).* Mankato, Minn.: Capstone Press, 2000.

Lambert-Eaton myasthia syndrome (LEMS) A rare disorder with symptoms very similar to those of MYASTHENIA GRAVIS. Muscle weakness is associated with disturbed communication between nerves and muscles. Unlike myasthenia gravis, where the neurotransmitter (the chemical that transmits impulses) is blocked because of antibodies to the receptors of the neurotransmitter (acetylcholine), Lambert-Eaton syndrome is caused by an insufficient release of neurotransmitter by the nerve cells. As muscle contraction is continued, the amount of neurotransmitter may build up in sufficient quantities and result in increased strength.

Reports show almost equal frequency in men and women, with it affecting primarily middle-aged and older adults. However, a few children younger than 17 years have been reported to have LEMS.

The true incidence of LEMS in the United States is unknown. Approximately 3 percent of patients with small-cell lung cancer are believed to be affected, or an estimated four per 1 million people in the U.S. This estimate does not consider the number of patients with LEMS who do not have small-cell lung carcinoma or any identifiable malignancy. About half the cases are associated with small-cell carcinoma of the lung. In fact, many malignancies may be involved, including such seemingly unrelated conditions as transitional-cell carcinoma of the bladder.

Causes

LEMS is the result of an autoimmune process in which antibodies develop to the voltage-gated calcium channels and impair the release of acetylcholine from the presynaptic terminal.

Clinical Features

Symptoms of LEMS include double vision, difficulty maintaining a steady gaze, swallowing diffi-

culty, a drooping head, poor posture, difficulty climbing stairs or lifting objects, needing help to get up out of a chair or bed, and difficulty talking or chewing. Although these symptoms are similar to those of myasthenia gravis, they will be less severe. There also may be muscle contractions or atrophy, fatigue, or facial paralysis. Any weakness or paralysis will improve with use of those muscles.

Complications

Difficulty breathing or swallowing.

Treatment

The goal of treatment is to improve muscle strength and treat tumors or other underlying disorders. Removing blood plasma and replacing it with fluid improves symptoms for some people. Prednisone or other medications that suppress the immune response may improve symptoms for some people. Other medications, with varying degrees of benefit include anticholinesterase medications such as Neostigmine or Pyridostigmine. Symptoms of Lambert-Eaton syndrome may improve with treatment, but not all people respond well to treatment.

lawsuits In a 1984 San Francisco case, a woman successfully sued Dow Corning, saying her silicone breast implants caused her several autoimmune disorders resulting in joint pains and chronic fatigue. The jury awarded her $211,000 in compensatory damages and $1.5 million in punitive damages. The evidence was then sealed by a court order.

In 1991, an Alabama jury awarded $5.4 million to a woman with breast implants who showed only preliminary symptoms of systemic autoimmune disease. Over the next seven years, more than 20,000 lawsuits were lodged against Dow Corning alone, plus many against other silicone implant manufacturers, with awards of as much as $30 million given out. More than 400,000 potential claims were facing the manufacturers, forcing Dow Corning to file for bankruptcy in 1995. Litigants claimed the implants had caused such autoimmune-related disorders as mixed connective-tissue disease, chronic fatigue, muscle pain, joint pain, atypical lupus, and multiple sclerosis-like symptoms.

During this time, several medical studies pointed away from such breast implant complications. In June 1994, *The New England Journal of Medicine* published a Mayo Clinic study that found no increased risk of connective-tissue disease and other disorders that were studied in women with silicone implants. The following year, the American College of Rheumatology issued a statement saying the evidence was "compelling" that implants did not cause systemic disease. In June 1995, the Harvard Nurses Epidemiologic Study was published in *The New England Journal of Medicine,* saying it found no increased risk of nor certain signs and symptoms of connective-tissue diseases in women with silicone implants. That was followed in 1997 by the American Academy of Neurology review of existing studies and report that "existing research shows no link between silicone breast implants and neurological disorders." In 1998, two large Scandinavian studies failed to show any link between silicone implants and neurological disease. Also during that year, a British panel of scientists reported no convincing evidence that implants cause disease.

Finally, in June 1999, after reviewing 17 broad epidemiological studies, examining other materials, and conducting public hearings, the U.S.'s most prestigious scientific organization, The Institute of Medicine (part of the National Academy of Sciences) released a 400-page report concluding that although silicone breast implants may cause local problems, such as hardening or scarring of breast tissue, they do not cause any systemic diseases such as lupus or rheumatoid arthritis.

leukocytes   The leukocytes, or white blood cells, defend the body against infecting organisms and foreign agents, both in the tissues and in the blood-stream itself. Human blood contains about 5,000 to 10,000 leukocytes per cubic millimeter; the number increases in the presence of infection. An extraordinary and prolonged proliferation of leukocytes is known as leukemia. This overproduction suppresses the production of normal blood cells. Conversely, a sharp decrease in the number of leukocytes (leukopenia) strips the blood of its defense against infection and is an equally serious condition. A dramatic fall in levels of certain white blood cells occurs in persons with AIDS. Leukocytes as well as erythrocytes are formed from stem cells in the bone marrow. Leukocytes have nuclei and are classified into two groups: granulocytes and agranulocytes.

leukoencephalitis, acute necrotizing hemorrhagic   A more rapid and severe onset variant of acute disseminated encephalomyelitis (ADEM) or postinfectious encephalitis, which is a demyelinating disease (neurological syndrome) that is thought to be of autoimmune origin. It usually occurs within two weeks after one of the childhood viral infections, such as measles or chicken pox, or following vaccination against rabies or smallpox. It affects mainly young adults and is the most severe form of demyelinating disease. It is frequently preceded by a respiratory infection. It has also been reported in association with chronic Epstein-Barr virus infection. Initial headaches, seizures, and drowsiness may progress to profound lethargy and even coma. Lesions are found in the white matter of the brain stem, cerebrum, and cerebellum and as a rule are asymmetric and few in number. Diagnosis is facilitated by CT scanning and MRI, which reveal the massive lesion in the cerebral white matter. Many cases terminate fatally in two or four days, but in others survival is longer. This is also known as Weston Hurst disease or Western Hurst syndrome.

Donnet, A., H. Dufour, D. Gambarelli, N. Bruder, J. F. Pellissier, and F. Grisoli. "Acute Weston Hurst Necrotizing Hemorrhagic Leukoencephalitis." *Revue Neurologique* 152, no. 12 (December 1996): 748–751.

lichen planus   An inflammatory autoimmune skin disease that affects the eyes, the skin, and the

mucosa lining of the mouth and genitalia. It may occur alone or with other autoimmune diseases, such as ocular cicatricial pemphigoid, an autoimmune eye disease; lupus, a systemic autoimmune disease that can involve any part or organ of the body; and sarcoidosis, also a systemic autoimmune disease. The disease is characterized by recurring inflammatory and itchy blisterlike eruptions on the skin or in the mucosa linings.

Lichen planus is not uncommon, accounting for approximately 5 percent of patients seen in an oral medicine clinic and about 1 percent of the general population. It usually affects persons between the ages of 30 to 65, although it can occur in children. It appears equally in males and females and in all races.

In most patients, the first attack may last several weeks or months, then clear up, but return within one or two years. Occasionally, it may become chronic and even disabling because of extreme itching and repetitious sores causing erosion of tissue and eventually disfigurement.

Causes

The exact cause is unknown, but lichen planus is believed to be related to an allergic or immune reaction. It has been known to develop after exposure to potential allergens such as medications, dyes, and other chemical substances. Symptoms increase with emotional stress, possibly because of changes in the immune system during stress. It also frequently occurs along with other disorders, most notably hepatitis C.

Clinical Features

Lichen planus presents as bumps that are reddish purple and flat across the top. They may appear anywhere on the body, but most usually locate on the inside of the wrists and ankles. There may be thick patches of these bumps wherever they occur, and the itching will range from mild to severe. Although the distinctive appearance of these lesions makes lichen planus relatively easy to recognize, the doctor or dentist may choose to confirm the diagnosis via a skin biopsy.

Complications

Oral lichen planus can lead to poor dental hygiene and gum disease. Long-standing mouth ulcers may develop into oral cancer. In some cases, changes will occur in the nails because of damage to the nail root. These changes include grooving, ridges, splitting, and thinning in a few fingernails or toenails; rarely, all nails are affected.

Treatment

At times, lichen planus of the skin will cause little problem and resolve itself with no treatment within two years. However, many times the itching is severe enough to require attention. Because no cure is known for lichen planus, any treatment is intended only to relieve the itching and to speed healing of the rash. If a medication can be determined to be triggering the outbreaks, identifying and discontinuing that medication usually clears up the condition within a few weeks.

Because every case of lichen planus is different, no one treatment will always work. Antihistamines may reduce discomfort. Anesthetic mouth washes may numb the area temporarily and make eating more comfortable if mouth lesions are present. Topical corticosteroids (such as triamcinolone acetonide cream) or oral corticosteroids (such as prednisone) are prescribed to reduce inflammation and suppress the immune/allergic response. Corticosteroids may be injected directly into a lesion. Topical retinoic acid (vitamin A) cream and other anti-inflammatory or antipruritic ointments or creams may reduce itching and inflammation and may aid healing. Ultraviolet light therapy may be beneficial in more severe cases.

Most cases clear up within 18 months. About one in five will reappear later.

Bhattacharya, M., I. Kaur, B. Kumar. "Lichen Planus: A Clinical and Epidemiological Study." *The Journal of Dermatology* 27, no. 9 (September 2000): 576–582.

Thornhill, M. H. "Immune Mechanisms in Oral Lichen Planus." *Acta Odontologica Scandinavica* 59, no. 3 (June 2001): 174–177.

Tosti, A., B. M. Piraccini, S. Cambiaghi, and M. Jorizzo. "Nail Lichen Planus in Children: Clinical Features, Response to Treatment, and Long-Term Follow-Up." *Archives of Dermatology* 137, no. 8 (August 2001): 1,027–1,052.

life expectancy The number of years that an average person of a given age may be expected to live. A few autoimmune diseases can significantly shorten one's life expectancy. For example, when autoimmune HEPATITIS escalates to cirrhosis of the liver, it can shorten the patient's life expectancy to 10 years. In most cases, though, because of increased knowledge about the diseases and their complications, autoimmune patients can expect close to a normal life span.

- Life expectancy for people with INSULIN-DEPENDENT DIABETES mellitus is shortened by an average of 15 years.
- Male RHEUMATOID ARTHRITIS (RA) suffers experience a reduced life expectancy of seven years; females with RA have a reduced life expectancy of three years.
- The prognosis for patients with SYSTEMIC LUPUS ERYTHEMATOSUS has greatly improved over the last few decades with at least 80 percent to 90 percent of all patients surviving 10 years. Thereafter, life expectancy approximates that of age-matched controls. According to the Lupus Foundation of Minnesota, with early diagnosis, appropriate medical care, and certain (often minor) lifestyle adjustments, the vast majority of individuals with lupus can expect to have a reasonably "normal" life expectancy. Lupus Canada adds that better methods of diagnosis, treatment, and follow-up have improved the life expectancy of lupus patients so that nowadays, lupus is seldom seen to be fatal.
- Most people with MULTIPLE SCLEROSIS (MS) now have a near-normal life expectancy, although this has not always been the case. Life expectancy from time of diagnosis has increased over time as management and control of complications improved. According to the National Women's Health Information Center, average life expectancy is 35 years after onset of symptoms. Most people with MS can function effectively; however, a rare form of acute MS can be fatal within weeks.
- Although MYASTHENIA GRAVIS (MG) can be fatal if a respiratory crisis is not immediately treated, normal life expectancy is the rule with proper treatment.

lymph   A transparent, slightly yellow fluid that carries lymphocytes, bathes the body tissues, and drains into the lymphatic vessels.

lymphatic organs   See LYMPHOID ORGANS.

lymphatic vessels   A body-wide network of channels, similar to the blood vessels, that transport lymph to the immune organs and into the bloodstream.

lymph glands   A popular name for LYMPH NODES.

lymph nodes   Small, bean-shaped organs of the immune system, distributed widely throughout the body, and linked by lymphatic vessels. Lymph nodes are garrisons of B, T, and other immune cells, and connect to each other via small channels called lymphatics.

The lymph nodes filter lymph fluid as it flows through them, trapping bacteria, viruses, and other foreign substances, which are then destroyed by special white blood cells called lymphocytes. Lymph nodes may be found singly or in groups. They may be as small as the head of a pin or as large as an olive. Groups of lymph nodes can be felt in the neck, groin, and underarms. Many lymph nodes in the body cannot be felt.

When a part of the body is infected, the nearby lymph nodes become swollen as they collect and destroy the infecting organisms. For example, if a person has a throat infection, the lymph nodes in the neck may swell and become tender.

lymphocytes   Small white blood cells produced in the lymphoid organs and paramount in the immune defenses. Under normal conditions, lymphocytes make up about 20 percent to 35 percent of all white cells but multiply rapidly in the face of infection. There are two basic types of lymphocytes: the B cells and the T cells. B cells tend to migrate into the connective tissue, where they develop into plasma cells that produce highly specific antibodies against foreign antigens (bacteria and toxins). Other B cells act as memory cells, ready for subsequent infection by the same organism. Some T lymphocytes kill invading cells directly; others interact with other immune system cells, regulating the immune response.

lymphoid organs   The organs of the immune system, where lymphocytes develop and congregate. They include the bone marrow, thymus, lymph nodes, spleen, and various other clusters of lymphoid tissue. The blood vessels and lymphatic vessels can also be considered lymphoid organs.

lymphokines   Powerful chemical substances secreted by lymphocytes. These soluble molecules help direct and regulate the immune responses.

lymph system   This system is made up of lymph nodes, the thymus in the first several decades of life, the lymphatic channels, lymphatic tissue of the marrow, the gastrointestinal tract, the skin, and the spleen. It also includes the T, B, and NK (natural killer) lymphocytes contained in those sites. It carries fluid (LYMPH), nutrients, and waste materials between the body tissues and the bloodstream. The lymphatic system is also an important part of the immune system, the body's defense system against disease.

macrophage A large and versatile immune cell that acts as a microbe-devouring phagocyte, an antigen-presenting cell, and an important source of immune secretions. Macrophages have the ability to recognize and ingest foreign antigens through receptors on the surface of their cell membranes.

major histocompatibility complex (MHC) A group of genes that controls several aspects of the immune response. MHC genes code for self markers on all body cells.

mast cell A granule-containing cell found in most body tissues but especially numerous in connective tissue, the innermost layer of the skin, and mucosal membranes of the respiratory system. The contents of mast cells, along with those of basophils, are responsible for the symptoms of allergy by making and releasing histamine and other mediators of inflammation.

Medicare/Medicaid Medicare and Medicaid, enacted as Title XIX of the Social Security Act in 1965, originally provided health care coverage to Americans over the age of 65. In 1972, Medicare was expanded to Americans living with disabilities. The joint federal-state Medicaid program provides health care coverage to low-income families with children under 21. These programs were administered by the Social Security Administration until 1977. That year, Medicare and Medicaid were transferred to the Department of Health and Human Services and to the Health Care Financing Administration (HCFA). In 1997, the State Children's Health Insurance Program (SCHIP) was included in the Balanced Budget Act.

In June 2001, as part of a package of reforms, HCFA was renamed the Centers for Medicare & Medicaid Services and refocused along its three primary lines of service: the Center for Medicare Management, Center for Beneficiary Choices, and the Center for Medicaid and State Operations.

Medicare

Medicare is an insurance program. Under the program, medical bills are paid from trust funds to which those covered have contributed. Medicare primarily serves people over 65, whatever their income, and younger disabled people and dialysis patients. Patients pay some costs through deductibles for hospital and other expenses. Small monthly premiums are required for nonhospital coverage. A federal program, Medicare coverage is basically the same everywhere in the United States. The Medicare 800 number (1-800-633-4227) provides service to beneficiaries 24 hours a day, seven days a week.

In 2002, the Centers for Medicare & Medicaid Services announced that Medicare will cover intravenous immune globulin treatments for some patients with five autoimmune mucocutaneous blistering diseases.

Medicaid

Medicaid is an assistance program. Medical bills are paid from federal, state, and local taxes. Medicaid assists low-income people of every age. Patients usually do not have to pay for authorized medical expenses. A small copayment is sometimes required. Within broad national guidelines, which the federal government provides, each of the states establishes its own eligibility standards; determines the type, amount, duration, and scope of services; sets the rate of payment for services; and administers its own program. Thus, the Medicaid program varies considerably from state to state, as well as within each state over time.

medication compliance The term refers to the extent to which a patient adheres to instructions regarding taking medication, including dosage, timing, and duration. Noncompliance is a problem with many sufferers of chronic illnesses, such as of autoimmune diseases, and may lead to worsening symptoms, hospitalization, and death.

Prescription drugs are a cornerstone of disease treatment; however, their effectiveness relies on reasonably good compliance with the prescribed regimen. That compliance is often lacking, according to studies, which have shown that only one in three patients stays on their correct drug regimen. Patients miss doses, fail to take their medicine as directed, or stop taking their medicine completely once they "feel better," despite directions to continue taking the medicine. Research has found that in the United States, noncompliance with prescription medication causes 125,000 deaths and costs an estimated $75.6 billion yearly.

Among the reasons patients give for not following physician or label directions are that the medication is not alleviating the symptoms; it is causing unpleasant side effects; or it is inconvenient to take, such as when traveling, at work, or on vacation. The patient sometimes decides he or she feels well enough not to take the medication any longer. Often, the medicine causes discomfort, such as insulin shots for diabetes. Studies have indicated that new drugs requiring less frequent administration may improve compliance.

Compliance is particularly important in the management of diseases such as RHEUMATOID ARTHRITIS (RA), in which the treatment options are heavily oriented toward medication therapies. Physicians must place extra emphasis on educating RA patients about the proper use of a medication—what to expect from the drug and in what time frame. Patients must inform their doctors if a drug is not working for them or if they are experiencing side effects, so the doctor can determine whether an alternate drug should be prescribed. It is especially important that RA patients

not stop taking medications simply because they are feeling better, because arthritis medications are usually prescribed for long-term and continuous use.

medications and autoimmune diseases Because the actual cause of autoimmune diseases is unknown, specific treatments have not been found to cure them. Instead, doctors help patients manage their diseases with various medications aimed at treating the symptoms that beset autoimmune patients.

In some diseases, such as lupus or rheumatoid arthritis, medication can occasionally slow, perhaps even stop, the immune system's destruction of the kidneys or joints. Medications or therapies that slow or suppress the immune system response in an attempt to stop the inflammation involved in the autoimmune attack are called immunosuppressive medications. These drugs include corticosteroids (prednisone), methotrexate, cyclophosphamide, azathioprine, and cyclosporin. Unfortunately, these medications also suppress the ability of the immune system to fight infection, among other severe side effects. Because of this potential for medication-caused complications, it is important for patients to keep their physicians informed of any additional problems or symptoms that might be caused by medications.

In some patients, a limited number of immunosuppressive medications may result in disease remission (abatement of a disease for a significant amount of time). Even if their disease goes into remission, patients are advised to discontinue taking their medication. The possibility that the disease may restart when medication is discontinued must be balanced with the long-term side effects from the immunosuppressive medication.

Medical scientists are striving to develop medications that produce remissions with fewer side effects. Much current research is focused on developing therapies that target various steps in the immune response. Ultimately, medical science's goal is to develop therapies that prevent autoimmune diseases. To this end, a significant amount of time and resources are spent studying the immune system and pathways of inflammation.

National Institutes of Health. "Understanding Autoimmune Disease," NIH Publication No. 98-4273, May 1998.

medication interactions   The combined effect of taking many medications at the same time or with other substances, such as food or alcohol. Certain combinations of medications may cause results different from any of the individual medications being taken alone. For example, one medication might reduce or increase the effects of another drug; two medications taken together may produce a new and dangerous interaction; or two similar medications taken together may produce an effect that is greater than would be expected from taking just one of the medications. Some medications work well with other medications (are synergistic); other combinations can be dangerous, even deadly.

Autoimmune patients may take several medications each day, and the chances of developing undesired drug interactions increase rapidly with each additional medication taken. According to *Taber's® Cyclopedic Medical Dictionary,* when eight or more medications are being taken, there is a 100 percent chance of interaction.

At times physicians may intentionally prescribe combinations of drugs to take advantage of their interactions in order to increase the effectiveness of treatment. Many medication interactions, however, are not planned and only serve to reduce the expected benefit or to cause adverse reactions.

Autoimmune patients who are on long-term or lifelong medication regimes often carry warning cards or bracelets to alert others, in the case of an emergency, to what medications the patient is currently taking. An example of this is the diabetes patient on insulin.

In addition to prescription medications, over-the-counter medications can interact with each other and with prescription medication. Examples include:

Antacids can interfere with drug absorption of antibiotics (i.e., tetracycline), thereby reducing the effectiveness of the drug in fighting infection.
Antihistamines, often used for allergies and colds, can increase the sedative effects of barbiturates, tranquilizers, and some prescription pain relievers.
Iron supplements taken with antibiotics can reduce or stop the ability of the antibiotics to fight infection. (The chemicals in the supplement and the antibiotic bind together in the stomach, instead of being absorbed into the bloodstream.)

Many medications can interact with alcohol. Alcohol-medication interactions are estimated to be a factor in at least 25 percent of all emergency-room admissions. In their publication *Alcohol Alert,* the National Institute on Alcohol Abuse and Alcoholism lists several specific interactions. Examples include

Antibiotics are used to treat autoimmune diseases such as BULLOUS PEMPHIGOID and CICATRICIAL PEMPHIGOID. In combination with acute alcohol consumption, some antibiotics may cause nausea, vomiting, headache, and possibly convulsions; among these antibiotics are furazolidone (Furoxone), griseofulvin (Grisactin and others), metronidazole (Flagyl), and the antimalarial quinacrine (Atabrine).
Antidiabetic medications. Oral hypoglycemic drugs are prescribed to help lower blood sugar levels in some patients with diabetes. Acute alcohol consumption prolongs, and chronic alcohol consumption decreases, the availability of tolbutamide (Orinase). Alcohol also interacts with some drugs of this class to produce symptoms of nausea and headache such as those described for metronidazole.

When medications and certain foods are taken at the same time, they can interact in ways that diminish the effectiveness of the ingested drug or reduce the absorption of food nutrients. Additionally, vitamin and herbal supplements taken with prescribed medication can result in adverse reactions. According to the Ohio State University Extension Senior Series, some examples of how foods and drugs can interact include the following:

• Speeding or slowing the action of a medication
• Impaired absorption of vitamins and minerals in the body

- Stimulation or suppression of the appetite
- Altering how nutrients are used in the body
- Interactions, caused by herbs, with anesthesia, beta-blockers, and anticoagulants

(See also EMERGENCY MEDICAL IDENTIFICATION.)

Copies of the *Alcohol Alert* are available free of charge from the Scientific Communications Branch, Office of Scientific Affairs, NIAAA, Willco Building, Suite 409, 6000 Executive Boulevard, Bethesda, MD 20892-7003. Telephone: (301) 443-3860.
Ohio State University Extension, Ohio Department of Aging. *Adverse Drug-Drug and Food-Drug Medication Interactions,* Senior Series #SS-129-97-R02, 2001.

men and autoimmune diseases   Overall, men contract autoimmune diseases at only about one-quarter the rate of women. Yet CARDIOMYOPATHY, CHRONIC INFLAMMATORY DEMYELINATING POLYNEU-ROPATHY, INCLUSION BODY MYOSITIS, and REITER'S SYN-DROME are more common in men. Other differences also exist between men and women in specific diseases. For example, men with multiple sclerosis begin to show symptoms later than women with the disease do. At the same time, the disease seems to progress faster in men than in women. Women tend to develop lupus during their childbearing years, while men are affected much later in life.

memory cell   An immune cell that responds immediately when it meets an antigen for the first time but then reverts to a small resting cell. When it is exposed to the antigen a second time, the memory cell does recognize it and starts an immune response.

Ménière's disease   A recurrent abnormality of the inner ear causing a usually progressive group of symptoms. These include vertigo or severe dizziness, tinnitus or a roaring sound in the ears, fluctuating hearing loss, and the sensation of pressure or pain in the affected ear. The disorder usually affects only one ear and is a common cause of hearing loss. Named after French physician Prosper Ménière who first described the syndrome in 1861, Ménière's disease is now also referred to as endolymphatic hydrops.

Based on a recent study, the National Institute on Deafness and Other Communication Disorders (NIDCD) estimates that currently approximately 615,000 individuals are with diagnosed Ménière's disease in the United States and 45,500 new cases are diagnosed each year. The disease occurs more frequently in males than in females, with the onset usually after the age of 50.

Causes
The cause of Ménière's disease is unknown, although edema, or swelling, of the membranous labyrinth has been found. Other possible causes are disturbance of the autonomic regulation of the endolymphatic system, local allergy of the inner ear, and vascular disturbance of a layer of fibrous vascular tissue covering the outer wall of the cochlear duct. Stress and emotional disturbances seem to contribute to attacks.

Many experts on Ménière's disease think that a rupture of the membranous labyrinth allows the endolymph to mix with perilymph, another inner ear fluid that occupies the space between the membranous labyrinth and the bony inner ear. This mixing, scientists believe, can cause the symptoms of Ménière's disease. Scientists are investigating several possible causes of the disease, including environmental factors, such as noise pollution and viral infections, as well as biological factors.

Clinical Features
The symptoms of Ménière's disease occur suddenly and can arise daily or as infrequently as once a year. Vertigo, often the most debilitating symptom of Ménière's disease, forces the sufferer to lie down. Vertigo attacks can lead to severe nausea, vomiting, and sweating and often come with little or no warning. Sometimes Ménière's disease can occur without vertigo. In this type of the disorder, the endolymphatic distension is limited to the cochlea, the snailshell-like spiral tube in the inner ear.

Some individuals with Ménière's disease have attacks that start with tinnitus, a loss of hearing, or a full feeling or pressure in the affected ear. It is important to remember that all of these symptoms are unpredictable. Typically, the attack is characterized by a combination of vertigo, tinnitus, and hearing loss lasting several hours. However, people experience these discomforts at varying frequencies, durations, and intensities. Some may feel slight vertigo a few times a year. Others may be occasionally disturbed by intense, uncontrollable tinnitus while sleeping. Still other Ménière's disease sufferers may notice a hearing loss and feel unsteady all day long for prolonged periods. Other occasional symptoms of Ménière's disease include headaches, abdominal discomfort, and diarrhea. A person's hearing tends to recover between attacks but over time becomes worse.

Properly diagnosing Ménière's disease entails several procedures. These include a medical history interview and a physical examination by a physician; hearing and balance tests; and medical imaging with magnetic resonance imaging (MRI). Accurate measurement and characterization of hearing loss are of critical importance in diagnosing Ménière's disease.

Through the use of several types of hearing tests, physicians can characterize hearing loss as being sensory, arising from the inner ear, or neural, arising from the hearing nerve. An auditory brain stem response, which measures electrical activity in the hearing nerve and brain stem, is useful in differentiating between these two types of hearing loss. Under certain circumstances, electrocochleography, recording the electrical activity of the inner ear in response to sound, helps confirm the diagnosis.

To test the vestibular or balance system, physicians irrigate the ears with warm and cool water. This flooding of the ears, known as caloric testing, results in nystagmus, rapid eye movements that can help a physician analyze a balance disorder. Because tumor growth can produce symptoms similar to Ménière's disease, magnetic resonance imaging is a useful test to determine whether a tumor is causing the patient's vertigo and hearing loss.

Treatment

No cure exists for Ménière's disease. Medical and behavioral therapy, however, are often helpful in managing its symptoms. Although many operations have been developed to reverse the disease process, their value has been difficult to establish.

Unfortunately, all operations on the ear carry a risk of hearing loss.

The most commonly performed surgical treatment for Ménière's disease is the insertion of a shunt, a tiny silicone tube that is positioned in the inner ear to drain off excess fluid.

In another more reliable operation is a vestibular neurectomy. In it, the vestibular nerve, which affect balance, is severed so that it no longer sends distorted messages to the brain. However, this balance nerve is very close to the hearing and facial nerves. Thus, the risk of affecting a patient's hearing or facial muscle control increases with this type of surgical treatment. Also, older patients often have difficulty recovering from this type of surgery.

A labyrinthectomy, the removal of the membranous labyrinth, is an irreversible procedure that is often successful in eliminating the dizziness associated with Ménière's disease. This procedure, however, results in a total loss of hearing in the operated ear—an important consideration since the second ear may one day be affected. Also, labyrinthectomies themselves may result in other balance problems.

Some physicians recommend a change of diet to help control Ménière's symptoms. Eliminating caffeine, alcohol, and salt may relieve the frequency and intensity of attacks in some people. Eliminating tobacco use and reducing stress levels may lessen the severity of the symptoms. Additionally, medications that control allergies, reduce fluid retention, or improve blood circulation in the inner ear may also help.

National Institute on Deafness and Other Communication Disorders, National Institutes of Health. *Because You Asked About Ménière's Disease,* NIH Publication No. 98-3404. July 1998, updated April 1999.

menopause Menopause may have a connection, either directly or indirectly, to several autoimmune diseases. Several reports have suggested that early menopause (which occurs in about 1 percent of women) has a strong positive association with autoimmunity. Approximately 20 percent to 40 percent of women with premature menopause (ovarian failure before age 40) also have autoimmune disorders, particularly autoimmune thyroid disease. In addition, circulating anti-ovarian autoantibodies have been observed with greater frequency among people who have experienced premature ovarian failure compared with healthy control subjects, even though they had no evidence of overt autoimmune disease. Still to be determined is whether the clustering of autoimmune diseases within individuals is an independent risk factor for earlier menopause. Among other autoimmune diseases that seem to be affected by menopause:

- It is common for SJÖGREN'S DISEASE to be misdiagnosed as allergies, aging, or symptoms of menopause.

- As a result of the Familial Autoimmune and Diabetes (FAD) Study, Dorman et al. determined that women with Type 1 diabetes (INSULIN-DEPENDENT DIABETES) were more likely to experience menopause at a younger age.

- Onset of RHEUMATOID ARTHRITIS tends occur later in life, with a peak around the age of menopause, when estrogen levels decline. However, the incidence rates for men and women become similar around the age of menopause, suggesting that aging is a more critical factor than hormone changes.

- Estrogen in the form of hormone replacement at menopause has been reported to exacerbate SYSTEMIC LUPUS ERYTHEMATOSUS (SLE) activity, but there are differing opinions on whether estrogen does indeed affect SLE. Similarly, there is a lack of clarity regarding the effects of estrogen on rheumatoid arthritis. There is no significant information on the effects of estrogen on other autoimmune diseases.

Dorman J. S., A. R. Steenkiste, T. P. Foley, E. S. Strotmeyer, J. P. Burke, L. H. Kuller, and C. K. Kwoh. "Menopause in Type 1 Diabetic Women: Is It Premature?" *Diabetes* 50, no. 8 (August 2001): 1,857–1,862.
"Hormones & Autoimmunity." *InFocus,* American Autoimmune Related Diseases Association, Inc. (AARDA). Available online. URL: http://www.aarda.org/hormone_art2.html. Downloaded on 18 July 2002.

menstruation Several autoimmune diseases can contribute to menstrual problems:

- Women with Type 1 diabetes (INSULIN-DEPENDENT DIABETES) have a delayed onset of menstruation and a greater prevalence of menstrual disorders than women without diabetes.

- In ADDISON'S DISEASE, menstrual periods may become irregular or stop.

- Patients with CELIAC DISEASE may experience missed menstrual periods (often because of excessive weight loss).

- Patients with HASHIMOTO'S THYROIDITIS may present with increased menstrual flow.

- Women with autoimmune HEPATITIS may stop having menstrual periods.

- Women with INTERSTITIAL CYSTITIS often have symptoms that get worse during menstruation.

microbes Minute living organisms, including bacteria, viruses, fungi, and protozoa.

mixed connective tissue disease (MCTD) A chronic inflammatory autoimmune disease. The term MCTD is used to describe overlapping groups of connective tissue disorders that cannot be diagnosed in more precise terms. Whether MCTD should be considered a distinct clinical entity is still a matter of debate. Diagnosis of MCTD as a different entity from lupus or rheumatoid arthritis is difficult. The syndrome is characterized by joint pain; muscle weakness; cardiac, lung and skin manifestations; kidney disease; and dysfunction of the esophagus. It is also referred to as undifferentiated connective tissue disease.

Mixed connective tissue disease can occur at any age, with the average age of onset in the third decade. Eight out of 10 patients are women. The disease occurs in all races and is found worldwide.

First described as a separate disease in 1972, mixed connective tissue disease has been used to cover those incidences of connective tissue disease that do not meet the criteria of any other specific connective tissue diseases. For example, when inheritance can be ruled out as a definite cause (as in Marfan's syndrome and Ehlers-Danlos syndrome) and when the classic connective tissue autoimmune diseases (systemic lupus erythematosus, rheumatoid arthritis, sclero-derma, polymyositis, and dermatomyositis), which have specific presentations and diagnostics, are not apparent but some of their characteristics are present, the doctor will usually refer to the condition as mixed or undifferentiated connective tissue disease. In some cases the individual's symptoms will gradually change until one of the classic diseases emerges as a full-blown disease. In other cases, the undifferentiated connective tissue disease may never develop into a fully definable condition.

Clinical Features

Diagnosis of actual mixed connective tissue disease is made when the patient exhibits features that overlap the classical autoimmune connective tissue diseases plus has high quantities of antinuclear antibodies and antibodies to ribonucleoprotein in his or her blood but does not have the antibodies that characterize systemic lupus erythematosus and scleroderma.

Treatment

Treatment of mixed connective tissue disease will generally be based on those features causing the symptoms and will generally use anti-inflammatory and immunosuppressive drugs to suppress the inflammation present in the tissues. These drugs include nonsteroidal anti-inflammatory drugs (NSAIDs), glucocorticosteroids (prednisone), and cytotoxic drugs (methotrexate, azathioprine, and cyclophosphamide).

molecular biology   The branch of biology that deals with the formation, structure, and function of macromolecules essential to life, such as nucleic acids and proteins, particularly as to their role in cell replication and the transmission of genetic information. Thus, molecular biologists are involved in the manipulation of DNA so that it can be sequenced or mutated.

molecule   The smallest amount of a specific chemical substance that can exist alone. (To break a molecule down into its constituent atoms is to change its character. A molecule of water, for instance, reverts to oxygen and hydrogen.)

monoclonal antibodies   Antibodies produced by a single cell or its identical progeny, specific for a given antigen. As a tool for binding to specific protein molecules, monoclonal antibodies are invaluable in research, medicine, and industry.

monocyte   A large phagocytic white blood cell that, when it enters tissue, develops into a macrophage.

monokines   Powerful chemical substances secreted by monocytes and macrophages. These soluble molecules help direct and regulate the immune responses.

Mooren's ulcer (MU)   A painful, relentless, chronic, but rare, peripheral lesion developing in the cornea of the eye. It is idiopathic, meaning it occurs in the complete absence of any diagnosable systemic disorder that could be responsible for the progressive destruction of the cornea. Mooren's ulcer typically occurs in healthy, adult men; however, it can occur at any age and in both sexes.

Mooren's ulcer was first described by Bowman in 1849 and McKenzie in 1854 as "chronic serpiginous ulcer of the cornea." It was the German opthalmologist Mooren, however, who first published several cases of this condition in 1863 and who was also the first to describe this corneal condition clearly and define it as a clinical entity.

Causes

The precise root cause of Mooren's ulcer remains unknown. However, evidence suggests that it is an autoimmune process, with both cell-mediated and humoral components. Plasma cells, neutrophils, mast cells, and eosinophils have been found in the involved areas. Researchers still do not know if cell-mediated and/or humoral immune mechanisms are involved directly in the origin or development of MU; they may simply accompany the corneal destruction that is caused by another mechanism. Scientists think that the conjunctiva adjacent to the ulcer contains inflammatory cells that may produce antibodies against the cornea and cytokines, which amplify the inflammation and recruit additional inflammatory cells.

Johns Hopkins researchers found a previously unknown protein in the eye that leads to "melt-down" of the cornea. The Hopkins team found evidence that part of the protein CO-Ag may resemble the surfaces of certain bacteria or viruses. Their belief is that in Mooren's ulcer, this similarity apparently fools the immune system into mistaking the protein for a germ. In the resulting attack on the protein, the cornea is destroyed. The researchers hope this finding will help them determine the cause of MU and why only certain groups of people get it.

Clinical Features

Patients with Mooren's ulcer typically present with redness and tearing of the eye as well as intolerance of light, but pain is the most outstanding feature. The pain is often incapacitating and may be out of proportion to the inflammation. There may be a decrease in visual acuity. Its most unique characteristics, according to Foster, "Include the 'eating away' of cornea central to the most obvious crescent or epithelial defect and stromal melting, likened to the gnawing away of tissue that perhaps one could visualize as having been accomplished by a rodent (hence the name in some circles as corneal ulcer rodens)."

Complications

Complications from MU may include iritis, hypopyon, glaucoma, and cataract. Perforation may occur in 35 percent to 40 percent of cases, often associated with minor trauma to the weakened cornea.

Treatment

Topical steroids (prednisolone acetate or prednisolone phosphate 1 percent) are the initial treatments of choice. Oral pulse therapy (prednisone) is often used when topical therapy is ineffective or not possible. Therapeutic soft contact lens or patching of the eye may be helpful in the beginning. If the ulcer progresses despite the steroid regimen, any of various types of eye surgery may be performed. According to Nguyen, cryotherapy, conjunctival resection, and thermocoagulation have all been found to give some relief at the site of the ulcers, but recurrence can occur at the same or other sites.

Cases of bilateral or progressive MU that fail to respond to therapeutic steroids and conjunctival resection will require systemic cytotoxic chemotherapy to bring a halt to the progressive corneal destruction. Nguyen wrote, "At the Immunology and Uveitis Service at the Massachusetts Eye and Ear Infirmary, we believe that the evidence for the efficacy of systemic immunosuppressive chemotherapy for progressive bilateral MU is quite strong, and that such treatment should be employed sooner rather than later in the care of such patients, before the corneal destruction has become too extensive to need surgery."

Bowman, W. *The Parts Concerned in the Operations of the Eye.* Cited by E. Nettleship in "Chronic Serpiginous Ulcer of the Cornea (Mooren's Ulcer)." *Transactions of the Ophthalmological Societies of the United Kingdom* 22:103–104, 1902.

Chow, C., and C. S. Foster. "Mooren's Ulcer." *International Ophthalmology Clinics* 36 (1996): 1–13.

Foster, C. Stephen. *Mooren's Ulcer.* Boston, Mass.: Massachusetts Eye and Ear Infirmary Immunological Service, 1998.

McKenzie, H. *Disease of the Eye.* 1854, p. 631.

Mooren, A. "Ulcus Rodens." *Ophthalmiatrische Beobachtungen.* (1867) 107–110.

Nguyen, Quan Dong. *Mooren's Ulcer: Diagnosis and Management.* Boston, Mass.: Massachusetts Eye and Ear Infirmary Immunology Service, 1997.

Watson, P. G. "Management of Mooren's Ulceration." *Eye* 11 (1997): 349–356.

multiple sclerosis (MS)   A lifelong chronic disease diagnosed primarily in young adults. During an MS attack, inflammation occurs in areas of the white matter of the central nervous system (nerve fibers that are the site of multiple sclerosis lesions) in random patches called plaques. This process is followed by destruction of myelin, which insulates nerve cell fibers in the brain and spinal cord. Myelin facilitates the smooth, high-speed transmission of electrochemical messages between the brain, the spinal cord, and the rest of the body. When it is damaged, neurological transmission of messages may be slowed or blocked completely, leading to diminished or lost function. The name *multiple sclerosis* signifies both the number (multiple) and condition (sclerosis, from the Greek term for scarring or hardening) of the demyelinated areas in the central nervous system.

Although multiple sclerosis was first diagnosed in 1849, the earliest known description of a person with possible MS dates from 14th-century Holland. An unpredictable disease, MS can range from relatively benign to somewhat disabling to devastating as communication between the brain and other parts of the body is disrupted.

The vast majority of patients are mildly affected. However, in the worst cases, multiple sclerosis can render a person unable to write, speak, or walk. A physician can diagnose MS in some patients soon after the onset of the illness. In others, however, physicians may not be able to identify the cause of the symptoms readily, leading to years of uncertainty and multiple diagnoses punctuated by baffling symptoms that mysteriously wax and wane.

No one knows exactly how many people have multiple sclerosis. It is believed that, currently, there are approximately 250,000 to 350,000 people in the United States with MS diagnosed by a physician. This estimate suggests that approximately 200 new cases are diagnosed each week.

Most people experience their first symptoms of multiple sclerosis between the ages of 20 and 40, but a diagnosis is often delayed. This is due to both the transitory nature of the disease and the lack of a specific diagnostic test—specific symptoms and changes in the brain must develop before the diagnosis is confirmed.

Although scientists have documented cases of MS in young children and elderly adults, symptoms rarely begin before age 15 or after age 60. Whites are more than twice as likely as other races to develop MS. In general, women are affected at almost twice the rate of men. However, among patients who develop the symptoms of MS at a later age, the gender ratio is more balanced.

MS is five times more prevalent in temperate climates—such as those found in the northern United States, Canada, and Europe—than in tropical regions. Furthermore, the age of 15 seems to be significant in terms of risk for developing the disease. Some studies indicate that a person moving from a high-risk (temperate) to a low-risk (tropical) area before the age of 15 tends to adopt the risk (in this case, low) of the new area and vice versa. Other studies suggest that people moving after age 15 maintain the risk of the area where they grew up.

These findings indicate a strong role for an environmental factor in the cause of multiple sclerosis. It is possible that at the time of or immediately following puberty, patients acquire an infection with a long latency period. Conversely, people in some areas may come into contact with an unknown protective agent during the time before puberty. Other studies suggest that the unknown geographic or climatic element may actually be simply a matter of genetic predilection and reflect racial and ethnic susceptibility factors.

Periodically, scientists receive reports of MS clusters. The most famous of these MS "epidemics" took place in the Faeroe Islands north of Scotland in the years following the arrival of British troops during World War II.

Despite intense study of this and other clusters, no direct environmental factor has been identified. Nor has any definitive evidence been found to link daily stress to MS attacks, although evidence indicates that the risk of worsening is greater after acute viral illnesses.

Clinical Features

Symptoms of MS may be mild or severe, may be of long duration or short, and may appear in various combinations, depending on the area of the nervous system affected. Complete or partial remission of symptoms, especially in the early stages of the disease, occurs in approximately 70 percent of MS patients.

The initial symptom of MS is often blurred or double vision, red-green color distortion, or even blindness in one eye. Inexplicably, visual problems tend to clear up in the later stages of MS. Inflammatory problems of the optic nerve may be diagnosed as retrobulbar or optic neuritis. Fifty-five percent of MS patients will have an attack of optic neuritis at some time or other, and it will be the first symptom of MS in approximately 15 percent. This has led to the general recognition of optic neuritis as an early sign of MS, especially if tests also reveal abnormalities in the patient's spinal fluid.

Most MS patients experience muscle weakness in their extremities and difficulty with coordination and balance at some time during the course of the disease. These symptoms may be severe enough to impair walking or even standing. In the worst cases, MS can produce partial or complete paralysis. Spasticity—the involuntary increased tone of muscles leading to stiffness and spasms—is common, as is fatigue. Fatigue may be triggered by physical exertion and improve with rest, or it may take the form of a constant and persistent tiredness.

Most people with MS also exhibits paresthesias, transitory abnormal sensory feelings such as numbness, prickling, or pins and needles sensations. Uncommonly, some may also experience pain. Loss of sensation sometimes occurs. Speech impediments, tremors, and dizziness are other frequent complaints. Occasionally, people with MS have hearing loss.

Approximately half of all people with MS experience cognitive impairments such as difficulties with concentration, attention, memory, and poor judgment, but such symptoms are usually mild and are frequently overlooked. In fact, they are often detectable only through comprehensive testing. Patients themselves may be unaware of their cognitive loss. Often a family member or friend first notices a deficit. Such impairments are usually mild and rarely disabling. Intellectual and language abilities are generally spared.

Cognitive symptoms occur when lesions develop in brain areas responsible for information processing. These deficits tend to become more apparent as the information to be processed becomes more complex. Fatigue may also add to processing difficulties. Scientists do not yet know whether altered cognition in MS reflects problems with information acquisition, retrieval, or a combination of both. Types of memory problems may differ depending on the individual's disease course (relapsing remitting, primary progressive) and so on. Apparently, though, no direct correlation exists between the duration of illness and the severity of cognitive dysfunction.

Depression, which is unrelated to cognitive problems, is another common feature of MS. In addition, about 10 percent of patients suffer from more severe psychotic disorders such as manic depression and paranoia. Five percent may experience episodes of inappropriate euphoria and despair—unrelated to the patient's actual emotional state—known as *laughing/weeping syndrome.* This syndrome is thought to be due to demyelina-

tion in the brain stem, the area of the brain that controls facial expression and emotions, and is usually seen only in severe cases.

In about 60 percent of MS patients, heat—whether generated by temperatures outside the body or by exercise—may cause temporary worsening of many MS symptoms. In these cases, eradicating the heat eliminates the problem. Some temperature-sensitive patients find that a cold bath may temporarily relieve their symptoms. For the same reason, swimming is often a good exercise choice for people with MS.

When faced with a patient whose symptoms, neurological examination, and medical history suggest MS, physicians use a variety of tools to rule out other possible disorders. They perform a series of laboratory tests that, if positive, confirm the diagnosis.

Imaging technologies such as magnetic resonance imaging (MRI)—often used in conjunction with the contrast agent gadolinium, which helps distinguish new plaques from old on MRI—can help locate central nervous system lesions resulting from myelin loss. However, because these lesions can also occur in several other neurological disorders, they are not absolute evidence of MS. Magnetic resonance spectroscopy (MRS) is a new tool being used to investigate MS. Unlike MRI, which provides an anatomical picture of lesions, MRS yields information about the biochemistry of the brain in MS.

Evoked potential tests, which measure the speed of the brain's response to visual, auditory, and sensory stimuli, can sometimes detect lesions the scanners miss. Like imaging technologies, evoked potentials are helpful but not conclusive because they cannot identify the cause of lesions.

The physician may also study the patient's cerebrospinal fluid (the colorless liquid that circulates throughout the brain and spinal cord) for cellular and chemical abnormalities often associated with MS. These abnormalities include increased numbers of white blood cells and higher-than-average amounts of protein, especially myelin basic protein and an antibody called immunoglobulin G. Physicians can use several different laboratory techniques to separate and graph the various proteins in MS patients' cerebrospinal fluid. This process often identifies the presence of a characteristic pattern called oligoclonal bands.

Because no single test unequivocally detects MS, it is often difficult for the physician to differentiate between an MS attack and symptoms that can follow a viral infection or even an immunization. Many doctors will tell their patients they have "possible MS." If, as time goes by, the patient's symptoms show the characteristic relapsing-remitting pattern or continue in a chronic and progressive fashion, and if laboratory tests rule out other likely causes, or if specific tests become positive, the diagnosis may eventually be changed to "probable MS."

A number of other diseases may produce symptoms similar to those seen in MS. Other conditions with an intermittent course and MS-like lesions of the brain's white matter include polyarteritis, lupus erythematosus, syringomyelia, tropical spastic paraparesis, some cancers, and certain tumors that compress the brain stem or spinal cord. Progressive multifocal leukoencephalopathy can mimic the acute stage of an MS attack. The physician will also need to rule out stroke, neurosyphilis, spinocerebellar ataxias, pernicious anemia, diabetes, Sjögren's disease, and vitamin B_{12} deficiency. Acute transverse myelitis may signal the first attack of MS, or it may indicate other problems such as infection with the Epstein-Barr or herpes simplex B viruses. Recent reports suggest that the neurological problems associated with Lyme disease may present a clinical picture much like MS.

Investigators are continuing their search for a definitive test for MS. Until one is developed, however, evidence of both multiple attacks and central nervous system lesions must be found—a process that can take months or even years—before a physician can make a definitive diagnosis of MS.

Causes

Even though scientists have learned a great deal about MS in recent years, its cause remains unknown. Investigators continue to look into the body's autoimmune system, infectious agents, and genetics as culprits. Studies into these areas strengthen the theory that MS is the result of a number of factors rather than a single gene or other agent. Such studies use magnetic resonance imaging to visualize the evolution of multiple sclerosis lesions in the white matter of the brain.

Components of myelin such as myelin basic protein have been the focus of much research because, when injected into laboratory animals, they can precipitate experimental allergic encephalomyelitis (EAE), a chronic relapsing brain and spinal cord disease that resembles MS. The injected myelin probably stimulates the immune system to produce antimyelin T cells that attack the animal's own myelin.

Investigators are also looking for abnormalities or malfunctions in the blood-brain barrier, a protective membrane that controls the passage of substances from the blood into the central nervous system. In MS, components of the immune system may possibly get through the barrier and cause nervous system damage.

Scientists have studied a number of infectious agents (such as viruses) that have been suspected of causing MS but have been unable to implicate any one particular agent. Viral infections are usually accompanied by inflammation and the production of gamma interferon, a naturally occurring body chemical that has been shown to worsen the clinical course of MS. It is possible that the immune response to viral infections may themselves precipitate an MS attack. There seems to be little doubt that something in the environment is involved in triggering MS.

Increasing scientific evidence suggests that genetics may play a role in determining a person's susceptibility to multiple sclerosis. Some populations, such as Gypsies, Eskimos, and Bantus, never get MS. Native Indians of North and South America, the Japanese, and other Asian peoples have very low incidence rates. It is unclear whether this is due mostly to genetic or environmental factors.

In the population at large, the chance of developing MS is less than $1/10$ percent. However, if one person in a family has MS, that person's first-degree relatives—parents, children, and siblings—have a 1 percent to 3 percent chance of getting the disease.

For identical twins, the likelihood that the second twin may develop MS if the first twin does is about 30 percent. For fraternal twins (who do not inherit identical gene pools), the likelihood is closer to that for nontwin siblings, or about 4 percent.

The fact that the rate for identical twins both developing MS is significantly less than 100 percent suggests that the disease is not entirely genetically controlled. Some (but definitely not all) of this effect may be due to shared exposure to something in the environment or to the fact that some people with MS lesions remain essentially asymptomatic throughout their lives.

Further indications that more than one gene is involved in MS susceptibility comes from studies of families in which more than one member has MS. Several research teams found that people with MS inherit certain regions on individual genes more frequently than people without MS. Of particular interest is the human leukocyte antigen (HLA) or major histocompatibility complex region on chromosome 6. HLAs are genetically determined proteins that influence the immune system.

The HLA patterns of MS patients tend to be different from those of people without the disease. Investigations in northern Europe and America have detected three HLAs that are more prevalent in people with MS than in the general population. Studies of American MS patients have shown that people with MS also tend to exhibit these HLAs in combination—that is, they have more than one of the three HLAs—more frequently than the rest of the population. Furthermore, evidence shows that different combinations of the HLAs may correspond to variations in disease severity and progression.

Studies of families with multiple cases of MS and research comparing genetic regions of humans to those of mice with experimental allergic encephalomyelitis suggest that another area related to MS susceptibility may be located on chromosome 5. Other regions on chromosomes 2, 3, 7, 11, 17, 19, and X have also been identified as possibly containing genes involved in the development of MS.

These studies strengthen the theory that MS is the result of a number of factors rather than a single gene or other agent. Development of MS is likely to be influenced by the interactions of a number of genes, each of which (individually) has only a modest effect. Additional studies are needed to pinpoint specifically which genes are involved, determine their function, and learn how each gene's interactions with other genes and with the environment make an individual susceptible to MS. In addition to leading to better ways to diagnose MS, such studies should yield clues to the underlying causes of MS and, eventually, to better treatments or a way to prevent the disease.

Studies have shown that MS has no adverse effects on the course of pregnancy, labor, or delivery. In fact, symptoms often stabilize or remit during pregnancy. This temporary improvement is thought to relate to changes in a woman's immune system that allow her body to carry a baby. Because every fetus has genetic material from the father as well as the mother, the mother's body should identify the growing fetus as foreign tissue and try to reject it in much the same way the body seeks to reject a transplanted organ. To prevent this from happening, a natural process takes place to suppress the mother's immune system in the uterus during pregnancy and not reject the developing baby.

Complications

As the disease progresses, sexual dysfunction may become a problem. Bowel and bladder control may also be lost.

Treatment

As yet, no cure is available for multiple sclerosis. Many patients do well with no therapy at all, especially because many medications have serious side effects and some carry significant risks. Naturally occurring or spontaneous remissions make it difficult to determine the therapeutic effects of experimental treatments. However, the emerging evidence that MRIs can chart the development of lesions is already helping scientists evaluate new therapies.

Until recently, the principal medications physicians used to treat MS were steroids possessing anti-inflammatory properties. These include adrenocorticotropic hormone (better known as ACTH), prednisone, prednisolone, methylprednisolone, betamethasone, and dexamethasone. Studies suggest that intravenous methylprednisolone may be superior to the more traditional intravenous ACTH for patients experiencing acute relapses; no strong evidence exists to support the use of these drugs to treat progressive forms of MS. Also, there is some indication that steroids may be more appropriate for people with movement, rather than sensory, symptoms.

Although steroids do not affect the course of MS over time, they can reduce the duration and severity of attacks in some patients. The mechanism behind this effect is not known; one study suggests the medications work by restoring the effectiveness of the blood-brain barrier. Because steroids can produce numerous adverse side effects (acne, weight gain, seizures, and psychosis), they are not recommended for long-term use.

One of the most promising MS research areas involves naturally occurring antiviral proteins known as interferons. Two forms of beta interferon (Avonex and Betaseron) have now been approved by the Food and Drug Administration for treatment of relapsing-remitting MS. A third form (Rebif) is marketed in Europe. Beta interferon has been shown to reduce the number of exacerbations and may slow the progression of physical disability. When attacks do occur, they tend to be shorter and less severe. In addition, MRI scans suggest that beta interferon can decrease myelin destruction.

Investigators speculate that the effects of beta interferon may be due to the drug's ability to correct an MS-related deficiency of certain white blood cells that suppress the immune system and/or its ability to inhibit gamma interferon, a substance believed to be involved in MS attacks. Alpha interferon is also being studied as a possible treatment for MS. Common side effects of interferons include fever, chills, sweating, muscle aches, fatigue, depression, and injection site reactions.

Scientists continue their extensive efforts to create new and better therapies for MS. The goals of therapy are threefold: to improve recovery from attacks, to prevent or lessen the number of relapses, and to halt disease progression. Some therapies currently under investigation include the following.

Immunotherapy   As evidence of immune system involvement in the development of MS has grown, trials of various new treatments to alter or suppress immune responses are being conducted. These therapies are, at this time, still considered experimental.

Results of recent clinical trials have shown that immunosuppressive agents and techniques can positively (if temporarily) affect the course of MS. However, toxic side effects often preclude their widespread use. In addition, generalized immunosuppression leaves the patient open to a variety of viral, bacterial, and fungal infections.

Over the years, MS investigators have studied a number of immunosuppressant treatments. Among the therapies being studied are cyclosporine (Sandimmune), cyclophosphamide (Cytoxan), methotrexate, azathioprine (Imuran), and total lymphoid irradiation. This last therapy is a process whereby the MS patient's lymph nodes are irradiated with X rays in small doses over a few weeks to destroy lymphoid tissue, which is actively involved in tissue destruction in autoimmune diseases. Inconclusive and/or contradictory results of these trials, combined with the therapies' potentially dangerous side effects, dictate that further research is necessary to determine what, if any, role they should play in the management of MS. Studies are also being conducted with the immune-system-modulating drugs linomide (Roquinimex), cladribine (Leustatin), and mitoxantrone.

In October 2000, the FDA approved Novantrone (mitoxantrone), an approved cancer drug, for treating patients with advanced or chronic multiple sclerosis. Two randomized, multicenter clinical studies, totaling about 200 patients, demonstrated that Novantrone could reduce the number of relapse episodes and decrease the progression of disability in patients with secondary (chronic) progressive, progressive-relapsing, or worsening relapsing-remitting MS (all forms of the disease in which patients become significantly more abnormal between relapses as time passes). The trials showed that Novantrone can help reduce the number of relapses and help patients keep their mobility longer.

Two other experimental treatments—one involving the use of monoclonal antibodies and the other involving plasma exchange, or plasmapheresis—may have fewer dangerous side effects. Monoclonal antibodies are identical, laboratory-produced antibodies that are highly specific for a single antigen. They are injected into the patient in the hope that they will alter the patient's immune response. Plasmapheresis is a procedure in which blood is removed from the patient, and the plasma is separated from other blood substances, which may contain antibodies and other immunologically active products. These other blood substances are discarded, and the plasma is then transfused back into the patient. Because their worth as treatments for MS has not yet been proven, these experimental treatments remain at the stage of clinical testing.

Bone marrow transplantation (a procedure in which bone marrow from a healthy donor is infused into patients who have undergone drug or radiation therapy to suppress their immune system so they will not reject the donated marrow) and injections of venom from honeybees are also being studied. Each of these therapies carries the risk of potentially severe side effects.

Therapy to improve nerve impulse conduction
Because the transmission of electrochemical messages between the brain and body is disrupted in MS, medications to improve the conduction of nerve impulses are being investigated. Since demyelinated nerves show abnormalities of potassium activity, scientists are studying drugs that block the channels through which potassium moves, thereby restoring conduction of the nerve impulse. In several small experimental trials, derivatives of a drug called aminopyridine temporarily improved vision, coordination, and strength when given to MS patients who suffered from both visual symptoms and heightened sensitivity to temperature. Possible side effects of these therapies include paresthesias (tingling sensations), dizziness, and seizures.

Therapies targeting an antigen   Trials of a synthetic form of myelin basic protein, called copolymer I (Copaxone), have shown promise in treating people in the early stages of relapsing-remitting MS. Copolymer I, unlike so many drugs tested for the treatment of MS, seems to have few side effects. Recent trial data indicate that copolymer I can reduce the relapse rate by almost one-third. In addition, patients given copolymer I were more likely to show neurological improvement than those given a placebo. The Food and Drug Administration has made the drug available to people with early relapsing-remitting MS through its Treatment IND program and is currently reviewing data from a large-scale study to determine whether or not to approve the drug for marketing.

Investigators are also looking at the possibility of developing an MS vaccine. Myelin-attacking T cells were removed, inactivated, and injected back into animals with experimental allergic encephalomyelitis (EAE). This procedure results in destruction of the immune system cells that were attacking myelin basic protein. In a couple of small trials, scientists have tested a similar vaccine in humans. The product was well tolerated and had no side effects, but the studies were too small to establish efficacy. Patients with progressive forms of MS did not appear to benefit. However, relapsing-remitting patients showed some neurological improvement and had fewer relapses and reduced numbers of lesions in one study. Unfortunately, the benefits did not last beyond two years.

A similar approach, known as peptide therapy, is based on evidence that the body can mount an immune response against the T cells that destroy myelin, but this response is not strong enough to overcome the disease. To induce this response, the investigator scans the myelin-attacking T cells for the myelin-recognizing receptors on the cells' surface. A fragment, or peptide, of those receptors is then injected into the body. The immune system recognizes the injected peptide as a foreign invader and launches an attack on any myelin-destroying T cells that carry the peptide. The injection of portions of T cell receptors may heighten the immune system reaction against the errant T cells much the same way a booster shot heightens immunity to tetanus. Alternatively, peptide therapy may jam the errant cells' receptors, preventing the cells from attacking myelin.

Despite these promising early results, there are some major obstacles to developing vaccine and peptide therapies. Individual patients' T cells vary so much that developing a standard vaccine or peptide therapy beneficial to all, or even most, MS patients may not be possible. At this time, each treatment involves extracting cells from each individual patient, purifying the cells, and then growing them in culture before inactivating and chemically altering them. This makes producing sufficient quantities for therapy extremely time consuming, labor intensive, and expensive. Further studies are necessary to determine whether universal inoculations can be developed to induce suppression of MS patients' overactive immune systems.

Protein-antigen feeding is similar to peptide therapy but is a potentially simpler means to the same end. Whenever people eat, the digestive system breaks each food or substance into its primary nonantigenic building blocks, thereby averting a potentially harmful immune attack. So, strange as it may seem, antigens that trigger an immune response when they are injected can encourage immune system tolerance when taken orally. Furthermore, this reaction is directed solely at the specific antigen being fed. Wholesale immunosuppression, which can leave the body open to a variety of infections, does not occur. Studies have shown that when rodents with EAE are fed myelin protein antigens, they experience fewer relapses. Data from a small, preliminary trial of antigen feeding in humans found limited suggestion of improvement, but the results were not statistically significant. A multicenter trial is being conducted to determine whether protein antigen feeding is effective.

Cytokines   As growing insight into the workings of the immune system gives researchers new knowledge about the function of cytokines, the powerful chemicals produced by T cells, the possibility of using them to manipulate the immune system becomes more attractive. Scientists are studying a variety of substances that may block harmful cytokines, such as those involved in inflammation, or that encourage the production of protective cytokines. A drug that has been tested as a depression treatment, rolipram, has been shown to reduce levels of several destructive cytokines in animal models of MS. Its potential as a therapy for MS is not known at this time, but side effects seem modest. Protein-antigen feeding, discussed above, may release transforming growth factor beta (TGF), a protective cytokine that inhibits or regulates the activity of certain immune cells. Preliminary tests indicate that it may reduce the number of immune cells commonly found in MS patients' spinal fluid. Side effects include anemia and altered kidney function.

Interleukin-4 (IL-4) is able to diminish demyelination and improve the clinical course of mice with EAE, apparently by influencing developing T cells

to become protective rather than harmful. This also appears to be true of a group of chemicals called retinoids. When fed to rodents with EAE, retinoids increase levels of TGF and IL-4, which encourage protective T cells while decreasing the numbers of harmful T cells. This results in improvement of the animals' clinical symptoms.

Remyelination   Some studies focus on strategies to reverse the damage to myelin and oligodendrocytes (the cells that make and maintain myelin in the central nervous system), both of which are destroyed during MS attacks. Scientists now know that oligodendrocytes may proliferate and form new myelin after an attack. Therefore, there is a great deal of interest in agents that may stimulate this reaction. To learn more about the process, investigators are looking at how drugs used in MS trials affect remyelination. Studies of animal models indicate that monoclonal antibodies and two immunosuppressant drugs, cyclophosphamide and azathioprine, may accelerate remyelination, while steroids may inhibit it. The ability of intravenous immunoglobulin (IVIg) to restore visual acuity and/or muscle strength is also being investigated.

Diet   Over the years, many people have tried to implicate diet as a cause of or treatment for MS. Some physicians have advocated a diet low in saturated fats; others have suggested increasing the patient's intake of linoleic acid, a polyunsaturated fat, via supplements of sunflower seed, safflower, or evening primrose oils. Other proposed dietary "remedies" include megavitamin therapy, including increased intake of vitamins B_{12} or C; various liquid diets; and sucrose-, tobacco-, or gluten-free diets. To date, clinical studies have not been able to confirm benefits from dietary changes.

Unproven therapies   Because MS is a disease with a natural tendency to remit spontaneously and for which there is no universally effective treatment and no known cause, it is a magnet for an array of unsubstantiated claims of cures. At one time or another, many ineffective and even potentially dangerous therapies have been promoted as treatments for MS. A partial list of these "therapies" includes: injections of snake venom, electrical stimulation of the spinal cord's dorsal column, removal of the thymus gland, breathing pressurized (hyperbaric) oxygen in a special chamber, injections of beef heart and hog pancreas extracts, intravenous or oral calcium orotate (calcium EAP), hysterectomy, removal of dental fillings containing silver or mercury amalgams, and surgical implantation of pig brain into the patient's abdomen. None of these treatments is an effective therapy for MS or any of its symptoms.

Treatment of Symptoms

While some scientists look for therapies that will affect the overall course of the disease, others are searching for new and better medications to control the symptoms of MS without triggering intolerable side effects.

Many people with MS have problems with *spasticity,* a condition that primarily affects the lower limbs. Spasticity can occur either as a sustained stiffness caused by increased muscle tone or as spasms that come and go, especially at night. It is usually treated with muscle relaxants and tranquilizers. Baclofen (Lioresal), the most commonly prescribed medication for this symptom, may be taken orally or, in severe cases, injected into the spinal cord. Tizanidine (Zanaflex), used for years in Europe and now approved in the United States, appears to function similarly to baclofen. Diazepam (Valium), clonazepam (Klonopin), and dantrolene (Dantrium) can also reduce spasticity. Although its beneficial effect is temporary, physical therapy may also be useful and can help prevent the irreversible shortening of muscles known as contractures. Surgery to reduce spasticity is rarely appropriate in MS.

Weakness and ataxia (incoordination) are also characteristic of MS. When weakness is a problem, some spasticity can actually be beneficial by lending support to weak limbs. In such cases, medication levels that completely alleviate spasticity may be inappropriate. Physical therapy and exercise can also help preserve remaining function. Patients may find that various aids—such as foot braces, canes, and walkers—can help them remain independent and mobile. Occasionally, physicians can provide temporary relief from weakness, spasms, and pain by injecting a drug called phenol into the spinal cord, muscles, or nerves in the arms or legs. Further research is needed to find or develop effec-

tive treatments for MS-related weakness and ataxia.

Although improvement of *optic* symptoms usually occurs even without treatment, a short course of treatment with intravenous methylprednisolone (Solu-Medrol) followed by treatment with oral steroids is sometimes used. A trial of oral prednisone in patients with visual problems suggests that this steroid is not only ineffective in speeding recovery but may also increase patients' risk for future MS attacks. Curiously, prednisone injected directly into the veins—at 10 times the oral dose—did seem to produce short-term recovery. Because of the link between optic neuritis and MS, the study's investigators believe these findings may hold true for the treatment of MS as well. A follow-up study of optic neuritis patients will address this and other questions.

Fatigue, especially in the legs, is a common symptom of MS and may be both physical and psychological. Avoiding excessive activity and heat are probably the most important measures patients can take to counter physiological fatigue. If psychological aspects of fatigue such as depression or apathy are evident, antidepressant medications may help. Other drugs that may reduce fatigue in some, but not all, patients include amantadine (Symmetrel), pemoline (Cylert), and the still-experimental drug aminopyridine.

People with MS may experience several types of *pain.* Muscle and back pain can be helped by aspirin or acetaminophen and by physical therapy to correct faulty posture and strengthen and stretch muscles. The sharp, stabbing facial pain known as trigeminal neuralgia is commonly treated with carbamazepine, anticonvulsant drugs, or occasionally, surgery. Intense tingling and burning sensations are harder to treat. Some people get relief with antidepressant drugs; others may respond to electrical stimulation of the nerves in the affected area. In some cases, the physician may recommend codeine.

As the disease progresses, some patients develop *bladder malfunctions.* Urinary problems are often the result of infections that can be treated with antibiotics. The physician may recommend that patients take vitamin C supplements or drink cranberry juice, as these measures acidify urine and may reduce the risk of further infections. Several medications are also available. The most common bladder problems encountered by MS patients are urinary frequency, urgency, or incontinence. A small number of patients, however, retain large amounts of urine. In these patients, catheterization may be necessary. In this procedure, a catheter or drainage tube is temporarily inserted (by the patient or a caretaker) into the urethra several times a day to drain urine from the bladder. Surgery may be indicated in severe, intractable cases. Scientists have developed a bladder pacemaker that has helped people with urinary incontinence in preliminary trials. The pacemaker, which is surgically implanted, is controlled by a handheld unit that allows the patient to stimulate the nerves electrically that control bladder function.

MS patients with urinary problems may be reluctant to drink enough fluids, leading to *constipation*. Drinking more water and adding fiber to the diet usually alleviates this condition. *Sexual dysfunction* may also occur, especially in patients with urinary problems. Men may experience occasional failure to attain an erection. Penile implants, injection of the drug papaverine, and electrostimulation are techniques used to resolve the problem. Women may experience insufficient lubrication or have difficulty reaching orgasm; in these cases, vaginal gels and vibrating devices may be helpful. Counseling is also beneficial, especially in the absence of urinary problems, since psychological factors can also cause these symptoms. For instance, *depression* can intensify symptoms of fatigue, pain, and sexual dysfunction. In addition to counseling, the physician may prescribe antidepressant or antianxiety medications. Amitriptyline is used to treat laughing/weeping syndrome.

Tremors are often resistant to therapy but can sometimes be treated with drugs or, in extreme cases, surgery. Investigators are currently examining a number of experimental treatments for tremors.

National Institute of Neurological Disorders and Stroke, National Institutes of Health. *Multiple Sclerosis: Hope Through Research,* 1996.

The National Institute of Neurological Disorders and Stroke, National Institutes of Health. *NINDS Multiple Sclerosis Information Page,* Available online. URL: http://www.ninds.nih.gov/health_and_medical/disorders/multiplesclerosis.htm. Downloaded on 18 July 2002.

myasthenia gravis (MG)   A chronic autoimmune neuromuscular disease characterized by varying degrees of weakness of the skeletal (voluntary) muscles of the body. It is characterized by reversible fatigability. The name *myasthenia gravis,* which is Latin and Greek in origin, literally means "grave muscle weakness." With current therapies, however, most cases of myasthenia gravis are not as grave as the name implies. In fact, for the majority of individuals with myasthenia gravis, life expectancy is not lessened by the disorder.

There are several forms of myasthenia gravis, and various clinical classifications have been suggested. One form, restricted ocular MG (ROMG) usually affects only the ocular (eye) muscles, resulting in weakness and a droopy or sleepy appearance. ROMG often develops into generalized myasthenia (GMG). ROMG is probably an autoimmune disease in which an antibody is directed at extraocular muscle. In persons with ROMG, detecting the autoantibodies that are the hallmark of generalized myasthenia gravis is usually difficult.

GMG is a chronic autoimmune neuromuscular disease that can affect all of the skeletal muscles, including the extraocular muscles. It may occur alone or in combination with other autoimmune disorders. There is also a drug-induced form of MG caused by the prescription drug D-penicillamine. Drug-induced MG usually remits when the drug is stopped.

The hallmark of myasthenia gravis is muscle weakness that increases during periods of activity and improves after periods of rest. Certain muscles such as those that control eye and eyelid movement, facial expression, chewing, talking, and swallowing are often, but not always, involved in the disorder. The muscles that control breathing and neck and limb movements may also be affected.

Myasthenia gravis occurs in all ethnic groups and both genders. It most commonly affects young adult women (under 40) and older men (over 60), but it can occur at any age. The age of the patient at the onset of MG is a factor is the classification of either early-onset or late-onset of MG. The usual patient with early-onset GMG is female, with the disease beginning before the age of 40 and an association with hyperplastic thymus. Late-onset GMG affects both males and females equally and occurs after the age of 40. It is associated with the presence of a thymoma.

Causes

Myasthenia gravis is caused by a defect in the transmission of nerve impulses to muscles. It occurs when normal communication between the nerve and muscle is interrupted at the neuromuscular junction—the place where nerve cells connect with the muscles they control. Normally, when impulses travel down the nerve, the nerve endings release a neurotransmitter substance called acetylcholine. Acetylcholine travels through the neuromuscular junction and binds to acetylcholine receptors that are then activated and generate a muscle contraction.

In myasthenia gravis, antibodies block, alter, or destroy the receptors for acetylcholine at the neuromuscular junction. This prevents the muscle contraction from occurring. These antibodies are produced by the body's own immune system. Thus, myasthenia gravis is an autoimmune disease because the immune system—which normally protects the body from foreign organisms—mistakenly attacks itself.

The thymus gland, which lies in the upper chest area beneath the breastbone, plays an important role in the development of the immune system in early life. Its cells form a part of the body's normal immune system. The gland is somewhat large in infants, grows gradually until puberty, and then gets smaller and is replaced by fat with age. In adults with myasthenia gravis, the thymus gland is abnormal. It contains certain clusters of immune cells indicative of lymphoid hyperplasia, a condition usually found only in the spleen and lymph nodes during an active immune response. Some individuals with myasthenia gravis develop thymomas or tumors on the thymus gland. Generally, thymomas are benign, but they can become malignant.

The relationship between the thymus gland and myasthenia gravis is not yet fully understood. Scientists believe the thymus gland may give incorrect instructions about the production of the acetylcholine receptor antibodies, thereby setting the stage for the attack on neuromuscular transmission.

In neonatal myasthenia gravis, the fetus may acquire immune proteins (antibodies) from a mother affected with myasthenia gravis. Generally, cases of neonatal myasthenia gravis are transient (temporary), and the child's symptoms usually disappear within a few weeks after birth. Other children develop myasthenia gravis indistinguishable from adults. Myasthenia gravis in juveniles is common.

Myasthenia gravis is not directly inherited nor is it contagious. Occasionally, the disease may occur in more than one member of the same family.

Rarely, children may show signs of congenital myasthenia gravis or congenital myasthenic syndrome. These are not autoimmune disorders but are caused by defective genes that control proteins in the acetylcholine receptor or in acetylcholinesterase.

Clinical Features

Although myasthenia gravis may affect any voluntary muscle, muscles that control eye and eyelid movement, facial expression, and swallowing are most frequently affected. The onset of the disorder may be sudden. Symptoms often are not immediately recognized as myasthenia gravis.

In most cases, the first noticeable symptom is weakness of the eye muscles. In others, difficulty in swallowing and slurred speech may be the first signs. The degree of muscle weakness involved in myasthenia gravis varies greatly among patients. It ranges from a localized form, limited to eye muscles (ocular myasthenia), to a severe or generalized form in which many muscles—sometimes including those that control breathing—are affected. Symptoms, which vary in type and severity may include a drooping of one or both eyelids (ptosis); blurred or double vision (diplopia) due to weakness of the muscles that control eye movements; unstable or waddling gait; weakness in arms, hands, fingers, legs, and neck; a change in facial expression; difficulty in swallowing and shortness of breath; and impaired speech (dysarthria).

Unfortunately, a delay in diagnosis of one or two years is not unusual in cases of myasthenia gravis.

Because weakness is a common symptom of many other disorders, the diagnosis is often missed in people who experience mild weakness or in those individuals whose weakness is restricted to only a few muscles.

The first steps in diagnosing myasthenia gravis include reviewing the individual's medical history and both physical and neurological examinations. The signs a physician must look for are impairment of eye movements or muscle weakness without any changes in the individual's ability to feel things. If the doctor suspects myasthenia gravis, several tests are available to confirm the diagnosis.

A special blood test can detect the presence of immune molecules or acetylcholine receptor antibodies. Most patients with myasthenia gravis have abnormally elevated levels of these antibodies. However, antibodies may not be detected in patients with only ocular forms of the disease.

Another test is called the edrophonium test. This approach requires the intravenous administration of edrophonium chloride or Tensilon, a drug that blocks the degradation (breakdown) of acetylcholine and temporarily increases the levels of acetylcholine at the neuromuscular junction. In people with myasthenia gravis involving the eye muscles, edrophonium chloride will briefly relieve weakness. Other methods to confirm the diagnosis include a version of a nerve conduction study that tests for specific muscle fatigue by repetitive nerve stimulation. This test records weakening muscle responses when the nerves are repetitively stimulated and helps to differentiate nerve disorders from muscle disorders. Repetitive stimulation of a nerve during a nerve conduction study may demonstrate decrements of the muscle action potential due to impaired nerve-to-muscle transmission.

A different test called single fiber electromyography (EMG), in which single muscle fibers are stimulated by electrical impulses, can also detect impaired nerve-to-muscle transmission. EMG measures the electrical potential of muscle cells. Muscle fibers in myasthenia gravis, as well as in other neuromuscular disorders, do not respond as well to repeated electrical stimulation when compared with muscles from normal individuals.

Computed tomography (CT) or magnetic resonance imaging (MRI) may be used to identify an abnormal thymus gland or the presence of a thymoma.

A special examination called pulmonary function testing—which measures breathing strength—helps to predict whether respiration may fail and lead to a myasthenic crisis.

Complications

In a few cases, the severe weakness of myasthenia gravis may cause a crisis (respiratory failure), which requires immediate emergency medical care. A myasthenic crisis occurs when weakness affects the muscles that control breathing, creating a medical emergency and requiring a respirator for assisted ventilation. In patients whose respiratory muscles are weak, crises—which generally call for immediate medical attention—may be triggered by infection, fever, an adverse reaction to medication, or emotional stress.

Treatment

Today, myasthenia gravis can be controlled. Several therapies are available to help reduce and improve muscle weakness. Medications used to treat the disorder include anticholinesterase agents such as neostigmine and pyridostigmine, which help improve neuromuscular transmission and increase muscle strength. Immunosuppressive drugs such as prednisone, cyclosporine, and azathioprine may also be used. These medications improve muscle strength by suppressing the production of abnormal antibodies. They must be used with careful medical follow-up because they may cause major side effects.

Thymectomy, the surgical removal of the thymus gland (which is abnormal in myasthenia gravis patients), improve symptoms in more than 50 percent of patients without thymoma and may cure some individuals, possibly by rebalancing the immune system. Other therapies used to treat myasthenia gravis include plasmapheresis, a procedure in which abnormal antibodies are removed from the blood, and high-dose intravenous immune globulin, which temporarily modifies the immune system and provides the body with normal antibodies from donated blood. These therapies may be used to help individuals during especially difficult periods of weakness. A neurologist, along with the primary care physician, will determine which treatment option is best for each individual depending on the severity of the weakness, which muscles are affected, the individual's age, and other associated medical problems.

With treatment, the outlook for most patients with myasthenia gravis is bright. They will have significant improvement of their muscle weakness, and they can expect to lead normal or nearly normal lives. Some cases of myasthenia gravis may go into remission temporarily, and muscle weakness may disappear completely so that medications can be discontinued. Stable, long-lasting complete remissions are the goal of thymectomy.

Christadoss, Premkumar, ed. *Myasthenia Gravis—Disease Mechanism and Immunointervention.* Dordrecht, The Netherlands: Kluwer Academic Publishers, 2000.
National Institute of Neurological Disorders and Stroke, National Institutes of Health. *Myasthenia Gravis Fact Sheet,* NIH Publication No. 99-768, August 1999.

myasthenia gravis research Today's myasthenia gravis research includes a broad spectrum of studies conducted and supported by the National Institute of Neurological Disorders and Stroke (NINDS). NINDS scientists are evaluating new and improving current treatments for the disorder. One such study is testing the efficacy of intravenous immune globulin in patients with myasthenia gravis. The goal of the study is to determine whether this treatment safely improves muscle strength. Another study seeks to understand the molecular basis of synaptic transmission in the nervous system. The objective of this study is to expand current knowledge of the function of receptors and to apply this knowledge to the treatment of myasthenia gravis.

myelin A fatty covering insulating nerve cell fibers in the brain and spinal cord, myelin facilitates the smooth, high-speed transmission of electrochemical messages between these components of the central nervous system and the rest of the body. In MULTIPLE SCLEROSIS, myelin is damaged through a process known as demyelination, which results in distorted or blocked signals.

myocarditis, autoimmune Myocarditis is an inflammation of the heart muscle. It is a principal cause of heart disease and sudden cardiac death in young adults. Sometimes it is diagnosed only after the death of a young person following vigorous exercise. Although it is uncommon, myocarditis occurs in people of all ages.

Causes

Myocarditis is often caused by infection from a coxsackie virus. Although most people recover from viral myocarditis with no ill effects, a small number of people develop autoimmune myocarditis, in which the body's own immune system attacks the heart muscle, eventually leading to heart failure. Myocarditis can result from interaction of the immune system with viral infections such as polio, measles, or influenza. The virus causes heart muscle cell proteins to enter the blood. The body's immune system attacks the protein in the blood and also in the heart, causing the heart tissue to become inflamed and damaged. The heart's electrical system and its ability to pump blood may then be impaired.

Sometimes, however, myocarditis is directly caused by a bacterial, viral, parasitic, or fungal infection. The strep infection known as rheumatic fever is well-known as a cause of heart defects. However, anything that produces inflammation of the heart muscle, including chemical poisoning, results in myocarditis.

Clinical Features

Mild cases may produce no symptoms. When symptoms do occur, they may vary from fatigue, shortness of breath, rapid or irregular heartbeat, or fever to strong chest pain or lung congestion in more severe cases. Myocarditis will often resemble a lingering flu. In cases of infectious illness accompanied by irregular heartbeat or chest pain, the physician will suspect myocarditis and order a chest X ray and an electrocardiogram (EEG). These tests will show whether the heart is enlarged or damaged and will also reveal any problems in the electrical activity of the heart. In some cases, an echocardiogram will be used to look at blood flow and pressures within the heart and show the strength of the contractions. In very severe cases, a heart biopsy may be needed, with a very small piece of heart muscle tissue surgically removed and then examined under a microscope.

Complications

If untreated, myocarditis may permanently damage heart muscle tissue and heart valves. It may also lead to congestive heart failure.

Treatment

Most cases clear up without treatment, although corticosteroid drugs may occasionally be prescribed to reduce inflammation. Antibiotics are often sufficient to eliminate the underlying cause in the case of a bacterial infection. When necessary, other drugs may be prescribed to restore the heart to a stable condition. If the heart has been severely damaged, valve replacements to repair it or even a heart transplant may be required.

myocarditis, autoimmune research Researchers at the Johns Hopkins Bloomberg School of Public Health have discovered that COMPLEMENT, a key protein of the innate immune system, is critical to the development of autoimmune myocarditis. According to the study, the researchers prevented autoimmune myocarditis in mice by blocking the production of complement and by blocking its interaction with two key complement receptors. The study examines the role of the innate immune system during the formation of autoimmune myocarditis, which may lead to better diagnosis and prevention of this deadly disease and other autoimmune disorders.

The research team wanted to know why myocarditis triggers an autoimmune response in a small group of people. Their research showed that complement and its receptors are key pieces of that puzzle. The body has two levels of defense in the immune system: the innate immune response, which people are born with, and the adaptive immune response, which people learn by experience. The innate immune system "holds the fort" with complement, which motivates T cells and cytokines of the adaptive immune system to mount a response and fight off the infection. During this learning phase, the researchers believe, complement plays a critical role in the development of autoimmune myocarditis.

Kaya Z., M. Afanasyeva, Y. Wang, K. M. Dohmen, J. Schlichting, T. Tretter, D. Fairweather, V. M. Holers, and N. R. Rose. "Contribution of the Innate Immune System to Autoimmune Myocarditis: A Role for Complement." *Nature Immunology* 2 (2001): 739–745.

myositis An inflammation or swelling of muscle tissue, especially of voluntary (skeletal) muscles. It is often caused by injury or infection, which leads to pain, tenderness, and weakness. Types of myositis include pleurodynia (a viral infection affecting muscles around the rib cage), myositis ossificans (the damaged muscle is replaced by bone), POLYMYOSITIS (inflammation of muscles throughout the body), and DERMATOMYOSITIS (inflammation of muscles and the presence of a rash). Polymyositis and dermatomyositis are rare autoimmune diseases.

Native Americans with autoimmune diseases

The impact of autoimmune diseases on Native Americans as a group varies. Native Americans are playing an important role in the ongoing study of autoimmune diseases, but health care is of particular concern among this population. Roughly 23 percent of American Indian/ALASKA NATIVES do not have health INSURANCE, compared to 13 percent of Caucasian Americans. The lack of comprehensive health insurance limits American Indian/Alaska Native women's access to regular health services for disease prevention, screening, diagnosis, treatment, and management of chronic conditions such as autoimmune diseases. Among autoimmune disease most affecting Native Americans:

- IGA NEPHROPATHY occurs significantly more often in Native Americans than in any other ethnic group tested.

- Incidence of INSULIN-DEPENDENT DIABETES is lower for Native Americans than American Caucasians, while nonautoimmune Type 2 diabetes has a much higher incidence among Native Americans and other minority groups.

- American Indian children are more affected by JUVENILE ARTHRITIS than children from other ethnic backgrounds.

- In June 2000, the Consortium of Multiple Sclerosis Centers/North American Research Committee on Multiple Sclerosis (MS) released demographic information showing 14,420 (89.0 percent) non-Hispanic whites with MS, while only 174 Native Americans (1.1 percent) had the disease.

- Although RHEUMATOID ARTHRITIS (RA) affects all racial and ethnic groups, the highest prevalence of RA has been reported in the Pima and Chippewa. In a *Lakota Times* article, Dr. James Jarvis of the University of Oklahoma, stated "There's some tantalizing archaeological evidence that rheumatoid arthritis may have a Native American origin. There's no evidence of it in Europe prior to 1492." However, he noted, ancient skeletal remains of Indians who lived in what is now Tennessee and Ohio show evidence of having swollen joints.

- SCLERODERMA occurs with greater frequency in the Choctaw. A study of Oklahoma Choctaw suggests that the gene for the protein fibrillin-1 is a possible susceptibility gene for scleroderma. This finding is particularly significant because this gene plays an important role in an animal model of scleroderma.

- SYSTEMIC LUPUS ERYTHEMATOSUS (SLE) is seen most commonly in African Americans and Afro-Caribbeans, Native Americans, Latin Americans, and Chinese. According to a Canadian study comparing 120,000 North American Indians to the non-Indian population, the prevalence of SLE among Indians was more than double that of the remainder of the population. Native Americans also had higher SLE Disease Activity Index Scores at diagnosis and more frequent vasculitis and renal involvement, required more treatment later in the disease course, accumulated more damage following diagnosis, and had increased fatality.

Klinka, Karen. "Pipe Ceremony Blesses Rheumatoid Arthritis Study." *Indian Country Today* (*Lakota Times*), 31 August 1998, p. 7.

Peschken, C. A., and Esdaile, J. M. "Systemic Lupus Erythematosus in North American Indians: A Population Based Study." *Journal of Rheumatology* 27, no. 8 (August 2000): 1,884–1,891.

natural immunity Immunity that individuals are born with, that is genetically determined in specific species, populations, or families. For example, the measles virus cannot reproduce in canine cells because dogs have a natural immunity to measles. It does not require prior exposure and is not enhanced by prior exposure in order to keep out invading organisms (pathogens) such as viruses, bacteria, and fungi. An alternative term is *innate immunity*.

natural killer (NK) cells Large, granule-filled lymphocytes that have the ability to kill tumor cells and virus-infected body cells. They are known as natural killers because they attack without first having to recognize specific antigens. They do not require the intervention of helper T cells. They have characteristic markers on their cell surface, so they can be recognized in the blood.

necrosis The death of cells, tissues, or organs. Necrosis can occur when not enough blood is supplied to the tissue, as a result of trauma, or from radiation or chemical agents.

neuropathies Diseases of the nervous system. (See also DEMYELINATING NEUROPATHIES, PERIPHERAL NEUROPATHY.)

neutropenia Severe chronic neutropenia is a rare blood disorder characterized by abnormally low levels of certain white blood cells (neutrophils) in the body. Neutrophils are blood cells that are produced in the marrow, or core of the bones. The absolute neutrophil count (ANC) is found by multiplying the percentage of bands and neutrophils on a differential by the total white blood count. The blood normally contains about 1,500 to 8,000 neutrophils per cubic millimeter (mm^3) (or often written as 1.5 to 8.0×10^9 per liter of blood). When the number of neutrophils in the blood falls below 1,500 cells per mm^3 (1.5×10^9 per liter), the condition is called neutropenia. The severity of neutropenia is categorized as mild with ANC of 1,000 to 1,500 cells per mm^3, moderate with ANC of 500 to 1,000 cells per mm^3, and severe with an ANC of fewer than 500 cells per mm^3. The risk of bacterial infection is related to the severity and duration of neutropenia.

Neutrophils play an essential role in fighting bacterial infections by surrounding and destroying invading bacteria (phagocytosis) or infection. When bacteria invade the body, a chemical signal is sent out. The neutrophils, like firefighters responding to a blaze, rush to the site of infection. The bone marrow also responds by speeding up its production of neutrophils to replace those involved in fighting the infection. If, however, production of new neutrophils is suppressed or slowed down, a shortage may develop, and any infection can overwhelm the few neutrophils available. Therefore, a person with only a few neutrophils is at particular risk for developing a serious bacterial infection.

Neutropenia occurs more commonly in females than in males. Elderly individuals have a higher incidence rate than younger individuals.

Causes

Drugs, chemical agents, physical agents (for example, X-ray treatments), and certain infections can affect the bone marrow's production of cells. Anti-cancer medications destroy normal cells as well as malignant cells, and they often suppress the bone marrow's production of neutrophils. In some patients, especially those with chronic neutropenia, the cause is unknown. Disease processes that affect the immune system, like cancers, HIV infection, or autoimmune disorders, lead to neutropenia. If neutropenia does develop, patients must take care to minimize the risk of infection and be prompt in notifying their doctor or other health care provider.

Clinical Features

Symptoms associated with severe chronic neutropenia include recurring fevers, mouth sores (ulcers), and/or inflammation of the tissues that surround and support the teeth (periodontitis). Due to low levels of neutrophils, affected individuals may be more susceptible to recurring infections that, in some cases, may result in life-threatening complications. Severe chronic neutropenia may last for months or years and can affect both children and adults. There are three main forms of the disorder: congenital, idiopathic, and cyclic neutropenia. Severe chronic neutropenia may be inherited or acquired, or it may occur for unknown reasons (idiopathic).

Treatment

Treatments for neutropenia now include antibiotics to fight the resultant infections and drugs that stimulate the bone marrow to make neutrophils and help restore the body's defenses against infection. These drugs are known as granulocyte-colony-stimulating factors. They help keep the number of neutrophils in the blood above the dan-

ger level all or most of the time. The shorter the time the neutrophil count is low, the less chance there is of developing fever or infection.

Shin, Daniel D., et al. "Neutropenia." *eMedicine Journal* 3, no. 2 (7 February 2002). Available online. URL: http://www.emedicine.com/med/topic1640.htm.

neutrophil   A white blood cell that is an abundant and important phagocyte.

nucleus   The central cell structure that houses the chromosomes.

ocular cicatricial pemphigoid (OCP) An uncommon autoimmune disease involving primarily the mouth and eye mucous membranes. This disorder is characterized by the development of blisters of mucous membranes, though the skin may also be involved. The initial presentation is often that of red, painful, tearing, and light-sensitive eyes in a patient 60 to 70 years of age. This condition causes intense inflammation and scarring of the conjunctiva. This causes inward turning of the lid or entropion. In addition to scarring, the inflammatory lesions of the eye surfaces may result in loss of tear film, adhesions of the lids to the eye, corneal ulceration and perforation, and in the most relentlessly progressive or untreated cases, loss of the eye. There is frequently tense blistering lesions or erosions of the mucous membranes in the mouth. The skin may also be affected by the development of blisters and dermatitis (reddened, inflamed skin).

Treatment is with corticosteroids and immunosuppressive agents. High doses of prednisone are often started if the disease state is severe, and immunosuppressive agents (Dapsone) are subsequently begun. This medicine halts the intense inflammatory component associated with the disease. Even if it halts the progression of the disease, it may not improve any previous damage. The ocular surface disease must be treated with lubrication therapy, perhaps antibiotics, and sometimes surgical procedures in an attempt to maintain vision. Nevertheless, many patients will experience severe visual loss due to ocular surface scarring, despite the most aggressive management.

Foster, C. Stephen. *The Ocular Cicatricial Pemphigoid Antigen*. Boston: MEEI Immunology Service, 1997.
"Ocular Cicatricial Pemphigoid (OCP)," EyeMDLink.com. Available online. URL: http://www.eyemdlink.com/Condition.asp?ConditionID=509. Posted on 25 September 2001.
"Ocular Cicatricial Pemphigoid Antigen: Partial Sequence and Biochemical Characterization." *Proceedings of the National Academy of Science* 93 (December 1996): 14,714–14,719.

opportunistic infection An infection in an immunosuppressed person caused by an organism that does not usually trouble people with healthy immune systems.

opsonization The action of coating an organism with antibodies or a complement protein so as to make it palatable to phagocytes.

pain In general, there are two kinds of pain: acute and chronic. Acute pain is a normal sensation triggered in the nervous system to alert you to possible injury and the need to take care of yourself. Chronic pain is different. It persists. Pain signals keep firing in the nervous system for weeks, months, even years. Autoimmune diseases often are associated with chronic pain. Examples of those where pain is a symptom include the following:

- ANKYLOSING SPONDYLITIS can cause inflammation of the iris, called iritis, which is characterized by extreme pain in the eye.

- CROHN'S DISEASE and ULCERATIVE COLITIS patients may have abdominal pain that can be difficult to control.

- In FIBROMYALGIA, the body's immune system attacks the muscles, tendons, and ligaments, causing pain and tiredness.

- MULTIPLE SCLEROSIS symptoms include eye pain.

- PSORIASIS may affect very small areas of skin or cover the entire body with a buildup of red scales called plaques. The plaques are of different sizes, shapes, and severity and may be painful as well as unattractive.

- RHEUMATOID ARTHRITIS makes the tissues swell up, which can cause pain and stiffness in the joints.

- SCLERODERMA symptoms can include pain in the fingers and toes, and muscle soreness.

- SYSTEMIC LUPUS ERYTHEMATOSUS common symptoms include pain in the joints and chest pain when breathing.

parasite A plant or animal that lives, grows, and feeds on or within another living organism (the host) without contributing to its survival.

pathogen A microorganism capable of producing a disease. *Blood-borne pathogens* are pathogenic microorganisms that are present in human blood and can cause disease in humans. Pathogens include, as examples, hepatitis B virus (HBV) and human immunodeficiency virus (HIV).

pathogenesis The origin and development of a disease along with the chain of events leading to that disease.

pathogenic Causing disease or capable of doing so. Pathogenic bacteria are disease-causing bacteria. For example, pathogenic *Escherichia coli* are *E. coli* that are not innocuous (like most *E. coli*) but can make people ill and even kill them.

pemphigus vulgaris (PV) Pemphigus is a group of rare chronic autoimmune skin diseases characterized by blister formations in the outer layer of the skin and the mucous membranes. The most common form of pemphigus—pemphigus vulgaris (*vulgaris* is Latin for "common" or "ordinary")—usually begins with painful blister formations (bullae) occurring in the mouth and on the scalp. The blisters are soft and are easily broken. The blistering can also affect the esophagus, rectum, nose, or lining of the eyelids. These bullae heal without scarring. The disease is progressive and chronic but remains limited to mucous membranes in many patients. The trunk and other areas of the skin may become involved as the condition progresses.

Pemphigus vulgaris predominately occurs in middle-aged patients (between 30 and 50 years old) of Jewish or Mediterranean descent. However, it has been known to affect people across racial and cultural lines and has been documented in young adults and children. Pemphigus vulgaris has been associated with other autoimmune diseases, such as myasthenia gravis and systemic lupus.

Causes

In an affected individual, the antibodies erroneously perceive the skin and/or mucous membrane tissue as foreign and attacks them. Specifically, pemphigus vulgaris is now believed to result from the action of antidesmoglein 3, IgG autoantibodies that bind to stratified squamous epithelium. Immunofluorescent testing for these autoantibodies indicates that patients who progress to skin involvement also produce antibodies against desmoglein 1. Pemphigus vulgaris is not contagious. What aggravates the flares of the disease is not known. In medical journals, case histories have been described of outbreaks being triggered by radiation, surgery, medications, emotional stress, and even certain foods.

Clinical Features

Patients present with symptoms that include recurrent or relapsing skin lesions that look like soft blisters, mouth or skin ulcers that may drain or ooze, and crust that may spread to other skin areas, show superficial skin peeling, or detach easily. Diagnosis of an autoimmune bullous disease should be suspect when there is no clear history of exposure to a drug or a contact allergen or when other studies for infectious origins, such as herpes or impetigo, are negative. To differentiate these diseases, a careful history and physical examination are important. A skin biopsy is often helpful.

Complications

Drugs used to treat pemphigus vulgaris can have serious side effects and account for the majority of complications. Thus blood and urine must be monitored regularly. Other complications can include secondary bacterial, viral, or fungal infection of the skin; the spread of infection through the bloodstream; loss of extensive amounts of body fluids; and electrolyte imbalance or disturbances.

Treatment

No cure is available, so treatment is aimed at reducing the synthesis of these autoantibodies. Combination systematic therapy with corticosteroids and immunosuppressive agents is usually required, although the side effects of these potent medications may contribute to the patient's problems. Prednisone alone controls some cases. If the dosage cannot be tapered to 5 to 10 mg on alternate days within a year of treatment, azathioprine or cyclophosphamide must be added. In severe cases, plasmapheresis will be used to remove autoantibodies from the circulation. Severe cases of pemphigus are treated similarly to severe burns. Treatment may require hospitalization, including care in a burn unit or intensive care unit. If not treated, pemphigus vulgaris is usually fatal within two months to five years because of complications. Generalized infection is the most frequent cause of death. The mortality rate in patients with pemphigus vulgaris is up to 10 percent.

Nousari, H. C. and G. J. Anhalt. "Pemphigus and Bullous Pemphigoid." *Lancet* 354 (August 21, 1999): 667–672.

peripheral neuropathy (PN)   A common neurological disorder resulting from damage to the peripheral nerves (those nerves outside the central nervous system—the brain and spinal cord). In neuronal (axonal) neuropathies, the damage is to the nerve cell (the axon) itself. In demyelinating neuropathies, the damage is to the sheath that surrounds the nerves. Peripheral neuropathy affects 2 million people in the United States, most commonly those of middle age and the elderly.

Causes

Peripheral neuropathy may be caused by diseases of the nerves or as the result of systemic illnesses. Many neuropathies have well-defined causes such as INSULIN-DEPENDENT DIABETES, uremia, AIDS, or nutritional deficiencies. In fact, diabetes is one of the most common causes of peripheral neuropathy. Other causes include mechanical pressure such as compression or entrapment, direct trauma, penetrating injuries, contusions, fractures, or dislocated bones; pressure involving the superficial nerves (ulna, radial, or peroneal) that can result from prolonged use of crutches, from staying in one position for too long, or from a tumor; intraneural hemorrhage; exposure to cold or radiation; and vascular or collagen disorders such as atherosclerosis, SYSTEMIC LUPUS ERYTHEMATOSUS, SCLERODERMA, SARCOIDOSIS, RHEUMATOID ARTHRITIS, and POLYARTERITIS NODOSA. A common example of entrapment neuropathy is carpal tunnel syndrome, which has become more common because of the increasing use of computers. Although the causes of peripheral neuropathy are diverse, they produce common symptoms including weakness, numbness, paresthesia (abnormal sensations such as burning, tickling, pricking, or tingling), and pain in the arms, hands, legs, and/or feet. A large number of cases are of unknown cause.

Treatment

Therapy for peripheral neuropathy differs depending on the cause. For example, therapy for peripheral neuropathy caused by diabetes involves control of the diabetes. In cases where a tumor or ruptured disk is the cause, therapy may involve surgery to remove the tumor or to repair the ruptured disk. In entrapment or compression neuropathy, treatment may consist of splinting or surgical decompression of the ulnar or median nerves. Peroneal and radial compression neuropathies may require avoidance of pressure. Physical therapy and/or splints may be useful in preventing contractures (a condition in which shortened muscles around joints cause abnormal and sometimes painful positioning of the joints).

Recovery from peripheral neuropathy is usually slow. Depending on the type of peripheral neuropathy, the patient may fully recover without residual effects or may partially recover and have sensory, motor, and vasomotor (blood vessel) deficits. If severely affected, the patient may develop chronic muscular atrophy. (See also GUILLAIN-BARRÉ SYNDROME.)

Dyck, P. J., and P. K. Thomas, eds. *Diabetic Neuropathy*, 2nd ed. Philadelphia: W. B. Saunders Co., 1999.
National Institute of Neurological Disorders and Stroke, National Institutes of Health. *NINDS Peripheral Neuropathy Information*, 2001.
Rowland, L. P., ed. *Merritt's Textbook of Neurology*, 9th ed. Media, Pa.: Williams and Wilkins, 1995.
Vaillancourt, P. D., and H. M. Langevin. "Painful Peripheral Neuropathies." *The Medical Clinics of North America* 83, no. 3 (1999): 627–642.

perivenous encephalomyelitis Also known as acute disseminated encephalomyelitis (ADEM), perivenous encephalomyelitis is an acute, rapidly progressing, demyelinating multifocal disorder usually preceded by an infectious rash (such as measles or smallpox) or vaccination. Therefore it is also known as postinfectious or postvaccinal encephalomyelitis. The preceding infection may be viral (such as measles, chicken pox, German measles, mumps, influenza, or infectious mononucleosis) or bacterial (such as mycoplasma infection or scarlet fever). Most vaccinations preceding infection have been those against smallpox and rabies.

This illness was first described 250 years ago by the distinguished English physician Clifton, who noted that it occurred occasionally in patients who had smallpox. The white matter of the brain is predominantly affected. Under the microscope can be seen an invasion around the small veins by white blood cells from the blood. Where these cells accumulate, myelin is destroyed. The disorder never occurs before the age of two years, and once it is over, further attacks rarely develop. Recent long-term studies of patients with ADEM have shown that a significant number later on develop multiple sclerosis.

Causes

The association of the disease with an antecedent infection or immunization suggests an immunological process. Detailed laboratory studies involving measurement of antibrain antibodies and of cellular immune responses to specific myelin antigens have shown that these patients indeed have mounted an allergic response against their own brain constituents. Indeed, these antigens to which they are sensitive, when injected into animals, including monkeys, are capable of reproducing experimentally clinical and pathological findings similar to ADEM.

Clinical Features

After a latent period of two days to three weeks, the disease starts suddenly with a headache, stiff neck, vomiting, and/or a decreased level of consciousness and fever, soon followed by focal neurological deficits (confusion, delirium), and occasional coma. During this early period, neurological examination usually shows focal neurological signs such as bilateral optic neuritis, ataxia of the hands, clumsiness in walking, and paralysis down one side. Additionally, Korsakoff's psychosis may occur, and rarely seizures may be present. The duration of these symptoms varies. Some nonfatal cases having a mild attack lasting a few days to a month, and other fatal cases have a rapid progressive course over a number of days. The clinical sign that correlates most closely with the prognosis is the level of consciousness.

Treatment

The treatment of choice is to alter immune responses immediately upon diagnosis of the disease. Giving high doses of steroids coupled with azathioprine can often lead to a very rapid resolution of symptoms with an excellent prognosis. Occasionally, the illness may present in the spinal cord. In this presentation more than in others, the earlier the diagnosis, the better the prognosis. Overall, the prognosis is good where the diagnosis is made early and the appropriate therapy instituted without delay. Most patients show a good recovery, some are left with permanent neurological deficits, and a certain number may die during the acute phase. There is up to a 20 percent fatality rate. With survival, recovery is usually complete and there are no recurrences.

Behan, Peter O. *Acute Disseminated Encephalomyelitis.* Glasgow, Scotland: Institute of Neurological Sciences, Southern General Hospital. Available online. URL: http://gloxocentre.merseyside.org/ladem.htm. Downloaded 18 July 2002.

pernicious anemia (PA)   An autoimmune disease that occurs as an end stage of autoimmune gastritis that results in the destruction of gastric mucosa (moist tissue that lines the stomach). It follows long-term autoimmune gastritis (inflammation of the mucosal lining of the stomach). The autoimmune process is limited to the body of the stomach and causes gastric atrophy (wasting of tissue). PA is also known as Addison's anemia.

The autoimmune reaction is against the gastric intrinsic factor (a substance normally in the stomach that makes the absorption of vitamin B_{12} possible) and complement-fixing antibodies to gastric parietal cells (the binding site for vitamin B_{12}). Vitamin B_{12} binds with intrinsic factor before it is absorbed and used by the body. Long-term destruction of the parietal cells of the gastric mucosa results in atrophy leading to the inability of the stomach to absorb and utilize vitamin B_{12}. Thus, an absence of intrinsic factor prevents normal absorption of B_{12}, causing pernicious anemia, and is the end result of autoimmune gastritis. The gastric atrophy is caused by chronic inflammation from the autoimmune attack on the lining of the stomach and precedes the development of pernicious anemia by many years.

Although a juvenile form of the disease can occur in children, pernicious anemia usually does not appear before the age of 30. The average age at diagnosis is 60 years. Slightly more women than men are affected. The disease can affect all racial groups, but the incidence is higher among people of Scandinavian or northern European descent. Pernicious anemia has been observed to cluster in families.

Anyone with pernicious anemia usually needs intramuscular (IM) injections of vitamin B_{12}. Pernicious anemia is a chronic condition that needs to be monitored by a physician. Anyone with pernicious anemia has to take lifelong supplemental vitamin B_{12}, but the disease is controllable with proper attention.

phagocytes   Large white blood cells (neutrophils, monocytes, and macrophages) that contribute to the immune defenses by engulfing and killing foreign invaders like bacteria and viruses.

phagocytosis   The process by which a cell engulfs and destroys particles such as bacteria, other microorganisms, aged red blood cells, and foreign matter for purposes of defense or sustenance. The principal phagocytes (cells that can engage in phagocytosis) include the neutrophils and monocytes. The prefix *phago-* comes from the Greek *phago,* meaning "to eat." Phagocytosis takes place in three stages. In the first, the particles are covered with antibodies or complement to initiate the binding. Then in the second stage, the particles are engulfed and enclosed in a phagosome. During the third stage, the phagosome merges with lysosomes, whose enzymes destroy the engulfed particle.

phenotype   The observable traits or characteristics of an organism, for example hair color, weight, or the presence or absence of a disease. Phenotypic traits are not necessarily genetic.

plasma   The liquid part of the blood and lymphatic fluid, which makes up about half of the blood's volume. Plasma is devoid of cells and, unlike serum, has not clotted. Blood plasma contains antibodies and other proteins. It serves as the medium to transport electrolytes, glucose, proteins, and other substances to various places. At the same time, plasma also carries waste products away to the lungs, liver, kidneys, and spleen. Plasma is taken from donors and made into medications for a variety of blood-related conditions. Some blood plasma is also used in nonmedical products.

plasma cells   Large antibody-producing cells that develop from B cells.

platelets   Granule-containing cellular fragments critical for blood clotting and sealing off wounds. Platelets also contribute to the immune response.

polyarteritis nodosa (PAN)   A chronic inflammatory vascular disease that is strongly suspected of having an underlying autoimmune factor. It causes an inflammation of the arteries resulting in damage to the walls of the arteries, thus creating a narrowing of the vessels. This may result in lack of blood supply to tissues; possible formation of blood clots (thrombosis); and weakening, ballooning (aneurysm), or possible rupturing of vessel walls. PAN affects small-to-medium-sized arteries usually within the kidney, liver, gastrointestinal tract, central nervous system, and skin. The disease can occur by itself or in conjunction with other autoimmune disorders, such as lupus, rheumatoid arthri-

tis, Wegener's granulomatosis, or giant cells arteritis. Polyarteritis nodosa may also be referred to as periarteritis or polyarteritis.

According to the Johns Hopkins Vasculitis Center, polyarteritis nodosa is the "grandfather" of the vasculitides, having first been described in 1866. For nearly 100 years after its description, almost all types of vasculitis were called PAN. Polyarteritis nodosa tends to involve medium-sized blood vessels that have muscular walls, particularly those supplying blood to the gastrointestinal tract and nerves. It rarely involves the lungs and is sometimes associated with hepatitis B infections. It usually appears in adult males between ages 40 and 50 but occurs in every age group. The male-to-female ratio is three to one. Without treatment, almost all affected patients die within two to five years.

Causes
The exact cause of polyarteritis is not known. Bacterial or viral infection may possibly be the cause. Allergic reactions and vaccines have been linked to the disorder. There is a well-documented association with hepatitis B surface antigen positivity as well as a preceding streptococcal infection. Autoimmune diseases related to polyarteritis are Wegener's granulomatosis, Churg-Strauss syndrome, Takayasu's arteritis, and temporal or giant cell arteritis.

Clinical Features
Symptoms include fever, weight loss, fatigue, arthralgia, and myalgia. Skin changes include purpura and ulceration, usually occurring on the lower extremities. Approximately 25 percent of cases of classic polyarteritis nodosa will have cutaneous involvement. The most common cutaneous presentations include nodules, ulcers, and a livedo reticularis pattern on the lower extremities. The nodules are usually deep and painful, and they may occur on the trunk and upper extremities. Occasionally, periosteal new bone formation may occur under the skin lesions.

Treatment
Before the use of glucocorticoids, the five-year survival of individuals with polyarteritis nodosa was 10 percent if untreated. Today, the five-year survival

rate approximates 96 percent with the use of glucocorticoids and other immunosuppressive agents, such as cyclophosphamide. Patients with systemic involvement usually require high-dose glucocorticoid therapy, frequently for years. Patients with primarily cutaneous involvement will often achieve remission within three to six months on lower doses of glucocorticoids.

Guillevin, L., and F. Lhote. "Treatment of Polyarteritis Nodosa and Microscopic Polyangiitis." *Arthritis and Rheumatism* 41, no. 12 (1998): 2,100–2,105.

Kim, Leonard H. "Polyarteritis Nodosa," Department of Dermatology, New York University, Dermatology Online Journal. Available online. URL: http://dermatology.cdlib.org. Downloaded 18 July 2002.

polychondritis   A rare, multisystem degenerative autoimmune disease characterized by recurrent inflammation of the cartilage in the body. Deterioration of the cartilage may affect any site of the body where cartilage is present. The ears, larynx, and trachea (windpipe) may become floppy; and the bridge of the nose can collapse into a saddle nose shape. The aortic heart valve may be involved as well, resulting in a leaky valve. When this is the case, the patient will likely become easily tired or exhausted. The eyes and blood vessels, which have a biochemical makeup similar to that of cartilage, can also be affected. Polychondritis can be life threatening, debilitating, and difficult to diagnose because its symptoms are common and varied. Polychondritis may also be referred to as chronic atrophic polychondritis, relapsing polychondritis, and systemic chondromalacia von Meyenburg disease.

Polychondritis affects males and females in equal numbers. Symptoms usually begin between 40 and 60 years of age, although cases have been reported in persons as young as 30 months and as old as 90 years. It is estimated to affect one in 250,000 persons.

Causes

The cause of polychondritis is unknown, but it is suspected to be caused by an immune system disorder. It is frequently diagnosed along with rheumatoid arthritis and systemic lupus erythematosus.

Clinical Features

Typically, onset of polychondritis results in sudden pain in the inflamed tissue and swelling of the external ear. The most common first symptom of polychondritis is pain and swelling of the external ear. Usually, both ears turn red or purple and are tender to the touch. The swelling can extend into the ear canal and beyond, causing ear infections, hearing loss, balance disturbances with vertigo and vomiting, and eventually a droopy ear. The nose is often afflicted as well and can deteriorate into a flattened nose bridge called saddle nose. Inflammation of the eye occurs less frequently but can lead to blindness.

The disease may occur in episodes with complete remission between, or it may smolder along for years, causing progressive destruction. Fever, fatigue, and weight loss often develop. Other symptoms appear wherever inflammation occurs. Inflammation of the trachea can lead to throat pain, hoarseness, and breathing difficulty. Joint inflammation (arthritis) can cause pain, swelling, and stiffness of the joints, including of the hands, knees, ankles, wrists, and feet. Eye inflammation can be mild or severe and can damage vision. Cataracts can be caused by the inflammation or from the cortisone used to treat polychondritis.

Treatment

Conventional treatment involves the use of prednisone and other corticosteroids if the patient is able to tolerate the toxic side effects of these drugs.

For patients with more mild disease, nonsteroidal anti-inflammatory medications (NSAIDs), including ibuprofen (Motrin), naproxen (Naprosyn), or aspirin, can be helpful to control the inflammation. Usually, however, cortisone-related medications (steroids such as prednisone and prednisolone) are required. High-dose steroids are frequently necessary initially, especially when the eyes or breathing airways are involved. Moreover, most patients require steroids for long-term use.

Methotrexate (Rheumatrex) has shown promise as a treatment for relapsing polychondritis in combination with steroids as well as a maintenance treatment. Studies have demonstrated that methotrexate can help reduce the steroid requirements.

Other medications that have been tried in small numbers of patients with some reports of success include cyclophosphamide (Cytoxan), dapsone, azathioprine (Imuran), penicillamine (Depen, Cuprimine), cyclosporine, and combinations of these drugs with steroids. A collapsed chest or airway may require surgical support, and a heart valve or aorta may need repair or replacing.

As the disease progresses over a period of years, the mortality rate increases. At five years duration, polychondritis has a 30 percent mortality rate.

Gilliland, Bruce C. "Relapsing Polychondritis and Other Arthritides." In *Harrison's Principles of Internal Medicine,* edited by Antony S. Fauci, et al. New York: McGraw-Hill, 1998.

Polsdorfer, J. Ricker. "Relapsing Polychondritis." In *Health Topics A–Z.* Blue Cross and Blue Shield of Massachusetts, Inc. Available online: http://blueprint.bluecrossmn.com. Posted 14 July 1999.

Schumacher, H. Ralph. "Relapsing Polychondritis." In *Cecil Textbook of Medicine,* edited by J. Claude Bennett and Fred Plum. Philadelphia: W. B. Saunders, 1996.

polyglandular autoimmune syndromes (PGAS)

This is also called autoimmune endocrine failure syndrome, polyglandular deficiency syndrome, autoimmune polyendocrine syndrome APS, and immunoendocrinopathy syndrome. PGAS is a group of autoimmune disorders that involve endocrine glands and that results in failure of the glands to produce their hormones. Polyglandular syndromes involve a group of symptoms and signs of disordered function related to one another by some anatomic, physiological, or biochemical peculiarity affecting many glands. These are referred to as associated endocrinopathies, that is, diseases resulting from a disorder of an endocrine gland or glands. The endocrine system is responsible for the release of hormones into the blood or lymph. Deficiencies in the endocrine system can be caused by infection, infarction, or a tumor destroying all or a large part of the gland. However, the activity of an endocrine organ is most often depressed as a result of an autoimmune reaction that ultimately results in partial or complete destruction of the gland. Autoimmune disease affecting one organ is frequently followed by the impairment of other glands, resulting in multiple endocrine failure. People who develop a polyglandular autoimmune syndrome probably have a genetic predisposition to it.

Three syndromes of associated endocrinopathies have been defined as the polyglandular syndromes. They are categorized according to which endocrine glands are affected and whether symptoms develop in childhood or adulthood.

Autoimmune Polyglandular Syndrome Type I (APS1)

A rare autosomal recessive disorder that maps to human chromosome 21. This syndrome involves an infection of the skin or mucous membranes with any special species of candida (yeast infection), chiefly *Candida albicans,* and associated endocrinopathies (for example, Addison's disease of the adrenal glands and hypoparathyroidism). These diseases begin in early childhood. Patients initially develop candidiasis and hypoparathyroidism (underfunction of the parathyroid glands, which control calcium), but more than half of the patients also develop Addison's disease. Associated disorders include ovarian failure, alopecia (hair loss), malabsorption, eye inflammation, underdevelopment of tooth enamel, and chronic hepatitis; 15 percent have insulin-dependent Type 1 diabetes. APS1 is also known as autoimmune polyendocrinopathy-candidiasis-ectodermal dystrophy (APECED).

Patients have organ-specific autoantibodies and poorly defined defects in cell-mediated immunity. There is no HLA association. The laboratory studies in APS1 attest to an immune disease with low gamma globulin antibodies in blood (hypogamma-globulinemia) and a low T4/T8 cell ratio (as in AIDS). There is specific evidence for autoimmunity with antibodies directed against the adrenal and thyroid glands and against cell nuclei (antiadrenal, antithyroid, and antinuclear antibodies).

At the end of 1997, researchers reported that they isolated a novel gene, which they called AIRE (*auto*immune *re*gulator). Database searches revealed that the protein product of this gene is a transcription factor—a protein that plays a role in the regulation of gene expression. The researchers showed that mutations in this gene are responsible for the pathogenesis of APS1. APS1 is the first systemic autoimmune disease whose cause has been attributable to a defect in a single gene.

The identification of the gene defective in APS1 is the first step toward developing tests will be able to diagnose the disease genetically. Further investigations of the gene and its function should also facilitate finding a potential treatment for the disease as well as increasing general understanding of the mechanisms underlying other autoimmune diseases.

Autoimmune Polyglandular Syndrome Type II (APS2)

The most common of the polyglandular syndromes in which two or more autoimmune conditions are found; however, its prevalence is only 15 to 20 cases per million population. Fifty percent show Type 1 autoimmune diabetes and another associated condition, which may include Addison's disease, the celiac syndrome, vitiligo, pernicious anemia, myasthenia gravis, Graves' disease, and others. The adrenal glands are always underactive, and the thyroid gland frequently is. It generally develops in adults, usually around age 30, and primarily in women. This type is also known as Schmidt's syndrome.

Autoimmune Polyglandular Syndrome Type III (APS3)

This develops in adults and is maybe considered a preliminary stage of the type II syndrome. The associations are between insulin-dependent diabetes mellitus, thyroid gland affection that could produce hyperthyroidism or hypothyroidism, and a nonendocrinological disease, which could be rheumatological or not, and could be accompanied by less common manifestations like pernicious anemia, vitiligo, and alopecia. Circulating organ-specific autoantibodies are detected in the blood and a lymphocyte infiltrate in the affected glands in association with HLA. Type III patients have no adrenal gland problems; if they develop, the syndrome becomes type II.

PGAS Clinical Features

Because the various endocrine glands may be affected to varying degrees, those less affected may not be noticed initially. The glandular dysfunction does not occur in a specific sequence. As other symptoms develop, it becomes more apparent that more than one endocrine gland is underactive. Blood tests can then confirm the diagnosis of polyglandular autoimmune syndrome.

PGAS Treatment

Although polyglandular autoimmune syndrome cannot be cured, the appropriate hormone replacement therapy can be used for the various glandular deficiencies. However, any gonadal or candidiasis problems usually do not respond to treatment.

Baker, J. R. "Autoimmune Endocrine Disease." *The Journal of the American Medical Association* 278, no. 22 (1997): 1,931–1,937.

Chung, A. D., and J. C. English III. "Cutaneous Hyperpigmentation and Polyglandular Autoimmune Syndrome Type II." *Cutis* 59, no. 2 (1997): 77–80.

Graber, M. A., and H. A. Freed. "Polyglandular Autoimmune Syndrome: A Cause of Multiple and Sequential Endocrine Emergencies." *The American Journal of Emergency Medicine* 10, no. 2 (1992): 130–132.

Leor, J., et al. "Polyglandular Autoimmune Syndrome, Type 2." *Southern Medical Journal* 82, no. 3 (1989): 374–376.

Meyerson, J., et al. "Polyglandular Autoimmune Syndrome: Current Concepts." *Canadian Medical Association Journal* 138, no. 7 (1998): 605–612.

Mohon, Melissa A. "An Airman with Schmidt's Syndrome." *The Federal Air Surgeon's Medical Bulletin* (Spring 2001): 5–6.

polymyalgia rheumatica A rheumatic (inflammatory) disorder that is associated with moderate-to-severe muscle pain and stiffness in the neck, shoulder, and hip area. Stiffness is most noticeable in the morning. This disorder may develop rapidly—in some patients, overnight. In other people, polymyalgia rheumatica develops more gradually. The cause of polymyalgia rheumatica is not known. However, possibilities include immune system abnormalities and genetic factors. The fact that polymyalgia rheumatica is rare in people under the age of 50 suggests it may be linked to the aging process.

Polymyalgia rheumatica may go away without treatment in one to several years. With treatment, the symptoms of polymyalgia rheumatica are quickly controlled but relapse if treatment is stopped too early.

Causes

Although an autoantigen has not yet been found, the syndrome is thought to be autoimmune in nature because of the syndrome's relationship with giant cell arteritis (temporal arteritis). How or why polymyalgia rheumatica and giant cell arteritis are related is unclear. However, an estimated 15 percent of people in the United States with polymyalgia rheumatica also develop giant cell arteritis. Patients can develop giant cell arteritis either at the same time as polymyalgia rheumatica or after the polymyalgia symptoms disappear. About half of the people affected by giant cell arteritis also have polymyalgia rheumatica.

When a person is diagnosed with polymyalgia rheumatica, the doctor also looks for symptoms of giant cell arteritis because of the risk of blindness.

Caucasian women over the age of 50 are most at risk of developing polymyalgia rheumatica. Women are twice as likely as men to develop the condition. It almost exclusively affects people over the age of 50. The average age at onset is 70 years. Polymyalgia rheumatica is quite common. In the United States, an estimated 700 per 100,000 people in the general population over 50 years of age develop polymyalgia rheumatica. The highest rate of the disease is found in Denmark and Sweden.

Clinical Features

The primary symptoms of polymyalgia rheumatica are moderate-to-severe stiffness and muscle pain near the neck, shoulders, or hips. The stiffness is more severe upon waking or after a period of inactivity, and it typically lasts longer than 30 minutes. People with this condition also may have flulike symptoms, including fever, weakness, and weight loss.

No single test is available to diagnose polymyalgia rheumatica definitively. To diagnose the condition, a physician considers the patient's medical history, including symptoms that the patient reports, and the results of laboratory tests that can rule out other possible diagnoses.

The most typical laboratory finding in people with polymyalgia rheumatica is an elevated erythrocyte sedimentation rate, commonly referred to as the sed rate. This test measures how quickly red blood cells fall to the bottom of a test tube of unclotted blood. Rapidly descending cells (an elevated sed rate) indicate inflammation in the body. While the sed rate measurement is a helpful diagnostic tool, it alone does not confirm polymyalgia rheumatica. An abnormal result indicates only that tissue is inflamed, which is also a symptom of many forms of arthritis and/or other rheumatic diseases. Before making a diagnosis of polymyalgia rheumatica, the doctor may perform additional tests to rule out other conditions, including rheumatoid arthritis, because symptoms of polymyalgia rheumatica and rheumatoid arthritis can be similar.

The doctor may recommend a test for rheumatoid factor (RF). RF is an antibody sometimes found in the blood. People with rheumatoid arthritis are likely to have RF in their blood, but most people with polymyalgia rheumatica do not. If the diagnosis is still unclear, a physician may conduct additional tests to rule out other disorders. The disease usually occurs by itself; however, it not uncommonly occurs in conjunction with other conditions, such as infections, neoplasms, and autoimmune connective tissue diseases. When a secondary illness is identified, the majority of the time it is giant cell arteritis. Giant cell arteritis is found in approximately one-half of the patients with polymyalgia. However, only a minority of patients with the disease, who have no evidence of arteritis, ever develop giant cell arteritis.

Treatment

Polymyalgia rheumatica usually disappears without treatment in one to several years. With treatment, however, symptoms disappear quickly, usually in 24 to 48 hours. If there is no improvement, the doctor is likely to consider other possible diagnoses.

The treatment of choice is corticosteroid medication, usually prednisone. Polymyalgia rheumatica responds to a low daily dose of prednisone. The dose is increased as needed until symptoms disappear. Once symptoms disappear, the doctor may gradually reduce the dosage to determine the lowest amount needed to alleviate symptoms. The amount of time that treatment is needed is different for each patient. Most patients can discontinue medication after six months to two years. If symptoms recur, prednisone treatment is required again.

Nonsteroidal anti-inflammatory drugs (NSAIDs) such as aspirin and ibuprofen may also be used to treat polymyalgia rheumatica. The medication must be taken daily, and long-term use may cause stomach irritation. For most patients, NSAIDs alone are not enough to relieve symptoms.

Most people with polymyalgia rheumatica and giant cell arteritis lead productive, active lives. The duration of drug treatment differs by patient. Once treatment is discontinued, polymyalgia may recur; but once again, symptoms respond rapidly to prednisone. When properly treated, giant cell arteritis rarely recurs. (See also TEMPORAL ARTERITIS.)

polymyositis   An inflammatory muscle disease that causes varying degrees of decreased muscle power. The disease has a gradual onset and rarely affects persons under the age of 18. It most commonly occurs in those between 50 to 70 years old. It affects women twice as often as men. A Nurse Health Study (1976–90) found that the incidence of polymyositis affects approximately 120 women per million.

Causes

The cause of polymyositis is unknown. It is thought that an autoimmune reaction or a viral infection of the skeletal muscle may be a cause. Autoimmune factors are felt to be important, because autoantibodies are present in most patients. Some of the antibodies found in myositis are anti-Jo-1, anti-PL-12, anti-EJ, anti-OJ, anti-Mi-2, anti-MAS, anti-Fer, and anti-SRP.

Clinical Features

The most common symptom is muscle weakness, usually affecting those muscles that are closest to the trunk of the body (proximal). Eventually, patients have difficulty rising from a sitting position, climbing stairs, lifting objects, or reaching overhead. In some cases, distal muscles (those not close to the trunk of the body) may also be affected later in the course of the disease. Trouble with swallowing (dysphagia) may occur. Occasionally, the muscles ache and are tender to touch. Patients may also feel fatigue and discomfort and may have weight loss or a low-grade fever.

Treatment

Treatment for polymyositis generally consists of a steroid drug called prednisone. For patients in whom prednisone is not effective, immunosuppressants such as azathioprine and methotrexate may be prescribed. Physical therapy is usually recommended to preserve muscle function and avoid muscle atrophy.

The prognosis for polymyositis varies. Some cases respond to therapy. The disease is usually more severe and resistant to therapy in patients with cardiac or pulmonary problems. Death is rare but may occur in patients with severe and progressive muscle weakness, dysphagia, malnutrition, pneumonia, or respiratory failure. (See also DERMATOMYOSITIS.)

National Institute of Neurological Disorders and Stroke, National Institutes of Health. *NINDS Polymyositis Information Page,* 2001.

postmyocardial infarction syndrome   This is also known as DRESSLER'S SYNDROME or postinfarction syndrome. It is an uncommon condition that may occur as soon as a few days or as late as 11 weeks following a heart attack or heart surgery. It causes inflammation of the pericardium (membranous sac surrounding the heart), pleura, and possibly the lung tissue.

Causes

The cause is unknown. However, it is thought to be due to an autoimmune response directed against the damaged areas of heart muscle.

Clinical Features

It is characterized by fever, malaise, chest pain, pericarditis (inflammation of the outer covering membrane or sac of the heart, and pleurisy (inflammation of the outer lining of the lungs). Pain occurs when the inflamed pericardium rubs on the heart and is typically worse during deep breathing, while swallowing, and when in a reclining position (but relieved by sitting upright). The pain of Dressler's syndrome is sometimes confused with angina or recurrent heart attack.

Treatment

It is usually treated with anti-inflammatory drugs such as aspirin or NSAIDs (nonsteroidal anti-inflammatory agents) such as ibuprofen, naprosyn, or indomethacin. In the rare cases when those are not effective, cortisone may be used. In a very few cases, where the problem becomes recurrent, the pericardium may need to be surgically removed.

postpericardiotomy syndrome (PPS)   An inflammation of the pericardium (the sac surrounding the heart) caused by the pooling of blood in that area after open-heart surgery. It is associated with the development of antiheart antibodies. PPS is uncommon in infants but occurs with increasing frequency in children and adults. Estimated frequencies vary from 2 percent to 30 percent of patients undergoing surgery that involves opening the pericardium.

Causes

Various viral agents, including coxsackie B, adenovirus, and cytomegalovirus, have been present in approximately two-thirds of patients with postpericardiotomy syndrome. This suggests an autoimmune response associated with a viral infection.

Clinical Features

Fever symptoms usually develop within one to six weeks following surgery involving pericardiotomy. Despite high fever, the patient may not appear ill. The fever usually subsides within two to three weeks. Malaise, chest pain, irritability, and decreased appetite are typical presenting symptoms. Patients might also complain of dyspnea and arthralgias. Children might complain of chest pain worsening with inspiration and when in the supine position.

Complications

Tamponade (compression of the heart) is a life-threatening condition that can result from PPS. Tamponade occurs in approximately 1 percent of patients with PPS. The inflammatory changes seen with PPS may cause pericardial adhesions resulting in a localized tamponade.

Treatment

The treatment of choice is anti-inflammatory agents, such as aspirin, ibuprofen, naprosyn, or indomethacin. Corticosteroids are often used in more severe or treatment-resistant cases. Corticos-

teroids have resulted in rapid improvement in clinical symptoms and a decrease in antiheart antibodies. Bed rest and otherwise restricted physical activity are usually prescribed, at least until the initial symptoms subside. Surgery may be necessary in patients with persistent symptoms or who relapse after medical therapy. Most cases resolve within a few weeks.

Bartels, C., R. Honig, G. Burger, et al. "The Significance of Anticardiolipin Antibodies and Anti-Heart Muscle Antibodies for the Diagnosis of Postpericardiotomy Syndrome." *European Heart Journal* 15, no. 11 (November 1994): 1,494–1,499.
Kronick-Mest, C. "Postpericardiotomy Syndrome: Etiology, Manifestations, and Interventions." *Heart & Lung: The Journal of Critical Care* 18, no. 2 (March 1989): 192–198.
Prince, S. E., and B. A. Cunha. "Postpericardiotomy Syndrome." *Heart & Lung: The Journal of Critical Care* 26, no. 2 (March–April 1997): 165–168.
Skoumal, K., J. Graneto, and D. A. Lewis. "Postpericardiotomy Syndrome." *eMedicine Journal* 2, no. 5 (May 2001). Available online. URL: http://emedicine.com/ped/topic1875.htm.

pregnancy   Some autoimmune diseases have little or no effect on pregnancy; others can greatly increase the risks for miscarriage and/or maternal or fetal illness. Likewise, pregnancy can affect several autoimmune diseases. Women with an autoimmune disease need special medical attention during pregnancy.

With autoimmune diseases predominantly attacking women, and especially during their childbearing years, it is not surprising that pregnancy may play a role. Scientists have recently discovered that during pregnancy, the mother and fetus exchange body cells that can remain in either of their circulations for years following birth. On rare occasions, these exchanged cells can produce an autoimmune reaction in either the mother of the child.

In addition, Angier stated that "the hormones of pregnancy clearly influence a number of autoimmune diseases." (Pregnancy is associated primarily with elevated progesterone and to a lesser extent estrogen). Trying to determine why autoimmune diseases often subside in women during pregnancy and then flare up again with increased severity after childbirth, researchers have cited the influence of hormones that assist in reacting to stressful body conditions. Certain stress hormones seem to increase greatly during late pregnancy and subside after childbirth. These stress hormones are known to hinder the production of cytokines, the chemical messengers of the immune system. And this mechanism is believed to play a role in preventing the mother's immune system from rejecting the embryo. But after birth, the levels of stress hormones drop sharply, and at the same time, the levels of immune system cytokines surge.

A few autoimmune diseases affected by pregnancy:

- HASHIMOTO'S THYROIDITIS, GRAVES' DISEASES, and RHEUMATOID ARTHRITIS: These conditions generally improve during pregnancy but tend to return after pregnancy ends.
- Type 1 diabetic women are more likely to have adverse pregnancy outcomes than nondiabetic women.
- SYSTEMIC LUPUS ERYTHEMATOSUS (SLE) tends to flare during pregnancy, but the overall course of the disease is not affected. Pregnant women who have SLE commonly encounter premature delivery and poor fetal growth. The occurrence of fetal complications correlates with the level of maternal disease activity and the presence of specific antibodies. Uncommon problems from SLE include congenital fetal heart block (very slow fetal heart rate) and transient lupus in the newborn baby. It is important to monitor immune activity in mothers (especially antiRo and antiphospholipid antibodies) and as early as possible detect bradycardia (bradyarrhythmia) in fetus because it can be a marker of the congenital heart block development.

Angier, Natalie. "Researchers Piecing Together Autoimmune Disease Puzzle." *New York Times,* 19 June 2001, F1.

Dombroski, R. A. "Autoimmune Disease in Pregnancy." *Medical Clinics of North America* 73, no. 3 (May 1989): 605–621.

Thomas, Jennifer. "Pregnancy Can Set Stage for Autoimmune Diseases." HealthScoutNews.com. Available online. URL: http://body.subportal.com/health/Womens/Childbirth/504731.html. Posted on 13 November 2001.

prevalence The proportion of individuals in a population having a disease, based on the total number of cases of that disease in existence at any given time in any given population (such as United States, sex, or race). It is often given as the number of cases per 100,000 people. Prevalence is used to illustrate the category of a disease. For example, if using 100,000 as the given population, fewer than 0.5 cases would categorize the disease as extremely rare, 0.5 to 5 would be very rare, 5 to 50 would be rare, 50 to 200 would be uncommon, 200 to 1,000 would be fairly common, 1,000 to 5,000 would be common, 5,000 to 25,000 would be very common, and more than 25,000 per 100,000 would be extremely common.

primary agammaglobulinemia An immune disorder related to insufficient antibodies (hypogammaglobulinemia or low gamma globulins). It is manifested in a variety of immune deficiency disorders in which the immune system is compromised. This group of immune deficiencies may be the consequence of an inherited condition, an impaired immune system from known or unknown causes, a relation to autoimmune diseases, or a malignancy.

Antibodies are composed of immunoglobulins, which are essential to the immune system. They are produced by specialized cells (i.e., B lymphocytes) that circulate in the lymphatic fluid and blood. Antibodies fight off bacteria, viruses, and other foreign substances that threaten the body. Agammaglobulinemias are characterized by the abnormal functioning of specialized white blood cells called B lymphocytes. The B lymphocytes are supposed to search out and identify bacteria, viruses, or other foreign substances in the body. T lymphocytes, also known as the killer cells, assist B lymphocytes in responding to infection and other antigens. However, in some forms of primary agammaglobulinemias, neither the B nor the T lymphocytes function normally.

Immunoglobulin deficiencies may be referred to by many different names, as there are several variables within the separate but related immune disorders and also many subgroups. Antibody deficiency, immunoglobulin deficiency, and gamma globulin deficiency are all synonyms for hypogammaglobulinemia. Hypogammaglobulinemias related to autoimmunity include common variable immunodeficiency disease (CVI), selective immunoglobulin IgA deficiency, and IgG deficiency with increased IgM (hyper-IgM syndrome).

Treatment

The goal of treatment is to reduce the number and severity of infections. Intramuscular injections of gamma globulins help to boost the immune system. Infusions of blood plasma into a vein gives a quick supplement to the immune system (plasma contains antibodies, including IgG, IgM, and IgA). Antibiotics are used for the treatment of bacterial infections, with high doses of high-titer gamma globulin needed for severe infections. Treatment with immune globulins has improved the health of people with agammaglobulinemia. Without treatment, most severe infections are fatal.

Common variable immunodeficiency (CVI) CVI is also called hypogammaglobulinemia, adult-onset agammaglobulinemia, late-onset hypogammaglobulinemia, and acquired agammaglobulinemia. CVI is relatively common. Infants sometimes have symptoms of CVI, though in most cases symptoms do not show up until the second or third decade of life.

CLINICAL FEATURES OF CVI Most patients with CVI get frequent bacterial infections of the ears, sinuses, bronchi, and lungs. Patients may develop painful swollen joints in the knee, ankle, elbow, or wrist. CVI patients frequently complain of symptoms involving the digestive tract. They also commonly have an enlarged spleen and swollen glands or lymph nodes. Along with other autoimmune problems, some patients develop autoantibodies that attack their own blood cells. CVI patients have an increased risk of developing some cancers.

Blood tests to measure the amount of immunoglobulins in the blood of CVI patients show below-normal levels of IgG and IgA. Patients may have absent or slightly low levels of IgG antibodies, while IgM levels are low to normal. Blood tests also will determine how well B cells produce antibodies following a common immunization like a measles or tetanus shot. Other tests show doctors

how well the T cells are working. Doctors will test patients with digestive symptoms for gastrointestinal infections.

CAUSES OF CVI CVI has no clear pattern of inheritance. The cause is unknown.

TREATMENTS FOR CVI CVI patients receive immunoglobulin injections, or IVIg, every three to four weeks to restore normal antibody levels. Infections are treated with antibiotics. Physical therapy and daily postural drainage may help clear clogged lungs.

Selective immunoglobulin IgA deficiency Approximately one out of 600 individuals have selective IgA deficiency. Among those with this disease, people of European ancestry greatly outnumber those of other ethnic groups. People with this deficiency lack immunoglobulin A (IgA), a type of antibody that protects against infections of the mucous membranes lining the mouth, airways, and digestive tract.

CLINICAL FEATURES OF IGA DEFICIENCY Many IgA-deficient patients are healthy, with no more than the usual number of infections. Those patients who do have symptoms typically have recurring ear, sinus, or lung infections that may not respond to standard courses of antibiotics. People with IgA deficiency are likely to have other problems, including allergies, asthma, chronic diarrhea, and autoimmune diseases.

People with IgA deficiency have low levels of IgA antibodies in their blood. In contrast, their levels of IgM and IgG immunoglobulins usually are normal. IgA-deficient people also have normal levels of other immune system cells, including T cells, phagocytes, and complement proteins.

Doctors diagnose IgA deficiency by doing tests to measure the amount of total immunoglobulin in the blood as well as the type of immunoglobulin known as IgG2. Other tests determine how well a person is producing antibodies against specific germs following immunization with a common vaccine, such as a tetanus shot.

CAUSES OF IGA DEFICIENCY IgA deficiency is caused by faulty white blood cells called B cells or B lymphocytes. While patients have normal numbers of B cells, these cells do not mature into normal IgA-producing cells. Scientists do not yet know the exact cause or causes for these immature B cells. Sometimes clusters of cases occur in families. IgA-deficient patients are more likely than the general population to be related to someone with combined variable immunodeficiency, another form of immunodeficiency (hyper-IgM syndrome). Research is under way to determine the location of the suspected genes on the involved chromosomes.

TREATMENTS FOR IGA DEFICIENCY No specific treatment is available for selective IgA deficiency. Doctors treat bacterial infections with antibiotics, and patients with giardiasis (an infection caused by a common intestinal parasite) receive metronidazole or quinacrine hydrochloride.

Hyper-IgM syndrome Hyper-IgM is a rare immunodeficiency disease in which the immune system fails to produce IgA and IgG antibodies.

SYMPTOMS OF HYPER-IGM SYNDROME Infants with this syndrome usually develop recurring upper and lower respiratory infections within the first year of life. Other signs of the disease include enlarged tonsils, liver, and spleen; chronic diarrhea; and an increased risk of unusual or opportunistic infections and non-Hodgkin's lymphoma.

Laboratory tests will show normal numbers of T and B cells, high levels of IgM, and very low levels of IgG and IgA. The doctor may question whether the family recalls other relatives who became sick in infancy. Patients may also have neutropenia, a low number of white blood cells.

CAUSES OF HYPER-IGM SYNDROME A flawed gene (or genes) in T cells is responsible for hyper-IgM syndrome. The faulty T cells do not give B cells a signal they need to switch from making IgM to IgA and IgG. Most cases of hyper-IgM syndrome are linked to the X chromosome. Because males do not have a second, healthy, X chromosome to offset the disease, boys far outnumber girls with this disease.

TREATMENTS FOR HYPER-IGM SYNDROME Patients receive injections of intravenous immunoglobulin (IVIg) every three to four weeks. For neutropenia, patients can take granulocyte colony-stimulating factor (G-CSF). Their doctor may also prescribe antibiotics to prevent the respiratory infection, pneumocystis carinii pneumonia.

In a mouse model of this disease, scientists have restored the animal's ability to make antibodies and improved their survival by administering human-

made CD40 ligand, the molecule that allows T cells to communicate with B cells. A study to determine whether this treatment will be effective in humans is under way.

National Institute of Allergy and Infectious Diseases, National Institutes of Health, *Primary Immune Deficiency Fact Sheet,* 2001.

primary biliary cirrhosis (PBC) A chronic autoimmune disease that primarily affects the bile ducts of the liver. PBC is characterized by inflammatory destruction of the intrahepatic biliary system, a liver disease that slowly destroys the bile ducts in the liver. Bile, a substance that helps digest fat, leaves the liver through these ducts. When the ducts are damaged, bile builds up in the liver and damages liver tissues. Over time, the disease can cause cirrhosis and may make the liver stop working.

PBC may also be described as chronic nonsuppurative destructive cholangitis or as primary autoimmune cholangitis. Cirrhosis is actually a late manifestation of the disease. PBC ranges from very mild, when it may not even be detected, to a life-threatening illness. Early diagnosis and treatment is important in the outcome of the illness.

Causes

The origin of the disease still remains an enigma. The disease affects women more often that men, and usually occurs between the ages of 30 and 60 years. Some research suggests that the disease might be caused by a problem within the immune system.

The first hint of autoimmune disorder in PBC came with the recognition that the blood of patients with the disease gave a high-titer reaction in the autoantibody test. Soon researchers recognized that antimitochondrial reactivity was highly specific for the disease. Subsequently, evidence accumulated for many autoimmune disorders in PBC and for the likelihood that the disease had a multisystem expression but with the intrahepatic biliary system as the main target. The autoimmune attack causes inflammation and, eventually, damage to the bile ducts of the liver. Chronic inflammation causes scar tissue to form in the bile ducts and results in interference with the necessary excretion of bile.

Clinical Features

The most common symptoms of primary biliary cirrhosis are itchy skin and fatigue. Other symptoms include jaundice (yellowing of the eyes and skin), cholesterol deposits on the skin, fluid retention, and dry eyes or mouth. Some people with primary biliary cirrhosis also have osteoporosis, arthritis, and thyroid problems. Primary biliary cirrhosis is diagnosed through laboratory tests, X rays, and in some cases, a liver biopsy (a simple operation to remove a small piece of liver tissue).

Treatment

Treatment may include taking vitamin and calcium supplements, hormone therapy, and medicines to relieve symptoms. A liver transplant may be necessary if the liver is severely damaged.

National Digestive Diseases Information Clearinghouse (NDDIC), National Institute of Diabetes and Digestive and Kidney Diseases (NIDDK). *Primary Biliary Cirrhosis,* NIH Publication No. 99-4625, 1999, updated February 2001.

primary immune response The body's immune response to a first encounter with an antigen. The primary response can take some time to learn the structure of the pathogens, clear the infection, and generate immunologic memory. Immune memory greatly speeds up the response to pathogens that have been previously encountered. (See also SECONDARY IMMUNE RESPONSE.)

proteins Organic compounds (large, complex molecules) made up of one or more chains of amino acids. Proteins are one of the major components of plant and animal cells and tissues. They perform a wide variety of activities and supportive functions in the cell.

psoriasis A common, chronic (long-lasting) skin disease characterized by scaling and inflammation. Scaling occurs when cells in the outer layer of the skin reproduce faster than normal and pile up on the skin's surface.

Psoriasis affects between 1 percent and 2 percent of the United States's population, or about 5.5 million people. Although the disease occurs in all age groups and about equally in men and women, it primarily affects adults. People with psoriasis may suffer discomfort, including pain and itching, restricted motion in their joints, and emotional distress.

In its most typical form, psoriasis results in patches of thick, red skin covered with silvery scales. These patches, which are sometimes referred to as plaques, usually itch and may burn. The skin at the joints may crack. Psoriasis most often occurs on the elbows, knees, scalp, lower back, face, palms, and soles of the feet, but it can affect any skin site. The disease may also affect the fingernails, the toenails, and the soft tissues inside the mouth and genitalia. About 15 percent of people with psoriasis have joint inflammation that produces arthritis symptoms. This condition is called PSORIATIC ARTHRITIS.

Causes

Recent research indicates that psoriasis is likely a disorder of the immune system. Although a specific autoantibody has not been identified, autoimmunity is strongly suspected as being an underlying factor in psoriasis. Scientists now think that in psoriasis, an abnormal immune system causes activity by T cells in the skin. These T cells trigger the inflammation and excessive skin cell reproduction seen in people with psoriasis.

Other autoimmune diseases are often seen in families where one member has psoriasis. In about one-third of psoriasis cases, the psoriasis is inherited. Researchers are studying large families affected by psoriasis to identify a gene or genes that cause the disease.

People with psoriasis may notice that there are times when their skin worsens and then improves. Conditions that may trigger attacks (cause flare-ups) include changes in climate, infections, stress, and dry skin. Also, certain medicines, most notably beta-blockers (used to treat high blood pressure) and lithium or drugs used to treat depression, may trigger an outbreak or worsen the disease. Hormonal factors and smoking may also be triggers.

Clinical Features

Doctors usually diagnose psoriasis after a careful examination of the skin. However, diagnosis may be difficult because psoriasis can look like other skin diseases. A pathologist may assist with making the diagnosis by examining a small skin sample (biopsy) under a microscope.

Psoriasis comes in several forms. The most common form is plaque psoriasis (its scientific name is psoriasis vulgaris). In plaque psoriasis, lesions have a reddened base covered by silvery scales. Other forms of psoriasis include the following.

Guttate psoriasis Small, droplike lesions appear on the trunk, limbs, and scalp. Guttate psoriasis is most often triggered by bacterial infections (for example, streptococcus).

Pustular psoriasis Blisters of noninfectious pus appear on the skin. Attacks of pustular psoriasis may be triggered by medications, infections, emotional stress, or exposure to certain chemicals. Pustular psoriasis may affect either small or large areas of the body.

Inverse psoriasis Large, dry, smooth, vividly red plaques occur in the folds of the skin near the genitals, under the breasts, or in the armpits. Inverse psoriasis is related to increased sensitivity to friction and sweating and may be painful or itchy.

Erythrodermic psoriasis Widespread reddening and scaling of the skin is often accompanied by itching or pain. Erythrodermic psoriasis may be precipitated by severe sunburn, use of oral steroids (such as cortisone), or a drug-related rash.

Treatment

Doctors generally treat psoriasis in steps based on the severity of the disease, the extent of the areas involved, the type of psoriasis, or the patient's responsiveness to initial treatments. This is sometimes called the one-two-three approach. In step one, medicines are applied to the skin (topical treatment). Step two focuses on light treatments (phototherapy). Step three involves taking medicines internally, usually by mouth (systemic treatment).

Over time, affected skin can become resistant to treatment, especially when topical corticosteroids are used. Also, a treatment that works very well in one person may have little effect in another. Thus, doctors commonly use a trial-and-error approach to find a treatment that works. They may switch treatments periodically (for example, every 12 to 24 months) if resistance or adverse reactions occur. Treatment depends on the location of lesions, their size, the amount of the skin affected, previous response to treatment, and patients' perceptions about their skin condition and preferences for treatment. In addition, treatment is often tailored to the specific form of the disorder.

Topical Treatment

Treatments applied directly to the skin are sometimes effective in clearing psoriasis. Doctors find that some patients respond well to sunlight, corticosteroid ointments, medicines derived from vitamin D3, vitamin A (retinoids), coal tar, or anthralin. Other topical measures, such as bath solutions and moisturizers, may be soothing but are seldom strong enough to clear lesions over the long term and may need to be combined with more potent remedies.

Sunlight Daily, regular, short doses of sunlight that do not produce a sunburn clear psoriasis in many people.

Corticosteroids Available in different strengths, corticosteroids (cortisone) are usually applied twice a day. Short-term treatment is often effective in improving but not completely clearing psoriasis. If less than 10 percent of the skin is involved, some doctors will begin treatment with a high-potency corticosteroid ointment (for example, Diprolene, Temovate, Ultravate, or Psorcon). High-potency steroids may also be used for treatment-resistant plaques, particularly those on the hands or feet. Long-term use or overuse of high-potency steroids can lead to worsening of the psoriasis, thinning of the skin, internal side effects, and resistance to the treatment's benefits. Medium-potency corticosteroids may be used on the torso or limbs; low-potency preparations are used on delicate skin areas.

Calcipotriene This drug is a synthetic form of vitamin D3. (It is not the same as vitamin D supplements.) Applying calcipotriene ointment (for example, Dovonex) twice a day controls excessive production of skin cells. Because calcipotriene can irritate the skin, however, it is not recommended for the face or genitals. After four months of treatment, about 60 percent of patients have a good-to-excellent response. The safety of using the drug for cases affecting more than 20 percent of the skin is unknown, and using it on widespread areas of the skin may raise the amount of calcium in the body to unhealthy levels.

Coal tar Coal tar may be applied directly to the skin, used in a bath solution, or used on the scalp as a shampoo. It is available in different strengths, but the most potent form may be irritating. It is sometimes combined with ultraviolet B (UVB) phototherapy. When compared with steroids, coal tar has fewer side effects. However, it is messy and less effective and thus is not popular with many patients. Other drawbacks include its failure to provide long-term help for most patients, its strong odor, and its tendency to stain skin or clothing.

Anthralin Doctors sometimes use a 15- to 30-minute application of anthralin ointment, cream, or paste to treat chronic psoriasis lesions. However, this treatment often fails to clear lesions adequately, it may irritate the skin, and it stains skin and clothing brown or purple. In addition, anthralin is unsuitable for acute or actively inflamed eruptions.

Topical retinoid The retinoid tazarotene (Tazorac) is a fast drying, clear gel that is applied to the surface of the skin. Although this preparation does not act as quickly as topical corticosteroids, it has fewer side effects. Because it is irritating to normal skin, it should be used with caution in skin folds. Women of childbearing age should use birth control when using tazarotene.

Salicylic acid Salicylic acid is used to remove scales. It is most effective when combined with topical steroids, anthralin, or coal tar.

Bath solutions People with psoriasis may find that bathing in water with an oil added and then applying a moisturizer can soothe their skin. Scales can be removed and itching reduced by soaking for 15 minutes in water containing a tar solution, oiled oatmeal, Epsom salts, or Dead Sea salts.

Moisturizers When applied regularly over a long period, moisturizers have a cosmetic and soothing effect. Preparations that are thick and greasy usually work best because they hold water in the skin, reducing the scales and the itching.

Phototherapy

Ultraviolet (UV) light from the Sun causes the activated T cells in the skin to die, a process called apoptosis. Apoptosis reduces inflammation and slows the overproduction of skin cells that causes scaling. Daily, short, nonburning exposure to sunlight clears or improves psoriasis in many people. Therefore, sunlight may be included among the initial treatments for the disease. A more controlled form of artificial light treatment may be used in mild psoriasis (UVB phototherapy) or in more severe or extensive psoriasis (psoralen and ultraviolet A [PUVA] therapy).

UVB phototherapy Some artificial sources of UVB light are similar to sunlight. Newer sources, called narrow-band UVB, emit the part of the ultraviolet spectrum band that is most helpful for psoriasis. Some physicians will start with UVB treatments instead of topical agents. UVB phototherapy is also used to treat widespread psoriasis and lesions that resist topical treatment. This type of phototherapy is normally administered in a doctor's office by using a light panel or light box, although some patients can use UVB light boxes at home with a doctor's guidance. Generally, at least three treatments a week for two or three months are needed. UVB phototherapy may be combined with other treatments as well. One combined therapy program, referred to as the Ingram regime, involves a coal tar bath, UVB phototherapy, and application of an anthralin-salicylic acid paste, which is left on the skin for six to 24 hours. A similar regime, the Goeckerman treatment, involves application of coal tar ointment and UVB phototherapy.

PUVA This treatment combines oral or topical administration of a medicine called psoralen with exposure to ultraviolet A (UVA) light. Psoralen makes the body more sensitive to this light. PUVA is normally used when more than 10 percent of the skin is affected or when rapid clearing is required because the disease interferes with a person's occupation (for example, when a model's face or a carpenter's hands are involved). When compared with UVB treatment, PUVA treatment taken two to three times a week clears psoriasis more consistently and in fewer treatments. However, it is associated with more short-term side effects, including nausea, headache, fatigue, burning, and itching. Long-term treatment is associated with an increased risk of squamous cell and melanoma skin cancers. PUVA can be combined with some oral medications (retinoids and hydroxyurea) to increase its effectiveness. Simultaneous use of drugs that suppress the immune system, such as cyclosporine, have little beneficial effect and increase the risk of cancer. In very rare cases, patients who must travel long distances for PUVA treatments may, with a physician's close supervision, be taught to administer this treatment at home.

Systemic Treatment

For more severe forms of psoriasis, doctors sometimes prescribe medicines that are taken internally.

Methotrexate This treatment, which can be taken by pill or injection, slows cell production by suppressing the immune system. Patients taking methotrexate must be closely monitored because it can cause liver damage and/or decrease the production of oxygen-carrying red blood cells, infection-fighting white blood cells, and clot-enhancing platelets. As a precaution, doctors do not prescribe the drug for people with long-term liver disease or anemia. Methotrexate should not be used by pregnant women, by women who are planning to get pregnant, or by their male partners.

Cyclosporine When taken orally, cyclosporine (Neoral) acts by suppressing the immune system in a way that slows the rapid turnover of skin cells. It may provide quick relief of symptoms, but it is usually effective only during the course of treatment. The best candidates for this therapy are those with severe psoriasis who have not responded to or cannot tolerate other systemic therapies. Cyclosporine may impair kidney function or cause high blood pressure (hypertension), so patients must be carefully monitored by a doctor. Also, cyclosporine is not recommended for patients who have a weak immune system, those who have had substantial exposure to UVB or PUVA in the past, or those who are pregnant or breast-feeding.

Hydroxyurea (Hydrea) When compared with methotrexate and cyclosporine, hydroxyurea is less toxic but also less effective. It is sometimes combined with PUVA or UVB. Possible side effects include anemia and a decrease in white blood cells and platelets. Like methotrexate and cyclosporine, hydroxyurea must be avoided by pregnant women or those who are planning to become pregnant.

Retinoids A retinoid, such as acitretin (Soriatane), is a compound with vitamin A-like properties that may be prescribed for severe cases of psoriasis that do not respond to other therapies. Because this treatment may also cause birth defects, women must protect themselves from pregnancy beginning one month before through three years after treatment. Most patients experience a recurrence of psoriasis after acitretin is discontinued.

Antibiotics Although not indicated in routine treatment, antibiotics may be employed when an infection, such as streptococcus, triggers the outbreak of psoriasis, as in certain cases of guttate psoriasis.

Camisa, Charles. *Handbook of Psoriasis.* Malden, Mass.: Blackwell Science Inc., 1998.
Cram, David L. and Zimmerman, Gail. *Coping with Psoriasis: A Patient's Guide to Treatment.* Omaha, Nebr.: Addicus Books, 2000.
National Institute of Arthritis and Musculoskeletal and Skin Diseases Information Clearinghouse, National Institutes of Health. *Questions and Answers About Psoriasis,* 1999, updated January 2002.

psoriatic arthritis Joint inflammation that occurs in about 10 percent of people with PSORIASIS. In most of these cases, joint involvement will occur after the onset of psoriasis lesions. The arthritis is usually mild, affecting only a few joints, and spontaneous remissions occur. In some cases, psoriatic arthritis affects the joints at the ends of the fingers and is accompanied by changes in the fingernails and toenails. In a few persons, the arthritis is severe and affects the spine in addition to other joints. In addition to the usual treatments for psoriasis, the arthritis is treated with nonsteroid anti-inflammatory medications (NSAIDS) or sodium salicylate to reduce the pain and inflammation of the joints. Occasionally, particularly painful joints may be injected with steroid medications.

quality of life A term with varying definitions for different people that changes over time. Generally, it refers to the meaning or satisfaction one derives from living. Flanagan offered five "domains" of life quality—physical and material well-being, relations with other people, social and community activities, personal development and fulfillment, and recreation—with a person's overall quality of life hinging on the degree of satisfaction and importance that person places on any and all of those domains.

Physical well-being—or health—as it applies to quality of life, includes the person's ability to perform normal daily activities required to meet basic needs and fulfill usual roles. One of doctors' primary goals when treating patients with chronic autoimmune diseases is to help them maintain as meaningful a quality of life as possible.

Flanagan, J. C. "A Research Approach to Improving Our Quality of Life." *American Psychologist* 33, no. 2. (February 1978): 138–147.

race/ethnicity   Just as gender plays a role in understanding, diagnosing, and treating autoimmune diseases, race, ethnicity, and culture also influence the body's organ systems, health status, and behaviors. For example, SYSTEMIC LUPUS ERYTHEMATOSUS, a chronic autoimmune disease of young women, has a higher incidence and prevalence in African Americans. The Hopkins Lupus Cohort, a prospective longitudinal study of SLE outcomes, has shown that race is a major predictor of clinical manifestations, laboratory and serologic tests, and disease-related morbidity. The effect of race on musculoskeletal morbidity remains even after adjustment for education, insurance status, and smoking.

Similarly, Andrews et al. assessed the influence of race, sex, and puberty on clinical features and outcome in 115 patients with autoimmune juvenile myasthenia gravis (JMG). These demographic variables influenced not only disease incidence but also disease severity, response to therapy, and outcome, despite comparable therapeutic strategies. (See also AFRICAN AMERICANS WITH AUTOIMMUNE DISEASES; ALASKA NATIVES AND AUTOIMMUNE DISEASES; ASIANS/PACIFIC ISLANDER AMERICANS; HISPANICS/LATINOS AND AUTOIMMUNE DISEASES; NATIVE AMERICANS WITH AUTOIMMUNE DISEASES.)

Andrews, P. I., J. M. Massey, J. F. Howard Jr., and D. B. Sanders. "Race, Sex, and Puberty Influence Onset, Severity, and Outcome in Juvenile Myasthenia Gravis." *Neurology* 44, no. 7 (July 1994): 208–214.
Petri M. "The Effect of Race on Incidence and Clinical Course in Systemic Lupus Erythematosus: The Hopkins Lupus Cohort." *Journal of the American Medical Women's Association* 53, no. 1 (Winter 1998): 9–12.

Raynaud's phenomenon (RP)   A disorder of the small blood vessels that feed the skin. During an attack of Raynaud's, these arteries contract briefly, limiting blood flow. This is called a vasospasm; the attacks are vasospastic attacks. When deprived of the blood's oxygen, the skin first turns white then blue. The skin turns red as the arteries relax and blood flows again. Extremities—hands and feet—are most commonly affected, but Raynaud's can attack other areas such as the nose and ears. Raynaud's phenomenon can occur on its own, or it can be secondary to another condition such as scleroderma or lupus.

Raynaud's phenomenon is considered to be a common condition. Although estimates vary, recent surveys show that Raynaud's phenomenon may affect 5 percent to 10 percent of the general population in the United States. Women are more likely than men to have the disorder. Those women between the ages of 15 and 50 are most often affected (as many as 25 percent of young women), but anyone can have the problem. Raynaud's phenomenon appears to be more common in people who live in colder climates. However, people with the disorder who live in milder climates may have more attacks during periods of colder weather.

Causes

Doctors do not completely understand the cause of Raynaud's. However, they believe the body's blood vessels overreact to cold.

When a person is exposed to cold, the hands and feet lose heat rapidly. The body's normal response is to slow the loss of heat and preserve its core temperature. To maintain this temperature, the blood vessels that control blood flow to the skin surface move blood from arteries near the surface to veins deeper in the body. For people who have Raynaud's phenomenon, this normal body response is intensified by the sudden spasmodic contractions of the small blood vessels (arterioles) that supply blood to the fingers and toes. The arteries of the fingers and toes may also collapse. As a result, the blood supply to the extremities is greatly decreased, causing a reaction that includes skin discoloration and other changes. In persons with Raynaud's, these small blood vessels overrespond to cold. For example, reaching into a refrigerator may trigger an attack.

Once the attack begins, a person may experience three phases of skin color changes (white, blue, and red) in the fingers or toes. The order of the color changes is not the same for all people, and not everyone has all three colors. Pallor (whiteness) may occur in response to spasm of the arterioles and the resulting collapse of the digital arteries. Cyanosis (blueness) may appear because the fingers or toes are not getting enough oxygen-rich blood. The fingers or toes may also feel cold and numb. Finally, as the arterioles dilate (relax) and blood returns to the digits, rubor (redness) may occur. As the attack ends, throbbing and tingling may occur in the fingers and toes. There is often a sense of hand clumsiness. It usually occurs as repeated attacks lasting an average of 15 to 20 minutes following rewarming, although an attack can last from less than a minute to several hours.

Cold temperatures are more likely to provoke an attack when the individual is physically or emotionally stressed. Rapidly changing temperature can be a prime cause of attack even in a warm environment. For some persons, exposure to cold is not even necessary; stress alone causes vessels to narrow.

The doctor must determine whether the patient has Raynaud's alone (called primary Raynaud's phenomenon) or if another disease or some aspect of the patient's lifestyle is causing the symptoms. If the problem is caused by another disease or risk factor, the patient is said to have secondary Raynaud's phenomenon. In medical literature, primary Raynaud's phenomenon may also be called Raynaud's disease, idiopathic Raynaud's phenomenon, or primary Raynaud's syndrome. In popular terms, the disease is sometimes called white finger, wax finger, or dead finger.

Primary Raynaud's phenomenon Most people who have Raynaud's phenomenon have the primary form (the milder version). A person who has primary Raynaud's phenomenon has no underlying disease or associated medical problems. More women than men are affected, and approximately 75 percent of all cases are diagnosed in women who are between 15 and 40 years old. Primary Raynaud's usually affects both hands and both feet.

People who have only vasospastic attacks for several years, without involvement of other body systems or organs, rarely have or will develop a secondary disease (that is, a connective tissue disorder such as scleroderma) later. Several researchers who studied people who appeared to have primary Raynaud's phenomenon over long periods of time found that less than 9 percent of these people developed a secondary disease.

Secondary Raynaud's phenomenon Although secondary Raynaud's phenomenon is less common than the primary form, it is often a more complex and serious disorder and usually affects either both hands or both feet. Secondary means that patients have an underlying disease or condition that causes Raynaud's phenomenon. Connective tissue diseases are the most common cause of secondary Raynaud's phenomenon. Some of these diseases reduce blood flow to the digits by causing blood vessel walls to thicken and the vessels to constrict too easily. Raynaud's phenomenon is seen in approximately 85 percent to 95 percent of patients with scleroderma and mixed connective tissue disease, and it is present in about one-third of patients with systemic lupus erythematosus (SLE). Most studies show that SLE patients with RP are not different from other SLE patients. However, some reports have suggested that those with RP have milder SLE but are more likely to develop bone complications (aseptic necrosis of bone) while on corticosteroid. Raynaud's phenomenon can also occur in patients who have other connective tissue diseases, including Sjögren's syndrome, dermatomyositis, polymyositis, and rheumatoid arthritis.

Possible causes of secondary Raynaud's phenomenon, other than connective tissue diseases, are carpal tunnel syndrome and obstructive arterial disease (blood vessel disease). Some drugs, including beta-blockers (used to treat high blood pressure), ergotamine preparations (used for migraine headaches), certain agents used in cancer chemotherapy, and drugs that cause vasoconstriction (such as some over-the-counter cold medications and narcotics), are linked to Raynaud's phenomenon. Smoking is also one cause.

People in certain occupations may be more vulnerable to secondary Raynaud's phenomenon. Some workers in the plastics industry (who are exposed to vinyl chloride) develop a scleroderma-like illness, of which Raynaud's phenomenon can be a part. Workers who operate vibrating tools can develop a type of Raynaud's phenomenon called vibration-induced white finger. In a Canadian study, 50 percent of 146 tree fellers examined in British Columbia had this type; it affected 75 percent of workers with more than 20 years of experience. Another study showed that 45 percent of 58 rock drillers had attacks of white finger, 25 percent of workers had less than five years of experience, but 80 percent of those with more than 16 years experience were affected.

People with secondary Raynaud's phenomenon often experience associated medical problems. The more serious problems are skin ulcers (sores) or gangrene (tissue death) in the fingers or toes. Painful ulcers and gangrene are fairly common and can be difficult to treat. In addition, a person may experience heartburn or difficulty in swallowing. These two problems are caused by weakness in the muscle of the esophagus (the tube that takes food and liquids from the mouth to the stomach) that can occur in people with connective tissue diseases.

Clinical Features

Symptoms include changes in skin color (white to blue to red) and skin temperature (the affected area feels cooler). Usually there is no pain. However, the affected area commonly feels numb or prickly, as if it has fallen asleep. Pain, sometimes with redness, will sometimes accompany the return of blood circulation—generally after 30 minutes to two hours.

An attack is usually temporary, so the doctor relies on the patient's description to diagnose the problem. If a doctor suspects Raynaud's phenomenon, he or she will ask the patient for a detailed medical history. The doctor will then examine the patient to rule out other medical problems. The patient might have a vasospastic attack during the office visit, which makes diagnosing Raynaud's phenomenon easier. Most doctors find diagnosing Raynaud's phenomenon fairly easy but identifying the form (primary or secondary) of the disorder more difficult.

Nail fold capillaroscopy (the study of capillaries under a microscope) can help the doctor distinguish between primary and secondary Raynaud's phenomenon. During this test, the doctor puts a drop of oil onto the patient's nail folds, the skin at the base of the fingernail. The doctor then examines the nail folds under a microscope to look for abnormalities of the tiny blood vessels called capillaries. If the capillaries are enlarged or deformed, the patient may have a connective tissue disease.

The doctor may also order two particular blood tests, an antinuclear antibody test (ANA) and an erythrocyte sedimentation rate (ESR). The ANA test determines whether the body is producing special proteins (antibodies) often found in people who have connective tissue diseases or other autoimmune disorders. The ESR test is a measure of inflammation in the body and tests how fast red blood cells settle out of unclotted blood. Inflammation in the body causes an elevated ESR.

Complications

In most people with secondary Raynaud's, the problem does not get worse. A rare but serious complication of primary Raynaud's is dry gangrene, or dead flesh. This may occur if the arteries stay contracted so that blood cannot bring oxygen to the area. Severe cases cause disability and may force workers to leave their jobs.

Treatment

The aims of treatment are to reduce the number and severity of attacks and to prevent tissue damage and loss in the fingers and toes. Most doctors are conservative in treating patients with primary and secondary Raynaud's phenomenon; that is, they recommend nondrug treatments and self-help measures first. Doctors may prescribe medications for some patients, usually those with secondary Raynaud's phenomenon. In addition, patients are treated for any underlying disease or condition that causes secondary Raynaud's phenomenon.

Nondrug treatments and self-help measures
Several nondrug treatments and self-help measures can decrease the severity of Raynaud's attacks and promote overall well-being. Between 40 to 60 percent of patients with primary Raynaud's respond to management techniques.

• Take action during an attack—an attack should not be ignored. Its length and severity can be lessened by a few simple actions. The first and most important action is to warm the hands or feet. In cold weather, people should go indoors. Running warm water over the fingers or toes or soaking them in a bowl of warm water will warm them. Taking time to relax will further help to end the attack. If a stressful situation triggers the attack, a person can help stop the attack by getting out of the stressful situation and relaxing. After several sessions of training, patients can often prevent or stop attacks using biofeedback, a technique in which patients are taught to think their fingers or toes warm. Biofeedback along with warming the hands or feet in water to help lessen the attack.

• Keep warm—it is important not only to keep the extremities warm but also to avoid chilling any part of the body. In cold weather, people with Raynaud's phenomenon must pay particular attention to dressing. Wearing several layers of loose clothing, warm socks, boots, hats, and gloves or mittens is recommended. A hat is important because a great deal of body heat is lost through the scalp. Feet should be kept dry and warm. People with Raynaud's should also wear wristlets to close the space between the sleeves and mitten. Chemical warmers, such as small heating pouches that can be placed into pockets, mittens, boots, or shoes, can give added protection during long periods outdoors. Some people find wearing mittens and socks to bed during winter helpful. People who have secondary Raynaud's phenomenon should talk to their doctors before exercising outdoors in cold weather.

• People with Raynaud's phenomenon should also be aware that air-conditioning can trigger attacks. Turning down the air-conditioning or wearing a sweater may help prevent attacks. Some people find it helpful to use insulated drinking glasses and to put on gloves or oven mitts, or to use potholders, before handling frozen or refrigerated foods.

• Quit smoking—the nicotine in cigarettes causes the skin temperature to drop, which may lead to an attack.

• Control stress—because stress and emotional upsets may trigger an attack, particularly for people who have primary Raynaud's phenomenon, learning to recognize and avoid stressful situations may help control the number of attacks. Many people have found that relaxation or biofeedback training can help decrease the number and severity of attacks. Local hospitals and other community organizations, such as schools, often offer programs in stress management.

• Exercise—many doctors encourage patients who have Raynaud's phenomenon, particularly the primary form, to exercise regularly. Most people find that exercise promotes overall well-being, increases energy level, helps control weight, and promotes restful sleep. Patients with Raynaud's phenomenon should talk to their doctors before starting an exercise program.

• Be cautious—patients with Raynaud's should guard against cuts, bruises, and other injuries to the affected areas. Activities such as sewing may have to be limited.

• See a doctor—people with Raynaud's phenomenon should see their doctors if they are worried or frightened about attacks or if they have questions about caring for themselves. They should always see their doctors if attacks occur only on one side of the body (one hand or one foot) and any time an attack results in sores or ulcers on the fingers or toes.

Treatment with medications People with secondary Raynaud's phenomenon are more likely than those with the primary form to be treated with medications. Many doctors believe that the most effective and safest drugs are calcium channel blockers, which relax smooth muscle and dilate the small blood vessels. These drugs decrease the frequency and severity of attacks in about two-thirds of patients who have primary and secondary Raynaud's phenomenon. These drugs can also help heal skin ulcers on the fingers or toes.

Other patients have found relief with drugs called alpha-blockers that counteract the actions of norepinephrine, a hormone that constricts blood vessels. Some doctors prescribe a nonspecific vasodilator (a drug that helps relax artery walls to improve blood flow), such as nitroglycerine paste, which is applied to the fingers, to help heal skin ulcers. Treatment for Raynaud's phenomenon is not always successful. Often, patients with the secondary form will not respond as well to treatment as those with the primary form of the disorder.

Patients may find that one drug works better than another. Some people may experience side effects that require stopping the medication. For other people, a drug may become less effective over time. Women of childbearing age should know that the medications used to treat Raynaud's phenomenon may affect the growing fetus. Therefore, women who are pregnant or are trying to become pregnant should avoid taking these medications if possible.

Coffman, Jay D. *Raynaud's Phenomenon*. New York, N.Y.: Oxford University Press, 1989.

National Heart, Lung, and Blood Institute, National Institutes of Health. *Facts About Raynaud's Phenomenon*, NIH Publication No. 93-2263, July 1993.

National Institute of Arthritis and Musculoskeletal and Skin Diseases, National Institutes of Health. *Questions and Answers about Raynaud's Phenomenon*, NIH Publication No. 01-4911, May 2001.

red blood cells   See ERYTHROCYTES/RED BLOOD CELLS.

Reiter's syndrome   A disorder that causes three seemingly unrelated symptoms: arthritis, redness of the eyes (conjunctivitis), and urinary tract signs (urethritis). Doctors sometimes refer to Reiter's syndrome as a seronegative spondyloarthropathy because it is one of a group of disorders that cause inflammation throughout the body, particularly in parts of the spine and at other joints where tendons attach to bones. (Examples of other seronegative spondyloarthropathies include psoriatic arthritis, ankylosing spondylitis, and inflammatory bowel syndrome arthritis.) Inflammation is a characteristic reaction of tissues to injury or disease and is marked by four signs: swelling, redness, heat, and pain.

Reiter's syndrome was first described by Hans Reiter in 1916, a German military physician. Urethritis usually appears first. A patient who has all three of these manifestations is said to have the complete syndrome. This disease was later shown to have an infectious cause, with chlamydia being the organism most frequently associated with Reiter's syndrome. Patients having an initiating infectious episode and the subsequent arthritis are said to have an incomplete syndrome. By the current definition, as proposed in 1981 by the American Arthritis Association, Reiter's syndrome is a type of arthritis that follows urethritis, cervicitis, or dysentery. Other possible effects are inflammatory eye lesions, oral ulcers, inflammation of the skin covering the end of the penis, and scaling lesions of the palms, soles, penis, area around the nails, and occasionally other areas.

Reiter's syndrome is also referred to as reactive arthritis, which means that the arthritis occurs as a reaction to an infection that started elsewhere in the body. In many patients, the infection begins in the genitourinary tract (bladder, urethra, penis, or vagina). The infection is most commonly passed from one person to another by sexual intercourse. This form of the disorder is sometimes called genitourinary or urogenital Reiter's syndrome. Another form of the disorder, called enteric or gastrointestinal Reiter's syndrome, develops when a person eats food or handles substances that are tainted with bacteria.

Men between the ages of 20 and 40 are most likely to develop Reiter's syndrome. It is the most common type of arthritis affecting young men. Among men under age 50, about 3.5 per 100,000 develop Reiter's syndrome each year. Three percent of all men with a sexually transmitted disease develop Reiter's syndrome. Women can also develop the disorder, though less often than men, with features that are often milder and more subtle.

Causes

When a preceding infection is recognized, symptoms of Reiter's syndrome appear about one to three weeks after the infection. *Chlamydia trachomatis* is the bacteria most often associated with Reiter's syndrome acquired through sexual contact. Several different bacteria are associated with Reiter's syndrome acquired through the digestive tract, including *Salmonella, Shigella, Yersinia,* and *Campylobacter.* People may become infected with these bacteria after eating or handling improperly prepared food, such as meats that are not stored at the correct temperature.

Doctors do not know exactly why some people exposed to these bacteria develop the disorder and others do not. However, they have identified a genetic factor (HLA-B27) that increases a person's chance of developing Reiter's syndrome. About 80 percent of people with Reiter's syndrome are HLA-B27 positive. Only 6 percent of people who do not have the syndrome have the HLA-B27 gene.

Reiter's syndrome is not contagious; that is, a person with the disorder cannot pass it to somebody else. However, the bacteria that can trigger it can be passed from one person to another, although not all people infected with the bacteria will develop Reiter's syndrome. Rather, people who develop the disease have likely inherited a trait that makes them susceptible.

Clinical Features

The symptoms can affect many different parts of the body but most typically affect the urogenital tract, the joints, and the eyes. Less common symptoms are mouth ulcers, skin rashes, and heart valve problems. The signs may be so mild that patients do not notice them. They usually come and go over a period of several weeks to several months.

Urogenital tract symptoms   Reiter's syndrome often affects the urogenital tract, including the prostate, urethra, and penis in men and the fallopian tubes, uterus, and vagina in women. Men may notice an increased need to urinate, a burning sensation when urinating, and a discharge from the penis. Some men with Reiter's syndrome develop prostatitis, inflammation of the prostate gland. Symptoms of prostatitis can include fever, chills, increased need to urinate, and a burning sensation when urinating.

Women with Reiter's syndrome also develop signs in the urogenital tract, such as inflammation of the cervix (cervicitis) or inflammation of the urethra (urethritis), which can cause a burning sensation during urination. In addition, some women also develop salpingitis (inflammation of the fallopian tubes) or vulvovaginitis (inflammation of the vulva and vagina). These conditions may or may not cause any symptoms.

Joint symptoms or arthritis   The arthritis associated with Reiter's syndrome typically affects the knees, ankles, and feet, causing pain and swelling. Wrists, fingers, and other joints are less often affected. Patients with Reiter's syndrome commonly develop inflammation where the tendon attaches to the bone, a condition called enthesopathy. Enthesopathy may result in heel pain and the shortening and thickening of fingers and toes. Some people with Reiter's syndrome also develop heel spurs, bony growths in the heel that cause chronic or long-lasting foot pain.

Arthritis in Reiter's syndrome can also affect the joints in the back and cause spondylitis (inflammation of the vertebrae in the spinal column) or sacroiliitis, inflammation of the joints in the lower back that connect the spine to the pelvis. People with Reiter's syndrome who have the HLA-B27 gene have a greater chance of developing sacroiliitis and spondylitis.

Eye involvement   Conjunctivitis, an inflammation of the mucous membrane that covers the eyeball and eyelid, develops in about 50 percent of people with urogenital Reiter's syndrome and 75 percent of people with enteric Reiter's syndrome. A few people may develop uveitis, an inflammation of the inner eye. Conjunctivitis and uveitis can cause redness of the eyes, eye pain and irritation, and blurred vision. Eye involvement typically occurs early in the course of Reiter's syndrome, and symptoms may come and go.

Other symptoms   About 20 percent to 40 percent of men with Reiter's syndrome develop small, shallow, painless sores or lesions, called balanitis circinata, on the end of the penis. A small percentage of men and women develop rashes of small hard nodules on the soles of the feet and less often on the palms of the hands or elsewhere. These rashes are called keratoderma blennorrhagica. In addition, some people with Reiter's syndrome develop mouth ulcers that come and go. In some cases, these ulcers are painless and go unnoticed.

Diagnosing Reiter's syndrome is often difficult because there is no specific test to confirm that a person has it. When a patient reports symptoms, the doctor must examine him or her carefully and rule out other causes of arthritis.

The doctor will take the patient's complete medical history, noting current symptoms as well as any previous diseases, problems, and infections. Because the symptoms of Reiter's syndrome can be vague, it is sometimes useful for the patient to keep a log of the symptoms that occur, when they occur, and for how long. It is especially important to report any flulike symptoms, such as fever, vomiting, or diarrhea, even if they were mild, because they may be associated with the initial bacterial infection.

The doctor may use various blood tests to help rule out other conditions and confirm a suspected diagnosis of Reiter's syndrome. Tests may be done to determine the presence of rheumatoid factor or antinuclear antibodies. Results of these tests are abnormal in patients with other types of arthritis such as rheumatoid arthritis or lupus, but they are typically normal in patients with Reiter's syndrome. Doctors may determine the erythrocyte sedimentation rate, or sed rate, which is the rate at which red blood cells settle at the bottom of a test tube of blood. An elevated sed rate indicates inflammation somewhere in the body. Typically, people with rheumatic diseases, including Reiter's syndrome, have an elevated sed rate. In some patients with suspected Reiter's syndrome, the doctor may do a blood test to determine the presence or absence of HLA-B27.

The doctor is also likely to perform tests for infections that might be associated with Reiter's syndrome. Patients are generally tested for a chlamydia infection because recent studies have shown that early treatment in chlamydia-induced Reiter's syndrome may ameliorate the course of the disease. In many people with Reiter's syndrome, there is no clear evidence of infection at the time they are seen, although antibodies may be detected

in the blood, indicating that an infection was present in the past. The doctor may test samples of cells taken from the patient's throat as well as the urethra in men or cervix in women. Urine and stool samples may also be tested. The synovial fluid (the fluid that lubricates the joints) or the membrane (synovium) that lines the joint may be removed from the joint affected by arthritis. Studies of the fluid or the synovium can help the doctor make certain there is no infection in the joint.

Doctors sometimes use X rays to help establish a diagnosis of Reiter's syndrome and rule out other causes of arthritis. Common findings on X rays of patients with Reiter's syndrome include spondylitis, sacroiliitis, swelling of soft tissues, damage to cartilage or bone margins of the joint, and bone deposits where the tendon attaches to the bone.

Complications

About 10 percent of people with Reiter's syndrome, usually those with prolonged disease, develop heart problems. These include aortic regurgitation (leakage of blood from the aorta into the heart chamber) and pericarditis (inflammation of the membrane that covers and protects the heart).

Treatment

Although no cure exists for Reiter's syndrome, treatments that effectively relieve the symptoms are available. Many symptoms may even disappear for long periods of time. The doctor is likely to use one or more of the following treatments.

Bed rest   Short periods of bed rest are sometimes effective in reducing the pain and inflammation of arthritis. Lying down can reduce the pressure of the body's weight on a painful joint and provide relief for some patients.

Exercise   Even before symptoms disappear, some strengthening and gentle range-of-motion exercises will maintain or improve joint function. Strengthening exercises build up the muscles around the joint to support it better. Isometric tightening of muscles without moving the joints can be used even in active, painful disease. Range-of-motion exercises improve movement and flexibility, and they reduce stiffness in the affected joint. Before beginning an exercise program, patients should talk to the doctor, who can recommend appropriate exercises.

Nonsteroidal anti-inflammatory drugs (NSAIDs) This type of medicine effectively reduces joint inflammation and is commonly used to treat patients with Reiter's syndrome. Some NSAIDs, such as aspirin and ibuprofen, are available without a prescription. Many others require a doctor's prescription.

Corticosteroid injections For people with severe joint inflammation, injections of corticosteroids directly into the affected joint may effectively reduce inflammation. Doctors typically use this treatment only after trying to control arthritis with NSAIDs. Corticosteroid injections are most commonly used for severe knee or ankle inflammation.

Topical corticosteroids This type of medicine can be put directly onto the skin lesions associated with Reiter's syndrome. Topical corticosteroids reduce inflammation and promote healing.

Antibiotics Antibiotics may be prescribed to eliminate the bacterial infection that triggered Reiter's syndrome. The specific antibiotic prescribed depends on the type of bacterial infection that has to be treated. Patients must carefully follow the doctor's instructions about how much medicine to take and for how long; if the medicine is not taken correctly, the infection may not go away. Often, an antibiotic is taken once or twice a day for seven to 10 days or longer. Some doctors may recommend that a person with Reiter's syndrome take antibiotics for a long period of time (up to three months). Current research shows that this practice usually has no effect on the course of the disease and is therefore unnecessary. However, in cases when chlamydia triggers Reiter's syndrome, prolonged antibiotic treatment is effective in shortening the length of time that a person has symptoms.

Immunosuppressive medicines A small percentage of patients with Reiter's syndrome have severe symptoms that cannot be controlled with the treatments described earlier. For these people, medicine that suppresses the immune system, such as sulfasalazine or methotrexate, may be effective.

Most people with Reiter's syndrome recover fully from the initial flare of symptoms and are able to return to regular activities within two to six months after the first symptoms appear. Arthritis may last up to six months, although the symptoms are usually very mild and do not interfere with daily activities. Only 20 percent of people with Reiter's syndrome will have chronic arthritis, which is usually mild. Some patients experience symptom recurrence. Studies show that about 15 percent to 50 percent of patients will develop symptoms sometime after the initial flare has disappeared. Back pain and arthritis are the symptoms that most commonly reappear. A small percentage of patients will have deforming arthritis and severe symptoms that are difficult to control with treatment.

National Arthritis and Musculoskeletal and Skin Diseases Information Clearinghouse (NAMSIC), National Institutes of Health. *Questions and Answers About Reiter's Syndrome,* 1999.

relapse The reappearance (recurrence) of a disease after apparent recovery or the return of symptoms after a REMISSION.

relative risk A statistical comparison between two groups of people in a well-defined population. Relative risk is used to determine if a specific risk factor or disease is associated with an increase, decrease, or no change in the disease rate in those populations. Relative risk for a disease is the ratio of the rates in exposed and unexposed populations.

religion/spirituality Various articles in the popular media have asserted that a growing number of studies are showing that spirituality and involvement in religious activities may be more involved in the healing process than previously thought. For example, according to Bruce S. Rabin, M.D., Ph.D, "The emotional feeling provided through religion—of greater satisfaction with life, personal happiness, and fewer negative psychosocial consequences associated with traumatic life events—are all likely to be important factors in the health-promoting influence of religion. Indeed, older adults, particularly women, who attend religious services at least once a week appear to have a survival advantage over those attending services less frequently."

Rabin defines the two terms thus: "Religion is something that can be measured in the sense of being able to count how many times an individual attends a place of worship or prays. Spirituality is something that is very personal, that cannot be measured, but which helps a person relax and calm their fears and anxieties. One may feel spiritual when they look at a beautiful painting, or a tree, or a waterfall, or read a book they enjoy, or pray. Individuals who are high in spirituality have a better quality of both mental and physical health than those who are not."

But some experts have cautioned that religious beliefs can be harmful when they encourage excessive guilt, fear, and lowered self-worth. A researcher at Bowling Green State University in Ohio found that religious people who view humans as "sinners in the hands of an angry God" tend to be more depressed and anxious than religious people without such beliefs. One author also noted that spirituality does not guarantee health. Members of some religions refuse medical treatment and rely solely on prayer for physical health—a practice that may result in illness and death.

Sloan and Bagiella refute the claims that "studies" show religion or spirituality as being health determinants.

Claims about religion, spirituality, and health have recently appeared with increasing frequency, in both the popular media and professional journals. These claims have asserted that there are a great many studies in the literature that have examined relations between religious involvement and health outcomes and that the majority of them have shown that religious people are healthier. We examined the validity of these claims in two ways: (a) To determine the percentage of articles in the literature that were potentially relevant to such a claim, we identified all English-language articles with published abstracts identified by a Medline search using the search term religion in the year 2000, and (b) to examine the quality of the data in articles cited as providing support for such a claim, we examined all articles in the area of cardiovascular disease and hypertension cited by two comprehensive reviews of the literature. Of the 266 articles published in the year 2000 and identified by the Medline search, only 17 percent were relevant to claims of health benefits associated with religious involvement. About half of the articles cited in the comprehensive reviews were irrelevant to these claims. Of those that actually were relevant, many either had significant methodological flaws or were misrepresented, leaving only a few articles that could truly be described as demonstrating beneficial effects of religious involvement. We conclude that there is little empirical basis for assertions that religious involvement or activity is associated with beneficial health outcomes.

Daaleman T. P., A. Kuckelman Cobb, and B. B. Frey. "Spirituality and Well-being: An Exploratory Study of the Patient Perspective." *Social Science and Medicine* 53, no. 11 (December 2001): 1,503–1,511.

Potter M. L., and J. A. Zauszniewski. "Spirituality, Resourcefulness, and Arthritis Impact on Health Perception of Elders with Rheumatoid Arthritis." *Journal of Holistic Nursing* 18, no. 4 (December 2000): 311–331; discussions 332–336.

Rabin, Bruce. "The Effect Of Stress On Health." KBCO.com Lifestyles Magazine. Available online: URL: http://www.kbco.com/lifestyles/features/features13.html. Downloaded on 19 July 2002.

Sloan, R. P., and E. Begiella. "Claims about Religious Involvement and Health Outcomes." *Annals of Behavioral Medicine* 24, no. 1 (Winter 2002): 14–21.

"Spirituality." iVillage.com. Available online. URL: http://www.ivillagehealth.com/library/onemed/content/0,7064,241012_248508,00.html. Downloaded on 19 July 2002.

remission   A temporary lessening or disappearance of the symptoms of a disease. Remissions are common in many chronic (long-term) disease. MULTIPLE SCLEROSIS is one such disease where a pattern of alternating remission and RELAPSE is the norm.

research   See CLINICAL STUDIES/RESEARCH.

rheumatic fever   A delayed consequence of an untreated upper respiratory infection with group A streptococci (streptococcal pharyngitis or strep throat). Rheumatic fever is an autoimmune disease in which there is a hypersensitive reaction of the immune system to group A beta-hemolytic streptococcal infection. Rheumatic fever is not a contagious disease but, rather, a complication of the strep throat infection. A small percentage, probably less than 0.3 percent, of all people who have streptococcal pharyngitis will develop acute rheumatic fever. The disease can cause serious, debilitating damage to the heart and involve other tissues.

The majority of cases of rheumatic fever occur in children, adolescents, and young adults. The peak age of incidence for rheumatic fever is five to 15 years, but cases do occur in adults. Acute rheumatic fever is rare in children less than four years of age.

Causes

Heart-reactive antibodies (HRAs), which attack one's own heart tissue, have long been known to play a role in the causation of rheumatic fever. Rheumatic fever and resulting heart disease are initiated by a throat infection with a group A beta-hemolytic streptococcus. As a consequence of this infection, some patients produce HRAs without developing the disease, some develop rheumatic heart disease, and some patients develop both. The majority of patients with group A beta-hemolytic streptococcal infections do not get rheumatic fever. Why some individuals are more susceptible to developing HRAs has been the subject of much research. An HRA-linked B cell alloantigen has been implicated in the increased susceptibility.

Clinical Features

Initially, rheumatic fever is acute. The major symptoms of rheumatic fever are carditis, polyarthritis, chorea, subcutaneous nodules, and a rash called erythema marginatum.

Carditis is the most significant manifestation of rheumatic fever because it may cause permanent organ damage or death. Carditis is frequently mild or asymptomatic and therefore difficult to detect. Although not fully understood, a person's immune system response to a streptococcal infection appears to cause tissue degeneration, most frequently heart valve tissue, and subsequently cardiac disability or death.

Polyarthritis is arthritis in a number of joints at a time. Chorea is a neurological syndrome that may appear after a latent period of several months. Chorea is seen as rapid, purposeless, involuntary movements in the extremities and the face. Subcu-

taneous nodules are firm, painless lesions that occur over bony surfaces just under the skin. Erythema marginatum is a rash that appears mostly on the trunk and extremities.

There is a latent period of one to five weeks (average 19 days) between streptococcal pharyngitis and the initial episode of acute rheumatic fever. The average duration of an attack of acute rheumatic fever is three months or longer. After the acute attack has subsided, many people are left with damaged heart valves (rheumatic heart disease). Some people will have recurrent acute attacks of rheumatic fever, frequently causing more damage to the heart valves.

Rheumatic fever may be difficult to diagnose. There are no specific laboratory tests to diagnose acute rheumatic fever. In general, rheumatic fever can be diagnosed with documentation of a recent infection with group A streptococcal infection and observation of one or more of the major symptoms.

Treatment

Antibiotics will not modify an acute rheumatic fever attack nor affect the subsequent development of carditis. However, a recommended regimen of antibiotics prescribed for treatment of streptococcal pharyngitis is recommended to eradicate any group A streptococci remaining in the patient and in part, to prevent spread of the organism to close contacts.

Those people who have already suffered a rheumatic fever attack are extremely susceptible to a recurrence if they are again infected with group A streptococci. Patients who have experienced a documented acute rheumatic fever attack should receive continuous antibiotic prophylaxis to prevent streptococcal infections at least until reaching adulthood or at least five years after their most recent attack. Patients whose acute rheumatic fever attack has left them with damaged heart tissue may need lifelong antibiotic prophylaxis. Invasive dental or surgical procedures may require additional antibiotic prophylaxis for patients with rheumatic valvular heart disease.

Prevention of rheumatic fever involves prompt, accurate diagnosis and effective treatment of streptococcal pharyngitis. This is especially so in school-aged children and others who live in crowded conditions such as the military and large house-holds.

English, Peter C. *Rheumatic Fever in America and Britain: A Biological, Epidemiological, and Medical History.* New Brunswick, N.J.: Rutgers University Press, 1999.

South Dakota Department of Health, Office of Disease Prevention. *Rheumatic Fever,* Pierre, S.D.: 2001.

rheumatoid arthritis (RA) An inflammatory disease that causes pain, swelling, stiffness, and loss of function in the joints. Rheumatoid arthritis is one of the more difficult of the autoimmune rheumatic diseases to control and can do the most damage to the joints. It has several special features that make it different from other kinds of arthritis. For example, rheumatoid arthritis generally occurs in a symmetrical pattern. This means that if one knee or hand is involved, the other one is also. The disease often affects the wrist joints and the finger joints closest to the hand. It can also affect other parts of the body besides the joints. In addition, people with the disease may have fatigue, occasional fever, and a general sense of not feeling well (malaise). In some cases, the internal organs and systems can become involved and ultimately damaged.

Scientists estimate that about 2.1 million people, or 1 percent of the U.S. adult population, have rheumatoid arthritis. Interestingly, some recent studies have suggested that the overall number of new cases of rheumatoid arthritis may actually be going down. Scientists are now investigating why this may be happening.

Rheumatoid arthritis occurs in all races and ethnic groups. Although the disease generally starts between the ages of 20 and 50 and occurs with increased frequency in older people, children and young adults also develop it. Like some other forms of arthritis, rheumatoid arthritis occurs much more frequently in women than in men. About two to three times as many women as men have the disease.

The severity of rheumatoid arthritis varies from person to person. For some people, it lasts only a few months or a year or two and goes away without causing any noticeable damage. In some cases, the disease may be mild, while in others it can be crippling. Its course is unpredictable. It can flare up

suddenly and just as quickly go into remission. Still others have severe disease that is active most of the time, lasts for many years, and leads to serious joint damage and disability. Emotional stress is not a direct cause of rheumatoid arthritis but can hasten progression of the disease and make it worse.

Although rheumatoid arthritis can have serious effects on a person's life and well-being, current treatment strategies—including pain relief and other medications, a balance between rest and exercise, and patient education and support programs—allow most people with the disease to lead active and productive lives. In recent years, research has led to a new understanding of rheumatoid arthritis and has increased the likelihood that, in time, researchers can find ways to reduce the impact of this disease greatly.

Complications

Daily joint pain is an inevitable consequence of the disease. Most patients also experience some degree of depression, anxiety, and feelings of helplessness. In some cases, rheumatoid arthritis can interfere with a person's ability to carry out normal daily activities, limit job opportunities, or disrupt the joys and responsibilities of family life.

Causes

A normal joint (the place where two bones meet) is surrounded by a joint capsule that protects and supports it. Cartilage covers and cushions the ends of the two bones. The joint capsule is lined with a type of tissue called synovium, which produces synovial fluid. This clear fluid lubricates and nourishes the cartilage and bones inside the joint capsule.

In rheumatoid arthritis, the immune system, for unknown reasons, attacks a person's own cells inside the joint capsule. White blood cells that are part of the normal immune system travel to the synovium and cause a reaction. This reaction, or inflammation, is called synovitis. It results in the warmth, redness, swelling, and pain that are typical symptoms of rheumatoid arthritis. During the inflammation process, the cells of the synovium grow and divide abnormally, making the normally thin synovium thick and resulting in a joint that is swollen and puffy to the touch.

As rheumatoid arthritis progresses, these abnormal synovial cells begin to invade and destroy the cartilage and bone within the joint. The surrounding muscles, ligaments, and tendons that support and stabilize the joint become weak and unable to work normally. All of these effects lead to the pain and deformities often seen in rheumatoid arthritis. Doctors studying rheumatoid arthritis now believe that damage to bones begins during the first year or two that a person has the disease. This is one reason early diagnosis and treatment are so important in the management of rheumatoid arthritis. Rheumatoid arthritis can also cause more generalized bone loss that may lead to osteoporosis (fragile bones that are prone to fracture).

Some people also experience the effects of rheumatoid arthritis in places other than the joints. About one-quarter develop rheumatoid nodules. These are bumps under the skin that often form close to the joints. Many people with rheumatoid arthritis develop anemia, or a decrease in the normal number of red blood cells. Other effects, which occur less often, include neck pain and dry eyes and mouth. Very rarely, people may have inflammation of the blood vessels, the lining of the lungs, or the sac enclosing the heart.

Genetic (inherited) factors Scientists have found that certain genes that play a role in the immune system are associated with a tendency to develop rheumatoid arthritis. At the same time, some people with rheumatoid arthritis do not have these particular genes, and other people have these genes but never develop the disease. This suggests that a person's genetic makeup is an important part of the story but not the whole answer. Clearly, however, more than one gene is involved in determining whether a person develops rheumatoid arthritis and, if so, how severe the disease will become.

Environmental factors Many scientists think that something must occur to trigger the disease process in people whose genetic makeup makes them susceptible to rheumatoid arthritis. An infectious agent such as a virus or bacterium appears likely, but the exact agent is not yet known. However, rheumatoid arthritis is not contagious. A person cannot catch it from someone else.

Other factors Some scientists also think that a variety of hormonal factors may be involved. These hormones, or possibly deficiencies or changes in certain hormones, may promote the development of rheumatoid arthritis in a genetically susceptible person who has been exposed to a triggering agent from the environment. Even though all the answers are not known, one thing is certain: rheumatoid arthritis develops as a result of an interaction of many factors. Much research is going on now to understand these factors and how they work together.

Clinical Features

Rheumatoid arthritis can be difficult to diagnose in its early stages for several reasons. First, there is no single test for the disease. In addition, symptoms differ from person to person and can be more severe in some people than in others. Also, symptoms can be similar to those of other types of arthritis and joint conditions, and some time may be needed for other conditions to be ruled out as possible diagnoses. Finally, the full range of symptoms develops over time, and only a few symptoms may be present in the early stages. As a result, doctors use a variety of tools to diagnose the disease and to rule out other conditions.

Medical history This is the patient's description of symptoms and when and how they began. Good communication between patient and doctor is especially important here. For example, the patient's description of pain, stiffness, and joint function and how these change over time is critical to the doctor's initial assessment of the disease and his or her assessment of how the disease changes.

Physical examination This includes the doctor's examination of the joints, skin, reflexes, and muscle strength.

Laboratory tests One common test is for rheumatoid factor, an antibody that is eventually present in the blood of most rheumatoid arthritis patients. Not all people with rheumatoid arthritis test positive for rheumatoid factor, however, especially early in the disease. Additionally, some others who do test positive never develop the disease. Other common tests include one that indicates the presence of inflammation in the body (the erythrocyte sedimentation rate), a white blood cell count, and a blood test for anemia.

X rays X rays are used to determine the degree of joint destruction. They are not useful in the early stages of rheumatoid arthritis before bone damage is evident, but they can be used later to monitor the progression of the disease.

Treatment

Doctors use a variety of approaches to treat rheumatoid arthritis. These are used in different combinations and at different times during the course of the disease. They are chosen according to the patient's individual situation. No matter what treatment the doctor and patient choose, however, the goals are the same: relieve pain, reduce inflammation, slow down or stop joint damage, and improve the person's sense of well-being and ability to function.

Lifestyle   This approach includes several activities that help improve a person's ability to function independently and maintain a positive outlook.

REST AND EXERCISE   Both rest and exercise help in important ways. People with rheumatoid arthritis need a good balance between the two, with more rest when the disease is active and more exercise when it is not. Rest helps to reduce active joint inflammation and pain and to fight fatigue. The length of time needed for rest will vary from person to person. In general, though, shorter rest breaks every now and then are more helpful than long times spent in bed.

Exercise is important for maintaining healthy and strong muscles, preserving joint mobility, and maintaining flexibility. Exercise can also help people sleep well, reduce pain, maintain a positive attitude, and lose weight. Exercise programs should be planned and carried out to take into account the person's physical abilities, limitations, and changing needs.

CARE OF JOINTS   Some people find that using a splint for a short time around a painful joint reduces pain and swelling by supporting the joint and letting it rest. Splints are used mostly on wrists and hands but also on ankles and feet. A doctor or a physical or occupational therapist can help a patient get a splint and ensure that it fits properly. Other ways to reduce stress on joints include self-help devices (for example, zipper pullers and long-handled shoe horns); devices to help with getting on and off chairs, toilet seats, and beds; and changes in the ways that a person carries out daily activities.

Stress reduction   People with rheumatoid arthritis face emotional challenges as well as physical ones. The emotions they feel because of the disease—fear, anger, and frustration—combined with any pain and physical limitations can increase their stress level. Although there is no evidence that stress plays a role in causing rheumatoid arthritis, it can make living with the disease difficult at times. Stress may also affect the amount of pain a person feels. A number of successful techniques can be used to cope with stress. Regular rest periods can help, as can relaxation, distraction, or visualization exercises. Exercise programs, participation in support groups, and good communication with the health care team are other ways to reduce stress.

HEALTHFUL DIET   With the exception of several specific types of oils, no scientific evidence indicates that any specific food or nutrient helps or harms most people with rheumatoid arthritis. However, an overall nutritious diet with enough—but not an excess of—calories, protein, and calcium is important. Some people may need to be careful about drinking alcoholic beverages because of the medications they take for rheumatoid arthritis. Those taking methotrexate may need to avoid alcohol altogether. Patients should ask their doctors for guidance on this issue.

CLIMATE   Some people notice that their arthritis gets worse when the weather suddenly changes. However, there is no evidence that a specific climate can prevent or reduce the effects of rheumatoid arthritis. Moving to a new place with a different climate usually does not make a long-term difference in a person's rheumatoid arthritis.

Medications   Most people who have rheumatoid arthritis take medications. Some medications are used only for pain relief; others are used to reduce inflammation. Still others—often called disease-modifying antirheumatic drugs, or DMARDs—are used to try to slow the course of the disease. The person's general condition, the current and predicted severity of the illness, the length of time he or she will take the drug, and the drug's effectiveness and potential side effects are important considerations in prescribing drugs for rheumatoid arthritis. (See table of "Medications Commonly Used to Treat Rheumatoid Arthritis" in

Appendix VI. It shows currently used rheumatoid arthritis medications, along with their effects, side effects, and monitoring requirements.)

Traditionally, rheumatoid arthritis therapy has involved an approach in which doctors prescribed aspirin or similar drugs, rest, and physical therapy, first and prescribed more powerful drugs later only if the disease became much worse. Recently, many doctors have changed their approach, especially for patients with severe, rapidly progressing rheumatoid arthritis. This change is based on the belief that early treatment with more powerful drugs and the use of drug combinations in place of single drugs may be more effective in halting the progression of the disease and reducing or preventing joint damage.

Two new research studies reflect a rheumatoid arthritis research effort moving at a breathtaking pace, according to experts in the field. One study has shown that a combination of the drugs infliximab (Remicade) and methotrexate significantly reduced the symptoms of RA and halted progression of joint damage over methotrexate treatment alone in a 54-week trial of 428 patients. The other reveals that etanercept (Enbrel), when compared with methotrexate alone, also arrested joint damage and more rapidly decreased symptoms in a 12-month trial of 632 patients.

Peter E. Lipsky, M.D., scientific director of the National Institute of Arthritis and Musculoskeletal and Skin Diseases (NIAMS) and lead author of the infliximab study, remarked that "in the last two years, rheumatoid arthritis research has moved further than in the last 30." There has been much excitement, he said, about the wealth of new treatments now becoming available and the potential to prevent and heal structural damage to the joints of people with RA.

Dr. Lipsky led the infliximab study while at the University of Texas Southwestern Medical Center in Dallas. According to the paper, nearly 52 percent of the patients taking the infliximab/methotrexate combination showed symptom reductions, compared with 17 percent of methotrexate-only patients. X-ray examination showed that joint damage was halted in those given the drug combination. In 40 to 55 percent of patients, joint damage decreased, implying that some damage had

been repaired. Joint damage proceeded in the group given only methotrexate. The combination, which was well tolerated, also significantly improved quality of life. The benefits of the drug combination was sustained during the second year of the study.

In the second study, led by Joan Bathon, M.D., at Johns Hopkins University, Baltimore, etanercept was compared with methotrexate in patients with early disease. Etanercept acted more rapidly than methotrexate and also resulted in fewer adverse events. The rate of joint damage, as measured by X rays, was significantly reduced in the etanercept group compared with the methotrexate-treated group. After one year of treatment, 72 percent of the etanercept patients had no progression in erosions compared with 60 percent of the methotrexate-treated patients.

Infliximab and etanercept belong to a class of drugs called *biological response modifiers* that neutralize the inflammatory protein tumor necrosis factor. The drugs act by blocking the activity of destructive inflammatory cells that cause the joint damage characteristic of RA.

Methotrexate is a drug that suppresses the immune system and has been used historically in higher doses for cancer therapy. It was approved over a decade ago for treating certain types of arthritis and skin conditions.

Surgery Several types of surgery are available to patients with severe joint damage. The primary purpose of these procedures is to reduce pain, improve the affected joint's function, and improve the patient's ability to perform daily activities. Surgery is not for everyone, however, and the decision should be made only after careful consideration by patient and doctor. Together they should discuss the patient's overall health, the condition of the joint or tendon that will be operated on, and the reason for and the risks and benefits of the surgical procedure. Cost may be another factor. Commonly performed surgical procedures include joint replacement, tendon reconstruction, and synovectomy.

JOINT REPLACEMENT This is the most frequently performed surgery for rheumatoid arthritis. It is done primarily to relieve pain and improve or preserve joint function. Artificial joints are not always permanent and may eventually have to be replaced. This may be an issue for younger people.

TENDON RECONSTRUCTION Rheumatoid arthritis can damage and even rupture tendons, the tissues that attach muscle to bone. This surgery, which is used most frequently on the hands, reconstructs the damaged tendon by attaching an intact tendon to it. This procedure can help to restore hand function, especially if the tendon is completely ruptured.

SYNOVECTOMY In this surgery, the doctor actually removes the inflamed synovial tissue. Synovectomy by itself is seldom performed now because not all of the tissue can be removed and the tissue eventually grows back. Synovectomy is done as part of reconstructive surgery, especially tendon reconstruction.

Routine monitoring and ongoing care Regular medical care is important to monitor the course of the disease, determine the effectiveness and any negative effects of medications, and change therapies as needed. Monitoring typically includes regular visits to the doctor. It may also include blood, urine, and other laboratory tests and also X rays.

Alternative and complementary therapies Special diets, vitamin supplements, and other alternative approaches have been suggested for the treatment of rheumatoid arthritis. Although many of these approaches may not be harmful in and of themselves, controlled scientific studies either have not been conducted or have found no definite benefit to these therapies. Some alternative or complementary approaches may help the patient cope or reduce some of the stress associated with living with a chronic illness. As with any therapy, patients should discuss the benefits and drawbacks with their doctors before beginning an alternative or new type of therapy. If the doctor feels the approach will not be harmful, it can be incorporated into a patient's treatment plan. However, not to neglecting regular health care is important. The Arthritis Foundation publishes material on alternative therapies as well as established therapies, and patients may want to contact this organization for information.(See also JUVENILE ARTHRITIS, RHEUMATOID ARTHRITIS RESEARCH.)

Bathon, J., R. Martin, R. Fleishmann et al. "A Comparison of Etanercept and Methotrexate in Patients with Early Rheumatoid Arthritis." *The New England Journal of Medicine* 343, no. 22 (2000): 1,586–1,593.

Henkel, Gretchen, et al. *The Arthritis Foundation's Guide to Good Living with Rheumatoid Arthritis.* Marietta, Ga.: Longstreet Press, Inc., 1998.

Lee, Thomas F. *Conquering Rheumatoid Arthritis: The Latest Breakthroughs and Treatments.* Amherst, N.Y.: Prometheus Books, 2001.

Lipsky, P., D. Van Der Heijde, E. St. Clair et al. "Infliximab and Methotrexate in the Treatment of Rheumatoid Arthritis." *The New England Journal of Medicine* 343, no. 22 (2000): 1,594–1,602.

National Institute of Arthritis and Musculoskeletal and Skin Diseases Information Clearinghouse (NIAMS), National Institutes of Health. *Handout on Health: Rheumatoid Arthritis,* 1998.

Shlotzhauer, Tammi L. and James L. McGuire, eds. *Living With Rheumatoid Arthritis,* Johns Hopkins Health Book. Baltimore, Md.: Johns Hopkins University Press, 1995.

rheumatoid arthritis research Over the past several decades, research has greatly increased researchers' understanding of immunology, genetics, and cellular and molecular biology. This foundation in basic science is now showing results in several areas important to rheumatoid arthritis. Scientists are thinking about rheumatoid arthritis in exciting ways that were not possible even 10 years ago.

The National Institutes of Health (NIH) funds a wide variety of medical research at its headquarters in Bethesda, Maryland, and at universities and medical centers across the United States. One of the NIH institutes, the National Institute of Arthritis and Musculoskeletal and Skin Diseases (NIAMS), is a major supporter of research and research training in rheumatoid arthritis through grants to individual scientists, specialized centers of research, and multipurpose arthritis and musculoskeletal diseases centers.

The following are examples of current research directions in rheumatoid arthritis supported by the federal government through the NIAMS and other parts of the NIH:

• Scientists are looking at basic abnormalities in the immune systems of people with rheumatoid arthritis and in some animal models of the disease to understand why and how the disease develops. Findings from these studies may lead to precise, targeted therapies that could stop the inflammatory process in its earliest stages. They may even lead to a vaccine that could prevent rheumatoid arthritis.

- Researchers are studying genetic factors that predispose some people to developing rheumatoid arthritis as well as factors connected with disease severity. Findings from these studies should increase understanding of the disease and will help develop new therapies as well as guide treatment decisions. In a major effort aimed at identifying genes involved in rheumatoid arthritis, the NIH and the Arthritis Foundation have joined together to support the North American Rheumatoid Arthritis Consortium. This group of 12 research centers around the United States is collecting medical information and genetic material from 1,000 families in which two or more siblings have rheumatoid arthritis. It will serve as a national resource for genetic studies of this disease.

- Scientists are also gaining insights into the genetic basis of rheumatoid arthritis by studying rats with autoimmune inflammatory arthritis that resembles human disease. NIAMS researchers have identified several genetic regions that affect arthritis susceptibility and severity in these animal models of the disease. They have found some striking similarities between rats and humans. Identifying disease genes in rats should provide important new information that may yield clues to the causes of rheumatoid arthritis in humans.

- Scientists are studying the complex relationships among the hormonal, nervous, and immune systems in rheumatoid arthritis. For example, they are exploring whether and how the normal changes in the levels of steroid hormones (such as estrogen and testosterone) during a person's lifetime may be related to the development, improvement, or flares of the disease. Scientists are also looking at how these systems interact with environmental and genetic factors. Results from these studies may suggest new treatment strategies.

- Researchers are exploring why so many more women than men develop rheumatoid arthritis. In hopes of finding clues, they are studying female and male hormones and other elements that differ between women and men, such as possible differences in their immune responses.

- To find clues to new treatments, researchers are examining why rheumatoid arthritis often improves during pregnancy. Results of one study suggest that the explanation may be related to differences in certain special proteins between a mother and her unborn child. These proteins help the immune system distinguish between the body's own cells and foreign cells. Such differences, the scientists speculate, may change the activity of the mother's immune system during pregnancy.

- A growing body of evidence indicates that infectious agents, such as viruses and bacteria, may trigger rheumatoid arthritis in people who have an inherited predisposition to the disease. Investigators are trying to discover which infectious agents may be responsible. More broadly, they are also working to understand the basic mechanisms by which these agents might trigger the development of rheumatoid arthritis. Identifying the agents and understanding how they work could lead to new therapies.

- Scientists are searching for new drugs or combinations of drugs that can reduce inflammation, can slow or stop the progression of rheumatoid arthritis, and also have few side effects. Studies in humans have shown that a number of compounds have such potential. For example, some studies are breaking new ground in the area of biopharmaceuticals, or biologics. These new drugs are based on compounds occurring naturally in the body and are designed to target specific aspects of the inflammatory process.

- Investigators have also shown that treatment of rheumatoid arthritis with minocycline, a drug in the tetracycline family, has a modest benefit. The effects of a related tetracycline called doxycycline are under investigation. Other studies have shown that the omega-3 fatty acids in certain fish or plant seed oils also may reduce rheumatoid arthritis inflammation. However, many people are not able to tolerate the large amount of oil necessary for any benefit.

- Investigators are examining many issues related to quality of life for rheumatoid arthritis patients and quality, cost, and effectiveness of health care services for these patients. Scientists have found that even a small improvement in a patient's sense of physical and mental well-being can have an impact on his or her quality of life and use of health care services. Results from studies like these will help health care providers design integrated treatment strategies that cover all of a patient's needs—emotional as well as physical.

Scientists are making rapid progress in understanding the complexities of rheumatoid arthritis—how and why it develops, why some people get it and others do not, and why some people get it more severely than others. Results from research are having an impact today, enabling people with rheumatoid arthritis to remain active in life, family, and work far longer than was possible 20 years ago. There is also hope for tomorrow, as researchers continue to explore ways of stopping the disease process early, before it becomes destructive, or even preventing rheumatoid arthritis altogether.

RNA (ribonucleic acid)   A chemical similar to a single strand of DNA. In RNA, the letter U, which stands for uracil, is substituted for T in the genetic code. RNA delivers DNA's genetic message to the cytoplasm of a cell, where proteins are made.

risk factors   Environmental, chemical, psychological, physiological, or genetic elements that cause a person to be more likely to develop a disease. Risk factors for many autoimmune diseases are still being determined, but some have been linked to genes, infections, and the environment. Risk factors for selected autoimmune diseases:

- RHEUMATOID ARTHRITIS—Infectious arthritis, gout, repeated injuries, obesity, age, occupational exposure to silica dust; strong genetic.

- SYSTEMIC LUPUS ERYTHEMATOSUS—Ultraviolet light, hormonal factors, industrial chemicals; strong genetic and black race; stress can cause a relapse.

- MULTIPLE SCLEROSIS—Exposure to a virus or bacteria, smoking; strong genetic.

- CROHN'S DISEASE—Lack of earlier exposure to infections; genetic, Jewish.

- ULCERATIVE COLITIS—Lack of earlier exposure to infections, genetic.

- FIBROMYALGIA—Injury, trauma, stress, or a virus.

- GRAVES' DISEASE—Physical or emotional stress. Environmental factors may trigger; strong familial.

- SCLERODERMA—Occupational exposure to silica dust or vinyl chloride, childbearing years, black race.

- HASHIMOTO'S THYROIDITIS—Iodine intake, lithium, age, strong familial; possibly a virus.

- SJÖGREN'S SYNDROME—Mid-adult years, strong familial.

- INSULIN-DEPENDENT DIABETES—Virus may trigger, strong genetic.

Source: Connecticut Women's Health, Hartford, Conn.: Connecticut Department of Public Health, 2001.

salivary glands Organs that secrete saliva, a watery or viscous substance that moistens and softens food, in the mouth. The salivary glands include three major pairs of glands—the parotid glands in front of the ear, the sublingual glands on the floor of the mouth under the tongue, and the submandibular glands below the lower jaw. Saliva helps an individual speak, eat, chew, and swallow, and it protects the teeth and gums from microbial infection. When saliva is insufficient, the mouth feels dry, a condition called XEROSTOMIA. The salivary glands are severely damaged and atrophy in a number of autoimmune disorders such as SJÖGREN'S DISEASE and SYSTEMIC LUPUS ERYTHEMATOSUS. The damage is done partly by the formation of immune complexes (antigen-antibody associations), which are precipitated in the gland and initiate the destruction or by the action of cytotoxic (cell-damaging) T cells. In these circumstances, the loss of saliva is permanent.

sarcoidosis A chronic disease that may affect many body systems. It can appear in almost any body organ but most often starts in the lungs or lymph nodes. It is characterized by small collections of cells called granulomas. Sarcoidosis may be misdiagnosed as tuberculosis, which is also characterized by granuloma formations. The disease varies in severity and may affect any part of the body.

Sarcoidosis was first identified over 100 years ago by two dermatologists working independently, Dr. Jonathan Hutchinson in England and Dr. Caesar Boeck in Norway. Sarcoidosis was originally called Hutchinson's disease or Boeck's disease. Dr. Boeck went on to fashion today's name for the disease from the Greek words "sark" and "oid," mean-

ing fleshlike. The term describes the skin eruptions that are frequently caused by the illness.

Sarcoidosis was once considered a rare disease. Scientists now know that it is a common chronic illness that appears all over the world. In Sweden, the disease affects 6.5 persons in 10,000. Not until the mid-1940s—when a large number of cases were identified during mass chest X-ray screening for the armed forces—was its high prevalence recognized in North America. It is the most common of the fibrotic lung disorders and occurs often enough in the United States for Congress to have declared a national Sarcoidosis Awareness Day in 1990.

Anyone can get sarcoidosis. It occurs in all races and in both sexes. Nevertheless, the risk is greater if one is a young African-American adult, especially an African-American woman, or of Scandinavian, German, Irish, or Puerto Rican origin. No one knows why.

Because sarcoidosis can escape diagnosis or be mistaken for several other diseases, scientists can only guess at how many people are affected. The best estimate today is that about five in 100,000 Caucasian people in the United States have sarcoidosis. Among African Americans, it occurs more frequently, in probably 40 out of 100,000 people.

There are about 25,000 cases in the United States, and the disease is most common in the southeast part of the United States. Overall, there appear to be 20 cases per 100,000 in cities on the East Coast and somewhat fewer in rural locations. Some scientists, however, believe these figures greatly underestimate the percentage of the U.S. population with sarcoidosis.

Sarcoidosis occurs predominantly between the ages of 20 and 40 years. Caucasian women are just as likely as Caucasian men to get sarcoidosis, but

African-American females get sarcoidosis two times as often as African-American males. Also, Caucasian patients are more likely to develop the milder form of the disease; African Americans tend to develop the more chronic and severe form.

Causes

The cause of sarcoidosis is suspected of being autoimmune and may be triggered by an agent such as a slow virus or possibly a variety of other toxic agents. Genetic predisposition may also be an important factor in the development of sarcoidosis.

Clinical Features

Not all cases of sarcoidosis are alike. Some patients have few if any symptoms, while others experience many. The disease can appear suddenly and disappear. Alternatively, it can develop gradually and go on to produce symptoms that come and go, sometimes for a lifetime. As sarcoidosis progresses, small lumps, or granulomas, appear in the affected tissues. In the majority of cases, these granulomas clear up, either with or without treatment. In the few cases where the granulomas do not heal and disappear, the tissues tend to remain inflamed and become scarred (fibrotic).

Shortness of breath (dyspnea) and a cough that will not go away can be among the first symptoms of sarcoidosis. However, sarcoidosis can also show up suddenly with the appearance of skin rashes. Red bumps (erythema nodosum) on the face, arms, or shins and inflammation of the eyes are also common symptoms. It is not unusual, however, for sarcoidosis symptoms to be more general. Weight loss, fatigue, night sweats, fever, or an overall feeling of ill health can also be clues to the disease.

The lungs are usually the first site involved in sarcoidosis. About nine out of 10 sarcoidosis patients have some type of lung problem, with nearly one-third of these patients showing some respiratory symptoms—usually coughing, either dry or with phlegm, and dyspnea. Occasionally, patients have chest pain and a feeling of tightness in the chest.

Sarcoidosis of the lungs is thought to begin with alveolitis (inflammation of the alveoli), the tiny saclike air spaces in the lungs where carbon dioxide and oxygen are exchanged. Alveolitis either clears up spontaneously or leads to granuloma formation. Eventually fibrosis can form, causing the lung to stiffen and making breathing even more difficult.

In addition to the lungs and lymph nodes, the body organs more likely than others to be affected by sarcoidosis are the liver, skin, heart, nervous system, and kidneys, in that order of frequency. Patients can have symptoms related to the specific organ affected, they can have only general symptoms, or they can be without any symptoms whatsoever. Symptoms can also vary according to how long the illness has been under way, where the granulomas are forming, how much tissue has become affected, and whether the granulomatous process is still active. Enlargement of the salivary or tear glands and cysts in bone tissue are also among sarcoidosis signals.

Eye disease occurs in about 20 to 30 percent of patients with sarcoidosis, particularly in children who get the disease. Almost any part of the eye can be affected—the membranes of the eyelids, cornea, outer coat of the eyeball (sclera), retina, and lens. The eye involvement can start with no symptoms at all or with reddening or watery eyes.

The skin is affected in about 20 percent of sarcoidosis patients. Skin sarcoidosis is usually marked by small, raised patches on the face. Occasionally, the patches are purplish in color and larger. Patches can also appear on limbs, the face, and buttocks.

In an occasional case (1 percent to 5 percent), sarcoidosis can lead to neurological problems. For example, sarcoid granulomas can appear in the brain, spinal cord, and facial and optic nerves. Facial paralysis and other symptoms of nerve damage call for prompt treatment.

Laboratory Tests

No single test can be relied on for a correct diagnosis of sarcoidosis. X rays and blood tests are usually the first procedures the doctor will order. Pulmonary function tests often provide clues to diagnosis. Other tests may also be used, some more often than others. Many of the tests used to diagnose sarcoidosis can also help the doctor follow the progress of the disease and determine whether the sarcoidosis is getting better or worse.

Chest X ray A picture of the lungs and heart, as well as the surrounding tissues containing lymph nodes, where infection-fighting white blood cells form, can give the first indication of sarcoidosis. For example, a swelling of the lymph glands between the two lungs can show up on an X ray. An X ray can also show which areas of the lung are affected.

Pulmonary function tests By performing a variety of tests called pulmonary function tests (PFT), the doctor can find out how well the lungs are doing their job of expanding and exchanging oxygen and carbon dioxide with the blood. The lungs of sarcoidosis patients cannot handle these tasks as well as they should. This is because granulomas and fibrosis of lung tissue decrease lung capacity and disturb the normal flow of gases between the lungs and the blood.

One PFT procedure calls for the patient to breathe into a machine, called a spirometer. It is a mechanical device that records changes in the lung size as air is inhaled and exhaled as well as the time the patient takes to do this.

Blood tests Blood analyses can evaluate the number and types of blood cells in the body and how well the cells are functioning. They can also measure the levels of various blood proteins known to be involved in immunological activities. They can show increases in serum calcium levels and abnormal liver function that often accompany sarcoidosis.

Blood tests can measure a blood substance called angiotensin-converting enzyme (ACE). Because the cells that make up granulomas secrete large amounts of ACE, the enzyme levels are often high in patients with sarcoidosis. ACE levels, however, are not always high in sarcoidosis patients, and increased ACE levels can also show up in other illnesses.

Bronchoalveolar lavage This test uses an instrument called a bronchoscope—a long, narrow tube with a light at the end—to wash out, or lavage, cells and other materials from inside the lungs. This wash fluid is then examined for the amount of various cells and other substances that reflect inflammation and immune activity in the lungs. A high number of white blood cells in this fluid usually indicates an inflammation in the lungs.

Biopsy Microscopic examination of specimens of lung tissue obtained with a bronchoscope, or of specimens of other tissues, can tell a doctor where granulomas have formed in the body.

Gallium scanning In this procedure, the doctor injects the radioactive chemical element gallium-67 into the patient's vein. The gallium collects at places in the body affected by sarcoidosis and other inflammatory conditions. Two days after the injection, the body is scanned for radioactivity.

Increases in gallium uptake at any site in the body indicate that inflammatory activity has developed at the site and also give an idea of which tissue, and how much tissue, has been affected. However, because any type of inflammation causes gallium uptake, a positive gallium scan does not necessarily mean that the patient has sarcoidosis.

Kveim test This test involves injecting a standardized preparation of sarcoid tissue material into the skin. On the one hand, a unique lump formed at the point of injection is considered positive for sarcoidosis. On the other hand, the test result is not always positive even if the patient has sarcoidosis.

The Kveim test is not used often in the United States because no test material has been approved for sale by the U.S. Food and Drug Administration. However, a few hospitals and clinics may have some standardized test preparation prepared privately for their own use.

Slit lamp examination An instrument called a slit lamp, which permits examination of the inside of the eye, can be used to detect silent damage from sarcoidosis.

Complications

From 20 percent to 30 percent of sarcoidosis patients are left with some permanent lung damage. In 10 percent to 15 percent of the patients, sarcoidosis can become chronic. When either the granulomas or fibrosis seriously affect the function of a vital organ—the lungs, heart, nervous system, liver, or kidneys, for example—sarcoidosis can be fatal. This occurs 5 percent to 10 percent of the time. In a few cases, cataracts, glaucoma, and blindness can result.

Although severe sarcoidosis can reduce the chances of becoming pregnant, particularly for older women, many young women with sarcoidosis have given birth to healthy babies while on treatment. Patients planning to have a baby should discuss the matter with their doctor. Medical checkups all through pregnancy and immediately thereafter are especially important for sarcoidosis patients. In some cases, bed rest is necessary during the last three months of pregnancy.

Treatment

Sarcoidosis often goes away by itself, with those cases healing in 24 to 36 months. Although sarcoidosis may go away spontaneously without treatment, many patients will have it for their lifetime. There is no cure at this time, but sarcoidosis can be controlled with medications.

When therapy is recommended, the main goal is to keep the lungs and other affected body organs working and to relieve symptoms. The disease is considered inactive once the symptoms fade. After many years of experience with treating the disease, corticosteroids remain the primary treatment for inflammation and granuloma formation. Prednisone is probably the corticosteroid most often prescribed today. No treatment is available at present to reverse the fibrosis that might be present in advanced sarcoidosis.

Occasionally, a blood test will show a high blood level of calcium accompanying sarcoidosis. The reasons for this are not clear. Some scientists believe that this condition is not common. When it does occur, the patient may be advised to avoid calcium-rich foods, vitamin D, or sunlight or to take prednisone; this corticosteroid quickly reverses the condition.

Because sarcoidosis can disappear even without therapy, doctors sometimes disagree on when to start the treatment, what dose to prescribe, and how long to continue the medicine. The doctor's decision depends on the organ system involved and how far the inflammation has progressed. If the disease appears to be severe—especially in the lungs, eyes, heart, nervous system, spleen, or kidneys—the doctor may prescribe corticosteroids.

Corticosteroid treatment usually results in improvement. Symptoms often start up again, however, when it is stopped. Treatment, therefore, may be necessary for several years, sometimes for as long as the disease remains active or to prevent relapse.

Frequent checkups are important so that the doctor can monitor the illness and, if necessary, adjust the treatment. Corticosteroids, for example,

can have side effects—mood swings, swelling, and weight gain because the treatment tends to make the body hold on to water; high blood pressure; high blood sugar; and craving for food. Long-term use can affect the stomach, skin, and bones. This situation can bring on stomach pain, an ulcer, or acne, or it can cause the loss of calcium from bones. However, if the corticosteroid is taken in carefully prescribed, low doses, the benefits from the treatment are usually far greater than the problems.

Besides corticosteroids, various other drugs have been tried, but their effectiveness has not been established in controlled studies. These drugs include chloroquine and D-penicillamine.

Several drugs such as chlorambucil, azathioprine, methotrexate, and cyclophosphamide, which might suppress alveolitis by killing the cells that produce granulomas, have also been used. None has been evaluated in controlled clinical trials, and the risk of using these drugs is high, especially in pregnant women.

Cyclosporine, a drug used widely in organ transplants to suppress immune reaction, has been evaluated in one controlled trial. It was found to be unsuccessful.

Baughman, R. P. et al. "Clinical Characteristics of Patients in a Case Control Study of Sarcoidosis." *American Journal of Respiratory and Critical Care Medicine* 164, no. 10 (November 2001): 1,885–1,889.

Freemer, M. and T. E. King. "The ACCESS Study. Characterization of Sarcoidosis in the United States." *American Journal of Respiratory and Critical Care Medicine* 164, no. 10 (November 2001): 1,754–1,755.

Luisetti, M., A. Beretta, and L. Casali. "Course and Prognosis of Sarcoidosis in African-Americans Versus Caucasians." *The European Respiratory Journal: Official Journal of the European Society for Clinical Respiratory Physiology* 18, no. 4 (October 2001): 738.

National Institutes of Health National Heart, Lung, and Blood Institute. *Sarcoidosis*, NIH Publication No. 95-3093, 1995.

Rybicki, B. A., et al. "Familial Aggregation of Sarcoidosis. A Case-Control Etiologic Study of Sarcoidosis (Access)." *American Journal of Respiratory and Critical Care Medicine* 164, no. 11 (December 2001): 2,085–2,091.

sarcoidosis research   Many questions about sarcoidosis remain unanswered. Identifying the agent that causes the illness, along with the inflammatory mechanisms that set the stage for the alveolitis, granuloma formation, and fibrosis that characterize the disease, is the major aim of the National Heart, Lung, and Blood Institute's program on sarcoidosis. Development of reliable methods of diagnosis, treatment, and eventually, the prevention of sarcoidosis is the ultimate goal.

Originally, scientists thought that sarcoidosis was caused by an acquired state of immunological inertness (anergy). This notion was revised a few years ago when the technique of bronchoalveolar lavage provided access to a vast array of cells and cell-derived mediators operating in the lungs of sarcoidosis patients. Sarcoidosis is now believed to be associated with a complex mix of immunological disturbances involving simultaneous activation, as well as depression, of certain immunological functions.

Immunological studies on sarcoidosis patients show that many of the immune functions associated with thymus-derived white blood cells, called T lymphocytes or T cells, are depressed. The depression of this cellular component of systemic immune response is expressed in the inability of the patients to evoke a delayed hypersensitivity skin reaction (a positive skin test) when tested by the appropriate foreign substance, or antigen, underneath the skin.

In addition, the blood of sarcoidosis patients contains a reduced number of T cells. These T cells do not seem capable of responding normally when treated with substances known to stimulate the growth of laboratory-cultured T cells. Neither do they produce their normal complement of immunological mediators, cytokines, through which the cells modify the behavior of other cells.

In contrast to the depression of the cellular immune response, the humoral immune response of sarcoidosis patients is often elevated. The humoral immune response is reflected by the production of circulating antibodies against a variety of exogenous antigens, including common viruses. This humoral component of systemic immune response is mediated by another class of lymphocytes known as B lymphocytes, or B cells, because they originate in the bone marrow.

In another indication of heightened humoral response, sarcoidosis patients seem prone to develop autoantibodies (antibodies against endogenous antigens) similar to rheumatoid factors.

With access to the cells and cell products in the lung tissue compartments through the bronchoalveolar technique, researchers can complement the above investigations at the blood level by analyzing local inflammatory and immune events in the lungs.

In contrast to what is seen at the systemic level, the cellular immune response in the lungs seems to be heightened rather than depressed. The heightened cellular immune response in the diseased tissue is characterized by significant increases in activated T lymphocytes with certain characteristic cell-surface antigens as well as in activated alveolar macrophages.

This pronounced, localized cellular response is also accompanied by the appearance in the lung of an array of mediators that are thought to contribute to the disease process. These include interleukin-1, interleukin-2, B cell growth factor, B cell differentiation factor, fibroblast growth factor, and fibronectin.

Because a number of lung diseases follow respiratory tract infections, ascertaining whether a virus can be implicated in the events leading to sarcoidosis remains an important area of research. Some recent observations seem to provide suggestive leads on this question. In these studies, the genes of cytomegalovirus (CMV), a common disease-causing virus, were introduced into lymphocytes, and the expression of the viral genes was studied. It was found that the viral genes were expressed both during acute infection of the cells and when the virus was not replicating in the cells. However, this expression seemed to take place only when the T cells were activated by some injurious event.

In addition, the product of a CMV gene was found capable of activating the gene in alveolar macrophages responsible for the production of interleukin-1. Since interleukin-1 levels are found to increase in alveolar macrophages from patients with sarcoidosis, this suggests that certain viral genes can enhance the production of inflammatory components associated with sarcoidosis. Whether these findings implicate viral infections in the disease process in sarcoidosis is unclear. Future research with viral models may provide clues to the molecular mechanisms that trigger alterations in lymphocyte and macrophage regulation leading to sarcoidosis.

In 1995, the National Heart, Lung, and Blood Institute started a multicenter case control study of the etiology of sarcoidosis. The investigation is collecting information and specimens for use in investigation of environmental, occupational, lifestyle, and genetic risk factors for sarcoidosis. Examination of the natural history of sarcoidosis is planned in patients at early and late stages of the disease. Such information should improve scientists' understanding of the cause(s) of sarcoidosis and provide insight into how to prevent and treat the disease better.

National Institutes of Health National Heart, Lung, and Blood Institute. *Sarcoidosis,* NIH Publication No. 95-3093, 1995.

scavenger cells   Any of a diverse group of cells that have the capacity to engulf and destroy foreign materials, dead tissues, or other cells. They include macrophages and polymorphonuclear neutrophils.

school, attending with autoimmune diseases   As expressed by Vetiska et al.:

Regular school attendance is important for a child's academic achievement, formation of peer relationships, and self-esteem. But children with chronic illnesses such as type 1 diabetes, juvenile rheumatoid arthritis, chronic fatigue syndrome, and other autoimmune diseases have greater school absenteeism rates than their healthier peers. Research suggests that chronic fatigue syndrome produces more long-term sickness absence than any other condition in schoolchildren. In their pilot study, Vetiska et al found that diabetic children miss, on average, a little more than one week per school year more than their non-diabetic siblings.

In addition to the attendance problem, diabetic children face other issues at school. According to Crawford, "There is a danger that teachers may think kids with diabetes sometimes pretend to feel low or high to get out of an activity they do not like. This is very unlikely. Most kids with diabetes don't want to be different, and they don't want their diabetes to cause them to be treated differently."

But in order to perform well in school, a child's blood sugar needs to remain in the acceptable range. Left untreated, both high- and low-blood-sugar levels can affect the child's ability to concentrate on schoolwork and participate in school activities. The results of one study suggest that the subtle cognitive deficits often documented in children with Type 1 diabetes may not significantly limit their academic abilities over time, but careful monitoring is still needed to ensure that episodes of hypoglycemia associated with seizures are not adversely affecting learning.

For some autoimmune diseases, such as juvenile arthritis or chronic fatigue syndrome, the family will need to request an Individual Education Plan from the school, likely incorporating home and/or distance learning for at least part of the school year. It may be necessary for the student's pediatrician to help set this up and monitor the child's progress.

Crawford, Eileen. *Recommendations for Management of Diabetes for Children in School.* Oklahoma City: Oklahoma Department of Health Diabetes Control Program, 1998.

McCarthy, A. M., S. Lindgren, M. A. Mengeling, E. Tsalikian, and J. C. Engvall. "Effects of Diabetes on Learning in Children." *Pediatrics* 109, no. 1 (January 2002): E9.

Spencer, C. H., R. Z. Fife, and C. E. Rabinovich. "The School Experience of Children With Arthritis." *Pediatric Clinics of North America* 42, no. 5 (October 1995): 1,285– 1,298.

Vetiska, J., L. Glaab, K. Perlman, and D. Daneman. "School Attendance of Children With Type 1 Diabetes." *Diabetes Care* 23, no. 11 (November 2000): 1,706–1,707.

SCID mouse   A laboratory animal that, lacking an enzyme necessary to fashion an immune system of its own, can be turned into a model of the human immune system when injected with human immune system cells.

scleritis   A potentially serious, severe, destructive, vision-threatening inflammation of the sclera (the white part of the eye). In over 50 percent of cases, it is associated with systemic autoimmune disease such as rheumatoid arthritis, ankylosing spondylitis, systemic lupus erythematosus, polyarteritis nodosa, and Wegener's granulomatosis.

Scleritis is most common between the ages of 30 and 60, and it affects women more often than men. Only rarely does it occur in children.

Causes

When not associated with autoimmune disease, scleritis can be caused by infections or chemical injuries. In some cases, the cause is unknown.

Clinical Features

Patients with scleritis will complain of very severe eye pain. Other symptoms include redness in the eye, which may turn into an intense purple. In a few cases, there will be blurred vision, sensitivity to light, or tearing of the eye. Bulging eyes may also be associated with this disease. Scleritis is usually confined to one eye but may appear in both.

Complications

If untreated, perforation of the eyeball may occur. Other complications may include keratitis (inflammation of the cornea), cataracts (scarring of the lens), uveitis (inflammation of the eye behind the pupil), and glaucoma (elevated pressure in the eye that may lead to vision loss).

Treatment

Treatment usually begins with eyedrops and a systemic corticosteroid such as prednisone. Non-steroidal anti-inflammatories such as ibuprofen may be used for pain relief. If the scleritis is unresponsive to systemic corticosteroids or when the patient has necrotizing scleritis (a more rare, serious type, which causes thinning of the sclera) and rheumatoid arthritis, systemic immunosuppression with drugs such as cyclophosphamide or azathioprine may be prescribed. Scleritis usually responds to treatment, but the condition may reappear.

scleroderma A chronic autoimmune disease that involves the skin and connective tissue. It was first described in medical literature in the 18th century. In localized scleroderma, the skin shows one or more patches of sclerosis (thickening and hardening). The systemic type involves the skin and the connective tissue, and it can affect the whole body. Both groups include subgroups. (See chart.)

Derived from the Greek words "sklerosis," meaning *hardness,* and "derma," meaning *skin,* scleroderma literally means hard skin. Though it is often referred to as if it were a single disease, scleroderma is really a symptom of a group of diseases that involve the abnormal growth of connective tissue, which supports the skin and internal organs. It is sometimes used, therefore, as an umbrella term for these disorders. In some forms of scleroderma, hard, tight skin is the extent of this abnormal process. In other forms, however, the problem goes much deeper, affecting blood vessels and internal organs, such as the heart, lungs, and kidneys.

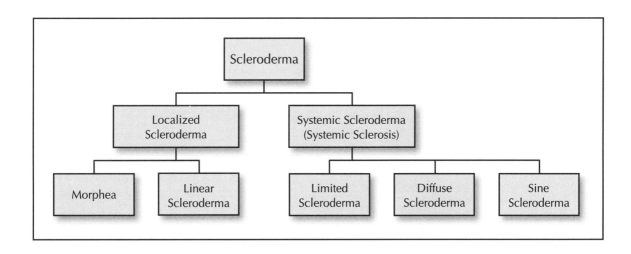

Scleroderma is called both a rheumatic disease and a connective tissue disease. The term *rheumatic disease* refers to a group of conditions characterized by inflammation and/or pain in the muscles, joints, or fibrous tissues. A connective tissue disease is one that affects the major connecting substance (collagen) in the skin, tendons, and bones.

There are different ways these groups and subgroups of scleroderma may be broken down or referred to and doctors may use different terms from what is shown in the figure. However, the following is a common way of classifying these diseases.

Localized Scleroderma

Localized types of scleroderma are those limited to the skin, related tissues, and, in some cases, the muscle below. Internal organs are not affected by localized scleroderma, and localized scleroderma can never progress to the systemic form of the disease. Often, localized conditions improve or go away on their own over time. However, the skin changes and damage that occur when the disease is active can be permanent. For some people, localized scleroderma is serious and disabling. There are two generally recognized types of localized scleroderma, morphea and linear scleroderma.

Morphea Morphea comes from a Greek word that means "form" or "structure." The word refers to local patches of scleroderma. The first signs of the disease are reddish patches of skin that thicken into firm, oval-shaped areas. The center of each patch becomes ivory colored with violet borders. These patches sweat very little and have little hair growth. Patches appear most often on the chest, stomach, and back. Sometimes they appear on the face, arms, and legs.

Morphea can be either localized or generalized. Localized morphea limits itself to one or several patches, ranging in size from 0.5 inches to 12 inches in diameter. The condition sometimes appears on areas treated by radiation therapy. Some people have both morphea and linear scleroderma. The disease is referred to as generalized morphea when the skin patches become very hard and dark and spread over larger areas of the body.

Regardless of the type, morphea generally fades out in three to five years. However, people are often left with darkened skin patches and, in rare cases, muscle weakness.

Linear scleroderma As suggested by its name, the disease has a single line or band of thickened and/or abnormally colored skin. Usually, the line runs down an arm or leg, but in some people, it runs down the forehead. People sometimes use the French term *en coup de sabre,* or "sword stroke," to describe this highly visible line.

Systemic Scleroderma

Systemic scleroderma, also known as systemic sclerosis, is the term for the disease that not only includes the skin but also involves the tissues beneath, including the blood vessels and major organs. Systemic sclerosis is typically broken down into diffuse and limited disease. People with systemic sclerosis often have all or some of the symptoms that some doctors call CREST, which stands for calcinosis, Raynaud's phenomenon, esophageal dysfunction, sclerodactyly, and telangiectasias.

Calcinosis The formation of calcium deposits in the connective tissues, which can be detected by X ray. They are typically found on the fingers, hands, face, and trunk and on the skin above the elbows and knees. When the deposits break through the skin, painful ulcers can result.

Raynaud's phenomenon A condition in which the small blood vessels of the hands and/or feet contract in response to cold or anxiety. As the vessels contract, the hands or feet turn white and cold, then blue. As blood flow returns, they become red. Fingertip tissues may suffer damage, leading to ulcers, scars, or gangrene.

Esophageal dysfunction Impaired function of the esophagus (the tube connecting the throat and the stomach) that occurs when smooth muscles in the esophagus lose normal movement. In the upper esophagus, the result can be swallowing difficulties; in the lower esophagus, the problem can cause chronic heartburn or inflammation.

Sclerodactyly Thick and tight skin on the fingers, resulting from deposits of excess collagen within skin layers. The condition makes bending or straightening the fingers harder. The skin may also appear shiny and darkened, with hair loss.

Telangiectasias Small red spots on the hands and face that are caused by the swelling of tiny blood vessels. While not painful, these red spots can create cosmetic problems.

Limited scleroderma Limited scleroderma typically comes on gradually and affects the skin only in certain areas: the fingers, hands, face, lower arms, and legs. Many people with limited disease have Raynaud's phenomenon for years before skin thickening starts. Others start out with skin problems over much of the body, which improves over time, leaving only the face and hands with tight, thickened skin. Telangiectasias and calcinosis often follow. Because of the predominance of CREST in people with limited disease, some doctors refer to limited disease as the CREST syndrome.

Diffuse scleroderma Diffuse scleroderma typically comes on suddenly. Skin thickening occurs quickly and over much of the body, affecting the hands, face, upper arms, upper legs, chest, and stomach in a symmetrical fashion (for example, if one arm or one side of the trunk is affected, the other is also affected). Some people may have more area of their skin affected than others. Internally, it can damage key organs such as the heart, lungs, and kidneys. People with diffuse disease are often tired, lose appetite and weight, and have joint swelling and/or pain. Skin changes can cause the skin to swell, appear shiny, and feel tight and itchy.

The damage of diffuse scleroderma typically occurs over a few years. After the first three to five years, people with diffuse disease often enter a stable phase lasting for varying lengths of time. During this phase, skin thickness and appearance stay about the same. Damage to internal organs progresses little if at all. Symptoms also subside; joint pain eases, fatigue lessens, and appetite returns.

Gradually, however, the skin starts to change again. Less collagen is made, and the body seems to get rid of the excess collagen. This process, called *softening*, tends to occur in reverse order of the thickening process; the last areas thickened are the first to begin softening. Some patients' skin returns to a somewhat normal state, while other patients are left with thin, fragile skin without hair or sweat glands. More serious damage to the heart, lungs, or kidneys is unlikely to occur unless previous damage leads to more advanced deterioration.

People with diffuse scleroderma face the most serious long-term outlook if they develop severe kidney, lung, digestive, or heart problems. Fortunately, less than one-third of patients with diffuse disease develop these problems. Early diagnosis and continual and careful monitoring are important.

Sine scleroderma Some doctors break systemic sclerosis down into a third subset called systemic sclerosis sine scleroderma. Sine may resemble either limited or diffuse systemic sclerosis, causing changes in the lungs, kidneys, and blood vessels. However, there is one key difference between sine and other forms of systemic sclerosis: it does not affect the skin.

Although scleroderma is more common in women, the disease also occurs in men and children. It affects people of all races and ethnic groups. However, there are some patterns by disease type:

- Localized forms of scleroderma are more common in people of European descent than in African Americans.

- Morphea usually appears between the ages of 20 and 40.

- Linear scleroderma usually occurs in children or teenagers.

- Systemic scleroderma, whether limited or diffuse, typically occurs in people from 30 to 50 years old. It affects more women of African-American than European descent.

Because scleroderma can be hard to diagnose and it overlaps with or resembles other diseases, scientists can only estimate how many cases there actually are. Estimates for the number of people in the United States with systemic sclerosis range from 40,000 to 165,000. By contrast, a survey that included all scleroderma-related disorders, including Raynaud's phenomenon, suggested a number between 250,000 and 992,500.

For some people, scleroderma (particularly the localized forms) is fairly mild and resolves with time. For others, though, living with the disease and its effects day to day has a significant impact on their quality of life.

Causes

Although scientists do not know exactly what causes scleroderma, they are certain that people cannot catch it from or transmit it to others. Studies of twins suggest it is also not inherited. Scientists suspect that scleroderma comes from several factors.

Abnormal immune or inflammatory activity Like many other rheumatic disorders, scleroderma is believed to be an autoimmune disease. In scleroderma, the immune system is thought to stimulate cells called fibroblasts to produce too much collagen. In scleroderma, collagen forms thick connective tissue that builds up around the cells of the skin and internal organs. In milder forms, the effects of this buildup are limited to the skin and blood vessels. In more serious forms, it also can interfere with normal functioning of skin, blood vessels, joints, and internal organs.

Genetic makeup While genes seem to put certain people at risk for scleroderma and play a role in its course, the disease is not passed from parent to child like some genetic diseases. However, some research suggests that having children may increase a woman's risk of scleroderma. Scientists have learned that when a woman is pregnant, cells from her baby can pass through the placenta, enter her bloodstream, and linger in her body—in some cases, for many years after the child's birth. Recently, scientists have found fetal cells from pregnancies of years past in the skin lesions of some women with scleroderma. They think that these cells, which are different from the woman's own cells, may either begin an immune reaction to the woman's own tissues or trigger a response by the woman's immune system to rid her body of those cells. Either way, the woman's healthy tissues may be damaged in the process. Further studies are needed to find out if fetal cells play a role in the disease.

Environmental triggers Research suggests that exposure to some environmental factors may trigger the disease in people who are genetically predisposed to it. Suspected triggers include viral infections, certain adhesive and coating materials, and organic solvents such as vinyl chloride or trichloroethylene. In the past, some people believed that silicone breast implants might have been a factor in developing connective tissue diseases such as scleroderma. However, several studies have not shown evidence of a connection.

Hormones By the middle-to-late childbearing years (ages 30 to 55), women develop scleroderma at a rate seven to 12 times higher than men. Because of female predominance at this and all ages, scientists suspect that something distinctly feminine, such as the hormone estrogen, plays a role in the disease. So far, the role of estrogen or other female hormones has not been proven.

Clinical Features

Finding one or more of the following factors can help a doctor diagnose a certain form of scleroderma:

- Changed skin appearance and texture, including swollen fingers and hands and tight skin around the hands, face, mouth, or elsewhere.
- Calcium deposits developing under the skin.
- Changes in the tiny blood vessels (capillaries) at the base of the fingernails.
- Thickened skin patches.

Lab tests help confirm a suspected diagnosis. At least two proteins, called antibodies, are commonly found in the blood of people with scleroderma:

- Antitopoisomerase-1 or anti-Scl-70 antibodies appear in the blood of up to 40 percent of people with diffuse systemic sclerosis.
- Anticentromere antibodies are found in the blood of as many as 90 percent of people with limited systemic sclerosis.

A number of other scleroderma-specific antibodies can occur in people with scleroderma, although less frequently. When present, however, they are helpful in making a clinical diagnosis.

Because not all people with scleroderma have these antibodies and because not all people with the antibodies have scleroderma, lab test results alone cannot confirm the diagnosis.

In some cases, the doctor may order a skin biopsy (the surgical removal of a small sample of skin for microscopic examination) to aid in or help confirm a diagnosis. However, skin biopsies, too, have their limitations. Biopsy results cannot distinguish between localized and systemic disease, for example.

Diagnosing scleroderma is easiest when a person has typical symptoms and rapid skin thickening. In other cases, a diagnosis may take months or even years as the disease unfolds and reveals itself and as the doctor is able to rule out some other potential causes of the symptoms. In some cases, a diagnosis is never made, because the symptoms that prompted the visit to the doctor go away on their own.

Complications

In diffuse systemic sclerosis, hand joints can stiffen because of hardened skin around the joints or inflammation of the joints themselves. Other joints can also become stiff and swollen.

When too much collagen builds up in the skin, it crowds out sweat and oil glands. This causes the skin to become dry and stiff.

Dental problems are common in people with scleroderma for a number of reasons. Tightening facial skin can make the mouth opening smaller and narrower, which makes caring for teeth difficult. Dry mouth due to salivary gland damage speeds up tooth decay. Damage to connective tissues in the mouth can lead to loose teeth.

Systemic sclerosis can affect any part of the digestive system. As a result, problems such as heartburn, difficulty swallowing, early satiety (the feeling of being full after barely starting to eat), or intestinal complaints such as diarrhea, constipation, and gas can occur. In cases where the intestines are damaged, the body may have difficulty absorbing nutrients from food.

About 10 percent to 15 percent of people with systemic sclerosis develop severe lung disease. This comes in two forms: pulmonary fibrosis (hardening or scarring of lung tissue because of excess collagen) and pulmonary hypertension (high blood pressure in the artery that carries blood from the heart to the lungs).

About 15 percent to 20 percent of people with systemic sclerosis develop heart problems. These include scarring and weakening of the heart (cardiomyopathy), inflamed heart muscle (myocarditis), and abnormal heartbeat (arrhythmia).

About 15 percent to 20 percent of people with diffuse systemic sclerosis develop severe kidney problems, including loss of kidney function.

Even if scleroderma does not cause any lasting physical disability, its effects on the skin's appearance—particularly on the face—can take their toll on the patient's self-esteem.

Treatment

Currently, no treatment controls or stops the underlying problem—the overproduction of collagen—in all forms of scleroderma. Thus, treatment and management focus on relieving symptoms and limiting damage from any complications.

Dunkin, Mary Anne. *Handout on Health: Scleroderma.* Bethesda, Md.: National Institute of Arthritis and Musculoskeletal and Skin Diseases, 2001.

Mayes, Maureen D. *The Scleroderma Book: A Guide for Patients and Families.* New York: Oxford University Press, 1999.

Melvin, Jeanne L. *Scleroderma: Caring for Your Hands & Face.* Bethesda, Md.: American Occupational Therapy Association, Inc., 1994.

Scammell, Henry. *Scleroderma: The Proven Therapy That Can Save Your Life.* New York: M. Evans & Co., 1998.

scleroderma research   Research is providing better ways to treat symptoms, prevent organ damage, and improve the quality of life for people with scleroderma. In the past two decades, multidisciplinary research has also provided new clues to understanding the disease, which is an important step toward prevention or cure.

Leading the way in funding this research is the National Institute of Arthritis and Musculoskeletal and Skin Diseases (NIAMS), a part of the National Institutes of Health (NIH). Other sources of funding for scleroderma research include pharmaceutical companies and organizations such as the Scleroderma Foundation, the Scleroderma Research Foundation, and the Arthritis Foundation. Scientists at universities and medical centers throughout the United States conduct much of this research.

Studies of the immune system, genetics, cell biology, and molecular biology have helped reveal the causes of scleroderma. This has improved existing treatment and created entirely new treatment approaches.

Research advances in recent years that have led to a better understanding of and/or treatment for the diseases include the following.

- The use of a hormone produced in pregnancy to soften skin lesions. Early studies suggest relaxin, a hormone that helps a woman's body to stretch to meet the demands of a growing pregnancy and delivery, may soften the connective tissues of women with scleroderma. The hormone is believed to work by blocking fibrosis, or the development of fibrous tissue between the body's cells.

- Finding a gene associated with scleroderma in Oklahoma Choctaw Native Americans. Scientists believe the gene, which codes for a protein called fibrillin-1, may put people at risk for the disease.

- The use of the drug iloprost for pulmonary hypertension. This drug has increased the quality of life and life expectancy for people with this dangerous form of lung damage.

- The use of the drug cyclophosphamide (Cytoxan) for lung fibrosis. One recent study suggested that treating lung problems early with this immunosuppressive drug may help prevent further damage and increase chances of survival.

- The increased use of ACE inhibitors for scleroderma-related kidney problems. For the past two decades, ACE inhibitors have greatly reduced the risk of kidney failure in people with scleroderma. Now evidence indicates that ACE inhibitors can actually heal the kidneys of people on dialysis for scleroderma-related kidney failure. As many as half of people who continue ACE inhibitors while on dialysis may be able to go off dialysis in 12 to 18 months.

Other studies are examining the following.

- Changes in the tiny blood vessels of people with scleroderma. By studying these changes, scientists hope to find the cause of cold sensitivity in Raynaud's phenomenon and how to control the problem.

- Immune system changes (and particularly how those changes affect the lungs) in people with early diffuse systemic sclerosis.

- The role of blood vessel malfunction, cell death, and autoimmunity in scleroderma.

- Skin changes in laboratory mice in which a genetic defect prevents the breakdown of collagen, leading to thick skin and patchy hair loss. Scientists hope that by studying these mice, they can answer many questions about skin changes in scleroderma.

- The effectiveness of various treatments, including methotrexate, a drug commonly used for rheumatoid arthritis and some other inflammatory forms of arthritis; collagen peptides administered orally; halofugione, a drug that inhibits the synthesis of type I collagen, which is the primary component of connective tissue; ultraviolet light therapy for localized forms of scleroderma; and stem cell transfusions, a form of bone marrow transplant that uses a patient's own cells, for early diffuse systemic sclerosis.

Scleroderma research continues to advance as scientists and doctors learn more about how the disease develops and its underlying mechanisms.

Recently, the NIAMS funded a Specialized Center of Research (SCOR) in scleroderma at the University of Texas-Houston. SCOR scientists are conducting laboratory and clinical research on the disease. The SCOR approach allows researchers to translate basic science findings quickly into improved treatment and patient care.

Dunkin, Mary Anne. *Handout on Health: Scleroderma.* Bethesda, Md.: National Institute of Arthritis and Musculoskeletal and Skin Diseases, 2001.

secondary immune response   If the body is reinfected with a previously encountered pathogen, it will have an adapted subpopulation of B cells and T cells to provide a very specific and rapid secondary response. This secondary response is usually so fast and efficient that people are not aware they have been reinfected. (See also PRIMARY IMMUNE RESPONSE.)

self-antigen   A substance or molecule that is recognized by the immune system but is from the same organism (one's own body).

self-tolerance   The absence of an immune response to one's own antigens.

serum The clear liquid that separates from the blood when it is allowed to clot. This fluid retains any antibodies that were present in the whole blood. It is used to provide immediate passive immunity for someone exposed to the same organism that elicited the antibodies contained in the serum.

sexuality and sexual problems Sexual relationships can be affected by autoimmune diseases. For men, diseases that affect blood vessels can lead to problems with erection. In women, damage to glands that produced moisture can lead to vaginal dryness. This makes intercourse painful. In both men and women, pain, weakness, or stiff joints may make it hard for them to move the way they once did. They may not be sure about how they look. Or they may be afraid that their partner will no longer find them attractive. With communication, good medical care, and perhaps counseling, many of these issues can be overcome or at least worked around.

Researchers from the University of Western Ontario looked at sexual function in male patients with rheumatoid arthritis and progressive systemic sclerosis (PSS) (see SCLERODERMA). Rates of impotence were higher in the group with PSS, which as a vascular disease can lead to constriction in blood vessels and resulting impotence. In the study, 81 percent of both the PSS and rheumatoid arthritis patients reported impotence as occurring after the onset of the disease. One hundred percent of PSS patients and 56 percent of rheumatoid arthritis patients also reported a change in their sexual function.

National Institute of Arthritis and Musculoskeletal and Skin Diseases (NIAMS), National Institutes of Health (NIH), *Questions and Answers about Autoimmunity,* NIH Publication No. 02-4858, 2002.

sign Any physical evidence or manifestation of an illness or disease of the body. Signs are apparent to trained medical personnel, as opposed to symptoms, which may be obvious only to the patient.

Sjögren's syndrome Pronounced SHOW-grins, this chronic inflammatory autoimmune disease

occurs when lymphocytes attack the glands in the body that produce moisture. The classic symptoms of Sjögren's syndrome are dry eyes and dry mouth; fatigue and joint pain are also common. Many parts of the body can be affected by Sjögren's syndrome, such as the lungs, brain, nerves, joints, kidneys, thyroid, and liver. In the majority of cases, the autoimmune response is confined to the tear ducts, salivary glands, and vagina.

In 1933, Swedish ophthalmologist Dr. Henrik Sjögren first reported that many of his female patients had dry eyes, dry mouth, and rheumatoid arthritis. Today, estimates are that 2 to 4 million Americans have Sjögren's syndrome. Sjögren's syndrome can affect both men and women at any age. However, the majority (90 percent) of patients are women, and the onset is most common in middle age or older. It can affect people of all races and ethnic backgrounds. It is rare in children, but it can occur.

A survey released in 2001 by the Sjögren's Syndrome Foundation showed that many women with the syndrome may be undiagnosed. According to the survey, women are disregarding or downplaying symptoms of the disease because, when the problem of dryness appears around the age of menopause, this symptom is often dismissed as "normal aging," one of the effects of menopause. The survey also revealed that physicians often misinterpret patients' concerns as menopause or age related.

Causes

In Sjögren's syndrome, the immune system produces B lymphocytes that produce self-reactive proteins called autoantibodies that may attack the tear, salivary, and other moisture-producing glands, thus destroying the glands and their ability to produce moisture. Self-reactive T lymphocytes may also play a role in producing tissue damage.

Researchers think Sjögren's syndrome is caused by a combination of genetic and environmental factors. Several different genes appear to be involved. However, scientists are not certain exactly which ones are linked to the disease since different genes seem to play a role in different people. For example, one gene predisposes Caucasians to the disease. Other genes are linked to Sjögren's in people of

Japanese, Chinese, and African-American descent. Simply having one of these genes will not cause a person to develop the disease, however. Some sort of trigger must activate the immune system.

Scientists think that the trigger may be a viral or bacterial infection. It might work like this: a person who has a Sjögren's-associated gene gets a viral infection. The virus stimulates the immune system to act, but the gene alters the attack, sending fighter cells (T lymphocytes) to the eye and mouth glands. Once there, the lymphocytes attack healthy cells, causing the inflammation that damages the glands and keeps them from working properly. These fighter cells are supposed to die after their attack in a natural process called apoptosis. However, in people with Sjögren's syndrome, they continue to attack, causing further damage. Scientists think that resistance to apoptosis may be genetic.

The possibility that the endocrine and nervous systems play a role is also under investigation.

Clinical Features

Some people with Sjögren's syndrome have a dry, gritty, or burning sensation in their eyes, and they may have trouble swallowing food or have to drink water often while talking. The dry mouth they experience feels like a mouth full of cotton. Their tongue may be sore or cracked, and they may experience an increase in dental cavities and mouth infections due to the lack of the protective effects of saliva. The sense of smell can change, and the person may develop a bad cough. Sjögren's can also cause dryness of the skin, nose, and vagina. It can also affect other major organs and systems of the body, including the kidneys, blood vessels, lungs, liver, and pancreas and the nervous and gastrointestinal systems. When Sjögren's affects other parts of the body, the condition is called extraglandular involvement because the problems extend beyond the tear and salivary glands.

Sjögren's syndrome can occur by itself, in which case it is called primary Sjögren's. It can, and often does, occur with other autoimmune disease, such as rheumatoid arthritis, lupus, polymyositis, or scleroderma—at which time it is called secondary Sjögren's. Both are systemic disorders, although the symptoms in primary are more restricted.

In primary Sjögren's syndrome, the doctor can trace the symptoms to problems with the tear and saliva glands. People with primary Sjögren's disease are likely to have characteristic autoantibodies, called anti-Ro (anti-SS-A) or anti-La (anti-SS-B), circulating in their blood. People with secondary Sjögren's also have antibodies characteristic of their underlying condition, such as ANA (in lupus), rheumatoid factor (in rheumatoid arthritis), or thyroglobulin autoantibodies (in Hashimoto's thyroiditis).

In secondary Sjögren's syndrome, the person had an autoimmune disease like rheumatoid arthritis or lupus before Sjögren's developed. People with this type tend to have more health problems because they have two diseases.

As with many autoimmune diseases, Sjögren's syndrome can be difficult to diagnose. In fact, studies show that Sjögren's patients suffer for an average of six years before obtaining an accurate diagnosis and effective treatment. No two people with the disease will have exactly the same set of symptoms or medical history. Furthermore, many of the symptoms overlap with those of other diseases. The symptoms may also come and go, causing a flare one day and going into remission on another. Also, not all dryness may be the result of Sjögren's syndrome. A number of medications, such as those used to treat allergies and depression, may cause dry eyes (called keratoconjunctivitis sicca or KCS) and dry mouth (called XEROSTOMIA). Finally, many individuals mistakenly assume that dryness is a normal part of aging and do not report the symptoms to their doctors.

A number of tests can help the doctor, usually a rheumatologist, make the diagnosis of Sjögren's syndrome. These include the Schirmer test to measure tear production and a biopsy of the minor salivary glands in the lip to determine the presence of lymphocytes. Blood tests for specific autoantibodies that may include Sjögren's include those for anti-SS-A (Sjögren's syndrome-associated antigen A or anti-Ro) and anti-SS-B (Sjögren's syndrome-associated antigen B or anti-La). However, not everyone with Sjögren's will test positive for these autoantibodies.

Complications

Lymphoma, a cancer of the lymph glands, occurs in approximately 5 percent of Sjögren's syndrome patients. Some women with Sjögren's may experience complications during pregnancy.

Treatment

Because there is no cure for Sjögren's syndrome, treatment is aimed at alleviating the symptoms. Artificial tears, a special kind of eye drop designed to treat dry eyes, and saliva substitutes are available in drug and grocery stores. A new prescription medication called pilocarpine (Salagen) can ease the symptoms of dry mouth. The doctor may prescribe nonsteroidal anti-inflammatory drugs (NSAIDS) for pain and discomfort, disease-modifying agents to try to slow down the progress of the disease, or immunosuppressant drugs to suppress the immune system. Most individuals with Sjögren's syndrome successfully manage the symptoms of their disease.

Carsons, Steven and Elaine Harns, eds. *The New Sjögren's Syndrome Handbook,* 2nd ed. N.Y.: Oxford University Press, 1998.

Clark, Cheri. *Questions and Answers: Sjögren's Syndrome.* Bethesda, Md.: National Institute of Arthritis and Musculoskeletal and Skin Diseases, 2001.

Dauphin, Sue. *Understanding Sjögren's Syndrome.* New York: Pixel Press, 1993.

smoking   Smoking has been determined to be a risk factor for several autoimmune diseases.

- In GOODPASTURE'S SYNDROME, smoking can lead to an increase in episodes of pulmonary bleeding.

- Smoking causes increased susceptibility to and increased severity of ophthalmopathy in GRAVES' DISEASE.

- In a Canadian study, a direct and significant association was observed between cigarette smoking and the risk of MULTIPLE SCLEROSIS.

- Results of a University of California study suggest that abstinence from smoking may reduce the risk of RHEUMATOID ARTHRITIS among postmenopausal women. Smoking also increases susceptibility and rheumatoid factor in rheumatoid arthritis.

- People with SCLERODERMA need to avoid smoking and being around smoke due to the risk of pulmonary fibrosis. Smoking can also worsen the scleroderma vascular and circulation problems, which can lead to more rapid progression of vascular disease and can increase the risks of digital ulcers and amputations.

Criswell L. A., L. A. Merlino, J. R. Cerhan, T. R. Mikuls, A. S. Mudano, M. Burma, A. R. Folsom, and K. G. Saag. "Cigarette Smoking and the Risk of Rheumatoid Arthritis Among Postmenopausal Women: Results from the Iowa Women's Health Study." *American Journal of Medicine* 112, no. 6 (April 15, 2002): 465–471.

Ghadirian P., B. Dadgostar, R. Azani, and P. Maisonneuve. "A Case-Control Study of the Association Between Socio-Demographic, Lifestyle and Medical History Factors and Multiple Sclerosis." *Canadian Journal of Public Health.* 92, no. 4 (July–August 2001): 281–285.

Harrison, B. J. "Influence of Cigarette Smoking on Disease Outcome in Rheumatoid Arthritis." *Current Opinions in Rheumatology* 14, no. 2 (March 2002): 93–97.

sperm (testicular) autoimmunity   A specific disorder that can interfere with the normal reproductive process and contribute to infertility but that is not usually an absolute cause of infertility. The larger the immunological response, the less likely that a pregnancy will occur. Experts estimate that autoimmunity may contribute to infertility in as many as 20 percent of couples who have no other known cause of the infertility. Sperm autoimmunity can occur in both men and women.

Sperm autoimmunity occurs at puberty. It is caused by the release of antibodies to sperm that come into contact with blood.

The process as explained by the Sher Institute for Reproductive Medicine:

Like any other kind of antibody manufactured by the body, sperm antibodies are formed in response to antigens. These antigens are proteins which appear on the outer sperm membranes as the young sperm cells develop within the male testes. Antigens can only stimulate antibody production when they come in contact with components of the blood. Under normal conditions, blood and sperm do not mix. Direct contact between the two is prevented by a cellular structure in the testes called the blood:testis barrier. This barrier is formed by Sertoli cells which abut very closely against each other, forming tight junctions that separate the developing sperm cells from the blood and prevent immunologic stimulation. However, the blood:testis barrier can be broken by physical or chemical injury or by infection. When this barrier is breached, sperm antigens escape from their immunologically protected environment and come in direct contact with blood elements that launch an immunologic attack.

In the female body, deposited sperm are regarded as foreign invader cells and as such would normally be targeted for attack and destruction by circulating antibodies. Yet sperm, which are immunologic aliens to the woman, do not usually cause an antibody response. Although a woman may be exposed to billions of sperm during her lifetime, few will develop sperm antibodies. Why this is so is not well understood. It is known that the cellular construction of the vagina provides a physical barricade somewhat similar to the blood:testis barrier in the male. Here, too, physical damage or infection will increase the likelihood of sperm and blood mixing and subsequent antibody production.

The result is that the antibodies kill or disable the sperm. Antibodies are protein molecules that bind (attach) to specific parts of the sperm (the head, the midpiece, or the tail) and cause problems in any of several ways.

- They may cause the sperm to stick together (agglutinate) in large masses. When this occurs, the clumped sperm are not able to migrate through the cervix and uterus.

- They may make it more difficult, if not impossible, to penetrate the cervical mucus (poor sperm transit) and gain access to the egg.

- They may interfere with the sperm's ability to penetrate the egg (blocked sperm-oocyte fusion) and thus not fertilize it.

Some experts believe that in most cases, the presence of these antibodies will not prevent conception unless a large percentage of sperm are affected.

Vasectomy, the primary sterility procedure in men, is the most common cause of sperm autoantibodies. Experts believe their typical development is as follows:

- Vasectomy works by severing the vas deferens (the sperm-carrying tube).

- After vasectomy, sperm continue to be produced but, instead of being confined to the reproductive passages, they leak out into the body.

- Here, the immune system may perceive them as foreign invaders and develops antibodies to attack them.

Such antibodies often persist, even if a man restores fertility by a successful reversal procedure (vasovasostomy). Even if the surgery successfully restores sperm flow, however, infertility may persist because of autoantibodies.

Antibodies to sperm can also appear in men without previous vasectomies and have been reported to be present in 5 percent to 10 percent of all subfertile men. Other conditions predisposing to sperm autoimmunity include testicular injury or inflammation, genital tract infection or obstruction, and family history of autoimmune disease. The causes of antibodies in these cases are usually not known.

Tests for Sperm Autoimmunity
Several tests are available to detect the presence of sperm antibodies. The immunobead binding test (IBT) is used to detect antibodies present in the blood serum, in cervical mucus (the primary site where the woman's immune system interacts with sperm), or on the sperm surface. The postcoital test, which is a standard part of infertility evaluation, may suggest the presence of sperm antibodies. Also, the mixed agglutination reaction (MAR) test uses antibodies bound to a small marker, which will attach to sperm that have antibodies on their surface. The results are read as a percentage of sperm bound by antibodies.

Treatment
Once sperm autoimmunity has been identified, several options are available.

Corticosteroids (prednisone) may be administered to suppress the immune system temporarily. However, in addition to a poor pregnancy rate with this treatment, the risk of serious side effects makes it a less desirable option.

Intrauterine insemination (IUI), also known as artificial insemination, with or without the use of fertility drugs, has been used as a treatment for infertility caused by sperm autoimmunity. However, it is not suggested for moderate or severe cases of male sperm autoimmunity.

In vitro fertilization (IVF) is considered the most effective treatment for sperm immunity, especially in cases with high levels of antibodies. According to the Sher Institute, the best option is a form of IVF known as intracytoplasmic sperm injection (ICSI), where each egg is injected with a single sperm; high pregnancy and birth rates have been reported.

Diekman, A. B., E. J. Norton, V. A. Westbrook, K. L. Klotz, S. Naaby-Hansen and J. C. Herr. "Anti-Sperm Antibodies from Infertile Patients and Their Cognate Sperm Antigens: A Review. Identity Between SAGA-1, the H6-3C4 Antigen, and CD52." *American Journal of Reproductive Immunology* 43, no. 4 (March 2002): 134–143.
Gehlbach, Dan and Gilbert G. Haas, Jr. "Immunological Factor and Infertility." The Fertility Network.
"Treatment of Infertility Associated with the Presence of Sperm Antibodies in the Man." Sher Institute for Reproductive Medicine.

spleen   A lymphoid organ in the abdominal cavity that is an important center for immune system activities.

stem cells   Cells from which all other cells of the body derive. Stem cells have the ability to divide for indefinite periods in culture and to give rise to specialized cells. They are best described in the context of normal human development. Human development begins when a sperm fertilizes an egg and creates a single cell that has the potential to form an entire organism. This fertilized egg is totipotent, meaning that its potential is total. In the first hours after fertilization, this cell divides into two identical totipotent cells. This means that either one of these cells, if placed into a woman's uterus, has the potential to develop into a fetus. In fact, identical twins develop when two totipotent cells separate and develop into two individual, genetically identical human beings. Approximately four days after fertilization and after several cycles of cell division, these totipotent cells begin to specialize, forming a hollow sphere of cells, called a blastocyst. The blastocyst has an outer layer of cells, and inside the hollow sphere is a cluster of cells called the inner cell mass.

The outer layer of cells will go on to form the placenta and other supporting tissues needed for fetal development in the uterus. The inner cell mass cells will go on to form virtually all of the tissues of the human body. Although the inner cell mass cells can form virtually every type of cell found in the human body, they cannot form an organism because they are unable to give rise to the placenta and supporting tissues necessary for development in the human uterus. These inner cell mass cells are pluripotent—they can give rise to many types of cells but not all types of cells necessary for fetal development. Because their potential is not total, they are not totipotent and they are not embryos. If an inner cell mass cell were placed into a woman's uterus, it would not develop into a fetus.

The pluripotent stem cells undergo further specialization into stem cells that are committed to give rise to cells that have a particular function. Examples of this include blood stem cells that give rise to red blood cells, white blood cells, and platelets and skin stem cells that give rise to the various types of skin cells. These more specialized stem cells are called multipotent.

Although stem cells are extraordinarily important in early human development, multipotent stem cells are also found in children and adults. For example, consider one of the best-understood stem cells, the blood stem cell. Blood stem cells reside in the bone marrow of every child and adult, and they can be found in very small numbers circulating in the bloodstream. Blood stem cells perform the critical role of continually replenishing the body's supply of blood cells—red blood cells, white blood cells, and platelets—throughout life. A person cannot survive without blood stem cells.

At present, human pluripotent cell lines have been developed from two sources with methods previously developed in work with animal models.

In the work done by Dr. James Thomson, pluripotent stem cells were isolated directly from the inner cell mass of human embryos at the blastocyst stage. Dr. Thomson received embryos from IVF (in vitro fertilization) clinics. These embryos were in excess of the clinical need for infertility treatment. The embryos were made for purposes of reproduction, not research. Informed consent was obtained from the donor couples. Dr. Thomson isolated the inner cell mass and cultured these cells producing a pluripotent stem cell line.

In contrast, Dr. John Gearhart isolated pluripotent stem cells from fetal tissue obtained from terminated pregnancies. Informed consent was obtained from the donors after they had independently made the decision to terminate their pregnancy. Dr. Gearhart took cells from the region of the fetus that was destined to develop into the testes or the ovaries. Although the cells developed in Dr. Gearhart's lab and Dr. Thomson's lab were derived from different sources, they appear to be very similar.

Perhaps the most far-reaching potential application of human pluripotent stem cells is the generation of cells and tissues that could be used for so-called cell therapies. Many diseases and disorders result from disruption of cellular function or destruction of tissues of the body. Today, donated organs and tissues are often used to replace ailing or destroyed tissue. Unfortunately, the number of people suffering from these disorders far outstrips the number of organs available for transplantation. Pluripotent stem cells, stimulated to develop into specialized cells, offer the possibility of a renewable source of replacement cells and tissues to treat a myriad of diseases, conditions, and disabilities including Parkinson's and Alzheimer's diseases, spinal cord injury, stroke, burns, heart disease, diabetes, osteoarthritis, and rheumatoid arthritis.

The development of stem cell lines, both pluripotent and multipotent, that may produce many tissues of the human body is an important scientific breakthrough. It is not too unrealistic to say that this research has the potential to revolutionize the practice of medicine and improve the quality and length of life.

National Institutes of Health. *Stem Cells: A Primer,* 2000.

Shamblott, Michael et al. "Derivation of Pluripotent Stem Cells from Cultured Human Primordial Germ Cells." *Proceedings of the National Academy of Sciences of the United States of America* 95 (November 1998): 13,726–13,731.

Thomson, James et al. "Embryonic Stem Cell Lines Derived from Human Blastocysts." *Science* (November 1998): 1,145–1,147.

stem cell transplant   Replacement of the patient's diseased bone marrow with healthy new stem cells. When physicians harvest bone marrow for use in a transplant, they look for the stem cells. It has been estimated that less than one in 100,000 cells in the bone marrow are stem cells.

Stem cell transplants are classified based on which individual donates the stem cells and from where the stem cells are collected. Stem cells may be collected from the bone marrow, peripheral blood, or umbilical cord. The type of transplant designates which of these was the source—bone marrow transplantation (BMT), peripheral blood stem cell transplantation, or umbilical cord transplantation. Each of these sources has its own important advantages and disadvantages.

The second part of stem cell transplant classification is determined by who donates the stem cells. Stem cells may come from the patient (autologous), an identical twin (syngeneic), or someone other than the patient (allogeneic). Allogeneic stem cells are further classified by whether the individual donating the stem cells is related or unrelated to the patient. Umbilical cord blood is also considered to be a type of allogeneic stem cell transplant.

Before infusing stem cells into a patient, processing may be necessary. If the donor and recipient have a major blood group incompatibility, red blood cells will be removed from the graft to prevent a transfusion reaction from occurring. Some transplant centers may also treat the stem cells to reduce the number of T cells. This is done because these immune system cells can trigger graft-versus-host disease (GVHD) in the recipient.

When the stem cell graft is ready, it is infused into the patient's bloodstream through an intravenous line. The stem cells pass from the bloodstream into the internal cavities of marrow-containing bones. Until the donated stem cells grow and rebuild the recipient's blood and immune systems, the recipient is susceptible to infections. In the days and weeks following transplantation, transplant centers take steps to reduce recipients' exposure to viruses and bacteria. The centers watch each recipient carefully for any signs of infection.

Engraftment takes place when the donated stem cells begin to function in the recipient's body. Engraftment is measured by noting the number of neutrophils (a type of white blood cell) and platelets in the recipient's bloodstream. The usual measure is 500 neutrophils per cubic millimeter of blood or 20,000 platelets per cubic millimeter. Neutrophils usually engraft several days before the platelets. Engraftment of both cell types is important for a successful transplant.

When stem cells are infused into a patient's bloodstream, they will migrate to the interior of certain bones, set up housekeeping or colonize, and begin producing immature cells called *committed progenitors*. These committed progenitors produce colonies of cells that eventually mature into red blood cells, white blood cells, or platelets.

Autologous hemopoietic stem-cell transplantation (AHSCT) has been suggested as a possible treatment for severe autoimmune disease that does not respond to conventional treatment. Nico Wulffraat et al. reported preliminary success with the first four children with severe forms of juvenile chronic arthritis to be treated with AHSCT. The treatment was well tolerated and induced a remission of the disease, which had been resistant to conventional treatment. The follow-up (range six to 18 months) was too short, though, for the researchers to conclude these children to be completely cured.

The patients showed a drug-free follow-up with a marked decrease in joint swelling, pain, and morning stiffness. Erythocyte sedimentation rate, C-reactive protein, and hemoglobin returned to almost normal values within six weeks. Despite T cell depletion, there was a rapid immune reconstitution in three out of four children. Two patients developed a limited varicella zoster virus eruption, which was treated by aciclovir.

Stewart, Susan K. *Bone Marrow Transplants.* Highland Park, Ill.: BMT Newsletter, 1992.

"The Transplant." National Marrow Donor Program. Available online. URL: http://www.marrow.org. Posted August 2000.

Wulffraat, Nico, Anne van Royen, Marc Bierings, Jaak Vossen, and Wietse Kuis. "Autologous Haemopoietic Stem-Cell Transplantation in Four Patients with Refractory Juvenile Chronic Arthritis." *Lancet* 353 (1999): 550–553.

stiff-man syndrome   Also referred to as Moersch-Woltmann syndrome and stiff-person syndrome, stiff-man syndrome is a rare, severe autoimmune neurologic disease involving the central nervous system. The disease is characterized by a progressive rigidity or stiffness of the body musculature. The stiffness is caused by a diffuse hypertonia (excess muscular tension or pressure) that involves the voluntary muscles of the neck, shoulders, trunk, arms, and legs. Constant painful contractions and spasms of voluntary muscles, particularly the muscles of the back and upper legs, may also be present. Unlike many autoimmune diseases that have a higher incidence in women, stiff-man syndrome is found more frequently in men. Approximately 70 percent of those afflicted are men.

Causes
Although the exact cause of stiff-man syndrome is not clear, autoimmunity is thought to be a factor. Genetic factors have not been established, although familial occurrences of the disease and/or other autoimmune disorders appear to point in this direction. The frequent occurrence of insulin-dependent diabetes mellitus (IDDM), also referred to as Type 1 diabetes, in stiff-man syndrome supports this hypothesis. Other autoimmune disorders such as pernicious anemia (a chronic, progressive blood disorder) and thyroiditis (inflammation of the thyroid gland) may also occur more frequently in patients with stiff-man syndrome.

Clinical Features
Symptoms may occur gradually, spreading from the back and legs to the arms and neck. Symptoms may worsen when the affected individual is anxious or exposed to sudden motion or noise. Affected muscles may become twisted and contracted, resulting in bone fractures in the most severe cases. Individuals with stiff-man syndrome may have difficulty

making sudden movements and may have a stiff-legged, unsteady gait. Sleep usually suppresses frequency of contractions. Stiffness may increase, and patients may develop a hunched posture (kyphosis) or a swayback (lordosis).

Treatment

The drug diazepam, which relaxes the muscles, provides improvement in most cases. Baclofen, phenytoin, clonidine, or tizanidine may provide additional benefit. Physical and rehabilitation therapy may also be needed.

There is no cure for stiff-man syndrome. The long-term prognosis for individuals with stiff-man syndrome is uncertain. Management of the disorder with drug therapy may provide significant improvements and relief of symptoms.

Barker, R., and C. Marsden. "Successful Treatment of Stiff Man Syndrome with Intravenous Immunoglobulin." *Journal of Neurology, Neurosurgery, and Neuropsychiatry,* 62 (1997): 426.

Levy, L., M. K. Floeter, and M. Dalakas. "Stiff-Person Syndrome—An Autoimmune Disorder Affecting Gamma-Aminobutyric Acid (GABA) Neurotransmission." *Annals of Internal Medicine* 131 (1999): 522–530.

National Institute of Neurological Disorders and Stroke, National Institutes of Health. *NINDS Stiff-Person Syndrome Information,* 2001.

Spada, P., and J. Spada. "Stiff-Man Syndrome: A Rare Disorder of the Central Nervous System." *Journal of Neuroscience Nursing* 26, no. 6 (December 1994): 364–366.

stress   One of the paradoxes of stress and immunity is that on the one hand stress is thought to suppress immunity and decrease resistance to infections and cancer, while on the other it is known to exacerbate autoimmune diseases that should be ameliorated by a suppression of immune function.

Rockefeller University research in 1999 began to provide some common basis for explaining some of these paradoxes, according to the authors. "If it's a 'good' immune response, like fighting a pathogen or cancer cell, then this acute response protects the body in the short run. If the immune response is dysregulated, for example, during allergy, asthma, or arthritis, acute stress may make it worse." McEwen points out that the irony of allergies, autoimmunity, and asthma is that very frequently they are treated with stress hormones. If adminis-

tered properly, for example locally in high doses, or using synthetic steroids like dexamethasone, these hormones mimic the effects of chronic stress and suppress immune function.

Dhabhar F. S., and McEwen, B. S. "Enhancing Versus Suppressive Effects of Stress Hormones on Skin Immune Function." *Proceedings of the National Academy of Sciences* 96, no. 3 (February 1999): 1,059–1,064.

subacute bacterial endocarditis (SBE)   A bacterial infection that produces growths on damaged heart valves and, if untreated, can become fatal within six weeks to a year. Among the risk factors are a heart valve damaged by rheumatic fever or a chronic medical condition that weakens the immune system.

Subacute bacterial endocarditis occurs when bacteria lodge on damaged heart valves and produce clusters or vegetations on the valves. Pieces of these vegetations may dislodge and travel through the blood as emboli to such areas as the brain, spleen, or kidneys.

Causes

An injury to the skin, lining of the mouth, or gums can allow a small number of bacteria to invade the bloodstream, increasing the risk of endocarditis. Certain surgical, dental, and medical procedures may also introduce bacteria into the bloodstream—for example, the use of intravenous lines to provide fluids, nutrition, or medications; cystoscopy (insertion of a viewing tube to examine the bladder); and colonoscopy (insertion of a viewing tube to examine the large intestine). In people with normal heart valves, no harm is done, and the body's white blood cells destroy these bacteria. Damaged heart valves, however, may trap the bacteria, which then lodge on the endocardium and start to multiply. For this reason, it is important for people who are high risk to take antibiotics prior to dental and surgical procedures.

Clinical Features

Frequently, symptoms of SBE are mild or vague, with the disease evolving slowly. A low-grade fever may be present on a daily basis for months before other symptoms appear. Other symptoms may be nonspecific such as persistent fatigue, malaise (general discomfort), confusion, headaches, chills, and night sweats. As the illness progresses, small dark lines, called splinter hemorrhages, may appear under the fingernails; similarly, small spots that resemble tiny freckles may appear on the skin and on the whites of the eyes. The examining physician may find a new heart murmur or a different sound if a heart murmur already exists, the murmur or sound caused when the vegetations collect on the heart valves. The examination may also detect an enlarged spleen and mild anemia. Other symptoms may include muscle and joint pain, blood in the urine, shortness of breath, poor appetite, or weight loss.

Complications

If bacterial endocarditis is not adequately treated, it can be fatal. Even when treated, further damage to a heart valve can lead to heart failure. In addition, blood clots can form and travel throughout the bloodstream to the brain or lungs.

Treatment

Eradication of all microorganisms from the vegetations on the heart valve usually requires hospitalization for antibiotic therapy, generally given intravenously, at least at the outset. In a few instances, oral antibiotics taken at home will be successful. In unusual cases, surgery may be necessary to repair or replace a damaged heart valve.

subunit vaccine   A vaccine that uses merely one component of an infectious agent, rather than the whole, to stimulate an immune response.

superantigens   A class of antigens, including certain viruses and bacterial toxins, that unleash a massive immune response because they activate a whole family of T cells.

suppressor T cells   A subset of T cells that turn off antibody production and other immune responses. (See also T SUPPRESSOR CELL.)

surface markers   Surface proteins that are unique to certain cell types and that can be detected by antibodies or other detection methods.

sympathetic ophthalmia (SO)   A rare, bilateral granulomatous UVEITIS, associated with either a perforating eye injury or a foreign body that remains in the eye. Inflammation of the uveal tract (middle layer of the eye) in one eye results from a similar inflammation in the other eye. It is believed to be an autoimmune disease.

According to *A Historical Tour of Ophthalmology*, sympathetic ophthalmia was first indicated by Duddell in 1729, who recorded that he had seen many cases in which both eyes were lost, though only one was originally injured. However, not until nearly 100 years later was any clear conception developed. Demours did much in that direction, but it was Wardrop who drew attention to the fact that veterinary surgeons destroy the injured eye of a horse with lime or a nail in order that the good eye may be saved. Both the writings of Demours and of Wardrop appeared in 1818. In both, the term *sympathetic involvement* is employed. The first comprehensive description appeared in the third edition of MacKenzie's textbook (1840), and thereafter the seriousness of the condition and its relationship to injuries and retained foreign bodies was well realized. MacKenzie gave a detailed clinical description of the disease in 1865; Fuchs established the pathological definition in 1905.

No reliable demographic data exists for sympathetic ophthalmia. The incidence has been reported to be higher in men than women, but the difference is suggested to result from the higher incidence of accidental penetrating wounds in men. Similarly, the frequency of occurrence is higher in children under 10 years of age because of the higher frequency of injuries. It also increases in those over the age of 60 years because of the increase in eye surgery.

Causes

The exact cause is unknown, but SO is believed to represent an autoimmune response to components of the retina, retinal pigment epithelium, or choroid. It has been known to follow uncomplicated surgery for cataracts or glaucoma. The injured eye becomes inflamed first, and the other eye follows (as in *sympathetic*). Whenever there is severe trauma to an eye (notably a puncture wound or a retained foreign object), sympathetic ophthalmia is a threat. Because it may occur 10 days to many years following the injury, the individual should seek medical attention immediately at the first sign of blurred vision, redness, or photophobia.

Clinical Features

Symptoms include intolerance of light, redness in the eye, and blurred vision; in some cases, there are also floaters and possibly pain. The history of trauma differentiates this condition from other types of granulomatous uveitis; other differentiating factors include its bilateral, diffuse, and acute nature.

Complications

Common complications include band keratopathy, cataract, glaucoma, macular edema and scarring, and retinal detachment. If untreated, sympathetic ophthalmia can progress to complete bilateral blindness over a period of months or years.

Treatment

The mainstay of the treatment is corticosteroids given topically, systemically, and by injections. Immunosuppressive medications like cyclosporine are used as a second line of treatment. In certain cases, the injured eye must be removed to prevent blindness in the other eye.

Chua, C. N. "A Historical Tour of Ophthalmology." Available online. URL: http://www.mrcophth.com/. Posted 17 July 2000.

Shindo Y., S. Ohno, M. Usui, H. Ideta, K. Harada, H. Masuda, and H. Inoko. "Immunogenetic Study of Sympathetic Ophthalmia." *Tissue Antigens* 49, no. 2 (February 1997): 111–115.

symptom   Any abnormal change in appearance, sensation, or function experienced by a patient that indicates a disease process. A symptom is considered a subjective complaint that the health practitioner is not able to see; thus he or she must rely on the patient's description.

syndrome   A group of symptoms that occur together but that can result from different causes. A syndrome is a medical condition characterized by a collection of symptoms (what the patient feels) and signs (what a doctor can observe or measure).

systemic   A condition involving the body as a whole, as opposed to limited conditions that affect particular parts of the body. Systemic diseases can affect many parts of the body.

systemic lupus erythematosus (SLE)   Lupus is a chronic autoimmune disease in which the body's immune system, instead of serving its normal protective function, forms antibodies that attack healthy tissues and organs. For most people, lupus is a mild disease affecting only a few body organs; for others, it may cause serious and even life-threatening problems.

Lupus means "wolf." *Erythematosus* means "redness." In 1851, doctors coined the name lupus for the disease because they thought the facial rash that frequently accompanies lupus looked like the bite of a wolf.

There are several types of lupus. DISCOID LUPUS affects the skin, causing a rash and lesions, usually across the face and upper part of the body. Drug-induced lupus refers to a form of lupus caused by specific medications. Symptoms are similar to those of SLE (arthritis, rash, fever, and chest pain) that typically go away when the drug is stopped.

Neonatal lupus is a rare form of lupus affecting newborn babies of women with SLE or certain other immune system disorders. At birth, the babies have a skin rash, liver abnormalities, or low blood counts, which entirely go away over several months. However, babies with neonatal lupus may have a serious heart defect. Physicians can now identify most at-risk mothers, allowing for prompt treatment of the infant at or before birth. Neonatal lupus is very rare, and most infants of mothers with SLE are entirely healthy.

Systemic lupus erythematosus is the form of the disease that most people are referring to when they say *lupus*. The symptoms of SLE may be mild or serious. Although SLE usually first affects people between the ages of 15 and 45 years, it can occur in childhood or later in life as well. Systemic lupus erythematosus is usually more severe than discoid lupus and can attack any body organ or system, such as joints, kidneys, brain, heart, and lungs. If not controlled, systemic lupus can be life threatening. The number of Americans diagnosed with lupus is estimated at 1 million.

Although people with systemic lupus may have many different symptoms, some of the most common ones include extreme fatigue, painful or swollen joints (arthritis), unexplained fever, skin rashes, and kidney problems.

At present, there is no cure for lupus. However, lupus can be very successfully treated with appropriate drugs, and most people with the disease can lead active, healthy lives. Lupus is characterized by periods of illness, called flares, and periods of wellness, or remission. Understanding how to prevent flares and how to treat them when they do occur helps people with lupus maintain better health. Intense research is under way, and scientists funded by the National Institutes of Health are continuing to make great strides in understanding the disease, which may ultimately lead to a cure.

Two of the questions researchers are studying are who gets lupus and why. Already known is that many more women than men have lupus. Lupus is three times more common in African-American women than in Caucasian women and is also more common in women of Hispanic, Asian, and Native-American descent. In addition, lupus can run in families, but the risk that a child, brother, or sister of a patient will also have lupus is still quite low. Estimating how many people in the United States have the disease is difficult because its symptoms vary widely and its onset is often hard to pinpoint.

Causes

Lupus is a complex disease whose cause is unknown. It is likely that there is no single cause but rather a combination of genetic, environmental, and possibly hormonal factors that work together to cause the disease. The exact cause may differ from one person to another. Scientists are making progress in understanding the processes leading to lupus. Research suggests that genetics plays an important role; however, no specific lupus gene has been identified. Instead, it appears that several genes may increase a person's susceptibility to the disease.

The fact that lupus can run in families indicates that its development has a genetic basis. In addition, studies of identical twins have shown that

lupus is much more likely to affect both members of a pair of identical twins, who share the exact same set of genes, than two nonidentical twins or other siblings. However, scientists think that genes alone cannot account for who gets lupus. Other factors must also play a role. Some of the factors that scientists are studying include sunlight, stress, certain drugs, and infectious agents such as viruses. Even though a virus might trigger the disease in susceptible individuals, a person cannot catch lupus from someone else.

In lupus, the body's immune system does not work as it should. A healthy immune system produces substances called antibodies that help fight and destroy viruses, bacteria, and other foreign substances that invade the body. In lupus, the immune system produces antibodies against the body's healthy cells and tissues. These antibodies, called autoantibodies (auto means "self"), contribute to the inflammation of various parts of the body, causing damage and altering the function of target organs and tissues. In addition, some autoantibodies join with substances from the body's own cells or tissues to form molecules called immune complexes. A buildup of these immune complexes in the body also contributes to inflammation and tissue injury in people with lupus. Researchers do not yet understand all of the factors that cause inflammation and tissue damage in lupus, and this is an active area of research.

Clinical Features

Each person's experience with lupus is different, although certain patterns permit accurate diagnosis. Symptoms can range from mild to severe and may come and go over time. Common symptoms of lupus include painful or swollen joints, unexplained fever, and skin rashes, along with extreme fatigue. A characteristic skin rash—the so-called butterfly or malar rash—may appear across the nose and cheeks. Other rashes occur elsewhere on the face and ears, upper arms, shoulders, chest, and hands.

Other symptoms of lupus include chest pain, hair loss, sensitivity to the Sun, anemia (a decrease in red blood cells), and pale or purple fingers and toes from cold and stress. Some people also experience headaches, dizziness, depression, or seizures. New symptoms may continue to appear years after the initial diagnosis, and different symptoms can occur at different times.

In some people with lupus, only one system of the body such as the skin or joints is affected. Other people experience symptoms in many parts of their body. Just how seriously a body system is affected also varies from person to person. Most commonly, joints and muscles are affected, causing arthritis and muscle pain. Skin rashes are quite common. The following systems in the body also can be affected by lupus.

Kidneys Inflammation of the kidneys (nephritis) can impair their ability to get rid of waste products and other toxins from the body effectively. Because the kidneys are so important to overall health, lupus affecting the kidneys generally requires intensive drug treatment to prevent permanent damage. There is usually no pain associated with kidney involvement, although some patients may notice that their ankles swell. Most often, the only indication of kidney disease is an abnormal urine or blood test.

Lungs Some people with lupus develop pleuritis, an inflammation of the lining of the chest cavity that causes chest pain, particularly with breathing. Patients with lupus may also get pneumonia.

Central nervous system In some patients, lupus affects the brain or central nervous system. This can cause headaches, dizziness, memory disturbances, vision problems, stroke, or changes in behavior.

Blood vessels Blood vessels may become inflamed (vasculitis), affecting the way blood circulates through the body. The inflammation may be mild and may not require treatment, or it may be severe and require immediate attention.

Blood People with lupus may develop anemia, leukopenia (a decreased number of white blood cells), or a decrease in the number of platelets (thrombocytopenia). Some people with lupus may have abnormalities that cause an increased risk for blood clots.

Heart In some people with lupus, inflammation can occur in the heart itself (myocarditis and endocarditis) or the membrane that surrounds it (pericarditis), causing chest pains or other symp-

toms. Lupus can also increase the risk of atherosclerosis.

Diagnosing lupus can be difficult. The doctors may take months or even years to piece together the symptoms to diagnose this complex disease accurately. Making a correct diagnosis of lupus requires knowledge and awareness on the part of the doctor and good communication on the part of the patient. Giving the doctor a complete, accurate medical history is critical to the process of diagnosis. This information, along with a physical examination and the results of laboratory tests, helps the doctor consider other diseases that may mimic lupus or determine if the patient truly has the disease. Reaching a diagnosis may take time and occur gradually as new symptoms appear.

No single test can determine whether a person has lupus, but several laboratory tests may help the doctor to make a diagnosis. The most useful tests identify certain autoantibodies often present in the blood of people with lupus. For example, the antinuclear antibody (ANA) test is commonly used to look for autoantibodies that react against components of the nucleus, or command center, of the patient's own cells. Most people with lupus test positive for ANA. However, there are a number of other causes of a positive ANA besides lupus, including infections, other rheumatic or immune diseases, and occasionally as a finding in normal healthy adults. The ANA test simply provides another clue for the doctor to consider in making a diagnosis. In addition, there are blood tests for individual types of autoantibodies that are more specific to people with lupus, although not all people with lupus test positive for these and not all people with these antibodies have lupus. These antibodies include anti-DNA, anti-Sm, anti-RNP, anti-Ro (SSA), and anti-La (SSB). A positive anti-Sm is highly specific for SLE; it is rarely found in patients with other rheumatic diseases. The doctor may use these antibody tests to help make a diagnosis of lupus.

Some tests are used less frequently but may be helpful if the cause of a person's symptoms remains unclear. The doctor may order a biopsy of the skin or kidneys if those body system are affected. Some doctors may order a syphilis test or a test for anti-cardiolipin antibody. A positive test does not mean that a patient has syphilis. However, the presence of this antibody may increase the risk of blood clotting and can increase the risk of miscarriages in pregnant women with lupus. Again, all these tests merely serve as tools to give the doctor clues and information in making a diagnosis. The doctor will look at the entire picture—medical history, symptoms, and test results—to determine if a person has lupus.

Other laboratory tests are used to monitor the progress of the disease once it has been diagnosed. A complete blood count, urinalysis, blood chemistries, and erythrocyte sedimentation rate (ESR) test can provide valuable information. Another common test measures the blood level of a group of substances called complement. People with lupus often have increased ESRs and low complement levels, especially during flares of the disease. Lupus flares usually are associated with an increase in the anti-DNA titer.

Treatment

Diagnosing and treating lupus is often a team effort between the patient and several types of health care professionals. A person with lupus can go to his or her family doctor or internist or can visit a rheumatologist. A rheumatologist is a doctor who specializes in rheumatic diseases (arthritis and other diseases of the joints, bones, and muscles). Clinical immunologists (doctors specializing in immune system disorders) may also treat people with lupus. As treatment progresses, other professionals often help. These may include nurses, psychologists, social workers, and specialists such as nephrologists (doctors who treat kidney disease), hematologists (doctors specializing in blood disorders), dermatologists (doctors who treat skin disease), and neurologists (doctors specializing in disorders of the nervous system).

A conservative regimen of physical and emotional rest, protection from direct sunlight, a healthful diet, prompt treatment of infections, and avoidance of known aggravating factors are the mainstays of lupus therapy. In addition, for female patients, pregnancy must be planned for times when the disease is in remission.

Photosensitivity is an abnormal reaction to the ultraviolet (UV) rays of the Sun and results in the development or exacerbation of a rash that is sometimes accompanied by systemic symptoms. About one-third of lupus patients are photosensitive. All lupus patients should avoid direct, prolonged exposure to the Sun. Sun-sensitive patients should frequently apply a sunscreen with a Sun protection factor (SPF) of at least 15, avoid unprotected exposure between 10 A.M. and 4 P.M., and wear protective clothing, such as wide-brimmed hats and long sleeves. Lupus patients should be aware that UV rays are reflected off water and snow and that glass, such as car windows, does not provide total protection from UV rays.

Lupus patients should also know that fluorescent and halogen lights may emit UV rays and can aggravate lupus. This may be an issue for patients who work in offices lit by these kinds of lights. Sunscreen and protective clothing can help minimize exposure, and plastic devices are available that block UV emissions from fluorescent or halogen lightbulbs.

The range and effectiveness of treatments for lupus have increased dramatically, giving doctors more choices in how to treat the disease. It is important for the patient to work closely with the doctor and take an active role in treatment. Once lupus has been diagnosed, the doctor will develop a treatment plan based on the patient's age, sex, health, symptoms, and lifestyle. Treatment plans are tailored to the individual's needs and may change over time. In developing a treatment plan, the doctor has several goals: to prevent flares, to treat them when they do occur, and to minimize organ damage and complications. The doctor and patient should reevaluate the plan regularly to ensure that it is as effective as possible.

Several types of drugs are used to treat lupus. The treatment the doctor chooses is based on the patient's individual symptoms and needs. For people with joint pain, chest pain, or fever, drugs that decrease inflammation, referred to as nonsteroidal anti-inflammatory drugs (NSAIDs), are often used. While some NSAIDs are available over-the-counter, a doctor's prescription is necessary for others. NSAIDs may be used alone or in combination with other types of drugs to control pain, swelling, and fever. Even though some NSAIDs may be purchased without a prescription, they must be taken under a doctor's direction. Common side effects of NSAIDs, including those available over-the-counter, can include stomach upset, heartburn, diarrhea, and fluid retention. Some patients with lupus also develop liver and kidney inflammation while taking NSAIDs, making it especially important to stay in close contact with the doctor while taking these medications.

A new class of anti-inflammatory drugs called COX-2 inhibitors (celecoxib [Celebrex], rofecoxib [Vioxx], and mobic [Meloxicam]) have all of the same effects as NSAIDs on pain and inflammation but have a much lower risk of significant gastrointestinal side effects. These agents have not been extensively studied in patients with lupus and have not been approved by the Food and Drug Administration for use specifically in treating lupus. However, they might provide benefits similar to NSAIDs.

Antimalarials are another type of drug commonly used to treat lupus. These drugs were originally used to treat malaria, but doctors have found that they also are useful for lupus. Exactly how antimalarials work in lupus is unclear, but scientists think that they may work by suppressing parts of the immune response. A common antimalarial used to treat lupus is hydroxychloroquine (Plaquenil). It may be used alone or in combination with other drugs and is generally used to treat fatigue, joint pain, skin rashes, and inflammation of the lungs.

Clinical studies have found that continuous treatment with antimalarials may prevent flares from recurring. Side effects of antimalarials can include stomach upset and, extremely rarely, damage to the retina of the eye.

The mainstay of lupus treatment involves the use of corticosteroid hormones, such as prednisone (Deltasone), hydrocortisone, methylprednisolone (Medrol), and dexamethasone (Decadron, Hexadrol). Corticosteroids are related to cortisol, which is a natural anti-inflammatory hormone. They work by rapidly suppressing inflammation. Corticosteroids can be given by mouth, in creams applied to the skin, or by injection. Because they are potent drugs, the doctor will seek the lowest dose with the greatest benefit. Short-term side effects of corticosteroids include swelling, increased

appetite, weight gain, and emotional ups and downs. These side effects generally stop when the drug is stopped. It can be dangerous to stop taking corticosteroids suddenly, so it is very important that the doctor and patient work together in changing the corticosteroid dose. Sometimes doctors give very large amounts of corticosteroids by vein over a brief period of time (days). This is called *bolus* or *pulse* therapy. With this treatment, the typical side effects are less likely and slow withdrawal is unnecessary.

Long-term side effects of corticosteroids can include stretch marks on the skin, excessive hair growth, weakened or damaged bones (osteoporosis and osteonecrosis), high blood pressure, damage to the arteries, high blood sugar, infections, and cataracts. Typically, the higher the dose of prolonged corticosteroids, the more severe the side effects. Also, the longer they are taken, the greater the risk of side effects. Researchers are working to develop alternative strategies to limit or offset the use of corticosteroids. For example, corticosteroids may be used in combination with other, less potent drugs, or the doctor may try to decrease the dose slowly once the disease is under control. People with lupus who are using corticosteroids should talk to their doctors about taking supplemental calcium and vitamin D or other drugs to reduce the risk of osteoporosis (weakened, fragile bones).

In special circumstances, patients may require stronger drugs to combat lupus symptoms. In some patients, methotrexate (Folex, Mexate, or Rheumatrex) may be used to help control the disease. Patients who have many body systems affected by the disease may receive intravenous gamma globulin (Gammagard S/D), a blood protein that increases immunity and helps fight infection. Gamma globulin may also be used to control acute bleeding in patients with thrombocytopenia or to prepare a person with lupus for surgery.

For patients whose kidneys or central nervous systems are affected by lupus, a type of drug called an immunosuppressive may be used. Immunosuppressives, such as azathioprine (Imuran) and cyclophosphamide (Cytoxan), restrain the overactive immune system by blocking the production of some immune cells and curbing the action of others. These drugs may be given by mouth or by infusion (dripping the drug into the vein through a small tube). Side effects may include nausea, vomiting, hair loss, bladder problems, decreased fertility, and increased risk of cancer and infection. The risk for side effects increases with the length of treatment. As with other treatments for lupus, there is a risk of relapse after the immunosuppressives have been stopped.

Because of the nature and cost of the medications used to treat lupus, their potentially serious side effects, and the lack of a cure, many patients seek other ways of treating the disease. Some alternative approaches that have been suggested include special diets, nutritional supplements, fish oils, ointments and creams, chiropractic treatment, and homeopathy. Although these methods may not be harmful in and of themselves and they may be associated with symptomatic or psychosocial benefit, no research to date shows that they affect the disease process or prevent organ damage. Some alternative or complementary approaches may help the patient cope or reduce some of the stress associated with living with a chronic illness. If the doctor feels the approach has value and will not be harmful, it can be incorporated into the patient's treatment plan. However, neglecting regular health care or treatment of serious symptoms is important. An open dialogue between the patient and the physician about the relative values of complementary, alternative, and more traditional therapy is essential in permitting the patient to make an informed choice about treatment options.

Lupus and Quality of Life

Despite the symptoms of lupus and the potential side effects of treatment, people with lupus can maintain a high quality of life overall. One key to managing lupus is to understand the disease and its impact. Learning to recognize the warning signs of a flare can help the patient take steps to ward it off or reduce its intensity. Many people with lupus experience increased fatigue, pain, a rash, fever, abdominal discomfort, headaches, or dizziness just before a flare. Developing strategies to prevent flares can also be helpful, such as learning to recognize one's warning signals and maintaining good communication with one's doctor.

People with lupus must also receive regular health care instead of seeking help only when symptoms worsen. Having a medical exam and laboratory work on a regular basis allows the doctor to note any changes and may help predict flares. The treatment plan, which is tailored to the individual's specific needs and circumstances, can be adjusted accordingly. If new symptoms are identified early, treatments may be more effective. Other concerns can also be addressed at regular checkups. The doctor can provide guidance about such issues as the use of sunscreens, stress reduction, and the importance of structured exercise and rest as well as birth control and family planning. Because people with lupus can be more susceptible to infections, the doctor may recommend yearly influenza vaccinations or pneumococcal vaccinations for some patients.

People with lupus should receive regular preventive health care, such as gynecological and breast examinations. Regular dental care will help avoid potentially dangerous infections. If a person is taking corticosteroids or antimalarial medications, a yearly eye exam should be done to screen for and treat eye problems.

Staying healthy requires extra effort and care for people with lupus, developing strategies for maintaining wellness becomes especially important. Wellness involves paying close attention to the body, mind, and spirit. One of the primary goals of wellness for people with lupus is coping with the stress of having a chronic disorder. Effective stress management varies from person to person. Some approaches that may help include exercise, relaxation techniques such as meditation, and setting priorities for spending time and energy.

Developing and maintaining a good support system is also important. A support system may include family, friends, medical professionals, community organizations, and organized support groups. Participating in a support group can provide emotional help, boost self-esteem and morale, and help develop or improve coping skills.

Learning more about lupus may also help. Studies have shown that patients who are well informed and participate actively in their own care experience less pain, make fewer visits to the doctor, build self-confidence, and remain more active.

Pregnancy for Women with Lupus

Although a lupus pregnancy is considered high risk, most women with lupus carry their babies safely to the end of their pregnancy. Experts disagree on the exact numbers, but 20 percent to 25 percent of lupus pregnancies end in miscarriage, compared with 10 percent to 15 percent of pregnancies in women without the disease. Pregnancy counseling and planning before pregnancy are important. Ideally, a woman should have no signs or symptoms of lupus and be taking no medications for at least six months before she becomes pregnant.

Some women may experience a mild-to-moderate flare during or after their pregnancy, others do not. Pregnant women with lupus, especially those taking corticosteroids, are also more likely to develop high blood pressure, diabetes, hyperglycemia (high blood sugar), and kidney complications, so regular care and good nutrition during pregnancy are essential. It is also advisable to have access to a neonatal (newborn) intensive care unit at the time of delivery in case the baby requires special medical attention. About 25 percent of babies of women with lupus are born prematurely but do not suffer from birth defects.

Aladjem, Henrietta. *Understanding Lupus.* N.Y.: Charles Scribner's Sons, 1985.

Blau, Sheldon, with D. Schultz. *Living with Lupus.* N.Y.: Addison Wesley, 1993.

Digeronimo, Theresa Foy, and Sara J. Henry. *New Hope for People with Lupus: Your Friendly, Authoritative Guide to the Latest in Traditional and Complementary Solutions.* Rocklin, Calif.: Prima Publishing, 2001.

Horowitz, Mark, with M. Brill. *Living with Lupus.* N.Y.: Plume, 1994.

National Institute of Arthritis and Musculoskeletal and Skin Diseases (NIAMS), National Institutes of Health (NIH). *Lupus: A Patient Care Guide for Nurses and Other Health Professionals,* 1999.

Novak, Debbie. *Handout on Health: Systemic Lupus Erythematosus.* Bethesda, Md.: National Institute of Arthritis and Musculoskeletal and Skin Diseases Information Clearinghouse, 1997.

Phillips, Robert H., Ronald I. Carr, and Harry Spiera. *Coping With Lupus: A Practical Guide to Alleviating the Challenges of Systemic Lupus Erythematosus,* 3rd ed. N.Y.: Avery Penguin Putnam, 2001.

Wallace, Daniel J., and Bevra Hannahs Hahn, eds. *Dubois' Lupus Erythematosus,* 6th ed. N.Y.: Lippincott Williams & Wilkins Publishers, 2002.

Wallace, Daniel J. *The Lupus Book: A Guide for Patients and Their Families,* revised and expanded ed. N.Y.: Oxford University Press, 2000.

systemic lupus erythematosus research   Lupus is the focus of intense research as scientists try to determine what causes the disease and how it can best be treated. Some of the questions they are working to answer include, Exactly who gets lupus, and why? Why are women more likely than men to have the disease? Why are there more cases of lupus in some racial and ethnic groups? What goes wrong in the immune system, and why? How can physicians correct the way the immune system functions once something goes wrong? What treatment approaches will work best to lessen or cure lupus symptoms?

To help answer these questions, scientists are developing new and better ways to study the disease. They are doing laboratory studies that compare various aspects of the immune systems of people with lupus with those of other people both with and without lupus. They also use mice with disorders resembling lupus to understand the abnormalities of the immune system that occur in lupus better and to identify possible new therapies.

The National Institute of Arthritis and Musculoskeletal and Skin Diseases (NIAMS), a component of the National Institutes of Health (NIH), has a major program of lupus research in its intramural program in Bethesda, Maryland, and funds many individual researchers across the United States who are studying lupus. To help scientists gain new knowledge, the NIAMS has also established specialized centers of research devoted specifically to lupus research. In addition, the NIAMS is funding several lupus registries that will gather medical information as well as blood and tissue samples from patients and their relatives. This will give researchers across the country access to information and materials they can use to help identify genes that determine susceptibility to the disease.

Identifying genes that play a role in the development of lupus is an active area of research. For example, researchers suspect a genetic defect in a cellular process called apoptosis, or programmed cell death, in people with lupus. Apoptosis is similar to the process that causes leaves to turn color in autumn and fall from trees; it allows the body to eliminate cells that have fulfilled their function and typically need to be replaced. If there is a problem in the apoptosis process, harmful cells may stay around and do damage to the body's own tissues. For example, in a mutant mouse strain that develops a lupuslike illness, one of the genes that controls apoptosis is defective. When it is replaced by a normal gene, the mice no longer develop signs of the disease. Scientists are studying what role genes involved in apoptosis may play in human disease development.

Studying genes for complement, a series of proteins in the blood that play an important part in the immune system, is another active area of lupus research. Complement acts as a backup for antibodies, helping them destroy foreign substances that invade the body. If complement levels decrease, the body is less able to fight or destroy foreign substances. If these foreign substances are not removed from the body, the immune system may become overactive and begin to make autoantibodies.

Recent large studies of families with lupus have identified a number of genetic regions that appear to confer risk of SLE. Although the specific genes and their function remain unknown, intensive work in delineating the entire human genome offers promise that these genes will be identified in the near future. This should provide knowledge of the fundamental nature of the risk factors that can lead to lupus and new insights into how these risks can be modified.

It is thought that autoimmune diseases, such as lupus, occur when a genetically susceptible individual encounters an unknown environmental agent or trigger. In this circumstance, an abnormal immune response can be initiated that leads to the signs and symptoms of lupus. Research has focused on both the genetic susceptibility and the environmental trigger. Although the environmental trigger remains unknown, microbial agents such as Epstein-Barr virus and others have been considered. Researchers are also studying other factors that may affect a person's susceptibility to lupus. For example, because lupus is more common in women than in men, some researchers are investigating the role of hormones and other male-female

differences in the development and course of the disease.

University of California San Diego scientists have identified a genetic defect in mice that triggers a disease remarkably similar to lupus in humans. They state that their finding suggests a whole new way that lupus may arise. The scientists have linked lupuslike symptoms in mice with a mutation in a gene that helps form carbohydrates that dwell on cell surfaces. The mutation may alter cell-surface carbohydrates to the point where the immune system believes they are foreign and then attacks. This is a completely new concept of how autoimmune diseases may arise. In recent years, other researchers have found that some patients with autoimmune disorders have abnormalities in the way their bodies process carbohydrates. One of the study's researchers said that if a carbohydrate gene defect is behind at least some cases of lupus, it might be possible to treat the disease with gene therapy or through more traditional drug treatment.

A current study funded by the NIH is focusing on the safety and effectiveness of oral contraceptives (birth control pills) and hormone replacement therapy in women with lupus. Doctors have worried about the wisdom of prescribing oral contraceptives or estrogen replacement therapy for women with lupus because of a widely held view that estrogens can make the disease worse. However, recent limited data suggest these drugs may be safe for some women with lupus. Researchers hope this study will yield options for safe, effective methods of birth control for young women with lupus and enable postmenopausal women with lupus to benefit from estrogen replacement therapy.

Researchers are also focusing on finding better treatments for lupus. A primary goal of this research is to develop treatments that can effectively minimize the use of corticosteroids. Scientists are trying to identify combination therapies that may be more effective than single-treatment approaches. Researchers are also interested in using male hormones, called androgens, as a possible treatment for the disease. Another goal is to improve the treatment and management of lupus in the kidneys and central nervous system. For example, a 20-year study supported by the NIAMS and the NIH found that combining cyclophosphamide with prednisone helped delay or prevent kidney failure, a serious complication of lupus.

On the basis of new information about the disease process, scientists are using novel biologic agents to block parts of the immune system selectively. Development and testing of these new drugs, which are based on compounds that occur naturally in the body, comprise an exciting and promising new area of lupus research. The hope is that these treatments will not only be effective but will also have fewer side effects. Other treatment options currently being explored include reconstructing the immune system by bone marrow transplantation. In the future, gene therapy may also play an important role in lupus treatment.

With research advances and a better understanding of lupus, the prognosis for people with lupus today is far brighter than it was even 20 years ago. It is possible to have lupus and remain active and involved with life, family, and work. As current research efforts unfold, there is continued hope for new treatments, improvements in quality of life; and, ultimately, a way to prevent or cure the disease. The research efforts of today may yield the answers of tomorrow as scientists continue to unravel the mysteries of lupus.

Chui, Daniel, Gayathri Sellakumar, Ryan S. Green, Mark Sutton-Smith, Tammie McQuistan, Kurt W. Marek, Howard R. Morris, Anne Dell, and Jamey D. Marth. "Genetic Remodeling of Protein Glycosylation In Vivo Induces Autoimmune Disease." *Proceedings of the National Academy of Sciences of the United States of America* 98 (2001): 1,142–1,147.

Novak, Debbie. *Handout on Health: Systemic Lupus Erythematosus,* Bethesda, Md.: National Institute of Arthritis and Musculoskeletal and Skin Diseases Information Clearinghouse, 1997.

Takayasu's arteritis (TA) A rare and chronic inflammatory disease that affects the aorta (the body's largest blood vessel), its large branches, and the pulmonary arteries. Although it has been reported worldwide, it shows a propensity for young women in Southeast Asia, especially Japanese women. Females with this disease outnumber males by nine to one. The age of onset is typically under 40, especially between 15 and 20 years. The estimated incidence rate in the United States is 2.6 cases per million. The incidence in the Orient, particularly Japan, is much higher. Much of the literature describing Takayasu's arteritis has originated from Asian countries, and the disease was once thought to be restricted to these regions. During the past few decades, patients with Takayasu's arteritis have been increasingly recognized in Africa, western Europe, and North America. However, experience with this disease in the Western Hemisphere remains anecdotal. It is also known as Takayasu arteritis, pulseless disease, giant cell arteritis, occlusive thromboaortopathy, aortic arch syndrome, reverse coarction, and young Oriental female arteritis.

The first case of Takayasu arteritis was described in 1908 by Dr. Mikoto Takayasu (1872–1938), a Japanese physician, who reported a "wreathlike" appearance of blood vessels in the retina of a 21-year-old Japanese woman. At the same time, two of his colleagues, Dr. Onishi and Dr. Kagoshima, reported similar manifestations in patients who also had absent wrist pulses.

Through study of the disease over the years, it is now known that the blood vessels in the eye's retina were due to narrowing of the arteries in the neck. These blood vessel malformations are rarely seen in patients outside Southeast Asia. The missing or diminished pulses that frequently occur in TA patients are due to the narrowing of blood vessels to the arms.

Causes

An increased incidence of certain HLA markers in affected subjects and the occurrence in monozygotic twins suggest disease influence by genetic factors. Multiple antigenic triggers, including mycobacteria and streptococci, have been inconclusively suggested to initiate the disease. One line of research is examining whether antibodies to the lining of blood vessels may be responsible.

Clinical Features

Initially, patients will often develop systemic illness with symptoms of malaise, fever, night sweats, weight loss, arthritis, and fatigue. Frequently, the patient will be anemic, with elevations of the ESR (erythrocyte sedimentation rate) during this initial stage. This systemic phase gradually subsides and is followed by a more chronic stage characterized by inflammation and occlusion of the affected arteries. Other patients with Takayasu's arteritis will show only the occlusive stage without first going through the systemic illness. In the late stage, weakness of the arterial walls may give rise to localized aneurysms.

The vessels of the aortic arch are particularly vulnerable, and any or all may be occluded. The inflammation of the aorta and its branch arteries can lead to poor blood supply to tissues of the body, which can cause pain (claudication) in the arms or legs during exertion or their repetitive use (as in the calves during walking). The diminished blood flow can also lead to cool extremities, dizziness upon standing up, headaches, visual problems, chest pain, and abdominal pain. Muscle mass may be lost from the face and arms.

Because patients with early Takayasu arteritis may have nonspecific symptoms and because the disease is so rare, a doctor may not suspect TA until symptoms of arterial narrowing develop. This could be months or even years into the course of the illness. In fact, a review of TA patients at one U.S. hospital showed that only 6 percent were correctly diagnosed when they were initially evaluated.

The examining medical practitioner may notice markedly diminished or absent pulses and low or unobtainable blood pressure in the involved arteries arising from the aortic arch. When using a stethoscope, the examiner may also hear an abnormal bruit sound over the partially narrowed arteries. In about 25 percent of cases, wreathlike blood vessels may be in the eyes. Takayasu arteritis is ultimately diagnosed with an angiogram of the arteries (arteriogram), which allows the doctor to see the abnormally narrowed and constricted arteries.

Complications

Where marked impairment of blood supply to the brain or spinal cord exists, there may occur strokes or paralysis. The disease is often fatal if not treated.

For patients who live long lives in spite of having Takayasu's disease, significant problems must be recognized. Having a chronic illness requires periodic evaluation and adjustment of medications whenever necessary. The medications for TA have side effects, and these must be monitored by a physician as well as by blood tests. The effects of illness on function may be significant.

Treatment

Takayasu's disease is treated by suppressing the inflammation with cortisone medication. While most patients can improve, some do not or relapse. In cortisone-resistant patients, stronger medications that suppress the immune system (immunosuppressive drugs), thereby further decreasing active inflammation of the arteries, have been used. Examples include prednisone, prednisolone, methotrexate (Rheumatrex), cyclosporine, cyclophosphamide (Cytoxan), and azathioprine (Imuran). Strict control of elevated blood pressure is important.

If significant narrowing occurs in an artery, it may require repair or widening. This may be done via traditional surgery, angioplasty, or implanting of a stent.

The duration of Takayasu arteritis varies from patient to patient. In many cases, the active illness lasts for years, causing persistent inflammation and ongoing damage to the blood vessels. If a patient does enter remission, either spontaneously or after treatment, relapses can occur, but arterial damage may be permanent. Narrowed vessels may continue to disrupt blood flow to organs, although the TA itself is no longer active.

Kerr, Gail S., Claire W. Hallahan, Joseph Giordano, Randy Y. Leavitt, Anthony S. Fauci, et al. "Takayasu Arteritis." *Annals of Internal Medicine* 120 (1994): 919–929.

T cell　Small white blood cells that orchestrate and/or directly participate in the immune defenses. Also known as T LYMPHOCYTES, they are processed in the thymus and secrete cytokines. A subpopulation of long-lived T cells contributes to immunologic memory.

T cell receptor (TCR)　Membrane-bound proteins found on T cells, which recognize and bind foreign antigens. T cell receptors differ from B cell antibodies in that they cannot bind free antigens. For a T cell receptor, the antigen must be digested, degraded, and presented on the surface of another cell (an antigen-presenting cell, or APC) such as a macrophage. In the case of helper T cells, the antigen peptides must be presented on class II major histocompatibility complexes (MHC) or specialized APCs. In the case of killer (cytotoxic) T cells, the antigen peptides must be presented on class I MHC or tissue cells.

The T cell antigen receptor consists of either an alpha/beta chain (TCR-2) or a gamma/delta chain (TCR-1) associated with the CD3 molecular complex.

T cytotoxic cell　*Cytotoxic* means destructive to cells. Cytotoxic T cells (killer T cells) kill virus-infected and transplanted cells. They may also be responsible for tissue damage in some autoimmune diseases.

temporal arteritis/GCV   A chronic inflammatory autoimmune disease characterized by a generalized vasculitis. It results in swelling of arteries in the head (most often the temporal arteries, which are located on the temples on each side of the head), neck, and arms. This swelling causes the arteries to narrow, reducing blood flow. The inflammatory process is primarily found in these arteries but can on occasion involve the larger arteries. Veins are not usually affected by the disease. Temporal arteritis/GCV can be localized in the temporal area or can have systemic involvement. It may occur alone or in conjunction with polymyalgia rheumatica. Early treatment is critical for good prognosis. Temporal arteritis/GCV may also be referred to as giant cell arteritis, granulomatosis arteritis, and cranial arteritis.

Caucasian women over the age of 50 are most at risk of developing giant cell arteritis. Women are twice as likely as men to develop the condition. The average age at onset is 70 years. Giant cell arteritis is quite common. In the United States, an estimated 200 per 100,000 people over the age of 50 develop giant cell arteritis.

Causes

The underlying cause of the inflammation is an autoimmune reaction to the lining of these arteries.

Clinical Features

Early symptoms of giant cell arteritis may resemble the flu. People are likely to experience headaches, pain in the temples, and blurred or double vision. Severe headaches, jaw pain, and vision problems are typical symptoms of giant cell arteritis. In addition, physical examination may reveal an abnormal temporal artery: tender to the touch, inflamed, and with reduced pulse. Because of the possibility of permanent blindness, a temporal artery biopsy is recommended if there is any suspicion of giant cell arteritis.

In a person with giant cell arteritis, the biopsy will show abnormal cells in the artery walls. Some patients showing symptoms of giant cell arteritis will have negative biopsy results. In such cases, the doctor may suggest a second biopsy.

Complications

It is unclear how or why polymyalgia rheumatica and giant cell arteritis are related, but an estimated 15 percent of people in the United States with polymyalgia rheumatica also develop giant cell arteritis. Patients can develop giant cell arteritis either at the same time as polymyalgia rheumatica or after the polymyalgia symptoms disappear. About half of the people affected by giant cell arteritis also have polymyalgia rheumatica. When a person is diagnosed with polymyalgia rheumatica, the doctor also looks for symptoms of giant cell arteritis because of the risk of blindness. With proper treatment, the disease is not threatening. If untreated, however, giant cell arteritis can lead to serious complications including permanent vision loss and stroke. Patients must learn to recognize the signs of giant cell arteritis because they can develop even after the symptoms of polymyalgia rheumatica disappear.

Treatment

Giant cell arteritis carries a small but definite risk of blindness. The blindness is permanent once it happens. A high dose of prednisone is needed to prevent blindness and should be started as soon as possible, perhaps even before the diagnosis is confirmed with a temporal artery biopsy. When treated, symptoms quickly disappear. Typically, people with giant cell arteritis must continue taking a high dose of prednisone for one month. Once symptoms disappear, the sed rate is normal, and there is no longer a risk of blindness, the doctor can begin to reduce the dose gradually. When treated properly, giant cell arteritis rarely recurs.

National Institute of Arthritis and Musculoskeletal and Skin Diseases. *Questions and Answers About Polymyalgia Rheumatica and Giant Cell Arteritis,* 2001.

T helper cell   A subset of T cells that typically carry the CD4 marker and are essential for turning on antibody production, activating cytotoxic T cells, and initiating many other immune responses. These T cells recognize specific antigens in conjunction with class II major histocompatability complexes. (See also T LYMPHOCYTES.)

thymus   A primary lymphoid organ or gland, located high in the chest or neck area, where T cells proliferate and mature.

tissue typing   A method of matching major tissue antigens (human leukocyte antigens, or HLAs) on the tissues of a transplant donor with those of the recipient. The closer the match, the better the chance that the transplant will take.

T lymphocytes (T cells)   Small white blood cells that orchestrate and/or directly participate in the immune defenses. They are processed in the thymus and secrete lymphokines. The T cell is one of the most important elements in the human immune system. Its role in directly destroying infected or cancerous cells is great, and it is the control center for the rest of the acquired and innate immune system. The numerous cytokines it produces and its array of surface molecules are critical for the control of all other immune elements.

tolerance   A state of nonresponsiveness to a particular antigen or group of antigens; the failure to make antibodies to an antigen.

toxins   Agents produced by plants and bacteria, normally very damaging to animal cells, that can be delivered directly to target cells by linking them to monoclonal antibodies or lymphokines.

transplant rejection   Since the first successful organ transplant was performed in the United States in 1954, one of the most serious problems facing transplant recipients has been the possibility that their own bodies will try to reject or destroy the transplant. Except for transplants between identical twins, all transplant donors and recipients are immunologically incompatible. Rejection is part of the body's natural reaction to foreign invaders. Cells are tagged with surface molecules called major histocompatibility antigens (MHA), or in human called human leukocyte antigen (HLA). Much like fingerprints, HLAs are unique to an individual. Thus, when a person receives a transplant, his or her immune system identifies the foreign tags (MHAs) on the transplant and proceeds to rid the body of, or reject, the transplant. To reduce the risk of rejection, physicians try to find donors whose HLAs are as genetically close to those of the recipient as possible. Nevertheless, most transplants, with the exception of those donated by identical twins, are recognized by the patient's immune system as foreign. This biologic incompatibility is a barrier that causes the recipient to try to destroy or reject the new organ, tissue, or cells. Rejected transplants need to be surgically removed. If the transplant is a life-sustaining organ such as a lung, liver, or heart, a patient may die before a replacement organ is found. As surgical methods to transplant grafts improve, rejection becomes the major cause of graft failure. Of those awaiting organ transplantation, more than one-fourth of patients have already had at least one graft failure.

In the past few decades, transplantation research has focused on identifying and understanding the mechanisms of transplant rejection so that it can be prevented and survival can be prolonged. Among the most important advances has been the development of drugs that help prevent transplant rejection by suppressing the patient's immune system. National Institute of Allergy and Infectious Diseases (NIAID)-supported research led to the discovery and licensing in 1983 of cyclosporine, the first immunosuppressive drug for transplant patients. Cyclosporine and other immunosuppressive drugs have greatly increased the short-term success rate, particularly of kidney and other solid organ transplants. Unfortunately, these drugs are highly toxic and require adherence to a lifelong regimen that suppresses the entire immune system, thereby increasing the susceptibility of patients for developing infections, cancer, and other complications. Moreover, immunosuppressive drugs have not had a significant effect on increasing long-term transplant survival. More than half of transplanted kidneys, the organ most often transplanted, are rejected within 10 years. The patient must then receive another kidney transplant or start dialysis treatments, which are uncomfortable, expensive, and time-consuming.

NIAID-supported basic researchers have made major contributions to advances in understanding and preventing transplant rejection. One new approach to promoting long-term survival is selectively blocking the immune response that leads to rejection of transplanted organs, tissue, or cells. Scientists recently discovered that in addition to the MHAs, other molecules, called costimulatory molecules, are involved in immune tolerance. By using knowledge gained through a series of basic discoveries involving these costimulatory molecules, scientists are working to develop strategies to induce tolerance to transplanted organs and tissues.

In 1991, NIAID-supported basic researchers identified a molecule (called CD28) on the surface of T cells that was involved in the immune response to transplanted tissues or organs. During the following four years, scientists demonstrated that blocking the activity of CD28 inhibited immune system responses crucial to transplant rejection. In 1994, researchers identified CD40 as another cell surface molecule involved in the immune system response to transplants. A strategy emerged for inducing transplant tolerance by blocking the signals that these costimulatory molecules deliver to initiate an attack on a foreign tissue or organ.

Building on the discovery of these and other costimulatory molecules, NIAID-supported scientists developed animal models to determine whether blocking the activation of CD28 and CD40 signals can prevent transplant rejection in vivo (in the living body of an animal). In 1996, researchers sponsored by NIAID succeeded in prolonging the survival of skin and heart transplants in mice using this strategy, without the need for standard continuous therapy that globally suppresses the immune system. The following year, investigators at the Department of Defense used the same approach to achieve tolerance to kidney transplants in monkeys, a model that closely resembles human transplantation. While this approach to controlling the immune system prevents rejection, it leaves intact the ability to fight infections and is much less toxic than conventional immunosuppressive therapy. Blocking immune cell signals has the potential for addressing other problems faced by transplant patients. For example, in 1998, NIAID-supported scientists found that a costimulation blockade prevented graft-versus-host disease (GVHD) in patients who received bone marrow transplants. GVHD occurs when transplanted immune cells attack the healthy cells of the recipient, causing life-threatening illness.

NIAID is supporting studies of other strategies for inducing immune tolerance. These approaches include manipulating immune system messenger molecules called cytokines and triggering the suicide of the specific immune cells that would normally attack the transplant. Additional research is needed to determine how long transplant survival can be extended by using these strategies. The next challenge is to translate the information on immune tolerance obtained from experimental models into the development of safe and effective therapies for humans. Promising results in animal models and early human studies suggest that therapies involving tolerance induction have the potential to prevent transplant rejection without the use of immunosuppressive drugs. The ability to induce immune tolerance also holds promise for treating immunologic disorders, including autoimmune diseases.

Immune Tolerance: Improving Transplantation Success, National Institute of Allergy and Infectious Diseases: Stories of Discovery. Available online. URL: http://www.nih.gov/publications/transplant.htm. Downloaded on 22 July 2002.

transverse myelitis A neurological disorder caused by inflammation across both sides of one level, or segment, of the spinal cord. The term *myelitis* refers to inflammation of the spinal cord; *transverse* simply describes the position of the inflammation, that is, across the width of the spinal cord. Attacks of inflammation can damage or destroy myelin, the fatty insulating substance that covers nerve cell fibers (thus it is also called a demyelinating disorder). This damage causes nervous system scars that interrupt communications between the nerves in the spinal cord and the rest of the body. It may occur alone or in combination with demyelination in other parts of the nervous system.

Symptoms of transverse myelitis include a loss of spinal cord function over several hours to several weeks. What usually begins as a sudden onset of lower back pain, muscle weakness, or abnormal sensations in the toes and feet can rapidly progress to more severe symptoms, including paralysis, urinary retention, and loss of bowel control. Although some patients recover from transverse myelitis with minor or no residual problems, others suffer permanent impairments that affect their ability to perform ordinary tasks of daily living. Most patients will have only one episode of transverse myelitis; a small percentage may have a recurrence.

The segment of the spinal cord at which the damage occurs determines which parts of the body are affected. Nerves in the cervical (neck) region control signals to the neck, arms, hands, and muscles of breathing (the diaphragm). Nerves in the thoracic (upper-back) region relay signals to the torso and some parts of the arms. Nerves at the lumbar (midback) level control signals to the hips and legs. Finally, sacral nerves, located within the lowest segment of the spinal cord, relay signals to the groin, toes, and some parts of the legs. Damage at one segment will affect function at that segment and the segments below it. In patients with transverse myelitis, demyelination usually occurs at the thoracic level, causing problems with leg movement and bowel and bladder control, which require signals from the lower segments of the spinal cord.

Transverse myelitis occurs in adults and children, in both genders, and in all races. No familial predisposition is apparent. A peak in incidence rates (the number of new cases per year) appears to occur between the ages of 10 and 19 years and 30 and 39 years. Although only a few studies have examined incidence rates, an estimated 1,400 new cases of transverse myelitis are diagnosed each year in the United States, and approximately 33,000 Americans have some type of disability resulting from the disorder.

Causes

Researchers are uncertain of the exact causes of transverse myelitis. The inflammation that causes such extensive damage to nerve fibers of the spinal cord may result from viral infections, abnormal immune reactions, or insufficient blood flow through the blood vessels located in the spinal cord. Transverse myelitis may also occur as a complication of syphilis, measles, Lyme disease, and some vaccinations, including those for chicken pox and rabies. Cases in which a cause cannot be identified are called idiopathic.

Transverse myelitis often develops following viral infections. Infectious agents suspected of causing transverse myelitis include varicella zoster (the virus that causes chicken pox and shingles), herpes simplex, cytomegalovirus, Epstein-Barr, influenza, echovirus, human immunodeficiency virus (HIV), hepatitis A, and rubella. Bacterial skin infections, middle-ear infections (otitis media), and *Mycoplasma pneumoniae* (bacterial pneumonia) have also been associated with the condition.

In postinfectious cases of transverse myelitis, immune system mechanisms rather than active viral or bacterial infections appear to play an important role in causing damage to spinal nerves. Although researchers have not yet identified the precise mechanisms of spinal cord injury in these cases, stimulation of the immune system in response to infection indicates that an autoimmune reaction may be responsible. In autoimmune diseases, the immune system, which normally protects the body from foreign organisms, mistakenly attacks the body's own tissue, causing inflammation and, in some cases, damage to myelin within the spinal cord.

Because some affected individuals also have autoimmune diseases such as systemic lupus erythematosus, Sjögren's syndrome, and sarcoidosis, some scientists suggest that transverse myelitis may also be an autoimmune disorder. In addition, some cancers may trigger an abnormal immune response that may lead to transverse myelitis.

An acute, rapidly progressing form of transverse myelitis sometimes signals the first attack of multiple sclerosis (MS). However, studies indicate that most people who develop transverse myelitis do not go on to develop MS. Patients with transverse myelitis should nonetheless be screened for MS because patients with this diagnosis will require different treatments.

Some cases of transverse myelitis result from spinal arteriovenous malformations (abnormalities that alter normal patterns of blood flow) or vascular diseases such as atherosclerosis that cause ischemia, a reduction in normal levels of oxygen in spinal cord tissues. Ischemia can result from bleeding (hemorrhage) within the spinal cord, blood vessel blockage or narrowing, or other less common factors. Blood vessels bring oxygen and nutrients to spinal cord tissues and remove metabolic waste products. When these vessels become narrowed or blocked, they cannot deliver sufficient amounts of oxygen-laden blood to spinal cord tissues. When a specific region of the spinal cord becomes starved of oxygen, or ischemic, nerve cells and fibers may begin to deteriorate relatively quickly. This damage may cause widespread inflammation, sometimes leading to transverse myelitis. Most people who develop the condition as a result of vascular disease are past the age of 50, have cardiac disease, or have recently undergone a chest or abdominal operation.

Clinical Features

Transverse myelitis may be either acute (developing over hours to several days) or subacute (developing over one to two weeks). Initial symptoms usually include localized lower-back pain, sudden paresthesias (abnormal sensations such as burning, tickling, pricking, or tingling) in the legs, sensory loss, and paraparesis (partial paralysis of the legs). Paraparesis often progresses to paraplegia (paralysis of the legs and lower part of the trunk). Urinary bladder and bowel dysfunction is common. Many patients also report experiencing muscle spasms, a general feeling of discomfort, headaches, fever, and loss of appetite. Depending on which segment of the spinal cord is involved, some patients may experience respiratory problems as well.

From this wide array of symptoms, four classic features of transverse myelitis emerge: weakness of the legs and arms, pain, sensory alteration, and bowel and bladder dysfunction. Most patients will experience weakness of varying degrees in their legs; some also experience it in their arms. Initially, people with transverse myelitis may notice that they are stumbling or dragging one foot or that their legs seem heavier than normal. Coordination of hand and arm movements as well as arm and hand strength may also be compromised. Progression of the disease over several weeks often leads to full paralysis of the legs, requiring the patient to use a wheelchair.

Pain is the primary presenting symptom of transverse myelitis in approximately one-third to one-half of all patients. The pain may be localized in the lower back or may consist of sharp, shooting sensations that radiate down the legs or arms or around the torso.

Patients who experience sensory disturbances often use terms such as numbness, tingling, coldness, or burning to describe their symptoms. Up to 80 percent of those with transverse myelitis report areas of heightened sensitivity to touch such that clothing or a light touch with a finger causes significant discomfort or pain (a condition called allodynia). Many also experience heightened sensitivity to changes in temperature or to extreme heat or cold.

Bladder and bowel problems may involve increased frequency of the urge to urinate or have bowel movements, incontinence, difficulty voiding, the sensation of incomplete evacuation, and constipation. Over the course of the disease, the majority of people with transverse myelitis will experience one or several of these symptoms.

Physicians diagnose transverse myelitis by taking a medical history and performing a thorough neurological examination. Because distinguishing between a patient with an idiopathic form of transverse myelitis and one who has an underlying condition is often difficult, physicians must first eliminate potentially treatable causes of the condition. If a spinal cord injury is suspected, physicians seek first to rule out lesions (damaged or abnormally functioning areas) that could cause spinal cord compression. Such potential lesions include tumors, herniated or slipped disks, stenosis (narrowing of the canal that holds the spinal cord), and abscesses. To rule out such lesions and check for inflammation of the spinal cord, patients often undergo magnetic resonance imaging (MRI), a procedure that provides a picture of the brain and spinal cord. Physicians may also perform myelography, which involves injecting a dye into the sac that surrounds the spinal cord. The patient is then tilted up and down to let the dye flow around and outline the spinal cord while X rays are taken.

Blood tests may be performed to rule out various disorders such as systemic lupus erythematosus, HIV infection, and vitamin B_{12} deficiency. In some patients with transverse myelitis, the cerebrospinal fluid that bathes the spinal cord and brain contains more protein than usual and an increased number of leukocytes (white blood cells), indicating possible infection. A spinal tap may be performed to obtain fluid to study these factors.

If none of these tests suggests a specific cause, the patient is presumed to have idiopathic transverse myelitis.

Complications

Commonly experienced permanent neurological deficits resulting from transverse myelitis include severe weakness, spasticity (painful muscle stiffness or contractions), or paralysis; incontinence; and chronic pain. Such deficits can substantially interfere with a person's ability to carry out everyday activities such as bathing, dressing, and performing household tasks.

Treatment

As with many disorders of the spinal cord, no effective cure currently exists for people with transverse myelitis. Treatments are designed to manage and alleviate symptoms, and they largely depend upon the severity of neurological involvement. Therapy generally begins when the patient first experiences symptoms. Physicians often prescribe corticosteroid therapy during the first few weeks of illness to decrease inflammation. Although no clinical trials have investigated whether corticosteroids alter the course of transverse myelitis, these drugs are often prescribed to reduce immune system activity because of the suspected autoimmune mechanisms involved in the disorder. Corticosteroid medications that might be prescribed may include methylprednisone or dexamethasone. General analgesia will likely be prescribed for any pain the patient may have. Bedrest is also often recommended during the initial days and weeks after onset of the disorder.

Following initial therapy, the most critical part of the treatment for this disorder consists of keeping the patient's body functioning while hoping for either complete or partial spontaneous recovery of the nervous system. This may sometimes require placing the patient onto a respirator. Patients with acute symptoms, such as paralysis, are most often treated in a hospital or in a rehabilitation facility where a specialized medical team can prevent or treat problems that afflict paralyzed patients. Often, even before recovery begins, caregivers may be instructed to move patients' limbs manually to help keep the muscles flexible and strong and to reduce the likelihood of pressure sores developing in immobilized areas. Later, if patients begin to recover limb control, physical therapy begins to help improve muscle strength, coordination, and range of motion.

Recovery from transverse myelitis usually begins within two to 12 weeks of the onset of symptoms and may continue for up to two years. However, if there is no improvement within the first three to six months, significant recovery is unlikely. About one-third of people affected with transverse myelitis experience good or full recovery from their symptoms. They regain the ability to walk normally and experience minimal urinary or bowel effects and paresthesias. Another one-third show only fair recovery and are left with significant deficits such as spastic gait, sensory dysfunction, and prominent urinary urgency or incontinence. The remaining one-third show no recovery at all, remaining wheelchair bound or bedridden with marked dependence on others for the basic functions of daily living. Unfortunately, making predictions about individual cases is difficult. However, research has shown that a rapid onset of symptoms generally results in poorer recovery outcomes.

The majority of people with this disorder experience only one episode, although in rare cases, recurrent or relapsing transverse myelitis does occur. Some patients recover completely then experience a relapse. Others begin to recover then suffer worsening of symptoms before recovery continues. In all cases of relapse, physicians will likely investigate possible underlying causes such as MS or systemic lupus erythematosus since most people who experience relapse have an underlying disorder.

Ganesan, V., and M. Borzyskowski. "Characteristics and Course of Urinary Tract Dysfunction After Acute Transverse Myelitis in Childhood." *Developmental Medicine and Child Neurology* 43, no. 7 (July 2001): 473–475.

Kalita, J., and U. K. Misra. "Neurophysiological Studies in Acute Transverse Myelitis." *Journal of Neurology* 247, no. 12 (December 2000): 943–948.

Kovacs, B., T. L. Lafferty, L. H. Brent, and R. J. DeHoratius. "Transverse Myelopathy in Systemic Lupus Erythematosus: An Analysis of 14 Cases and Review of the Literature." *Annals of the Rheumatic Diseases* 59, no. 2 (February 2000): 120–124.

Transverse Myelitis Fact Sheet. Prepared by the Office of Communications and Public Liaison. Bethesda, Md.: National Institute of Neurological Disorders and Stroke, National Institutes of Health. NIH Publication No. 01-4841, 2001.

tri-molecular complex The critical step in the initiation of the immune response is the presentation by the antigen-presenting cell (APC) through the major histocompatibility complex (MHC) of a peptide to the T cell receptor (TCR). This is called the tri-molecular complex. If the accessory molecules are also active (B7 and CD28), the T cell is activated and proliferates. If these accessory molecules are absent or blocked, the T cell receives a message to become inactive (termed anergic) or to commit suicide through apoptosis.

T suppressor cell According to the Health on the Net Foundation (HON), the existence of these cells is a relatively recent discovery, so their functioning is still under debate. The basic concept of suppressor T cells is a cell type that specifically suppresses the action of other cells in the immune system, notably B cells and T cells, thereby preventing the establishment of an immune response. How this is done is not known with certainty, but it seems that certain specific antigens can stimulate the activation of the suppressor T cells. This suppression is believed to be mediated by some inhibitory factor secreted by suppressor T cells. It is not any of the known lymphokines.

tumor necrosis factor (TNF) A protein (cytokine) that mediates tumor cell necrosis and destroys cancer cells. TNF is released primarily by macrophages and T lymphocytes. Although it was initially discovered because of its cancer-killing activity, it has since been found that immune system cells produce this molecule during a wide range of active infections and also employ it to help regulate the normal immune response. In this way, it is a key chemical messenger of the immune system.

ulcerative colitis A nonspecific disease of the bowel that causes chronic inflammation and sores, called ulcers, in the top layers of the lining of the large intestine. The ulcers are caused by an acute inflammation of the colon characterized by several asymmetrical, superficial ulcerated areas (lesions). The inflammation usually occurs in the rectum and lower part of the colon, but it may affect the entire colon. Ulcerative colitis rarely affects the small intestine except for the lower section, called the ileum. Ulcerative colitis may also be called colitis, ileitis, or proctitis.

The inflammation makes the colon empty frequently, causing chronic, bloody diarrhea. Ulcers form in places where the inflammation has killed colon-lining cells; the ulcers bleed and produce pus and mucus. Because of the chronic inflammation of the wall of the colon, it may become thickened and develop scar tissue. The patient may develop polyplike structures as a result of the extended chronic inflammatory response.

Ulcerative colitis is an inflammatory bowel disease (IBD), the general name for diseases that cause inflammation in the intestines. Ulcerative colitis can be difficult to diagnose because its symptoms are similar to other intestinal disorders such as irritable bowel syndrome and another type of IBD called Crohn's disease. In Crohn's disease, the inflammation extends deeper within the intestinal wall. Crohn's disease usually occurs in the small intestine, but it can also occur in the mouth, esophagus, stomach, duodenum, large intestine, appendix, and anus.

The first sign of ulcerative colitis may begin at any age. However, the highest incidence is between ages 18 and 30 years of age, with an appreciable increase in frequency during the fifth and sixth decades of life. Children sometimes develop the disease. Ulcerative colitis affects men and women equally and appears to run in some families. Although all ethnic groups may develop the disease, it is most prevalent among people of Jewish descent.

Causes

Theories about what causes ulcerative colitis abound, but none have been proven. The disorder may be related to an autoimmune response or other immunological factors, or it may be caused by an unknown environmental agent. The most popular theory is that the body's immune system reacts to a virus or a bacterium by causing ongoing inflammation in the intestinal wall.

People with ulcerative colitis have abnormalities of the immune system, but doctors do not know whether these abnormalities are a cause or a result of the disease. Ulcerative colitis is not caused by emotional distress or sensitivity to certain foods or food products, but these factors may trigger symptoms in some people. Ulcerative colitis seems to run in families. A family member of a person with inflammatory bowel disease has an increased risk of developing the disease, suggesting a genetic predisposition.

Clinical Features

The most common symptoms of ulcerative colitis are abdominal pain and bloody diarrhea. Patients may also experience fatigue, weight loss, loss of appetite, rectal bleeding, and/or loss of body fluids and nutrients.

About half of patients have mild symptoms. Others suffer frequent fever, bloody diarrhea, nausea, and severe abdominal cramps. Ulcerative colitis may also cause problems such as arthritis, inflammation of the eye, liver disease (fatty liver, hepatitis, cirrhosis, and primary sclerosing cholangitis), osteoporosis, skin rashes, anemia, and kidney stones. No one knows for sure why problems occur outside the colon. Scientists think these complications may occur when the immune system triggers inflammation in other parts of the body. These problems are usually mild and go away when the colitis is treated.

A thorough physical exam and a series of tests may be required to diagnose ulcerative colitis. Blood tests may be done to check for anemia, which could indicate bleeding in the colon or rectum. Blood tests may also uncover a high white blood cell count, which is a sign of inflammation somewhere in the body. By testing a stool sample, the doctor can tell if there is bleeding or infection in the colon or rectum.

The doctor may do a colonoscopy. For this test, the doctor inserts an endoscope—a long, flexible, lighted tube connected to a computer and TV monitor—into the anus to see the inside of the colon and rectum. The doctor will be able to see any inflammation, bleeding, or ulcers on the colon wall. During the exam, the doctor may do a biopsy, which involves taking a sample of tissue from the lining of the colon to view with a microscope. A barium enema X ray of the colon may also be required. This procedure involves filling the colon with barium, a chalky white solution. The barium shows up white on X-ray film, allowing the doctor a clear view of the colon, including any ulcers or other abnormalities that might be there.

Complications

About 5 percent of people with ulcerative colitis develop colon cancer. The risk of cancer increases with the duration and the extent of involvement of the colon. For example, if only the lower colon and rectum are involved, the risk of cancer is not higher than normal. However, if the entire colon is involved, the risk of cancer may be as great as 32 times the normal rate.

Sometimes precancerous changes occur in the cells lining the colon. These changes are called *dysplasia.* People who have dysplasia are more likely to develop cancer than those who do not.

Treatment

Treatment for ulcerative colitis depends on the seriousness of the disease. Most people are treated with medication. In severe cases, a patient may need surgery to remove the diseased colon. Surgery is the only cure for ulcerative colitis.

Some people whose symptoms are triggered by certain foods are able to control the symptoms by avoiding foods that upset their intestines, like highly seasoned foods or milk sugar (lactose). Each person may experience ulcerative colitis differently, so treatment is adjusted for each individual. Emotional and psychological support is important.

Some people have remissions—periods when the symptoms go away—that last for months or even years. However, most patients' symptoms eventually return. This changing pattern of the disease means one cannot always tell when a treatment has helped.

Someone with ulcerative colitis may need medical care for some time. Regular doctor visits are necessary to monitor the condition.

Drug therapy   Most patients with mild or moderate disease are first treated with 5-ASA agents, a combination of the drugs sulfonamide, sulfapyridine, and salicylate that helps controls inflammation. Sulfasalazine is the most commonly used of these drugs. Sulfasalazine can be used for as long as needed and can be given along with other drugs. Patients who do not do well on sulfasalazine may respond to newer 5-ASA agents. Possible side effects of 5-ASA preparations include nausea, vomiting, heartburn, diarrhea, and headaches.

People with severe disease and those who do not respond to mesalamine preparations may be treated with corticosteroids. Prednisone and hydrocortisone are two corticosteroids used to reduce inflammation. They can be given orally, intravenously, through an enema, or in a suppository, depending on the location of the inflammation. Corticosteroids can cause side effects such as weight gain, acne, facial hair, hypertension, mood swings, and increased risk of infection, so doctors carefully watch patients taking these drugs.

Other drugs may be given to relax the patient or to relieve pain, diarrhea, or infection.

Occasionally, symptoms are severe enough that the person must be hospitalized. For example, a person may have severe bleeding or severe diarrhea that causes dehydration. In such cases, the doctor will try to stop diarrhea and loss of blood, fluids, and mineral salts. The patient may need a special diet, feeding through a vein, medications, or sometimes surgery.

Surgery About 25 percent to 40 percent of ulcerative colitis patients must eventually have their colons removed because of massive bleeding, severe illness, rupture of the colon, or risk of cancer. Sometimes the doctor will recommend removing the colon if medical treatment fails or if the side effects of corticosteroids or other drugs threaten the patient's health.

One of several surgeries may be done. The most common surgery is a proctocolectomy with ileostomy, which is done in two stages. In the proctocolectomy, the surgeon removes the colon and rectum. In the ileostomy, the surgeon creates a small opening in the abdomen, called a stoma, and attaches the end of the small intestine, called the ileum, to it. This type of ileostomy is called a Brooke ileostomy. Waste will travel through the small intestine and exit the body through the stoma. The stoma is about the size of a quarter and is usually located in the lower right part of the abdomen near the belt line. A pouch is worn over the opening to collect waste, and the patient empties the pouch as needed.

An alternative to the Brooke ileostomy is the continent ileostomy. In this operation, the surgeon uses the ileum to create a pouch inside the lower abdomen. Waste empties into this pouch, and the patient drains the pouch by inserting a tube into it through a small, leakproof opening in his or her side. The patient must wear an external pouch for only the first few months after the operation. Possible complications of the continent ileostomy include malfunctioning of the leakproof opening, which requires surgical repair, and inflammation of the pouch (pouchitis), which is treated with antibiotics.

An ileoanal anastomosis, or pull-through operation, allows the patient to have normal bowel movements because it preserves part of the rectum. This procedure is becoming increasingly common for ulcerative colitis. In this operation, the surgeon removes the diseased part of the colon and the inside of the rectum, leaving the outer muscles of the rectum. The surgeon then attaches the ileum to the inside of the rectum and the anus, creating a

pouch. Waste is stored in the pouch and passed through the anus in the usual manner. Bowel movements may be more frequent and watery than usual. Pouchitis is a possible complication of this procedure.

Not every operation is appropriate for every person. Which surgery to have depends on the severity of the disease and the patient's needs, expectations, and lifestyle. Most people with ulcerative colitis will never need to have surgery. If surgery ever does become necessary, however, some people find comfort in knowing that after the surgery, the colitis is cured and most people go on to live normal, active lives.

New Treatments

Researchers are always looking for new treatments for ulcerative colitis. Several drugs are being tested to see whether they might be useful in treating the disease.

Budesonide A corticosteroid called budesonide may be nearly as effective as prednisone in treating mild ulcerative colitis, and it has fewer side effects.

Cyclosporine Cyclosporine, a drug that suppresses the immune system, may be a promising treatment for people who do not respond to 5-ASA preparations or corticosteriods.

Nicotine In an early study, symptoms improved in some patients who were given nicotine through a patch or an enema. (*Caution:* Using nicotine as a treatment is still experimental—the findings do not mean that people should go out and buy nicotine patches or start smoking.)

Heparin Researchers overseas are examining whether the anticoagulant heparin can help control colitis by preventing blood clots.

National Institute of Diabetes and Digestive and Kidney Diseases. *Ulcerative Colitis,* NIH Publication No. 95-1597, 1992, updated 2000.

uveitis An inflammation inside the eye that affects one or more of the three parts of the eye that make up the uvea. As the American Autoimmune Diseases Association explains, "The eye is shaped much like a tennis ball, hollow inside with three different layers of tissue surrounding a central cavity. The outermost layer is the sclera (white coat of the eye), and the innermost layer is the retina (image-fathering tissue in the back of the eye much like the film in a camera). The middle layer between the sclera and retina is called the uvea, from the Greek word 'uva' meaning grape. In the laboratory, it looks much like a peeled grape. When the uvea becomes inflamed, the condition is called uveitis."

The uvea (or uveal tract) consists of three parts: the iris (the color of the eye, for example blue or brown), the ciliary body and its muscle (which focuses the lens), and the choroid (the coat or lining of the eye underneath the retina that contains many blood vessels). Uveitis may involve any of these three parts of the uvea but not necessarily all of them. When uveitis affects the iris, it is called iritis or anterior uveitis; when it affects the ciliary body, it is called cyclitis or intermediate uveitis; and when it affects the choroid, it is called choroiditis or posterior uveitis.

Iritis (anterior uveitis) is the most common form of the disease, which may affect one or both eyes. It is most common in young and middle-aged people.

Causes

Uveitis has many different causes. It may result from a virus (such as shingles, mumps, or herpes), a fungus (such as histoplasmosis), or a parasite (such as toxoplasmosis). It may follow eye trauma or surgery. In most cases, uveitis is not associated with these traceable causes and is called endoge-nous uveitis. In these cases, is thought to be due to an autoimmune disease. Inflammation in one eye can result from a severe injury to the opposite eye (sympathetic uveitis).

Clinical Features

Symptoms may include any combination of redness of the eye, sensitivity to light, a burning or itching in the eye, floaters (dark, floating spots in the vision), blurred vision, pain in the eye, and reduced pupils. These symptoms may develop suddenly and sometimes without the pain.

Complications

Because the uvea borders many important parts of the eye, inflammation of this layer may be sight threatening and more serious than the more common inflammations of the outside layers of the eye. It may lead to severe and permanent loss of vision. In addition, uveitis can lead to other impairments of the eye that may involve loss of vision, such as glaucoma, cataracts, or retinal damage.

Treatment

Treatment may include corticosteroid drugs, most often given in the form of eyedrops but sometimes in the form of pills or by injection. Eyedrops are used to dilate the pupil and reduce pain. Severe cases of uveitis may require treatment with chemotherapeutic agents to suppress the immune system.

vaccination A form of immunization in which killed or weakened infectious microorganisms are placed into the body, where antibodies against them are developed. If the same types of microorganisms enter the body again, they will be destroyed by the antibodies.

vaccine A substance that contains antigenic components from an infectious organism. By stimulating an immune response (but not disease), it protects against subsequent infection by that organism by producing immunity. Vaccines are administered through needle injections, by mouth, and by aerosol.

vasculitis An inflammation of the blood vessel system, which includes the veins, arteries, and capillaries. Vasculitis may affect blood vessels of any type, size, or location and therefore can cause dysfunction in any organ system, including the central and peripheral nervous systems. The symptoms of vasculitis depend on which blood vessels are involved and what organs in the body are affected. The disorder may occur alone or with other disorders such as TEMPORAL ARTERITIS. Vasculitis can occur alone, in conjunction with an allergic reaction, or with autoimmune diseases.

Vasculitis is a common disorder in many of the autoimmune diseases. It is the result of chronic inflammation of the blood vessel walls. Chronic inflammation causes a narrowing of the inside of the vessel and can obstruct the flow of blood to the tissue (ischemia). The lack of blood may cause damage to the tissues (necrosis), possible formation of blood clots (thrombosis), and a weakening or ballooning that can possibly cause a rupture of the vessel wall (aneurysm).

Arteries and veins of all sizes and in all parts of the body may be affected. Vasculitis may be localized or systemic, affecting many different parts of the body including major organs like the lungs, kidneys, heart, and brain. It may occur as an autoimmune disease itself or as a complication of many other autoimmune diseases.

Causes
Some forms of vasculitis may be caused by allergy or hypersensitivity to medications such as sulfa or penicillin, other drugs, toxins, and other inhaled environmental irritants. Other forms may be due to infection, parasites, or viral infections. These causes need to be ruled out before considering an underlying autoimmune disorder.

Treatment
Treatment for vasculitis depends on the severity of the disorder and the individual's general health. Treatment may include cortisone or cytotoxic drugs. Other treatments may include plasmapheresis (the removal and reinfusion of blood plasma), intravenous gammaglobulin, and cyclosporine. Some cases of vasculitis may not require treatment.

The prognosis for individuals with vasculitis varies depending on the severity of the disorder. Mild cases of vasculitis are generally not life-threatening. Severe cases (involving major organ systems), though, may be permanently disabling or fatal.

vesiculobullous dermatoses Skin diseases characterized by local or general distributions of blisters. They are classified according to the site and mode of blister formation. Lesions can appear spontaneously or be precipitated by infection, trauma, or sunlight. Etiologies include immunological and genetic factors.

veterans Since the Persian Gulf War ended in 1991, veterans have reported diverse, unexplained symptoms. Some have wondered if their development of systemic lupus erythematosus or fibromyalgia might be related to Gulf War service. In a Department of Defense (DOD) study, researchers determined that Gulf War veterans were not at increased risk of postwar hospitalization due to systemic lupus erythematosus. Gulf War veterans were slightly at risk of postwar hospitalization for fibromyalgia; however, this risk difference "was probably due to the Gulf War veteran clinical evaluation program beginning in 1994. These data do not support Gulf War service and disease associations."

In 1994, an immunologist from the private sector notified the Defense Science Board that some symptoms being reported by Gulf War–era veterans were very similar to those of her patients with autoimmune diseases. These patients had a range of symptoms affecting more than one of the body systems, and the immunologist believed they were associated with exposure to vaccine adjuvant formulations. In October 1995, the DOD, before a meeting of the Presidential Advisory Commission on Gulf War illnesses, dismissed this hypothesis on the grounds that it had administered only vaccines with aluminum salts (alum) as adjuvants. Alum has been used safely in millions of subjects for more than half a century.

A later Tulane Medical School study of 144 Gulf War–era veterans or military employees, which measured serum antibodies to squalene, found that the substantial majority (95 percent) of overtly ill deployed Gulf War Syndrome (GWS) patients had antibodies to squalene. These results, however, have not been confirmed by other investigators.

Moss wrote:

> Gulf War–related illnesses are mostly common ailments, but with incidence rates that exceed those expected in the population of Gulf War veterans. These illnesses may be the result of combinations of chemical and physiological stressors which may

have caused acute cellular effects sufficient to initiate processes of autoimmunity to various organs, tissues or types of cells. Two main suspects in the Gulf War cluster of illnesses are the "Nerve Gas Pill" (pyridostigmine bromide, PB, NAPS) and stress. One component of stress, beta-adrenergic load, potentiates the toxicity of PB. While similar types of chemical and physiological stressors are present in the general population, the Gulf War veteran population received these stressors in a short time, with greater intensity, and at a higher percentage exposure than normal for the general population.

Asa, P. B., Y. Cao, and R. F. Garry. "Antibodies to Squalene in Gulf War Syndrome." *Experimental and Molecular Pathology* 68, no. 1 (February 2000): 55–64.

Moss, J. I. "Many Gulf War Illnesses May Be Autoimmune Disorders Caused by the Chemical and Biological Stressors Pyridostigmine, Bromide, and Adrenaline." *Medical Hypotheses* 56, no. 2 (February 2001); 155–157.

Smith, T. C., G. C. Gray, and J. D. Knoke. "Is Systemic Lupus Erythematosus, Amyotrophic Lateral Sclerosis, or Fibromyalgia Associated with Persian Gulf War Service? An Examination of Department of Defense Hospitalization Data." *American Journal of Epidemiology* 151, no. 11 (June 2000): 1,053–1059.

Vikings Because MULTIPLE SCLEROSIS is most frequently found in Scandinavia, Iceland, the British Isles, and the countries settled by their inhabitants and their descendants, scientific historians have postulated that the Vikings may have been instrumental in disseminating genetic susceptibility to the disease in those areas, as well as in other parts of the world where they raided and engaged in trade.

Poser, C. M. "Viking Voyages: The Origin of Multiple Sclerosis? An Essay in Medical History." *Acta Neurologica Scandinavica* Supp. 161 (1995): 11–22.

virus Submicroscopic microbe that multiplies within living cells and causes disease such as chicken pox, measles, mumps, rubella, pertussis, and hepatitis. Viruses are not affected by antibiotics, the drugs used to kill bacteria.

vitiligo An autoimmune skin disease in which melanocytes (the cells that make pigment) in the skin, the mucous membranes (tissues that line the inside of the mouth, nose, and genital and rectal areas), and the retina (inner layer of the eyeball) are destroyed. As a result, white patches of skin appear on different parts of the body. The hair that grows in areas affected by vitiligo usually turns white.

Vitiligo is 10 to 15 times more common in patients with other autoimmune diseases, such as Addison's disease, diabetes mellitus, pernicious anemia, discoid lupus, and abnormal thyroid function. This disorder has only recently been identified as an autoimmune disease because organ-specific antibodies have now been detected in patients with vitiligo. Vitiligo has a tendency to run in families and may follow unusual trauma, especially to the head. Some people have reported that a single event such as sunburn or emotional distress triggered vitiligo; however, these events have not been scientifically proven to cause vitiligo. The disease may also be referred to as leukoderma.

About 1 percent to 2 percent of the world's population, or 40 to 50 million people, have vitiligo. In the United States, 2 to 5 million people have the disorder. Ninety-five percent of people who have vitiligo develop it before their 40th birthday. The disorder affects all races and both sexes equally.

Complications

The change in appearance caused by vitiligo can affect a person's emotional and psychological well-being and may create difficulty in getting or keeping a job. People with this disorder can experience emotional stress, particularly if vitiligo develops on visible areas of the body, such as the face, hands, arms, feet, or genitals. Adolescents, who are often particularly concerned about their appearance, can be devastated by widespread vitiligo. Some people who have vitiligo feel embarrassed, ashamed, depressed, or worried about how others will react.

Clinical Features

People who develop vitiligo usually first notice white patches (depigmentation) on their skin. These patches are more common in Sun-exposed areas, including the hands, feet, arms, face, and lips. Other common areas for white patches to appear are the armpits, groin, and around the mouth, eyes, nostrils, navel, and genitals.

Vitiligo generally appears in one of three patterns. In one pattern (focal pattern), the depigmentation is limited to one or only a few areas. In another pattern, some people develop depigmented patches on only one side of their bodies (segmental pattern). For most people who have vitiligo, though, depigmentation occurs on different parts of the body (generalized pattern). In addition to white patches on the skin, people with vitiligo may have premature graying of the scalp hair, eyelashes, eyebrows, and beard. People with dark skin may notice a loss of color inside their mouths.

There is no way to predict if vitiligo will spread. For some people, the depigmented patches do not spread. The disorder is usually progressive, however, and over time the white patches will spread to other areas of the body. For some people, vitiligo spreads slowly, over many years. For other people, spreading occurs rapidly. Some people have reported additional depigmentation following periods of physical or emotional stress.

Treatments

The goal of treating vitiligo is to restore the function of the skin and to improve the patient's appearance. Therapy for vitiligo takes a long time—it usually must be continued for six to 18 months. The choice of therapy depends on the number of white patches and how widespread they are and on the patient's preference for treatment. Each patient responds differently to therapy, and a particular treatment may not work for everyone. Current treatment options for vitiligo include medical, surgical, and adjunctive therapies (therapies that can be used along with surgical or medical treatments). All surgical therapies, though, are viewed as experimental because their effectiveness and side effects remain to be fully defined. The following describes available therapies.

Topical steroid therapy   Steroids may be helpful in repigmenting the skin (returning the color to white patches), particularly if started early in the disease. Corticosteroids are a group of drugs similar to the hormones produced by the adrenal glands (such as cortisone). Doctors often prescribe a mild topical corticosteroid cream for children under 10 years old and a stronger one for adults. Patients must apply the cream to the white patches on their skin for at least three months before seeing any results. It is the simplest and safest treatment but not as effective as psoralen photochemotherapy. The doctor will closely monitor the patient for side effects such as skin shrinkage and skin striae (streaks or lines on the skin).

Psoralen photochemotherapy Psoralen photochemotherapy (psoralen and ultraviolet A therapy, or PUVA) is probably the most beneficial treatment for vitiligo available in the United States. The goal of PUVA therapy is to repigment the white patches. However, it is time consuming, and care must be taken to avoid side effects, which can sometimes be severe. Psoralens are drugs that contain chemicals that react with ultraviolet light to cause darkening of the skin. The treatment involves taking psoralen by mouth (orally) or applying it to the skin (topically). This is followed by carefully timed exposure to ultraviolet A (UVA) light from a special lamp or to sunlight. Patients usually receive treatments in their doctors' offices so they can be carefully watched for any side effects. Patients must minimize exposure to sunlight at other times.

Topical psoralen photochemotherapy Topical psoralen photochemotherapy is often used for people with a small number of depigmented patches (affecting less than 20 percent of the body). It is also used for children two years old and older who have localized patches of vitiligo. Treatments are done in a doctor's office under artificial UVA light once or twice a week. The doctor or nurse applies a thin coat of psoralen to the patient's depigmented patches about 30 minutes before UVA light exposure. The patient is then exposed to an amount of UVA light that turns the affected area pink. The doctor usually increases the dose of UVA light slowly over many weeks. Eventually, the pink areas fade and a more normal skin color appears. After each treatment, the patient washes his or her skin with soap and water and applies a sunscreen before leaving the doctor's office.

There are two major potential side effects of topical PUVA therapy: severe sunburn and blistering, and too much repigmentation or darkening of the treated patches or the normal skin surrounding the vitiligo (hyperpigmentation). Patients can minimize their chances of sunburn if they avoid exposure to direct sunlight after each treatment. Hyperpigmentation is usually a temporary problem and eventually disappears when treatment is stopped.

Oral psoralen photochemotherapy Oral PUVA therapy is used for people with more extensive vitiligo (affecting greater than 20 percent of the body) or for people who do not respond to topical PUVA therapy. Oral psoralen is not recommended for children under 10 years of age because of an increased risk of damage to the eyes, such as cataracts. For oral PUVA therapy, the patient takes a prescribed dose of psoralen by mouth about two hours before exposure to artificial UVA light or sunlight. The doctor adjusts the dose of light until the skin areas being treated become pink. Treatments are usually given two or three times a week, but never two days in a row.

For patients who cannot go to a PUVA facility, the doctor may prescribe psoralen to be used with natural sunlight exposure. The doctor will give the patient careful instructions on carrying out treatment at home and monitor the patient during scheduled checkups.

Known side effects of oral psoralen include sunburn, nausea and vomiting, itching, abnormal hair growth, and hyperpigmentation. Oral psoralen photochemotherapy may increase the risk of skin cancer. To avoid sunburn and reduce the risk of skin cancer, patients undergoing oral PUVA therapy should apply sunscreen and avoid direct sunlight for 24 to 48 hours after each treatment. Patients should also wear protective UVA sunglasses for 18 to 24 hours after each treatment to avoid eye damage, particularly cataracts.

Depigmentation Depigmentation involves fading the rest of the skin on the body to match the already white areas. For people who have vitiligo on more than 50 percent of their bodies, depigmentation may be the best treatment option. Patients apply the drug monobenzylether of hydroquinone (monobenzone or Benoquin) twice a day to pigmented areas until they match the already depigmented areas. Patients must avoid direct skin-to-skin contact with other people for at least two hours after applying the drug.

The major side effect of depigmentation therapy is inflammation (redness and swelling) of the skin.

Patients may experience itching, dry skin, or abnormal darkening of the membrane that covers the white of the eye. Depigmentation is permanent and cannot be reversed. In addition, a person who undergoes depigmentation will always be abnormally sensitive to sunlight.

Autologous skin grafts In an autologous (use of a person's own tissues) skin graft, the doctor removes skin from one area of a patient's body and attaches it to another area. This type of skin grafting is sometimes used for patients with small patches of vitiligo. The doctor removes sections of the normal, pigmented skin (donor sites) and places them onto the depigmented areas (recipient sites). Autologous skin grafting has several possible complications. Infections may occur at the donor or recipient sites. The recipient and donor sites may develop scarring, a cobblestone appearance, or a spotty pigmentation, or they may fail to repigment at all. Treatment with grafting takes time and is costly, and most people find it neither acceptable nor affordable.

Skin grafts using blisters In this procedure, the doctor creates blisters on the patient's pigmented skin by using heat, suction, or freezing cold. The tops of the blisters are then cut out and transplanted to a depigmented skin area. The risks of blister grafting include the development of a cobblestone appearance, scarring, and lack of repigmentation. However, there is less risk of scarring with this procedure than with other types of grafting.

Micropigmentation (tattooing) Tattooing implants pigment into the skin with a special surgical instrument. This procedure works best for the lip area, particularly in people with dark skin; however, it is difficult for the doctor to match perfectly the color of the skin of the surrounding area. Tattooing tends to fade over time. In addition, tattooing of the lips may lead to episodes of blister outbreaks caused by the herpes simplex virus.

Autologous melanocyte transplants In this procedure, the doctor takes a sample of the patient's normal pigmented skin and places it into a laboratory dish containing a special cell culture solution to grow melanocytes. When the melanocytes in the culture solution have multiplied, the doctor transplants them to the patient's depigmented skin patches. This procedure is currently experimental and is impractical for the routine care of people with vitiligo.

Sunscreens People who have vitiligo, particularly those with fair skin, should use a sunscreen that provides protection from both the UVA and UVB forms of ultraviolet light. Sunscreen helps protect the skin from sunburn and long-term damage. Sunscreen also minimizes tanning, which makes the contrast between normal and depigmented skin less noticeable.

Cosmetics Some patients with vitiligo cover depigmented patches with stains, makeup, or self-tanning lotions. These cosmetic products can be particularly effective for people whose vitiligo is limited to exposed areas of the body. Dermablend, Lydia O'Leary, Clinique, Fashion Flair, Vitadye, and Chromelin offer makeup or dyes that patients may find helpful for covering up depigmented patches.

Counseling and support groups Many people with vitiligo find it helpful to get counseling from a mental health professional. People often find they can talk to their counselor about issues that are difficult to discuss with anyone else. A mental health counselor can also offer patients support and help in coping with vitiligo. In addition, attending a vitiligo support group may be helpful.

National Institute of Arthritis and Musculoskeletal and Skin Diseases. *Questions and Answers About Vitiligo,* NIH Publication No. 01-4909, 2001.

waning immunity   The loss of protective antibodies over time.

Wegener's granulomatosis   An uncommon disease characterized by inflammation of the blood vessels (VASCULITIS). This inflammation results in a reduction of oxygen in the blood and damages vital organs of the body by restricting blood flow to those organs and destroying normal tissue. Although vasculitis can damage any organ system, Wegener's granulomatosis primarily affects the respiratory tract (sinuses, nose, trachea [windpipe], and lungs) and the kidneys.

This disorder strikes men and women equally. Although it is more common in persons in their middle age, it can affect persons of any age. It is rare in African Americans and more common in Caucasians.

Causes
The vasculitis is the result of an autoimmune reaction in the wall of small and medium-sized blood vessels. In Wegener's granulomatosis, an autoantibody is directed toward components in the cytoplasm of certain white cells.

Complications
Chronic vasculitis causes a narrowing of the inside of the blood vessels and can result in obstruction of the flow of blood to the tissues. This situation may cause damage to the tissues (necrosis).

Clinical Features
The initial manifestations generally involve the upper and lower respiratory tract, with a chronic, progressive inflammation. The inflammation may form lumps or granulomas in the tissues or in the skin. It may progress into generalized inflammation of the blood vessels (vasculitis) and kidneys (glomerulonephritis). A limited form of the disease that does not involve the kidneys may occur.

The initial symptoms of Wegener's granulomatosis are often vague or nonspecific. They frequently include upper respiratory tract symptoms, joint pains, weakness, and fatigue.

Upper respiratory tract   The most common sign of Wegener's granulomatosis is involvement of the upper respiratory tract, which occurs in nearly all patients. Symptoms include sinus pain, discolored or bloody nasal drainage, and, occasionally, nasal ulcerations. A common manifestation of the disease is persistent rhinorrhea (runny nose) or other cold symptoms that do not respond to standard treatment or that become progressively worse. Rhinorrhea can result from nasal inflammation or sinus drainage and can cause pain. A hole or perforation of the nasal septum may develop, and collapse of the nasal bridge (called saddle nose deformity) may occur in some individuals. Blockage of the eustachian tubes, which are important for normal ear function, may cause chronic ear problems and hearing loss. A secondary bacterial infection can cause Wegener's-related sinusitis (inflammation of the sinuses) with congestion and chronic sinus pain.

Lungs   The lungs are affected in most patients with Wegener's granulomatosis, although no symptoms may be present. If symptoms are present, they include cough, hemoptysis (coughing up of blood), shortness of breath, and chest discomfort.

Kidneys   Kidney involvement, which occurs in more than three-fourths of patients, usually does not cause symptoms. If detected by blood tests, proper treatment can be started, preventing long-term damage to the kidneys.

Musculoskeletal system Pain in the muscles and joints or, occasionally, joint swelling affects two-thirds of patients with Wegener's granulomatosis. Although joint pain can be very uncomfortable, it does not lead to permanent joint damage or deformities.

Eyes Wegener's granulomatosis can affect the eyes in several ways. Patients may develop conjunctivitis (inflammation of the conjunctiva, the inner lining of the eyelid), scleritis (inflammation of the scleral layer, the white part of the eyeball), episcleritis (inflammation of the episcleral layer, the outer surface of the sclera), or an orbital mass lesion (a sore behind the eye globe). The symptoms of eye involvement include redness, burning, or pain in the eye. Double vision or a decrease in vision are serious symptoms requiring immediate medical attention.

Skin lesions Nearly half of all people with Wegener's granulomatosis develop skin lesions. These small red or purple raised areas or blisterlike lesions, ulcers, or nodules may or may not be painful.

Other symptoms Some patients experience narrowing of the trachea (subglottic stenosis). The symptoms can include voice changes, hoarseness, shortness of breath, or coughing.

The nervous system and heart may occasionally be affected. Fever and night sweats may also occur. However, fever may also signal an underlying infection, often of the upper respiratory tract.

To treat people with Wegener's granulomatosis most effectively, doctors must diagnose the disease early in its course. There are no blood tests that a doctor can use to diagnose Wegener's granulomatosis, but blood tests are important to rule out other causes of illness and to determine which organ sites may be affected. Most blood tests are nonspecific and can only suggest that a person has an inflammatory process. Anemia (low red blood cell count), elevated white blood cell count and platelet count, and an elevated sedimentation rate are commonly found in people with Wegener's granulomatosis. If the kidneys are involved, red blood cells and structures called red blood cell casts are visible in the urine when viewed under a microscope. The blood tests measuring kidney function (creatinine and BUN) may also show abnormalities.

X-ray results can be very helpful in diagnosing Wegener's granulomatosis. People with lung involvement will have abnormal chest X rays, which may show one or many fluffy infiltrates, solid nodules, or cavities. Sinus X rays or computed tomography (CT) scans in people with sinus involvement may show thickening of the sinus lining.

Many patients with active Wegener's granulomatosis have a blood test that reveals the presence of a specific type of antibody called antineutrophil cytoplasmic antibodies (ANCA) (an antibody is a disease-fighting protein). Although a positive ANCA test is useful in supporting a suspected diagnosis of Wegener's granulomatosis, in most instances it is not used by itself to make a diagnosis of this disorder. The ANCA test may be negative in some patients with active Wegener's granulomatosis.

Currently, the only definite way to diagnose Wegener's granulomatosis is by performing a biopsy of an involved organ site (usually the sinuses, lung, or kidney). The tissue is examined under the microscope to confirm the presence of vasculitis and granulomas (a specific type of inflammation), which together are diagnostic features of the disease. A biopsy is very important both to confirm the presence of Wegener's granulomatosis and also to assure the absence of other disorders that may have similar signs and symptoms.

Treatments

With the appropriate treatment, the outlook is good for patients with Wegener's granulomatosis. In a study of 158 patients who were treated at the National Institutes of Health (NIH), 91 percent of them markedly improved. After six months to 24 years of follow-up, 80 percent of the patients survived.

In most cases, standard therapy consists of a combination of a glucocorticoid drug that reduces inflammation and a cytotoxic drug that interferes with the abnormal growth of cells.

Prednisone is the most common glucocorticoid drug (a steroid) used. Prednisone is similar to hydrocortisone, the natural glucocorticoid hormone produced by the body. It is chemically different from the anabolic steroids that have been used by athletes and is given in doses much higher than the body normally produces. Prednisone is usually administered as a single morning dose in an attempt to imitate how the body normally secretes hydrocortisone. When the person's illness improves, the prednisone dose is gradually decreased and converted to an every other day dosing schedule, usually over a period of three to four months. With further improvement in the disease, the prednisone is very gradually decreased and discontinued completely after approximately six to 12 months. When prednisone is taken by mouth, the body stops making its own natural hydrocortisone. As the prednisone dose is gradually reduced, the body will resume making hydrocortisone again. Prednisone must never be stopped suddenly because the body requires prednisone (or hydrocortisone) for to function and may not be able to make what it needs immediately.

Cyclophosphamide (Cytoxan) is the most commonly used cytotoxic drug. Cyclophosphamide is taken once a day by mouth. The patient must take the drug all at once in the morning followed by drinking a large amount of fluids. Although the initial dose of cyclophosphamide is based on the patient's weight and kidney function, the doctor may adjust the dosage based on the blood counts, which are monitored closely to be sure that the white blood cell count is maintained at a safe level. Cyclophosphamide is continued for a full year beyond that point at which the disease is in remission. The dose of cyclophosphamide is then decreased gradually and eventually discontinued.

Cyclophosphamide and prednisone are both powerful drugs that suppress the immune system. Although these medications are beneficial in treating Wegener's granulomatosis, they have potentially serious side effects. Because these drugs suppress the immune system, they can affect the body's ability to fight off infection. Prednisone can cause weight gain, cataracts, brittle bones, diabetes, and alterations in mood and personality. Cyclo-

phosphamide can cause bone marrow suppression (lowering of blood counts), sterility, hemorrhagic cystitis (bleeding from the bladder), as well as other serious side effects.

Approximately half of all people with Wegener's granulomatosis may experience a return (relapse) of their disease. This occurs most frequently within two years of stopping medication but can potentially occur at any point both during treatment or after stopping treatment. Thus, it is extremely important that patients continue to see their physicians regularly, both while they are on these medications as well as after the medications have been stopped. Even while on medication, many patients are able to lead relatively normal lives and will remain in remission after therapy has been stopped completely.

National Institute of Allergy and Infectious Diseases, National Institutes of Health *Fact Sheet: Wegener's Granulomatosis,* 1997.

weight   Autoimmunity can affect weight in both directions. If the thyroid gland is the autoimmune target, you may gain weight. Yet Crohn's disease causes excessive weight loss, and Graves' disease causes unexplained weight loss.

white blood cells   See LEUKOCYTES.

women and autoimmune diseases   Women are especially hard hit by autoimmune diseases. Of the estimated 50 million Americans—one in five —who suffer from an autoimmune disease, three-quarters are women, many in their childbearing years. Scientists are investigating whether the female hormone estrogen may make a woman more susceptible to developing an autoimmune disease. Researchers at the New England Medical Center in Boston have found evidence suggesting that fetal cells that remain in a woman's blood many years after a pregnancy may trigger an autoimmune disease. They speculate the woman's immune system may recognize the fetal cells as foreign and mount an attack that leads to SCLERO-DERMA or another similar disease. (See the accompanying table.)

FEMALE TO MALE RATIOS IN AUTOIMMUNE DISEASES

Disease	Ratio	Disease	Ratio
Hashimoto's disease/hypothyroiditis	9:1	Graves' disease/hyperthyroidism	7:1
Systemic lupus erythematosus	9:1	Rheumatoid arthritis	4:1
Sjögren's syndrome	9:1	Scleroderma	3:1
Antiphospholipid syndrome	9:1	Myasthenia gravis	2:1
Primary biliary cirrhosis	9:1	Multiple sclerosis	2:1
Mixed connective tissue disease	8:1	Chronic idiopathic thrombocytopenic purpura	2:1
Chronic active hepatitis	8:1	Type 1 diabetes	1:1

(Source: American Autoimmune Related Diseases Association)

xenograft A surgical graft of tissue from an individual of one species to an individual of a different species.

xerostomia The medical term for dry mouth, which may indicate a malfunction of the salivary glands. Dry mouth is a fairly common condition that can result from certain medications (such as those used to treat allergies and depression), radiation treatments, and diseases such as Sjögren's syndrome and diabetes. Dry mouth is more than an inconvenience. Because of the important role that saliva plays in protecting the teeth and oral surfaces and in aiding digestion, dry mouth is an important condition to diagnose and treat. Chewing sugar-free gum, sipping water, and using saliva substitutes helps. A new oral medication called pilocarpine (Salagen) may provide long-lasting relief from some forms of xerostomia.

APPENDIXES

APPENDIX I
LIST OF AUTOIMMUNE DISEASES

Addison's disease (also called primary adrenal insufficiency, hypocortisolism, adrenal insuffiency, adrenocortical hypofunction, chronic adrenocortical insufficiency)

allergic asthma (also called bronchial asthma)

allergic rhinitis (also known as hay fever, nasal allergies, and pollinosis)

alopecia areata (also called alopecia totalis or alopecia universalis)

ankylosing spondylitis (AS) (also known as rheumatoid spondylitis, spondylitis, spondylarthropathy)

antiglomerular basement membrane (anti-GBM) disease

antiphospholipid syndrome (APS) (also referred to as antiphospholipid antibody syndrome, Hughes syndrome, and sticky blood)

autoimmune hemolytic anemia (AIHA) (also called idiopathic autoimmune hemolytic anemia, immunohemolytic anemia, and Coombs positive hemolytic anemia)

autoimmune inner ear disease (AIED)

autoimmune lymphoproliferative syndrome (ALPS) (also called Canale-Smith syndrome)

Behçet's disease

bullous pemphigoid (BP)

cardiomyopathy

celiac disease (also called nontropical sprue, celiac sprue, and gluten-sensitive enteropathy)

Chagas' disease (also called American trypanosomiasis)

chronic fatigue syndrome (CFS) (also known as myalgic encephalomyelitis [ME], postviral fatigue syndrome, and chronic fatigue and immune dysfunction syndrome [CFID])

chronic inflammatory demyelinating polyneuropathy (CIDP)

Churg-Strauss syndrome (also known as allergic granulomatosis)

cicatricial pemphigoid (CP) (also known as mucous membrane pemphigoid [MMP] or benign pemphigoid)

Cogan's syndrome

cold agglutinin disease (also called cold agglutinins, Weil-Felix reaction, Widal's test)

congenital heart block (also called atrioventricular [AV] block)

coxsackie myocarditis

CREST syndrome

Crohn's disease (also called ileitis, enteritis, regional enteritis, inflammatory bowel disease, granulomatous ileocolitis)

demyelinating neuropathies

dermatitis herpetiformis (DH)

discoid lupus

Dressler's syndrome (also called post-MI pericarditis, postcardiac injury syndrome, postcardiotomy pericarditis)

endometriosis

essential mixed cryoglobulinemia

Evans' syndrome (ES)

experimental allergic encephalomyelitis (EAE) (also called experimental autoimmune encephalomyelitic)

fibromyalgia (FMS)

Goodpasture's syndrome (GP) (also called antiglomerular basement membrane antibody disease, glomerulonephritis-pulmonary hemorrhage, lung purpura-glomerulonephritis, pulmonary-renal syndrome, rapidly progressive glomerulonephritis with pulmonary hemorrhage)

Graves' disease

Guillain-Barré syndrome (GBS) (also known as acute autoimmune neuropathy, acute inflammatory demyelinating polyradiculoneuropathy [AIDP], acute inflammatory polyneuropathy, Landry-Guillain-Barré syndrome, polyradiculoneuropathy, acute inflammatory)

Hashimoto's thyroiditis (also referred to as autoimmune thyroiditis, chronic lymphocytic thyroiditis, struma lymphomatosa, lymphadenoid goiter)

hepatitis, autoimmune (AIH) (also known as autoimmune chronic active hepatitis [CAH], idiopathic chronic active hepatitis, lupoid hepatitis)

herpes gestationis (HG) (also known as pemphigoid gestationis [PG])

idiopathic pulmonary fibrosis (IPF) (also known as idiopathic diffuse interstitial pulmonary fibrosis, pulmonary fibrosis, cryptogenic fibrosing alveolitis [CFA], fibrosing alveolitis, usual interstitial pneumonia [UIP])

idiopathic thrombocytopenic purpura (ITP) (also called immune thrombocytopenic purpura)

IgA nephropathy (IgAN) (also called nephropathy-IgA, Berger's disease)

inclusion body myositis (IBM) (also called inflammatory myopathy)

insulin-dependent diabetes mellitus (IDDM) (also known as Type 1 diabetes and juvenile onset diabetes)

interstitial cystitis (IC)

juvenile arthritis (JA) (also known as juvenile chronic arthritis [JCA], juvenile rheumatoid arthritis [JRA], juvenile chronic polyarthritis, Still's disease)

Lambert-Eaton syndrome (LEMS) (also known as myasthenic syndrome, Lambert-Eaton myasthenic syndrome)

lichen planus (LP)

leukoencephalitis, acute necrotizing hemorrhagic (also known as Weston Hurst disease, Western Hurst syndrome)

Ménière's disease (also referred to as endolymphatic hydrops)

mixed connective tissue disease (MCTD) (also referred to as undifferentiated connective tissue disease)

Mooren's ulcer

multiple sclerosis (MS)

myasthenia gravis (MG)

myocarditis, autoimmune

myositis

neutropenia

ocular cicatricial pemphigoid (OCP)

pemphigus vulgaris (PV)

peripheral neuropathy (PN) (also known as neuropathy,

sensory peripheral neuropathy, peripheral neuritis)

perivenous encephalomyelitis (also known as acute disseminated encephalomyelitis [ADEM], postinfectious or postvaccinal encephalomyelitis)

pernicious anemia (PA) (also known as Addison's anemia, Biermer's anemia, macrocytic achylic anemia, congenital pernicious anemia, juvenile pernicious anemia, vitamin B_{12} deficiency [malabsorption])

polyarteritis nodosa (PAN) (also referred to as periarteritis, polyarteritis, periarteritis nodosa)

polychondritis (also referred to as chronic atrophic polychondritis, relapsing polychondritis, systemic chondromalacia von Meyenburg disease)

polyglandular autoimmune syndromes (PGAS) (also called autoimmune endocrine failure syndrome, polyglandular deficiency syndrome, autoimmune polyendocrine syndrome [APS], immunoendocrinopathy syndrome)

autoimmune polyglandular syndrome type I (APS1) (also known as autoimmune polyendocrinopathy-candidiasis-ectodermal dystrophy [APECED])

autoimmune polyglandular syndrome type II (also known as Schmidt's syndrome)

polymyalgia rheumatica (PMR)

polymyositis

postmyocardial infarction syndrome (also known as Dressler's syndrome, postinfarction syndrome)

postpericardiotomy syndrome (PPS)

primary agammaglobulinemia

primary biliary cirrhosis (PBC)

psoriasis

psoriatic arthritis (PA)

Raynaud's phenomenon (RP) (also called Raynaud's disease, idiopathic Raynaud's phenomenon, primary Raynaud's syndrome, white finger, wax finger, dead finger)

Reiter's syndrome (also referred to as reactive arthritis)

rheumatic fever (RF) (also referred to as acute rheumatic fever)

rheumatoid arthritis (RA)

sarcoidosis

scleritis

scleroderma (SCL)

Sjögren's syndrome

sperm autoimmunity

stiff-man syndrome (also referred to as Moersch-Woltmann syndrome, stiff-person syndrome [SPS])

subacute bacterial endocarditis (SBE)

sympathetic ophthalmia (also called sympathetic uveitis)

systemic lupus erythematosus (SLE) (also referred to as disseminated lupus erythematosus, lupus, lupus erythematosus)

Takayasu's arteritis (TA) (also known as Takayasu arteritis, pulseless disease, giant cell arteritis, occlusive thrombo-aortopathy, aortic arch syndrome, reverse coarction, young Oriental female arteritis)

temporal arteritis (GCV) (also referred to as giant cell arteritis, granulomatosis arteritis, cranial arteritis)

transverse myelitis

ulcerative colitis (also called colitis, ileitis, proctitis)

uveitis (also referred to as iritis, pars planitis, chroiditis, chorioretinitis, anterior uveitis, posterior uveitis)

vasculitis

vesiculobullous dermatoses

vitiligo (also referred to as leukoderma)

Wegener's granulomatosis (also called midline granulomatosis)

APPENDIX II
MAJOR AUTOIMMUNE DISEASES LISTED BY MAIN TARGET ORGANS

NERVOUS SYSTEM

Multiple sclerosis
Myasthenia gravis
Autoimmune neuropathies such as Guillain-Barré
Autoimmune ureitis

BLOOD

Autoimmune hemolytic anemia
Pernicious anemia
Autoimmune thrombocytopenia

BLOOD VESSELS

Temporal arteritis
Antiphospholipid syndrome
Vasculitides such as Wegener's granulomatosis
Behçet's disease

SKIN

Psoriasis
Dermatitis herpetiformis
Pemphigus vulgaris
Vitiligo

GASTROINTESTINAL SYSTEM

Crohn's disease
Ulcerative colitis

Primary biliary cirrhosis
Autoimmune hepatitis

ENDOCRINE GLANDS

Type 1 or immune-mediated diabetes mellitus
Grave's disease
Hashimoto's thyroiditis
Autoimmune oophoritis and orchitis
Autoimmune disease of the adrenal gland

MULTIPLE ORGANS INCLUDING THE MUSCULOSKELETAL SYSTEMS[*]

Rheumatoid arthritis
Systemic lupus erythematosus
Scleroderma
Polymyositis, dermatomyositis
Spondyloarthropathies such as ankylosing spondylitis
Sjögren's syndrome

[*]These diseases are also called connective tissue (muscle, skeleton, tendons, fascia, and so on) diseases.
Source: National Institute of Allergy and Infectious Diseases

APPENDIX III
ORGANIZATIONS AND HELP GROUPS

American Association of Immunologists (AAI)
9650 Rockville Pike
Bethesda, MD 20814-3994
(301) 530-7178
(301) 571-1816 (Fax)

American Autoimmune Related Diseases Association, Inc. (AARDA)
National Office
22100 Gratiot Ave.
E. Detroit, MI 48021
(586) 776-3900

Washington Office
750 17th Street, N.W.
Suite 1100
Washington, DC 20006
(202) 466-8511
(800) 598-4668 (Toll free/Literature requests)

American Chronic Pain Association (ACPA)
P.O. Box 850
Rocklin, CA 95677-0850
ACPA@pacbell.net
(916) 632-0922
(916) 632-3208 (Fax)

American Pain Society
5700 Old Orchard Road
Skokie, IL 60077
(708) 966-5595

International Pain Foundation
909 Northeast 43rd Street
Suite 306
Seattle, WA 98105-6020
(206) 547-2157

Medic Alert Foundation International
2323 Colorado
Turlock, CA 95381
(209) 668-3333

National Chronic Pain Outreach Association
7979 Old Georgetown Road
Suite 100
Bethesda, MD 20814
(301) 652-4948

National Organization of Social Security Claimants Representatives
(NOSSCR—a lawyer referral source)
(800) 431-2804

U.S. Social Security Administration
Call your local social security office or
(800) 772-1213 (7:00 A.M.–7:00 P.M. ET weekdays)
http://www.ssa.gov

ADDISON'S DISEASE

Australian Addison's Disease Association Inc.
P.O. Box 2436
Coffs Harbour, NSW 2450, Australia

National Adrenal Diseases Foundation
505 Northern Boulevard
Suite 200
Great Neck, New York 11021
(516) 487-4992

ALLERGIC ASTHMA & ALLERGIC RHINITIS

Allergy & Asthma Network Mothers of Asthmatics (AANMA)
2751 Prosperity Ave.
Suite 150
Fairfax, VA 22031
(800) 878-4403
(703) 573-7794 (Fax)

American Academy of Allergy, Asthma & Immunology
611 East Wells Street
Milwaukee, WI 53202
(414) 272-6071

**American College of Allergy, Asthma &
Immunology**
85 West Algonquin Road
Suite 550
Arlington Heights, IL 60005
(847) 427-1200
(847) 427-1294 (Fax)

**Asthma and Allergy Foundation of America
(AAFA)**
1233 20th Street, NW
Suite 402
Washington, DC 20036
(202) 466-7643
(202) 466-8940 (Fax)

Food Allergy & Anaphylaxis Network
10400 Eaton Place
Suite 107
Fairfax, VA 22030
(800) 929-4040

**National Institute of Allergy and Infectious
Diseases (NIAID)**
NIAID Office of Communications and Public Liaison
Building 31, Room 7A-50
31 Center Drive, MSC 2520
Bethesda, MD 20892

ALOPECIA AREATA

Canadian Alopecia Areata Association
Box 42084, RP.O. Millbourne
Edmonton, Alberta, Canada T6K 4C4

Locks of Love
1640 S. Congress Ave.
Suite 104
Palm Springs, FL 33461
(561) 963-1677
(888) 896-1588 (Toll-free info)
(561) 963-9914 (Fax)

National Alopecia Areata Foundation (NAAF)
P.O. Box 150760
San Rafael, CA 94915-0760
(415) 472-3780
(415) 472-5343 (Fax)

National Alopecia Network
Box 21776
Detroit, MI 48221
(313) 861-0331

ANKYLOSING SPONDYLITIS

**Ankylosing Spondylitis International
Federation**
P.O. Box 179
Mayfield, East Sussex, TN20 6ZL, Great Britain
(+44-1435) 87 35 27
(+44-1435) 87 30 27 (Fax)

Spondylitis Association of America (SAA)
14827 Ventura Blvd. #222
Sherman Oaks, CA 91403
(818) 981-1616
(800) 777-8189 (Toll free)

ANTIGLOMERULAR BASEMENT MEMBRANE (ANTI-GBM) DISEASE

See GOODPASTURE'S SYNDROME

ANTIPHOSPHOLIPID SYNDROME (APS)

The Hughes Syndrome Foundation
The Rayne Institute
St. Thomas' Hospital
London, SE1 7EH, United Kingdom
020 7960 5561
020 7633 0462 (Fax)

AUTOIMMUNE INNER EAR DISEASE (AIED)

League for the Hard of Hearing
71 West 23rd Street
New York, NY 10010-4162
(917) 305-7700
(917) 305-7999 (TTY)
(917) 305-7888 (Fax)

Self Help for Hard of Hearing People, Inc.
7910 Woodmont Ave.
Suite 1200
Bethesda, MD 20814
(301) 657-2248
(301) 657-2249 (TTY)
(301) 913-9413 (Fax)

BEHÇET'S DISEASE

American Behçet's Disease Association
P.O. Box 15247
Chattanooga, TN 37415-0247
(800) 723-4238 (Toll free)

Behçets Organization Worldwide (BOW)
Head Office
P.O. Box 27
Watchet, Somerset, TA23 0YJ, United Kingdom

BOW-Australia
P.O. Box 5004
Falcon, WA 6210, Australia

BOW-USA
P.O. Box 49565
Blaine, MN 55449-0565

Behçet's Syndrome Society
3 Church Close
Lambourn
Hungerford
Berks RG17 8PU
United Kingdom
01 488 71116

BULLOUS PEMPHIGOID

The National Pemphigus Foundation
Atrium Plaza
Suite 203
828 San Pablo Avenue
Albany, CA 94706
(510) 527-4970

CARDIOMYOPATHY

American Heart Association
National Center
7272 Greenville Avenue
Dallas, TX 75231
(800) 242-8721 (Toll free)

Cardiomyopathy Association
40 The Metro Centre
Tolpits Lane
Watford
Herts WD1 8SB
United Kingdom
+44 (0) 1923 249 977
+44 (0) 1923 249 987 (Fax)

Cardiomyopathy Association of Australia Ltd.
26 Clanalpine Street
Mosman, NSW, 2088, Australia

Hypertrophic Cardiomyopathy Association
P.O. Box 306
Hibernia, NJ 07842
(973) 983-7429

Hypertrophic Cardiomyopathy Association of Canada
305-4625 Varsity Drive N.W.
Suite 65
Calgary, Alberta, Canada, T3A 0Z9

CELIAC DISEASE

American Celiac Society
59 Crystal Avenue
West Orange, NJ 07052
(973) 325-8837

Celiac Disease Foundation
13251 Ventura Blvd. #1
Studio City, CA 91604
(818) 990-2354
(818) 990-2379 (Fax)

Celiac Sprue Association/USA, Inc.
P.O. Box 31700
Omaha, NE 68131-0700
(402) 558-0600

Friends of Celiac Disease Research, Inc.
8832 North Port Washington Road
#204
Milwaukee, WI 53217
(414) 540-6679
(414) 540-0587 (Fax)

Gluten Intolerance Group of North America
15110 10th Avenue, SW
Suite A
Seattle, WA 98166-1820
(206) 246-6652

CHRONIC FATIGUE SYNDROME

American Association for Chronic Fatigue Syndrome
515 Minor Ave
Suite 18
Seattle, WA 98104
(206) 781-3544
(206) 749-9052 (Fax)

CFIDS Association of America
P.O. Box 220398
Charlotte, NC 28222-0398
(800) 442-3437 (Toll free)
(704) 365-2343 (Resource line)
(704) 365-9755 (Fax)

CFIDS Emergency Relief Services, Inc.
4714 Northwood Lake Drive
East Northport, AL 35473
(205) 339-2637

The ME Association
4 Top Angel
Buckingham Industrial Park
Buckingham
Buckinghamshire MK18 1TH
United Kingdom
(01) 280 816115
(01) 280 821602 (Fax)

National CFIDS Foundation
103 Aletha Rd.
Needham, MA 02492
(781) 449-3535
(781) 449-8606 (Fax)

CHRONIC INFLAMMATORY DEMYELINATING POLYNEUROPATHY (CIDP)

Canadian Neuropathy Association
c/o Garry Cyr
9273 Snoddon Road
Pefferlaw, Ontario L0E 1N0, Canada
(705) 437-3881

The Neuropathy Association
60 E. 42nd Street
Suite 942
New York, NY 10165
(212) 692-0662

CHURG-STRAUSS SYNDROME

Churg-Strauss Syndrome International Support Group
2 Saint Andrews Court
St. Augustine, FL 32084
(904) 824-1083

CICATRICIAL PEMPHIGOID (CP)

The National Pemphigus Foundation
Atrium Plaza
Suite 203
828 San Pablo Avenue
Albany, CA 94706
(510) 527-4970

CROHN'S DISEASE

Crohn's & Colitis Foundation of America, Inc.
386 Park Avenue South, 17th Floor
New York, NY 10016
(800) 932-2423
(212) 779-4098 (Fax)

Crohn's and Colitis Foundation of Canada
60 St. Clair Avenue East
Suite 600
Toronto, Ontario M4T 1N5, Canada
(416) 920-5035
(800) 387-1479 (Toll free)
(416) 929-0364 (Fax)

National Association for Colitis and Crohn's Disease (NACC)
4 Beaumont House
Sutton Road
St. Albans, Hertfordshire
AL1 5HH
United Kingdom

Pediatric Crohn's & Colitis Association, Inc.
P.O. Box 188
Newton, MA 02468
(617) 489-5854

Reach Out for Youth with Ileitis and Colitis, Inc.
15 Chemung Place
Jericho, NY 11753
(516) 822-8010

COGAN'S SYNDROME

Alexander Graham Bell Association for the Deaf and Hard of Hearing
3417 Volta Place, NW
Washington, DC 20007
(202) 337-5220 (TTY)
(800) HEAR-KID (Toll free)
(202) 337-8314 (Fax)

Association of Late Deafened Adults (ALDA)
10310 Main Street
Box 274
Fairfax, VA 22030
(708) 524-0025
(404) 289-1596 (TTY)
(404) 284-6862 (Fax)

Self Help for Hard of Hearing People, Inc. (SHHH)
7910 Woodmont Avenue
Suite 1200
Bethesda, MD 20814
(301) 657-2248
(301) 657-2249 (TTY)
(301) 913-9413 (Fax)

UPPA/Cogan's Contact Network
P.O. Box 415
Freehold, NJ 07728-0145
(732) 761-9809

CONGENITAL HEART BLOCK

American Heart Association
National Center
7272 Greenville Avenue
Dallas, TX 75231-4596
(214) 373-6300
(800) 242-8721 (Toll free)
(214) 373-0268 (Fax)

Congenital Heart Anomalies, Support, Education, & Resources
2112 North Wilkins Road
Swanton, OH 43558
(419) 825-5575
(419) 825-2880 (Fax)

International Bundle Branch Block Association
6631 West 83rd Street
Los Angeles, CA 90045-2899
(310) 670-9132

DISABILITY BENEFITS

Clearinghouse on Disability Information
Office of Special Education and Rehab Services
U.S. Department of Education
Room 3132, Switzer Building
Washington, DC 20202
(212) 205-8241

DISCOID LUPUS

Lupus Foundation of America, Inc.
1300 Piccard Drive
Suite 200
Rockville, MD 20850-4303

(301) 670-9292
(800) 558-0121 (Toll free)

ENDOMETRIOSIS

Endometriosis Association International Headquarters
8585 North 76th Place
Milwaukee, WI 53223
(414) 355-2200
(800) 992-3636 (Toll free)
(414) 355-6065 (Fax)

Endometriosis Association of Victoria (Australia)
37 Andrew Crescent
South Croydon, Victoria 3136, Australia
+61 3 9870 0536
+61 3 9870 3007

Endometriosis Research Center
630 Ibis Drive
Delray Beach, FL 33444
(561) 274-7442
(800) 239-7280 (Toll free)
(561) 274-9117 (Fax)

The Institute for the Study and Treatment of Endometriosis (ISTE)
2425 West 22nd Street
Oak Brook, IL 60523
(630) 954-0054
(630) 954-0064 (Fax)

National Endometriosis Society
50 Westminster Palace Gardens
Artillery Row
London
SW1P 1RL
United Kingdom

EVANS' SYNDROME

Evans' Syndrome Research and Support Group
P.O. Box 290203
Port Orange, FL 32119
or
5630 Devon St.
Port Orange, FL 32127
(386) 322-2655
(386) 788-0902 (Fax)

FIBROMYALGIA

American Fibromyalgia Syndrome Association, Inc.
6380 E. Tanque Verde
Suite D
Tucson, AZ 85715
(520) 733-1570

Fibromyalgia Network
P.O. Box 31750
Tucson, AZ 85751
(800) 853-2929 (Toll free)

National Fibromyalgia Awareness Campaign (NFAC)
2415 N. River Trail Road
Suite 200
Orange, CA 92865
(714) 921-0150
(714) 921-8139 (Fax)

National Fibromyalgia Partnership
140 Zinn Way
Linden, VA 22642-5609
(866) 725-4404 (Toll free)
(866) 666-2727 (Toll-free fax)

Oregon Fibromyalgia Foundation (OFF)
1221 S.W. Yamhill
Suite 303
Portland, OR 97205
(503) 892-8811

GOODPASTURE'S SYNDROME

American Kidney Fund
6110 Executive Boulevard
Suite 1010
Rockville, MD 20852
(800) 638-8299 (Toll free)

National Kidney Foundation
30 East 33rd Street
New York, NY 10016
(800) 622-9010 (Toll free)

GRAVES' DISEASE

National Graves' Disease Foundation
P.O. Box 1969
Brevard, NC 28712
(828) 877-5251

The Thyroid Society
7515 South Main Street
Suite 545
Houston, TX 77030
(713) 799-9909
(800) 849-7643 (Toll free)

GUILLAIN-BARRÉ SYNDROME (GBS)

Guillain-Barré Syndrome Association of New South Wales
P.O. Box 572
Epping, NSW 1710, Australia

Guillain-Barré Syndrome Foundation International
P.O. Box 262
Wynnewood, PA 19096
(610) 667-0131

Guillain-Barré Syndrome Support Group
LCC Offices
Eastgate, Sleaford
NG34 7EB
United Kingdom

HASHIMOTO'S THYROIDITIS

Thyroid Foundation of Canada
P.O. Box/CP 1919 Stn Main
Kingston, ON K7L 5J7, Canada
(613) 544-8364
(613) 544-9731 (Fax)

Thyroid Society For Education & Research
7515 South Main Street
Suite 545
Houston, TX 77030
(713) 799-9909
(800) 849-7643 (Toll free)

HEPATITIS (AUTOIMMUNE)

American Liver Foundation
75 Maiden Lane
Suite 603
New York, NY 10038
(800) 465-4837 (Toll free)

IDIOPATHIC PULMONARY FIBROSIS (IPF)

The American Lung Association
1740 Broadway
New York, NY 10019
(212) 315-8700

Coalition for Pulmonary Fibrosis
350 California Street
Suite 1600
San Francisco, CA 94104
(888) 222-8541 (Toll free)

IGA NEPHROPATHY

American Kidney Fund
6110 Executive Boulevard
Suite 1010
Rockville, MD 20852
(800) 638-8299 (Toll free)

IgA Nephropathy Foundation
One Johnson Pier #36
Half Moon Bay, CA 94019

IgA Nephropathy Support Network
400B Main Road
Gill, MA 01376
(413) 863-8663

International IgA Nephropathy Network
Centre for Kidney Research
The Children's Hospital at Westmead
Locked Bag 4001
Westmead, NSW 2145, Australia
+61 2 9845 3037
+61 2 9845 3038 (Fax)

National Kidney Foundation
30 East 33rd Street
New York, NY 10016
(800) 622-9010 (Toll free)

INCLUSION BODY MYOSITIS (IBM)

Myositis Association of America
755 Cantrell Avenue
Suite C
Harrisonburg, VA 22801
(540) 433-7686
(540) 432-0206 (Fax)

INSULIN-DEPENDENT DIABETES (TYPE 1)

American Association of Diabetes Educators
444 N. Michigan Avenue
Suite 1240
Chicago, IL 60611
(800) 832-6874 (Toll free)

American Diabetes Association
ADA National Service Center
1660 Duke Street
Alexandria, VA 22314
(800) 232-3472 (Toll free)

American Dietetic Association
216 W. Jackson Blvd.
Chicago, IL 60606-6995
(800) 366-1655 (Toll free)

Juvenile Diabetes Foundation International
120 Wall Street
New York, NY 10005-4001
(212) 785-9500
(800) JDF-CURE (Toll free)
(212) 785-9595 (Fax)

INTERSTITIAL CYSTITIS

American Foundation for Urologic Disease
The Bladder Health Council
1128 North Charles Street
Baltimore, MD 21201
(410) 468-1800
(800) 242-2383 (Toll free)

Interstitial Cystitis Association (ICA)
110 North Washington Street
Suite 340
Rockville, MD 20850
(301) 610-5300
(800) HELP-ICA (Toll free)
(301) 610-5308 (Fax)

Interstitial Cystitis Information Center (ICIC)
1706 Briery Road
Farmville, VA 23901

Interstitial Cystitis Network
5636 Del Monte Court
Santa Rosa, CA 95409
(707) 538-9442
(707) 538-9444 (Fax)

National Kidney Foundation
30 East 33rd Street
New York, NY 10016
(212) 889-2210
(800) 622-9010 (Toll free)

United Ostomy Association
36 Executive Park
Suite 120
Irvine, CA 92714
(714) 660-8624

JUVENILE ARTHRITIS

American College of Rheumatology
1800 Century Place
Suite 250
Atlanta, GA 30345
(404) 633-3777
(404) 633-1870 (Fax)

**American Juvenile Arthritis Organization
  (AJAO)**
Arthritis Foundation
P.O. Box 7669
Atlanta, GA 30357-0669
(404) 872-7100
(800) 283-7800 (Toll free)

Kids on the Block, Inc.
9385-C Gerwig Lane
Columbia, MD 21046
(410) 290-9095
(800) 368-5437 (Toll free)

MÉNIÈRE'S DISEASE

**American Academy of Otolaryngology-Head
  and Neck Surgery**
One Prince Street
Alexandria, VA 22314
(703) 519-1589
(703) 519-1585 (TTY)

Deafness Research Foundation
1050 17th Street NW
Suite 701
Washington, DC 20036
(800) 535-3313 (Toll free)
(202) 289-5850 (TTY)

Ear Foundation
1817 Patterson Street
Nashville, TN 37203

(615) 329-7807
(800) 545-HEAR (Toll free)
(615) 329-7849 (TTY)

The Ménière's Society
98 Maybury Road, Woking
Surrey
GU21 5HX
United Kingdom
(01483) 740597
(01483) 755441 (Fax)

Vestibular Disorders Association
P.O. Box 4467
Portland, OR 97208-4467
(503) 229-7706
(800) 837-8428 (Toll free)

MULTIPLE SCLEROSIS

International MS Support Foundation
9420 E. Golf Links Road
PMB #291
Tucson, AZ 85720-1340
(520) 579-9473 (Fax)

International Tremor Foundation
7046 West 105th Street
Overland Park, KS 66212-1803
(913) 341-3880
(888) 387-3667 (Toll free)
(913) 341-1296 (Fax)

Multiple Sclerosis Association of America
706 Haddonfield Road
Cherry Hill, NJ 08002
(856) 488-4500
(800) 532-7667 (Toll free)

Multiple Sclerosis Foundation
6350 North Andrews Avenue
Fort Lauderdale, FL 33309-2130
(954) 776-6805
888-MSFOCUS (Toll free)
(954) 351-0630 (Fax)

Multiple Sclerosis International Federation
3rd Floor Skyline House
200 Union Street
London SE1 0LX, United Kingdom
+44 (0) 20 7620 1911
+44 (0) 20 7620 1922 (Fax)

Multiple Sclerosis Society

MS National Centre
372 Edgware Road
Staples Corner
London, NW2 6ND, United Kingdom
020 8438 0700

Multiple Sclerosis Society of Canada

250 Bloor Street East
Suite 1000
Toronto, Ontario M4W 3P9, Canada
Phone: (416) 922-6065
(416) 922-7538 (Fax)

National Ataxia Foundation (NAF)

2600 Fernbrook Lane
Suite 119
Minneapolis, MN 55447-4752
(763) 553-0020
(763) 553-0167 (Fax)

National Multiple Sclerosis Society

733 Third Avenue
New York, NY 10017
(800) 344-4867 (Toll free)

MYASTHENIA GRAVIS

Muscular Dystrophy Association

3300 East Sunrise Drive
Tucson, AZ 85718-3208
(520) 529-2000
(800) 572-1717 (Toll free)
(520) 529-5300 (Fax)

Myasthenia Gravis Association

Keynes House
Chester Park
Alfreton Road
Derby
DE21 4AS
United Kingdom
01332-290219
01332-293641 (Fax)

Myasthenia Gravis Foundation of America

5841 Cedar Lake Road
Suite 204
Minneapolis, MN 55416
(952) 545-9438
(800) 541-5454 (Toll free)
(952) 545-6073 (Fax)

MYOSITIS

Myositis Association

755 Cantrell Avenue
Suite C
Harrisonburg, VA 22801
(540) 433-7686
(540) 432-0206 (Fax)

NEUTROPENIA

Neutropenia Support Association Inc.

P.O. Box 243, 905 Corydon
Winnipeg, Manitoba R3M 3S7, Canada
(204) 489-8454

PEMPHIGUS VULGARIS (PV)

International Pemphigus Foundation

Atrium Plaza
Suite 203
828 San Pablo Avenue
Albany, CA 94706
(510) 527-4970

PERIPHERAL NEUROPATHY (PN)

Canadian Neuropathy Association

c/o Garry Cyr
9273 Snoddon Road
Pefferlaw, Ontario L0E 1N0, Canada
(705) 437-3881

Neuropathy Association

60 E. 42nd Street
Suite 942
New York, NY 10165
(212) 692-0662

Neuropathy Trust

P.O. Box 26
Nantwich
Cheshire
CW5 5FP
United Kingdom
+44 (0)1270 611 828
+44 (0)1270 611 828 (Fax)

POLYCHONDRITIS

Relapsing Polychondritis Foundation

775 Bounty Place
Manteca, CA 95337

POLYMYOSITIS

Dermatomyositis and Polymyositis Support Group
146 Newtown Road
Woolston
Southampton
Hampshire
SO29HR
United Kingdom
01703-449708
01703-396402 (Fax)

Myositis Association of America, Inc.
755 Cantrell Avenue
Suite C
Harrisonburg, VA 22801
(540) 433-7686

PRIMARY AGAMMAGLOBULINEMIA

Immune Deficiency Foundation
40 W. Chesapeake Avenue
Suite 308
Towson, MD 21204
(800) 296-4433 (Toll free)
(410) 321-9165 (Fax)

International Patient Organization for Primary Immunodeficiencies
David Watters
The IPOPI Secretariat
C/o PiA
Alliance House
12 Caxton Street
London
SW1H 0QS
United Kingdom
+44 207 222 3545

Jeffrey Modell Foundation
747 Third Avenue, 34th Floor
New York, NY 10017
(800) JEFF-844 (Toll free)

PRIMARY BILIARY CIRRHOSIS

American Liver Foundation
75 Maiden Lane, Suite 603
New York, NY 10038
(800) GO-LIVER (465-4837) (Toll free)

PBC Foundation
11 Glenfinlas Street
Edinburgh, Scotland EH3 6AQ
0131 225 8586
0131 225 7579 (Fax)

PSORIASIS

National Psoriasis Foundation
6600 SW 92nd Avenue, Suite 300
Portland, OR 97223-7195
(503) 244-7404
(800) 723-9166 (Toll free)
(503) 245-0626 (Fax)

PSORIATIC ARTHRITIS

National Psoriasis Foundation
6600 SW 92nd Avenue
Suite 300
Portland, OR 97223-7195
(503) 244-7404
(800) 723-9166 (Toll free)
(503) 245-0626 (Fax)

RAYNAUD'S PHENOMENON

Raynaud's Association, Inc.
94 Mercer Avenue
Hartsdale, NY 10530
(914) 682-8341

Raynaud's Foundation
P.O. Box 346176
Chicago, IL 60634-6176
(773) 622-9220
(773) 622-9221 (Fax)

Raynaud's & Scleroderma Association
112 Crewe Road, Alsager
Cheshire ST7 2JA
United Kingdom
01-270-872776
01-270-883556 (Fax)

REITER'S SYNDROME

Arthritis Foundation
1330 West Peachtree Street
Atlanta, GA 30309
(404) 872-7100
(800) 283-7800 (Toll free)

Reiter's Information & Support Group Inc.
1105 D 15th Avenue #172
Longview, WA 98632-3068
(603) 696-0789 (Fax)

Spondylitis Association of America
P.O. Box 5872
Sherman Oaks, CA 91413
(818) 981-1616
(800) 777-8189 (Toll free)

RHEUMATOID ARTHRITIS

Arthritis Foundation
P.O. Box 7669
Atlanta, GA 30357-0669
(800) 283-7800 (Toll free)

ArthritisSupport.com (Pro Health)
2040 Alameda Padre Serra
Suite 101
Santa Barbara, CA 93103
(800) 733-1658 (Toll free)
(805) 965-0042 (Fax)

SARCOIDOSIS

Foundation for Sarcoidosis Research
P.O. Box 146229
Chicago, IL 60614
(773) 665-2400
(733) 665-0805 (Fax)

National Sarcoidosis Resource Center
P.O. Box 1593
Piscataway, NJ 08855-1593
(732) 699-0733
(732) 699-0882 (Fax)

**Sarcoidosis Family Aid and Research
   Foundation**
460A Central Avenue
East Orange, NJ 07018
Sarcoidosis Networking
13925 80th Street East
Puyallup, WA 98372
(206) 845-3108

Sarcoidosis Research Institute
3475 Central Avenue
Memphis, TN 38111
(901) 327-5454

SCLERODERMA

Juvenile Scleroderma Network, Inc.
1204 W. 13th Street
San Pedro, CA 90731
(310) 519-9511 (Phone/fax)
(800) 369-8309 (Toll free)

Raynaud's & Scleroderma Association
112 Crewe Road
Alsager
Cheshire
ST7 2JA
United Kingdom
01-270-872776
01-270-883556 (Fax)

Scleroderma Foundation
12 Kent Way
Suite 101
Byfield, MA 01922
(978) 463-5843
(800) 722-HOPE (4673) (Toll free)
(978) 463-5809 (Fax)

Scleroderma Research Foundation
2320 Bath Street
Suite 315
Santa Barbara, CA 93105
(805) 563-9133
(800) 441-CURE (Toll free)
(805) 563-2402 (Fax)

SJÖGREN'S SYNDROME

British Sjögren's Syndrome Association
Unit 1, Manor Workshops
West End, NAILSEA
Bristol
BS48 4DD
United Kingdom
44(0)1275-854215

Sjögren's Syndrome Foundation
366 North Broadway
Suite PH-W2
Jericho, NY 11753
(516) 933-6365
(800) 475-6473 (Toll free)
(516) 933-6368 (Fax)

Sjögren's Syndrome New Zealand
P.O. Box 25153
St. Heliers, Auckland

New Zealand
+64 9 528 6384
+64 9 528 6320 (Fax)

SYSTEMIC LUPUS ERYTHEMATOSUS (SLE)

Alliance for Lupus Research, Inc.
1270 Avenue of the Americas, Suite 609
New York, NY 10020
(212) 218-2840

Lupus Foundation of America
1300 Piccard Drive
Suite 200
Rockville, MD 20850-4303
(301) 670-9292
(800) 558-0121 (Toll free)

SLE Foundation, Inc.
149 Madison Avenue
Suite 205
New York, NY 10016
(212) 685-4118
(212) 545-1843 (Fax)

TAKAYASU'S ARTERITIS

Takayasu's Arteritis Association
16 Rose Lane
Bedford, NH 03110
(603) 641-2774
(603) 641-2774 (Fax)

Takayasu's Arteritis Foundation International
1500 Meeting House Road
Sea Girt, NJ 08750
(732) 449-0550
(732) 974-6726 (Fax)

Takayasu's Arteritis Research Association (TARA)
2030 County Line Road
Suite 199
Huntingdon Valley, PA 19006-1739
(800) 575-9390 (Toll free)

TRANSVERSE MYELITIS

Transverse Myelitis Association
1787 Sutter Parkway
Powell, OH 43065-8806
(614) 766-1806

ULCERATIVE COLITIS

Australian Crohn's & Colitis Association (ACCA)
P.O. Box 201
Mooroolbark, VIC 3138
61-3-9726-9008
61-3-9726-9914 (Fax)

Crohn's & Colitis Foundation of America Inc.
386 Park Avenue South, 17th floor
New York, NY 10016-8804
(212) 685-3440
(800) 932-2423 (Toll free)

National Association for Colitis and Crohn's Disease (NACC)
4 Beaumont House
Sutton Road
St. Albans, Hertfordshire
AL1 5HH
United Kingdom

Pediatric Crohn's & Colitis Association Inc.
P.O. Box 188
Newton, MA 02168
(617) 489-5854

Reach Out for Youth with Ileitis and Colitis Inc.
15 Chemung Place
Jericho, NY 11753
(516) 822-8010

United Ostomy Association, Inc.
19772 MacArthur Boulevard #200
Irvine, CA 92612-2405
(949) 660-8624
(800) 826-0826 (Toll free)
(949) 660-9262 (Fax)

UVEITIS

Uveitis Information Group
South House
Sweening
Vidlin
Shetland Isles
ZE2 9QE
Scotland
01806 577310

VITILIGO

American Vitiligo Research Foundation, Inc.
P.O. Box 7540
Clearwater, FL 33758
(727) 461-3899
(727) 461-4796 (Fax)

National Vitiligo Foundation
611 South Fleishel Avenue
Tyler, TX 75701
(903) 531-0074
(903) 525-1234 (Fax)

Vitiligo Society
125 Kennington Road
London
SE11 6SF
England

WEGENER'S GRANULOMATOSIS

Wegener's Foundation, Inc.
3705 South George Mason Drive
Suite 1813 South
Falls Church, VA 22041
(703) 931-5852

Wegener's Granulomatosis Association
(formerly Wegener's Granulomatosis Support Group,
    Inc. International)
P.O. Box 28660
Kansas City, MO 64188-8660
(816) 436-8211 (Phone/fax)
(800) 277-WGSG (9474) (Toll free)

**Wegener's Granulomatosis Support Group of
    Australia, Inc.**
P.O. Box 393
Greensborough, Victoria, Australia, 3088

**Wegener's Granulomatosis Support Group
    of Canada**
446-425 Hespeler Road
Cambridge, Ontario N1R 8J6, Canada
(877) 572-WGSG (9474)

APPENDIX IV
MEDICAL ALERT JEWELRY

About Me Jewelry
P.O. Box 20794
Tampa, FL 33622-0794
(877) 639-1004
jsulten1@tampabay.rr.com
http://www.aboutmejewelry.com/

Allergy Watch
Conrad Concepts, Inc.
1505 Fairfax Lane
Bartlett, IL 60103
(630) 483-8997
(630) 483-9501 (Fax)
conradconcepts@allergywatch99.com
http://www.allergywatch99.com/chronic.html

Beverly Hills Collar Company
34611 Camino Capistrano
Capistrano Beach, CA 92624
(949) 240-3825
(800) 891-2663 (Toll free)
(949) 496-0941 (Fax)
Kidsid@cox.net
http://www.id-tags.com/orderpg.htm

Custom ID Products
P.O. Box 19279
Seattle, WA 98109
(800) 439-8899 (Toll free)
(206) 287-9828 (Fax)

Deco Watch Accessories
P.O. Box 37034
Saint-Hubert, Quebec
Canada J3Y 8N3
(450) 443-0556
info@decowatch.com

Diabetes Research and Wellness Foundation
1206 Potomac Street NW
Washington, DC 20007

http://www.diabeteswellness.net/NewFiles/
alertidentification.html

Fax Factor
P.O. Box 6312
Lynnwood, WA 98036-0312
(206) 776-5879

ID-SOS Distributors
9920 S. Rural Road
#108
PMB 66
Tempe, AZ 85284
(480) 940-6236
http://www.id-sos.com/home2.htm

ID Technology
117 Nelson Road
Baltimore, MD 21208-1111
support@id-technology.com
http://www.id-technology.com/

Life Alert
Tinman Medical Identification
P.O. Box 386
Lynden, WA 98264
(888) 543-3253 (Toll free)
http://www.tinman.com/life/lamodels.html

LifeTag
7500 N. Mesa
Suite 216
El Paso, TX 79912
(915) 584-0022
(888) LIFETAG (Toll free)
(915) 584-9245 (Fax)
Lifetag@worldnet.att.net
http://www.susaneisen.com/lifetag.htm

MedicAlert
2323 Colorado Avenue
Turlock, CA 95382

(209) 668-3333
(888) 633-4298 (Toll free)
http://www.medicalert.org/

Medic Assist
10907 Shady Trail
104-B
Dallas, TX 75011-7627
(214) 357-0359
(214) 654-0697 (Fax)
http://www.medicassist.com/

Medic ID's International
P.O. Box 571687
Tarzana, CA 91357

(818) 705-0595
(800) 926-3342 (Toll free)
(818) 705-0773 (Fax)
http://www.medicid.com/

MedIDs.com
M.Stephens-MedIds.com
2400 Cypress Street
Suite 50, PMB 211
West Monroe, LA 71291
info@medids.com
http://www.medids.com/

APPENDIX V
WEBSITES OF INTEREST

American Association of Immunologists (AAI)
http://www.aai.org

American Autoimmune Related Diseases Association, Inc. (AARDA)
http://www.aarda.org/

American Chronic Pain Association (ACPA)
http://www.theacpa.org

AMFI—Autoimmune Diseases
http://www.amfoundation.org/autoimmune.htm

Autoimmune Diseases Online
http://www.autoimmune-disease.com/

Immune Web—Support and Information Network
http://www.immuneweb.org/

Johns Hopkins Autoimmune Disease Research Center
http://autoimmune.pathology.jhmi.edu/OurLab.html

Yahoo Health
http://dir.yahoo.com/Health/Diseases_and_Conditions/Autoimmune_Diseases/

ADDISON'S DISEASE

Addison and Cushing International Federation (ACIF)
http://www.nvacp.nl/page.php?main=5

Australian Addison's Disease Association Inc.
http://www.addisons.org.au/core.htm

ALLERGIC ASTHMA

Allergy and Asthma Disease Management Center
http://www.aaaai.org/aadmc/default.htm

Allergy & Asthma Network Mothers of Asthmatics (AANMA)
http://www.aanma.org/headquarters/

Allergy, Asthma & Immunology Online
http://www.allergy.mcg.edu/

Asthma and Allergy Foundation of America (AAFA)
http://www.aafa.org/

AsthmaMoms
http://www.asthmamoms.com/

Asthma Research at National Institute of Environmental Health Sciences
http://www.niehs.nih.gov/airborne/home.htm

The Center for Asthma and Allergic Disease
http://www-med.stanford.edu/school/pediatrics/Asthma_Center/

Clearbreathing—Asthma & Allergy Information
http://www.clearbreathing.com/index.asp

Focus on Allergy
http://www.niaid.nih.gov/newsroom/focuson/allergy99/allergyspot.htm

Food Allergy & Anaphylaxis Network
http://www.foodallergy.org/

FreeBreather—Allergies & Asthma
http://www.freebreather.com/asthma/allergies/allergies.html

Global Initiative for Asthma
http://www.ginasthma.com/

ibreathe.com—a respiratory resource site
http://gsk.ibreathe.com/ibreathe_pages/index.htm

Surrey Allergy Clinic
http://www.allergy-clinic.co.uk/allergic_asthma.htm

278

Web Sources For Consumer Information on Asthma
http://library.niehs.nih.gov/consumer/asthma.htm

ALLERGIC RHINITIS

AllergyUSA
http://www.allergyusa.com/allergicrhinitis.htm

ClearBreathing.com
http://www.clearbreathing.com/disease/rhinitis.asp

ALOPECIA AREATA

Alopecia Areata Information
http://www.keratin.com/ad/adindex.shtml

Alopecia Areata Support Community
http://alopeciaareata.resourcez.com/

Alopecia Areata Support Group
http://groups.yahoo.com/group/
   alopeciaareatasupportgroup

alopeciaKIDS
http://www.alopeciakids.org/

American Academy of Dermatology White Paper on Alopecia Areata
http://npntserver.mcg.edu/html/alopecia/
   documents/WhitePaper.html

The Bald Spot
http://www.islandnet.com/~sheilaj/

Harry's Alopecia Page in the Netherlands
http://www.alopecia.myweb.nl/

Locks of Love
http://www.locksoflove.org/

National Alopecia Areata Foundation (NAAF)
http://www.alopeciaareata.com/

Newsgroup
Alt.Baldspot

The Skin Site
http://www.skinsite.com/info_alopecia_areata.htm

ANKYLOSING SPONDYLITIS

Ankylosing Spondylitis International Federation
http://www.asif.rheumanet.org/

Ankylosing Spondylitis Internet Mailing List
http://www.familyvillage.wisc.edu/lists/as.html

KickAS Support Group
http://www.kickas.org/

National Ankylosing Spondylitis Society (NASS)
http://www.nass.co.uk/

Patrick's AS Web pages
http://website.lineone.net/~pgarvey/myweb/index.
   htm

Spondylitis Association of America (SAA)
http://www.spondylitis.org/

ANTIGLOMERULAR BASEMENT MEMBRANE (ANTI-GBM) DISEASE

See GOODPASTURE'S SYNDROME

ANTIPHOSPHOLIPID SYNDROME (APS)

Antiphospholipid Antibody Syndrome (APS) On The Net
http://www.mindspring.com/~waxman/

The Hughes Syndrome Foundation
http://www.hughes-syndrome.org/

Newsgroup/Chat Line
http://forums.delphiforums.com/apsantibody

Thrombosis Interest Group of Canada (T.I.G.C)
http://www.tigc.org/english.htm

AUTOIMMUNE INNER EAR DISEASE (AIED)

League for the Hard of Hearing
http://www.lhh.org/index.htm

Self Help for Hard of Hearing People
http://www.shhh.org/index.cfm

BEHÇET'S DISEASE

American Behçet's Disease Association
http://www.behcets.com/

Behçet's Organization Worldwide
http://www.behcets.org/

Behçet's Syndrome Society
http://www.behcets-society.fsnet.co.uk/index.html

BULLOUS PEMPHIGOID

The National Pemphigus Foundation
http://www.pemphigus.org/index.htm

CARDIOMYOPATHY

Cardiomyopathy Association
http://www.cardiomyopathy.org/

Cardiomyopathy Association of Australia Ltd.
http://www.cmaa.org.au/

Hypertrophic Cardiomyopathy Association
http://www.hcma-heart.com/

Hypertrophic Cardiomyopathy Association of Canada
http://hcmac-heart.ca/index.html

CELIAC DISEASE

Celiac Disease & Gluten-Free Diet Support Page
http://www.celiac.com/

Celiac Disease Foundation
http://www.celiac.org/

Friends of Celiac Disease Research, Inc.
http://www.friendsofceliac.com/

Gluten Intolerance Group of North America
http://www.gluten.net/

Yahoo! Health
http://dir.yahoo.com/Health/Diseases_and_
Conditions/Celiac_Disease/

CHRONIC FATIGUE SYNDROME

About Chronic Fatigue Syndrome & Fibromyalgia
http://chronicfatigue.about.com/

American Association for Chronic Fatigue Syndrome
http://www.aacfs.org/

CFIDS Association of America
http://www.cfids.org

CFIDS Emergency Relief Services, Inc.
http://www.cfidsers.org

Chronic Fatigue Syndrome & Fibromyalgia Information Exchange Forum
http://www.co-cure.org/

Chronic Fatigue Syndrome/Myalgic Encephalomyelitis
http://www.cfs-news.org/

The ME Association
http://www.meassociation.org.uk/

National CFIDS Foundation
http://www.ncf-net.org/

National ME/FM Action Network
http://www3.sympatico.ca/me-fm.action/

Yahoo! Health
http://dir.yahoo.com/Health/Diseases_and_
Conditions/Chronic_Fatigue_Syndrome/

CHRONIC INFLAMMATORY DEMYELINATING POLYNEUROPATHY (CIDP)

Canadian Neuropathy Association
http://www.canadianneuropathyassociation.org/

Eric's CIDP Information Page
http://www.geocities.com/ericvance/

The Neuropathy Association
http://www.neuropathy.org/association.asp

CHURG-STRAUSS SYNDROME

Churg-Strauss Syndrome International Support Group
http://www.churg-strauss.com/

A Savvy Vasculitis: Internet Resources for Churg-Strauss and Related Illnesses
http://www.blackandwhite.org/savvy/index.shtml

CICATRICIAL PEMPHIGOID (CP)

The National Pemphigus Foundation
http://www.pemphigus.org/k_pemph_cicatr.htm

CROHN'S DISEASE

Annie's Crohn's Disease Page
http://mycrohns.freeservers.com/

Crohn's & Colitis Foundation of America, Inc.
http://www.ccfa.org/

Crohn's and Colitis Foundation of Canada
http://www.ccfc.ca/

Crohn's/Colitis Home Page
http://qurlyjoe.bu.edu/cduchome.html

Crohn's Disease in the UK
http://communities.msn.co.uk/
    CrohnsDiseaseintheUK

Crohn's Disease Resource Center
http://www.healingwell.com/ibd/

Crohn's 4 Kids
http://www.geocities.com/crohnsdisease/

**Michael's Homepage—A Place for People with
    Crohn's**
http://www.geocities.com/HotSprings/Spa/5509/
    index2.html

**National Association for Colitis and Crohn's
    Disease (NACC)**
http://www.nacc.org.uk/

Pediatric Crohn's & Colitis Association, Inc.
http://pcca.hypermart.net

Teens With Crohn's Disease Website
http://pages.prodigy.net/mattgreen/

COGAN'S SYNDROME

**Cogan's Syndrome Educational Community
    Link**
http://www.geocities.com/cogans_syndrome/CSEC_L
    ink.html

Self Help for Hard of Hearing People
http://www.shhh.org/index.cfm

CONGENITAL HEART BLOCK

American Heart Association
http://www.americanheart.org

**Congenital Heart Anomalies, Support, Educa-
    tion, & Resources**
http://www.csun.edu/~hfmth006/chaser/

Congenital Heart Disease Resource Page
http://www.bamdad.com/sheri/

CREST SYNDROME

Coping with Crest
http://members.aol.com/REDAPRIL4/

Living and Enjoying Life With Crest Syndrome
http://www.geocities.com/crestsyndrome/

Scleroderma Overview: Crest Syndrome
http://sclerodermasupport.com/medical/overview/
    crest.htm

DERMATITIS HERPETIFORMIS (DH)

Dermatitis Herpetiformis Online Community
http://www.dhcondition.plus.com/

DISCOID LUPUS

Just for Discoid Lupus Forum
http://forums.delphiforums.com/lesion/start

Skin Disease in Lupus
http://www.lupus.org/topics/skin.html

See also SYSTEMIC LUPUS ERYTHEMATOSUS (SLE)

ENDOMETRIOSIS

Endometriosis Association
http://www.endometriosisassn.org/

**Endometriosis Association of Victoria
    (Australia)**
http://www.endometriosis.org.au/

Endometriosis.org
http://www.endometriosis.org/

Endometriosis Research Center (ERC)
http://www.endocenter.org/

Endometriosis ZONE
http://www.endozone.org/

**The Institute for the Study and Treatment of
    Endometriosis**
http://www.endometriosisinstitute.com/

National Endometriosis Society
http://www.endo.org.uk/

Yahoo! Health
http://dir.yahoo.com/Health/Diseases_and_
    Conditions/Endometriosis/

EVANS' SYNDROME

Evans' Syndrome Mailing List
http://groups.yahoo.com/group/EvansSyndrome/

Evans' Syndrome Research and Support
http://legalnurseassociates.com/evans.htm

FIBROMYALGIA

American Fibromyalgia Syndrome Association, Inc.
http://www.afsafund.org/

Fibrohugs Fibromyalgia Support Site
http://www.fibrohugs.com/

Fibromyalgia Community
http://www.fibrom-l.org/

Fibromyalgia Information
http://www.myalgia.com/

Fibromyalgia Information & Local Support
http://www.ncf.carleton.ca/fibromyalgia/

Fibromyalgia Links
http://www.angelfire.com/on/teenfms/fmslinks.html

Fibromyalgia Network
http://www.fmnetnews.com/

Fibromyalgia Patient Support Center
http://www.fmpsc.org/wall/wallinks.htm

Fibromyalgia Research and Information Library
http://www.coloradohealthnet.org/fibro/fibro_lib.html

FMS: An Iowa Nonprofit Support Group
http://www.angelfire.com/ia/cjmachine/fibro.html

Forum Fibromyalgia
http://www.fibromyalgie.com/fmsgb.html

Living With FMS
http://www.tidalweb.com/fms/

Missouri Arthritis Rehabilitation Research and Training Center
http://www.muhealth.org/~fibro/

National Fibromyalgia Partnership, Inc. (NFP)
http://www.fmpartnership.org/

Resource Site for Fibromyalgia Survivors
http://www.plaidrabbit.com/fms/index.html

Yahoo! Health
http://dir.yahoo.com/Health/Diseases_and_Conditions/Fibromyalgia/

GOODPASTURE'S SYNDROME

Goodpasture's Syndrome
http://www.geocities.com/CapeCanaveral/Lab/1075/

Personal Site and Mail List
http://www.geocities.com/HotSprings/Spa/1388/

GRAVES' DISEASE

Daisy's Graves' Disease Educational Site
http://daisyelaine_co.tripod.com/gravesdisease/

Dianne Wiley's Homepage
http://netnow.micron.net/~deecee/

National Graves' Disease Foundation
http://www.ngdf.org/

The Thyroid Society
http://the-thyroid-society.org/graves.html

GUILLAIN-BARRÉ SYNDROME (GBS)

gbs.org
http://www.gbs.org/

Guillain-Barré Syndrome
http://www.gbsyndrome.com/

Guillain-Barré Syndrome Association of New South Wales
http://members.ozemail.com.au/~guillain/

Guillain-Barré Syndrome Foundation International
http://www.guillain-barre.com/

Guillain-Barré Syndrome Support Group
http://www.gbs.org.uk/

Yahoo! Health
http://uk.dir.yahoo.com/health/Diseases_and_Conditions/Guillain_Barre_Syndrome/

HASHIMOTO'S THYROIDITIS

Hashimoto's Thyroiditis Activist Page
http://bonika53.tripod.com/hashmoto53/

HEPATITIS (AUTOIMMUNE)

American Liver Foundation
http://www.liverfoundation.org/html/livheal.dir/lhl3dox.fol/lhl4dox.fol/_lnh002os.htm

Autoimmune Hepatitis.com
http://autoimmunehepatitis.homestead.com/files/home.html

Hepatitis Central
http://hepatitis-central.com/hcv/autoimmune/toc.
  html

Women and Autoimmune Hepatitis
http://www.liverlifeline.com/wah.html

IDIOPATHIC PULMONARY FIBROSIS (IPF)

American Lung Association
http://www.lungusa.org/diseases/pulmfibrosis.html

Coalition for Pulmonary Fibrosis
http://www.coalitionforpf.org/

The dailylung.com Guide
http://www.dailylung.com/Interstial.htm

No Air To Go!
http://noairtogo.tripod.com/ild.htm

IDIOPATHIC THROMBOCYTOPENIC PURPURA (ITP)

ITP Support Association
http://www.itpsupport.org.uk/

Patient Support Groups
http://moon.ouhsc.edu/jgeorge/ITP1.html

IGA NEPHROPATHY

Australian Kidney Fact Sheets
http://www.kidney.org.au/renalresources/igAN.htm

IgA Nephropathy Foundation
http://www.igan.org/

IgA Nephropathy Support Group
http://groups.yahoo.com/group/iga-nephropathy/

International IgA Nephropathy Network
http://www.igan.net/

INCLUSION BODY MYOSITIS (IBM)

Inclusion Body Myositis (IBM) by Bill Tillier
http://members.shaw.ca/btillieribm/

Inclusion Body Myositis Discussion Board
http://www.myositissupportgroup.org/IBM/

Inclusion Body Myositis/MDA
http://www.mdausa.org/disease/ibm.html

Myositis Support Group
http://www.myositis.org.uk/

INSULIN-DEPENDENT DIABETES (TYPE 1)

Insulin Dependent Diabetes Trust—International
http://www.iddtinternational.org/iddt.html

On-line Community for Kids, Families and Adults with Diabetes
http://www.childrenwithdiabetes.com/index_
  cwd.htm

Type I Diabetes Center
http://www.healthatoz.com/atoz/Diabetes1/dia-
  betesindex1.asp

INTERSTITIAL CYSTITIS

Cystitis Research Center
http://pw1.netcom.com/~jewel3/uti/bacteria.html

IC Hope For Interstitial Cystitis
http://www.ic-hope.com/

Intercyst.org
http://www.intercyst.org/

International Interstitial Cystitis Network
http://www.interstitial-cystitis.org/

Interstitial Cystitis Association (ICA)
http://www.ichelp.com/

Interstitial Cystitis Information Center (ICIC)
http://www.moonstar.com/~icickay/

Interstitial Cystitis Network
http://www.ic-network.com/

Interstitial Cystitis Success Stories
http://www.icsuccessonline.com/

Interstitial Cystitis Support Group
http://www.interstitialcystitis.co.uk/

WebCompass—104 Articles About Interstitial Cystitis
http://www.incontinet.com/webcompass-ic.htm

JUVENILE ARTHRITIS

About the AJAO
http://www.arthritis.org/communities/about_ajao.asp

American College of Rheumatology
http://www.rheumatology.org

Juvenile Arthritis Awareness
http://www.fyldecoast.co.uk/grace/grace.htm

Juvenile Arthritis in the News
http://www.muhealth.org/~arthritis/ja/

Juvenile Chronic Arthritis
http://www.arthritis.co.za/jra.htm

LICHEN PLANUS

Lichen Planus Treatment Program on the Internet
http://www.lichenplanus.com/

MÉNIÈRE'S DISEASE

Ménière's.org
http://www.menieres.org/

Ménière's Society of the UK
http://www.menieres.co.uk/intro.html

Ménière's Support Group of Victoria
http://www.menieres.org.au/msgv.htm

Yahoo! Health
http://dir.yahoo.com/Health/Diseases_and_Conditions/Meniere_s/

MULTIPLE SCLEROSIS

All About Multiple Sclerosis
http://www.mult-sclerosis.org/

Consortium of Multiple Sclerosis Centers
http://www.mscare.org/

International Federation of MS Societies
http://www.infosci.org/

International MS Support Foundation
http://www.msnews.org/

International Tremor Foundation
http://www.essentialtremor.org

MS Crossroads
http://www.mscrossroads.org/

MSonly
http://www.msonly.com/

Multiple Sclerosis Association of America
http://www.msaa.com/

Multiple Sclerosis Foundation
http://www.msfacts.org/

Multiple Sclerosis Information & Support
http://www.msworld.org/

Multiple Sclerosis International Federation
http://www.msif.org

Multiple Sclerosis Society
http://www.mssociety.org.uk/index.html

Multiple Sclerosis Society of Canada
http://www.mssociety.ca/

National Ataxia Foundation (NAF)
http://www.ataxia.org

National Multiple Sclerosis Society
http://www.nmss.org/
http://www.nationalmssociety.org/

Patient Resources: Multiple Sclerosis
http://www.docguide.com/news/content.nsf/PatientResAllCateg/Multiple%20Sclerosis?OpenDocument

MYASTHENIA GRAVIS

Muscular Dystrophy Association
http://www.mdausa.org/

Myasthenia Gravis Association
http://www.mgauk.org/

Myasthenia Gravis Foundation of America
http://www.myasthenia.org/

MYOCARDITIS, AUTOIMMUNE

Cardiac Myosin-Induced Autoimmune Myocarditis
http://www.jhsph.edu/mmi/faculty/rose/rose.html

MYOSITIS

Myositis Association
http://www.myositis.org/

Myositis.com
http://www.myositis.com
(may still be under construction)

Myositis NW
http://www.myositisnw.org/

Myositis Support Group
http://www.myositissupportgroup.org/

Myositis Support Group—UK
http://www.myositis.org.uk/

NEUTROPENIA

Neutropenia Support Association Inc.
http://www.neutropenia.ca/

PEMPHIGUS VULGARIS (PV)

International Pemphigus Foundation
http://www.pemphigus.org/

Pemphigus.com
http://www.pemphigus.com/

PERIPHERAL NEUROPATHY (PN)

Canadian Neuropathy Association
http://www.canadianneuropathyassociation.org/

Jack Miller Center for Peripheral Neuropathy
http://peripheralneuropathy.bsd.uchicago.edu/

Neurology Channel
http://www.neurologychannel.com/neuropathy/

Neuropathy Association
http://www.neuropathy.org/association.asp

Neuropathy Trust
http://www.neuropathy-trust.org/

Peripheral Neuropathy Forum
http://neuro-www.mgh.harvard.edu:16080/forum/
    PeripheralNeuropathyMenu.html

POLYATERITIS NODOSA

Polyarteritis Nodosa (PAN) Support Site
http://www.angelfire.com/pa2/autoimmunesite/
    polyarteritis.html

POLYCHONDRITIS

How I Beat Relapsing Polychondritis
http://relapsingpolychondritis.com/

Polychondritis Educational Society, Ltd.
http://www.polychondritis.com/

Polychondritis Group
http://rpolychondritis.tripod.com/

POLYMYOSITIS

Myositis Association of America, Inc.
http://www.myositis.org

Polymyositis Discussion Board
http://www.myositissupportgroup.org/PM/

PRIMARY AGAMMAGLOBULINEMIA

Immune Deficiency Foundation
http://www.primaryimmune.org

**International Patient Organization for Primary
    Immunodeficiencies**
http://www.ipopi.org/

Jeffrey Modell Foundation
http://www.jmfworld.com/

PRIMARY BILIARY CIRRHOSIS

American Liver Foundation
http://www.liverfoundation.org

**Australian Primary Biliary Cirrhosis
    Support Group**
http://home.vicnet.net.au/~ozpbc/

PBCers Organization
http://pbcers.org/

PBC Foundation
http://www.nhtech.demon.co.uk/pbc/

PSORIASIS

Dave's Psoriasis Info
http://members.aol.com/psorsite/

National Psoriasis Foundation
http://www.psoriasis.org/

Psoriasis Genetics Laboratory
http://www.psoriasis.umich.edu/

Psoriasis Research
http://www.netlink.uk.com/psoriasis/

Yahoo! Health
http://dir.yahoo.com/Health/Diseases_and_
    Conditions/Psoriasis/

PSORIATIC ARTHRITIS

Psoriatic Arthritis List
http://groups.yahoo.com/group/PsoriaticArthritis/

Psoriatic Arthritis Support
http://www.wpunj.edu/icip/pa/

RAYNAUD'S PHENOMENON

Raynaud's & Scleroderma Association
http://www.raynauds.demon.co.uk/

Raynaud's Association
http://www.raynauds.org/index.htm

Raynaud's Foundation
http://members.aol.com/Raynauds/

Yahoo! Health
http://dir.yahoo.com/Health/Diseases_and_
    Conditions/Raynaud_s_Phenomenon/

REITER'S SYNDROME

Arthritis Foundation
http://www.arthritis.org/

Reiter's Information & Support Group Inc.
http://www.risg.org/

Spondylitis Association of America
http://www.spondylitis.org/

RHEUMATOID ARTHRITIS

Arthritis Foundation
http://www.arthritis.org/default.asp

Johns Hopkins Arthritis Presents Information on Rheumatoid Arthritis
http://www.hopkins-arthritis.som.jhmi.edu/
    rheumatoid/rheum.html

Rheumatoid Arthritis Information Network (RAIN)
http://www.healthtalk.com/rain/

Understanding Rheumatoid Arthritis
http://www.arthritissupport.com/understanding/
    rheumatoid/

SARCOIDOSIS

Foundation for Sarcoidosis Research (FSR)
http://www.fightsarcoidosis.org/

Joseph McLaurin Sarcoidosis Website
http://dolphin.upenn.edu/~jmclauri/

National Sarcoidosis Resource Center
http://www.nsrc-global.net/

Sarcoidosis Awareness Webring
http://www.geocities.com/ddplace/sarcwebring.html

Sarcoidosis Center
http://www.sarcoidcenter.com/

Sarcoidosis Online Sites
http://blueflamingo.net/sarcoid/

World Sarcoidosis Society
http://www.worldsarcsociety.com/

SCLERODERMA

I Have Scleroderma
http://www.ihavescleroderma.com/

Juvenile Scleroderma Network
http://www.jsdn.org/

Raynaud's & Scleroderma Association
http://www.raynauds.demon.co.uk/

Scleroderma Foundation
http://www.scleroderma.org/

Scleroderma from A-to-Z
http://www.sclero.org/

Scleroderma Research Foundation
http://www.srfcure.org/

Scleroderma Support
http://sclerodermasupport.com/

SJÖGREN'S SYNDROME

British Sjögren's Syndrome Association
http://ourworld.compuserve.com/homepages/
    bssassociation/

Internet Resources for Sjögren's Syndrome
http://dry.org/welcome.html

Sjögren's Syndrome Foundation
http://www.sjogrens.org

Sjögren's Syndrome New Zealand
http://www.sjogrensnewzealand.co.nz/

Sjögren's Syndrome Online Support
http://www.sjsworld.org/

STIFF-MAN SYNDROME

Stiff-Man Syndrome Discussion List
http://www.stiff-man.org/

BrainTalk Communities—Neurology Support Groups—Stiff-Person Syndrome Forum
http://neuro-mancer.mgh.harvard.edu/cgi-bin/forumdisplay.cgi?action=topics&number=132&SUBMIT=Go

SYSTEMIC LUPUS ERYTHEMATOSUS (SLE)

Lupus Foundation of America
http://www.lupus.org/

Lupus Links
http://www.silcom.com/~sblc/lupuslinks.html

SLE Clinical Trials
http://www.centerwatch.com/patient/studies/cat144.html

SLE Foundation, Inc.
http://www.lupusny.org/

TAKAYASU'S ARTERITIS

Takayasu's Arteritis Association
http://www.takayasus.com/

Takayasu's Arteritis Foundation International
http://www.takayasu.org/

Takayasu's Arteritis Research Association (TARA)
http://www.takayasus.org/

TRANSVERSE MYELITIS

Transverse Myelitis Association
http://www.myelitis.org/

Transverse Myelitis Bulletin Board
http://www.escribe.com/health/tmic/bb/

ULCERATIVE COLITIS

Australian Crohn's & Colitis Association (ACCA)
http://www.acca.net.au/

Crohn's & Colitis Foundation of America
http://www.ccfa.org/

Living With Ulcerative Colitis
http://www.living-better.com/

National Association for Colitis and Crohn's Disease (NACC)
http://www.nacc.org.uk/

Yahoo! Health
http://dir.yahoo.com/Health/Diseases_and_Conditions/Crohn_s_Disease_and_Ulcerative_Colitis/

UVEITIS

Uveitis and Immunology Service at Massachusetts Eye and Ear Infirmary
http://www.uveitis.org/

Uveitis and Other Eye Conditions
http://www.unykornz.com/uveitis/

Uveitis Information Group
http://www.uveitis.net/

Uveitis Support Online
http://www.geocities.com/uveitisonline/

VASCULITIS

Johns Hopkins Vasculitis Center
http://vasculitis.med.jhu.edu/

Vasculitis Update
http://www.vasculitis.org/

VITILIGO

American Vitiligo Research Foundation, Inc.
http://www.avrf.org/

National Vitiligo Foundation
http://www.nvfi.org/

Vitiligo.Net
http://www.vitiligo.net/

Vitiligo Society UK
http://www.vitiligosociety.org.uk/

Vitiligo Support
http://www.vitiligosupport.com/

Vitiligo Treatment Clinic
http://www.vitiligo-treatment.com/

WEGENER'S GRANULOMATOSIS

Wegener's Granulomatosis Association
http://www.wgsg.org/

Wegener's Granulomatosis Site
http://www.angelfire.com/ga/wegeners/

Wegeners Granulomatosis Support Group of Australia
http://users.netcon.net.au/ttp/content1.htm

Wegener's Granulomatosis Support Group of Canada
http://www.wgsg.ca/

APPENDIX VI
MEDICATIONS COMMONLY USED TO TREAT RHEUMATOID ARTHRITIS

Medications	Examples	Uses/Effects	Side Effects	Monitoring
Aspirin and other nonsteroidal anti-inflammatory drugs (NSAIDs)	Plain aspirin Buffered aspirin Ibuprofen (Advil,* Motrin IB) Ketoprofen (Orudis) Naproxen (Naprosyn) Celecoxib (Celebrex) Rofecoxib (Vioxx)	Used to reduce pain, swelling, and inflammation, allowing patients to move more easily and carry out normal activities Generally part of early and continuing therapy	Upset stomach Tendency to bruise easily Fluid retention (NSAIDs other than aspirin) Ulcers Possible kidney and liver damage (rare)	Patients should have periodic blood tests
Disease-modifying antirheumatic drugs (DMARDs) (also called slow-acting antirheumatic drugs [SAARDs] or second-line drugs)	Gold, injectable or oral (Myochrysine, Ridaura) Antimalarials, such as hydroxychloroquine (Plaquenil) Penicillamine (Cuprimine, Depen) Sulfasalazine (Azulfidine)	Used to alter the course of the disease and prevent joint and cartilage destruction May produce significant improvement for many patients Exactly how they work still unknown Generally take a few weeks or months to have an effect Patients may use several over the course of the disease	Toxicity is an issue DMARDs can have serious side effects: Gold—skin rash, mouth sores, upset stomach, kidney problems, low blood count Antimalarials—upset stomach, eye problems (rare) Penicillamine—skin rashes, upset stomach, blood abnormalities, kidney problems Sulfasalazine—upset stomach	Patients should be monitored carefully for continued effectiveness of medication and for side effects: Gold—blood and urine test monthly, more often in early use of drug Antimalarials—eye exam every six months Penicillamine—blood and urine test monthly more often in early use of drug Sulfasalazine—periodic blood and urine tests
Immunosuppressants (also considered DMARDs)	Methotrexate (Rheumatrex) Azathioprine (Imuran) Cyclosporine (Sandimmune, Neoral) Leflunomide (Arava)	Used to restrain the overly active immune system, which is key to the disease process Same concerns as with other DMARDs: Potential toxicity and diminishing effectiveness over time Methotrexate can result in rapid improvement, appears to be very effective	Toxicity is an issue immunosuppressants can have serious side effects: Methotrexate—upset stomach, potential liver problems, low white blood cell count Azathioprine—potential blood abnormalities, low white blood cell count, possible increased cancer risk	Patients should be carefully monitored for continued effectiveness of medication and for side effects: Methotrexate—regular blood tests, including liver function test, baseline chest X ray

Medications	Examples	Uses/Effects	Side Effects	Monitoring
		Azathioprine—first used in higher doses in cancer chemotherapy and organ transplantation, used in patients who have not responded to other drugs, used in combination therapy Cyclosporine—first used in organ transplantation to prevent rejection used in patients who have not responded to other drugs Leflunomide—reduces signs and symptoms as well as retards structural damage to joints caused by arthritis	Cyclosporine—high blood pressure, hair growth, tremors, loss of kidney function Leflunomide—diarrhea, skin rashes, hair loss, liver problems	Azathioprine—regular blood and liver function tests Cyclosporine—regular blood tests, including kidney function, and blood pressure Leflunomide—regular blood tests, including liver function tests
Corticosteroids (also known as glucocorticoids)	Prednisone (Deltasone, Orasone) Methylprednisolone (Medrol)	Used for their anti-inflammatory and immuno-suppressive effects Given either in pill form or as an injection into a joint Dramatic improvements in a very short time Potential for serious side effects, especially at high doses Often used early while waiting for DMARDs to work Also used for severe flares and when the disease does not respond to NSAIDs and DMARDs	Osteoporosis Mood changes Fragile skin, easy bruising Fluid retention Weight gain Muscle weakness Onset or worsening of diabetes Cataracts Increased risk of infection Hypertension (high blood pressure)	Patients should be monitored carefully for continued effectiveness of medication and for side effects
Biologic Response Modifiers	Etanercept (Enbrel)	Effective in patients with mild-to-moderate rheumatoid arthritis who have failed other drug therapies and, in addition, in patients with juvenile rheumatoid arthritis Given as a twice-a-week injection into the skin	Skin reactions at injection sites Headaches	Patients should be monitored closely for signs of infection

*Brand names included in this table are provided as examples only, and their inclusion does not mean that these products are endorsed by the National Institutes of Health or any other government agency. Also, if a particular brand name is not mentioned, this does not mean or imply that the product is unsatisfactory.

Source: National Institute of Arthritis and Musculoskeletal and Skin Diseases, Information Clearinghouse, NIAMS/National Institutes of Health

APPENDIX VII
PATIENT RESEARCH REGISTRIES

ALOPECIA AREATA

National Alopecia Areata Registry
University of Texas M.D. Anderson Cancer Center
Houston, TX
Principal Investigator: Dr. Madeleine Duvic
Registry Contact: Madeleine Duvic, M.D.
(713) 792-5999
(713) 794-1491 (Fax)
alopeciaregistry@mdanderson.org

> *This registry aims to seek out and classify medical and family history data for patients with three major forms of alopecia areata: alopecia areata, alopecia totalis, and alopecia universalis. Families with multiple affected members will be especially helpful to further research studies. The project will offer a future central information source where researchers can obtain statistical data associated with the disease.*

ANKYLOSING SPONDYLITIS

North American Spondylitis Consortium
University of Texas-Houston Health
   Science Center
Houston, TX
Principal Investigator: Dr. John D. Reveille
Registry Contact: Spondylitis Association of America
   Family Genetic Research Project
(888) 777-1594 (Toll free)

> *The consortium hopes to learn more about genes that play a role in the disease. They plan to collect medical information and genetic material (DNA) from 400 families nationwide in which two or more siblings have AS. Through genetic typing methods, researchers will search for genes that may contribute to a predisposition of AS. They also hope to identify, from newly mapped candidate genes, mutations and their effect on disease severity.*

ANTIPHOSPHOLIPID SYNDROME

**National Registry on Antiphospholipid
   Syndrome**
University of North Carolina
Chapel Hill, NC
Principal Investigator: Dr. Robert Roubey
Registry Contact: Robert A.S. Roubey, M.D.
(919) 966-0572
apscore@med.unc.edu

> *This registry will collect and update clinical, demographic, and laboratory information from patients with antiphospholipid syndrome (APS) and make it available to researchers and medical practitioners concerned with diagnosis and treatment. Registry scientists will collect data on patients with clinical signs of APS and on asymptomatic individuals who have antibodies but have not yet developed any clinical signs.*

FIBROMYALGIA

Fibromyalgia Family Study Registry
Case Western Reserve University
Cleveland, OH
Principal Investigator: Dr. Jane Olson
Registry Contact: Dr. Jane Olson
(216) 778-4589
ffs@darwin.cwru.edu

> *This research registry is aimed at the collection of multicase fibromyalgia syndrome (FMS) pedigrees. It involves the collection and validation of clinical, demographic, and laboratory data on FMS patients from families with at least two FMS-affected individuals and their family members. DNA is also being collected, stored, and genotyped so that that genetic linkage studies may be performed. Families are eligible for participation in this study if at least two closely related family members have FMS and if at least one of these has no other major rheumatologic disease.*

GENETICS OF RHEUMATOID ARTHRITIS REGISTRY

North Shore University Hospital
Manhasset, NY
Principal Investigator: Dr. Peter K. Gregersen
Registry Contact: Dr. Peter Gregersen
(800) 382-4827
narac@nshs.edu
www.medicine.ucsf.edu/divisions/rheum/narac

This is a national registry and repository dedicated to the collection and characterization of sibling pairs with rheumatoid arthritis (RA). The goal of the registry is to collect at least 1,000 families in which two or more siblings are affected with rheumatoid arthritis. The underlying scientific goal is to search for genes that predispose individuals to rheumatoid arthritis with the ultimate goal of understanding the cause of this disease, leading to better diagnosis and treatments. Each participant with rheumatoid arthritis is visited by a study coordinator at his or her doctor's office or other location convenient for the participant. An interview and brief physical exam will be performed, and a blood specimen obtained. In addition, a hand X ray will be done if one has not been taken within the last two years. Blood samples will be requested from the parents (if available) of the participating rheumatoid arthritis patients. As of May 2000, over 750 families have agreed to participate in this study. For a family to participate in the study, the following criteria must be met:

Two or more siblings with rheumatoid arthritis in the family
At least one sibling with documented erosions on hand X rays
At least one sibling with onset of rheumatoid arthritis between the ages of 18 and 60.

JUVENILE RHEUMATOID ARTHRITIS

Research Registry for Juvenile Rheumatoid Arthritis (JRA)
Children's Hospital Medical Center
Cincinnati, OH
Principal Investigator: Dr. David N. Glass
Co-Principal Investigator: Dr. Edward Giannini
Registry Contact: Edith Shear
(800) 559-7011
(513) 636-5990 (Fax)

The primary objective of the Juvenile Rheumatoid Arthritis Registry is the continued support of the

registry function with a focus on multicase families with affected sibling pairs and the development of a related genomics program to identify all of the genes for susceptibility. DNA will be obtained and stored on all registry patients and family members. Genome-wide screening will be carried out on the DNA in conjunction with collaborators from Stanford and Wake Forest Universities.

LUPUS

Lupus Registry and Repository
Oklahoma Medical Research Foundation
Oklahoma City, OK
Principal Investigator: Dr. John Harley
Registry Contact: John B. Harley, M.D., Ph.D.
(888) 655-8787
(405) 271-3045 (Fax)
john-harley@omrf.ouhsc.edu
www.omrf.ouhsc.edu/lupus

The objective of this registry is to support a core facility dedicated to the collection and characterization of multiplex lupus pedigrees. Clinical information, genotypes at over 300 loci, and family relationships structure are available from 102 pedigrees containing 592 family members. An additional 25 pedigrees are made available each succeeding year. Limited amounts of DNA, plasma, and serum are also available from these pedigrees. Investigators interested in using these data or materials should visit the website and/or contact Dr. Harley (Oklahoma Medical Research Foundation, 825 N.E. 13th Street, Oklahoma City, OK 73104).

RHEUMATOID ARTHRITIS

Rheumatoid Arthritis in African Americans Registry
University of Alabama
Birmingham, AL
Principal Investigator: Dr. Larry Moreland
Registry Contact:
Tina Parkhill
(205) 934-9368
tina.parkhill@ccc.uab.edu
or
Fannie Johnson, R.N.
(205) 934-7427
205-975-5554 (Fax)
fannie.johnson@ccc.uab.edu

This registry, Consortium for the Longitudinal Evaluations of African Americans with Early Rheumatoid

Arthritis (CLEAR), aims to collect clinical data, X-ray data, and DNA to help scientists analyze genetic and nongenetic factors that might predict disease course and outcomes of rheumatoid arthritis. Academic centers in the southeast United States will recruit African Americans to join the registry.

SCLERODERMA

Scleroderma Registry
Wayne State University
Detroit, MI
Principal Investigator: Dr. Maureen Mayes
Registry Contact: Dr. Maureen D. Mayes

(313) 966-7777
(313) 966-7778 (Fax)
www.tir.com/~silonet/homepage/semsf/registry.htm
The aim of the registry is to identify cases of systemic sclerosis; verify all diagnoses; establish a computer database; provide a continuous update of the prevalence, incidence, and mortality rates of scleroderma in this population; and establish prospectively the average annual mortality. A major focus of the registry is to establish a cohort of incident cases for early intervention trials and genetic studies as well as for basic science and other clinical and epidemiological studies.

Source: National Institute of Arthritis and Musculoskeletal and Skin Diseases

APPENDIX VIII

THE NATIONAL INSTITUTES OF HEALTH (NIH) INVESTMENT IN RESEARCH ON AUTOIMMUNE DISEASES

During the last two decades of the 20th century, intensive and highly productive research on the immune system resulted in a wealth of new information and extraordinary growth in conceptual understanding. These accomplishments now provide promising opportunities for major advances in the diagnosis, treatment, and prevention of autoimmune diseases. The National Institutes of Health (NIH) stands at the forefront of many of these accomplishments. Because autoimmune diseases span many organ systems and clinical disciplines, multiple NIH institutes, offices, and centers support research in this area in collaboration with a wide range of professional and patient advocacy organizations. NIH has placed a high priority on coordination to ensure the effective participation of public and private organizations and the efficient use of research resources.

To facilitate collaboration among those NIH components, other federal agencies, and private organizations with an interest in autoimmune diseases, the NIH established the Autoimmune Diseases Coordinating Committee in 1998, under the direction of the National Institute of Allergy and Infectious Diseases. Since its inception, the Committee has analyzed a wide range of ongoing and planned research programs and has developed cross-cutting initiatives to address key aspects of autoimmunity. In addition, the Committee has established work groups to foster scientific collaborations and to develop research initiatives in a variety of promising areas, including new therapeutic approaches such as the induction of immune tolerance, disease pre-vention, and the role of gender, genetics, infectious agents, and environmental factors in disease susceptibility, onset, and progression.

AUTOIMMUNE DISEASES COORDINATING COMMITTEE

NIH INSTITUTES, CENTERS, AND OFFICES

The National Institute of Allergy and Infectious Diseases (NIAID) conducts and supports research to elucidate the etiopathology of all autoimmune diseases and to develop new approaches to prevent and treat these immune-mediated diseases.

The National Institute of Arthritis and Musculoskeletal and Skin Diseases (NIAMS) conducts and supports research into the causes, treatment, and prevention of autoimmune components of rheumatic and skin diseases; the training of basic and clinical scientists to carry out this research; and the dissemination of information on research progress in these diseases.

The National Cancer Institute (NCI) conducts and supports autoimmunity research in paraneoplastic syndromes, in which autoimmune diseases are symptoms of an underlying malignancy, and in the deliberate induction of tumor-specific autoimmune responses for immunotherapeutic approaches to the treatment and cure of cancer.

The National Institute of Child Health and Human Development (NICHD) conducts and supports research in the prevention and treatment of Type 1 diabetes and in the reproductive sciences including premature ovarian failure of autoimmune etiology and uterine changes that occur in women with autoimmunity.

The National Institute on Deafness and Other Communication Disorders (NIDCD) conducts and supports research in the impact of autoimmune diseases on hearing, balance, smell, taste, voice, speech, and language.

The National Institute of Dental and Craniofacial Research (NIDCR) conducts and supports research in autoimmune diseases of the oral cavity, such as Sjögren's syndrome.

The National Institute of Diabetes and Digestive and Kidney Diseases (NIDDK) has broad interests in the area of autoimmunity and autoimmune diseases, including endocrine diseases, such as Type 1 diabetes and thyroiditis; digestive track and nutritional diseases, such as inflammatory bowel disease, celiac disease, primary biliary cirrhosis, and other autoimmune liver diseases; and kidney and blood/bone diseases, such as glomerulonephritis. A new "joint" branch within NIDDK, the Navy/NIDDK Transplant and Autoimmunity Branch, will study autoimmune pathogenesis of Type 1 diabetes and perform translational research leading to islet transplants for Type 1 diabetics.

The National Institute on Drug Abuse (NIDA) supports more than 85 percent of the world's research on health aspects of drug abuse and addiction. It also supports research on infections, including HIV/AIDS, and associated medical and health consequences, including immunosuppression in drug users. Research areas within NIDA's mission include the effects of drug abuse in patients with rheumatoid arthritis, diabetes-related metabolic disorders, lupus, and other autoimmune disorders.

The National Institute of Environmental Health Sciences (NIEHS) conducts and supports research to elucidate the role of environmental factors in the etiopathology of autoimmune diseases.

The National Eye Institute (NEI) conducts and supports autoimmunity research in immunosuppression, tolerance, anterior chamber-associated immune deviation, ocular complications from autoimmune diseases, and autoimmune uveitis.

The National Heart, Lung, and Blood Institute (NHLBI) supports investigations of the contribution of autoimmunity to diseases under its purview and in transfusion medicine and the use of autoimmune reagents and responses in disease diagnosis, treatment, and prevention.

The National Institute of Mental Health (NIMH) conducts and supports research in the contribution of central nervous system autoimmunity to the development of neuropsychiatric and behavioral disorders, such as autism, bulimia nervosa, and pediatric autoimmune neuropsychiatric disorders (PANDAS).

The National Institute of Neurological Disorders and Stroke (NINDS) conducts and supports research in autoimmune disorders of nerve and muscle such as multiple sclerosis, acute and chronic neurodegenerative diseases involving inflammatory mechanisms, and the impact of autoimmunity on the blood-brain barrier.

The National Institute of Nursing Research (NINR) supports research of establish a scientific basis for the care of individuals across the life span—from management of patients during illness and recovery to the reduction of risks for disease and disability and the promotion of healthy lifestyles. Research extends to problems encountered by patients, families, and caregivers and emphasizes the special needs of at-risk and underserved populations. Autoimmunity research aims to develop strategies to promote self-management, cope with chronic illness, promote adherence to treatment, and prevent complications in conditions such as diabetes, rheumatoid arthritis, and irritable bowel syndrome.

The Fogarty International Center (FIC) promotes international cooperation in biomedical sciences by encouraging collaboration between U.S. and foreign scientists.

The National Center for Research Resources (NCRR) provides a comprehensive range of resources and technologies to support biomedical research. Scientists use these resources to better understand, prevent, and treat autoimmune diseases.

The Office of Research on Women's Health (ORWH) works with the NIH Institutes and Centers to ensure that NIH-supported research focuses on issues important to women's health, to ensure that women and minorities are included in NIH-supported clinical research, and to enhance career opportunities for women in biomedical research.

FEDERAL AGENCIES

The **U.S. Food and Drug Administration (FDA)** regulates biological products, including blood, vaccines, therapeutics, and related drugs and devices, according to statutory authorities; assures that safe and effective drugs are available to Americans; ensures the safety and effectiveness of medical devices; and eliminates unnecessary human exposure to human-made radiation from medical, occupational, and consumer products.

The Office of Research and Development at the **U.S. Department of Veterans Affairs (VA)** National Headquarters improves the effectiveness, efficiency, and accessibility of health care services for veterans by supporting research on the pathology, diagnosis, and treatment of autoimmune diseases.

PRIVATE ORGANIZATIONS

The **American Autoimmune Related Diseases Association (AARDA)** is a nonprofit organization that fosters and facilitates collaboration in education, public awareness, research, patient services, information dissemination, and research in all autoimmune diseases.

The **American College of Rheumatology (ACR),** a nonprofit organization of physicians, health professionals, and scientists, advances rheumatology through programs of education, research, and advocacy and fosters excellence in the care of people with rheumatic and musculoskeletal diseases.

The **Crohn's and Colitis Foundation of America (CCFA)** is a nonprofit research organization that seeks the cause of and cure for Crohn's disease and ulcerative colitis, collectively known as inflammatory bowel disease.

The **National Multiple Sclerosis Society (NMSS),** a nonprofit organization, researches the cause and impact of MS and seeks to identify effective preventions, treatments, and a cure for this disease by obtaining and applying scientifically gathered basic, clinical, and health services knowledge.

The **Sjögren's Syndrome Foundation** is a nonprofit organization that educates patients, their families, the public, and health care providers about Sjögren's syndrome and encourages research for new treatments and a cure for this disease.

The **Systemic Lupus Erythematosus Foundation,** a nonprofit organization, seeks the cause, improved treatment, and a cure for lupus by funding medical research and providing services to assist patients, families, and friends.

MAJOR RESEARCH PROGRAMS BY THEMATIC AREAS

The development of autoimmune diseases reflects complex interactions between the immune system, genetic background, and environmental factors. Therefore, NIH-supported research is broad in scope, ranging from understanding the determinants of disease to developing effective therapies and strategies for preventing disease. The members of the NIH Autoimmune Diseases Coordinating Committee code the research that they support according to the thematic areas of *therapeutics, prevention, genetics, infectious agents and environmental factors; pathogenesis and immune dysfunction; epidemiology and risk factors; organ specificity; animal models; nursing; behavioral and health services research;* and *research resources.* Within this framework, NIH Institutes, Centers, and Offices and nonfederal partners coordinate efforts through research partnerships, sponsorship of workshops, and establishment of databases and other research resources accessible to the research community.

THERAPEUTICS

The NIH investment in basic research has yielded the knowledge necessary to develop new therapeutic strategies for the treatment of immune-mediated diseases. These preclinical research advances have provided an impetus for established pharmaceutical and emerging biotechnology companies to develop novel agents that may more selectively inhibit the deleterious immune responses in autoimmune diseases. The NIH is capitalizing on these advances through increased sponsorship of clinical trials, often in partnership with industry. Major ongoing and new clinical research programs include the following:

- **Immune Tolerance Network** The successful induction of immune tolerance is a major therapeutic goal for the treatment of many immune-mediated diseases. Tolerogenic approaches seek to modulate or block deleterious immune responses critical in the development and progression of disease and in the rejection of transplanted organs, tissues, and cells. In 1998, NIAID published a long-term research plan to accelerate the study of immune tolerance, particularly in the clinical setting (http://www.niaid.nih.gov/publications/immune/contents.htm). A major new clinical research program emanating from this research plan was established in September 1999, under the joint sponsorship of NIAID, the National Institute of Diabetes and Digestive and Kidney Diseases (NIDDK), and the JDFI. This unique consortium of more than 40 institutions in the United States, Canada, western Europe, and Australia is dedicated to the clinical evaluation of promising tolerance induction therapies in four areas: kidney transplantation, islet transplantation for Type 1 diabetes, autoimmune disorders, and asthma and allergic diseases (http://www.immunetolerance.org). The network will also develop assays and biomarkers to measure the induction, maintenance, and loss of immune tolerance in humans. Various clinical studies are in development for many autoimmune diseases, including MS, RA, Type 1 diabetes, and SLE.

- **Stem Cell Transplantation for the Treatment of Autoimmune Diseases** Stem cell transplantation is currently under evaluation for treatment of multiple autoimmune diseases. Several studies of safety have been completed; however, case-controlled studies of efficacy have not yet been conducted. In FY 1999, NIH initiated a coordinated research effort to study the safety and effectiveness of these treatment regimens for several autoimmune disorders.

- **Pilot Clinical Trials on Innovative Therapies for Rheumatic and Skin Diseases** This research initiative was implemented in FY 1999, under the leadership of the National Institute of Arthritis and Musculoskeletal and Skin Diseases (NIAMS), with several NIH Institutes, to develop innovative therapies for the treatment of rheumatic and skin diseases. Awards were made for research on the following diseases: Wegener's granulomatosis, RA, scleroderma, SLE, and ankylosing spondylitis (AS).

- **Autoimmunity Centers of Excellence** Four research centers were established in FY 1999 to support collaborative basic and clinical research on autoimmune diseases, including single-site or multisite clinical trials of immunomodulatory therapies. The centers bring together many different subspecialists (e.g., neurologists, gastroenterologists, and rheumatologists), as well as basic scientists, increasing clinical and research collaborations in autoimmunity.

- **Clinical Trials and Clinical Markers in Immunologic Diseases** In FY 2000, NIAID with several NIH components began a new research program focused on orphan clinical trials of immunomodulatory treatments for immune-mediated diseases, including autoimmune disorders, and the development of biological markers to measure disease activity, risk, and therapeutic effect.

- **Hyperaccelerated Awards for Mechanistic Studies of Immune Disease Trials** This existing research program supports mechanistic studies in conjunction with clinical trials of immunomodulatory interventions for immune-mediated diseases. Multiple NIH Institutes, Centers, and Offices are cosponsoring this program, which incorporates expedited procedures for review and award of meritorious great applications within 13 weeks of submission.

- **Cyclophosphamide in Scleroderma Pulmonary Disease** In FY 1999, the National Heart, Lung, and Blood Institute (NHLBI) began an investigator-initiated clinical trial of cyclophosphamide in the treatment of the pulmonary fibrosis associated with systemic sclerosis. In systemic sclerosis, interstitial pulmonary fibrosis is frequent (80 percent) and is now the leading cause of death. The mortality rate of patients with impaired pulmonary function is 40 percent to 45 percent within 10 years of onset.

Uncontrolled studies suggest that cyclophosphamide may stabilize or improve lung function in systemic sclerosis patients. The study is a five-year, 13-center, parallel-group, double-blind, randomized, controlled, phase III clinical trial of oral cyclophosphamide versus placebo to assess the efficacy of cyclophosphamide in stabilizing or improving the course of pulmonary disease in scleroderma. NIAMS also contributes to the support of this study.

- **Human Islet Transplantation into Humans** This program will support clinical studies using new methods to induce immune tolerance to prevent recurrence of the autoimmune destruction of beta cells in the islet and to prevent transplant rejection. The NIDDK, NIAID, and JDFI support this program.
- **New Strategies for the Treatment of Type 1 Diabetes** In FY 2000, the NIDDK, NIAID, and National Institute of Child Health and Development (NICHD) began a new program supporting clinical studies to test new approaches to treat Type 1 diabetes, including studies of immunomodulation.

PREVENTION

Knowledge of the genetic and environmental determinants of disease, coupled with a better understanding of human immunology, will provide the basis for the development of preventive approaches. Prevention or delay of disease onset for certain autoimmune diseases has been demonstrated in animal models.

- **Diabetes Prevention Trial—Type 1** Under the sponsorship of the NIDDK, NIAID, NICHD, CDC, JDFI, and the American Diabetes Association (ADA), this national multisite cooperative clinical trial is evaluating the use of parenteral and oral insulin for prevention of Type 1 diabetes in high-risk and intermediate-risk relatives of patients with Type 1 diabetes.
- **Basic Immunology Vaccine Research Centers** In FY 2000, NIAID established a new research program to support fundamental research relevant to the design and development of improved vaccines for immunologic and infectious diseases. This effort will enable the application of basic immunologic principles to the rational design of prevention strategies.

GENETICS

Certain autoimmune diseases have been linked to a particular set of genes called the major histocompatibility complex (MHC), known to be important in controlling immune responses. Recent findings suggest that other families of genes that regulate immune responses may be involved in the pathogenesis of autoimmune diseases.

- **North American Rheumatoid Arthritis Consortium** In FY 1997, the North American Rheumatoid Arthritis Consortium was established as part of a collaborative effort among NIAID, NIAMS, and the Arthritis Foundation (AF). Through this consortium, a registry and repository of clinical and genetic data has been developed as a research resource for the discovery of RA susceptibility genes.
- **Multiple Autoimmune Diseases Genetics Consortium** Under this FY 1999 research initiative, a repository of genetic and clinical data and samples is being developed from families in which two or more individuals are affected by two or more autoimmune diseases. This resource will promote research to advance the discovery of human immune response genes involved in autoimmunity.
- **Functional Genomics of the Developing Pancreas** This NIDDK research initiative will support the production, sequencing, and distribution of cDNA libraries for discovery and functional studies of genes regulating development of the normal and diabetic pancreas.
- **International Histocompatibility Working Group (IHWG)** The National Cancer Institute (NCI), NHLBI, NIDDK, and NIAID support the IHWG to develop, standardize, and distribute highly sensitive reagents for tissue typing worldwide. These efforts enhance identification of healthy individuals at risk for development of autoimmune disorders and ensure that transplant recipients will receive optimally matched donor organs and tissues.
- **North American Spondylitis Consortium** NIAMS established this consortium in FY 1999

to identify susceptibility genes for AS, a rare but painful disease of the spine primarily affecting men. Ten research centers and the Spondylitis Association of America are participating in this activity.

- **Juvenile Rheumatoid Arthritis Study** NIAMS expanded this registry in FY 1999 to collect DNA and to identify susceptibility genes for juvenile rheumatoid arthritis.

- **Lupus Registries and Repository** NIAMS established a registry and repository to collect clinical data and samples from patients with SLE and their families. This resource should assist investigators in identifying genes that determine susceptibility to lupus. A separate Registry for Neonatal Lupus will enhance the search for basic defects in neonatal lupus and may lead to improved diagnosis, treatment, and prevention methods. This registry also supported by NIAMS.

- **Vitiligo Genetic Linkage Project** Vitiligo is an autoimmune disease resulting in patchy depigmentation of the skin, which is particularly disfiguring in dark-skinned individuals. The aggregation of the disease in families is being utilized by Dr. Richard Spritz at the University of Colorado to map the vitiligo gene(s) in a U.S. and a United Kingdom cohort of vitiligo families. This project is supported by NIAMS.

INFECTIOUS AGENTS AND ENVIRONMENTAL FACTORS

A growing body of research concerns the role of infectious agents in triggering certain chronic diseases, including autoimmune disorders. Recently, several mechanisms have been proposed for this association and have proven to be operative in animal models.

- **Environmental/Infectious/Genetic Interactions in Autoimmune Disease** In FY 1999, under the leadership of the National Institute of Environmental Health Sciences (NIEHS) with multiple collaborating NIH Institutes, Centers, and Offices, a research program was established to support innovative studies to elucidate the role of environmental and infectious agents in autoimmune diseases and to clarify their interaction with genes in modulating immune res-

ponses. Enhanced knowledge in this area will contribute to the discovery of new therapeutic and preventive strategies.

- **Carolina Lupus Study** The NIEHS Division of Intramural Research supports the Carolina Lupus Study to identify the role of infectious agents and environmental exposures in the development of lupus, with a particular focus on African-American women, who are disproportionately affected by this disease.

PATHOGENESIS AND IMMUNE DYSFUNCTION

Research in this area focuses on understanding the disease process, particularly the defects in the immune response that cause the body to attack its own tissues and cells.

- **Diabetes Centers of Excellence** This continuation of a long-standing basic research program is supported jointly by the NIDDK, NIAID, and JDFI and focuses on increasing understanding of the fundamental disease processes and mechanisms involved in diabetes. A majority of the projects supported under this program address Type 1 diabetes.

- **NIAID-JDFI Interdisciplinary Programs in Autoimmunity** Five multidisciplinary projects are supported under this program to investigate the molecular, immunologic, and genetic mechanisms in the pathogenesis of autoimmunity.

- **Human Immunology Centers of Excellence** In FY 1999, NIAID established four new research centers focused on multidisciplinary approaches to define the mechanisms responsible for normal and pathologic human immune responses.

- **Innovative Research on Human Mucosal Immunity** The CCFA joined NIAID and the National Institute of Dental and Craniofacial Research (NIDCR) in sponsoring this FY 2000 research initiative to promote innovative investigations of the human mucosal immune system and its role in the pathogenesis of autoimmune diseases, including IBD.

- **Innovative Research on Immune Tolerance** NIAID and NIDDK cosponsor this initiative to support innovative research on mechanisms underlying long-term immune tolerance and to identify novel targets for future drug development. These projects began in FY 2001.

- **Diabetes and Endrocrinology Research Centers and Diabetes Research Training Centers** A portion of these centers supports basic and clinical research on Type 1 diabetes and other autoimmune diseases.
- **Veterans Administration (VA) Medical Centers** Basic and clinical research on autoimmune diseases is supported by the VA Medical Research Service through merit review grants. A distinctive feature of VA-sponsored research is the high proportion of medical doctorate investigators supported at VA Medical Centers across the United States.

EPIDEMIOLOGY AND RISK FACTORS

The incidence and prevalence of some autoimmune diseases appear to be increased in certain ethnic groups; for example, SLE, RA, and MS are increased in African-American, certain Native-American, and Caucasian populations, respectively. For many autoimmune diseases, relatively little is known about natural history preceding the onset of overt disease or about the genetic, behavioral, and environmental factors that contribute to disease progression. An expanded knowledge base in these areas would facilitate the design, implementation, and evaluation of prevention efforts.

- **DAISY (Diabetes Autoimmunity Study in the Young)** This long-term study, supported by NIDDK and NIAID, includes collection and follow-up of two cohorts: (1) healthy siblings and offspring of people with Type 1 diabetes and (2) healthy newborns with Type 1 diabetes-associated MHC genes but without a family history of diabetes. The study is collecting and analyzing data on infections, vaccination, diet, MHC genes, and autoantibodies to beta cell antigens in these cohorts.

ORGAN SPECIFICITY

Research in this area seeks to explain why the immune attack is limited to a specific organ in some autoimmune diseases (e.g., the central nervous system in MS), whereas in others, the tissue injury is widespread (e.g., SLE). Recent findings suggest that the target organ may play a more active role than previously thought in molding the tissue-specific immune responses.

- **Target Organ Damage in Autoimmune Diseases** Under the leadership of NIAMS, multiple NIH components, including NIAID, NIDCR, NIDDK, NHLBI, National Eye Institute (NEI), National Institute of Neurological Disorders and Stroke (NINDS), National Institute on Deafness and Communication Disorders (NIDCD), National Institute of Mental Health (NIMH), and Office of Research on Women's Health (ORWH), developed a FY 1999 research initiative to stimulate innovative and multidisciplinary studies of the involvement of target organs in autoimmune diseases. Knowledge gained in this area will make it possible to construct a more comprehensive picture of disease pathogenesis and will provide a scientific basis for new therapeutic interventions.

ANIMAL MODELS

The development of improved animal models will enhance studies in all of the above areas. In particular, models that more faithfully mimic human disease are essential in the preclinical evaluation of new therapeutic approaches and the application of such approaches in the clinical setting.

- **Nonhuman Primate Transplant Tolerance Cooperative Study Group** In FY 1998 and FY 1999, NIAID and NIDDK established this cooperative research program to evaluate the safety and efficacy of promising tolerance induction treatment regimens in nonhuman primate models of kidney and islet transplantation. The knowledge gained from this research effort will be critical to moving tolerance induction strategies into clinical trials.
- **Immunological Phenotyping of Mouse Mutants** In FY 1999, the National Center for Research Resources (NCRR) joined NIAID, NEI, NIEHS, NHLBI, NIDDK, and ORWH to cosponsor the development of new technologies for rapid immunologic screening of normal and mutagenized mice. These efforts will enable the detection and characterization of abnormal immune responses, with an emphasis on immune dysfunction associated with autoimmune diseases.

- **NIH Autoimmune Rat Model Repository and Development Center** This collaborative effort of multiple NIH Institutes organized by NIAMS and the NIH Office of Research Services' Veterinary Resources Program will develop and make available to researchers genetically characterized and disease-free laboratory rats for autoimmune disease research.

NURSING, BEHAVIORAL, AND HEALTH SERVICES RESEARCH

Quality of life can be severely compromised for those suffering from autoimmune diseases. The NIH supports a variety of unsolicited research, intervention, and education programs aimed at improving disease management and quality of life for patients with chronic illness, their families, and their caregivers. To promote the recruitment and development of health care professionals who treat patients with chronic illnesses, the NIH supports training programs and scientific and professional meetings in this area.

- **General Clinical Research Centers (GCRC)** The GCRCs, a NCRR-supported resource for clinical research, study the effect of stress, mood, and pain on disease pathology and develop new strategies to monitor disease activity and novel approaches for management of disease. Programs include Intensive Therapy for Youth with IDDM (insulin-dependent diabetes mellitus) at Washington University, St. Louis, MO; Biobehavioral Model of Stress and Multiple Sclerosis at the University of Pittsburgh, PA; and Psychosocial Aspects of Scleroderma at the University of California, San Diego.

- **Adolescent Diabetes Control and Quality of Life Improved by Combining Intensive Diabetes Therapy With Coping Skills Training** Interventions to improve metabolic control and quality of life in children with diabetes are of critical importance to reduce or prevent the onset of a number of long-term complications, e.g., blindness, heart disease, stroke, kidney failure, amputations, and nerve damage. National Institute of Nursing Research (NINR)-funded research is determining whether a coping skills training program, in conjunction with intensive

therapy, will enhance quality of life, increase metabolic control (which is extremely difficult to control in diabetic children), and reduce adverse diabetes events in adolescents. An NIH clinical trial has shown that intensive diabetes therapy can reduce the number and severity of diabetes complications in adolescents and young adults.

RESEARCH RESOURCES

Research resources include support for the training of basic and clinical researchers and a broad range of equipment and infrastructure needs.

- **JDFI Islet Production Network** The JDFI supports seven institutions in the United States and western Europe to produce islet cells for research. As part of the foundation's cosponsorship of the Immune Tolerance Network, islets for clinical trials in transplantation for Type 1 diabetes are being provided to qualified network investigators.

- **NIAID Repository of Transgenic and Gene-Targeted Mutant Mice** NIAID supports a repository of genetically manipulated mice and provides for the importation, verification, cryopreservation, breeding, and distribution of novel strains of transgenic or gene knockout mice for use by the extramural research community. This resource includes mouse models relevant for preclinical studies of autoimmunity.

- **NIAID MHC Tetramer Core Facility** In FY 1998, NIAID established a national facility to provide researchers with peptide-MHC tetrameric molecules for analyzing antigen-specific T cell responses. This methodology replaces and greatly improves upon cumbersome, insensitive, and time-consuming assays. Furthermore, by centralizing the production of these tetramers, reagents can be produced economically and can be made available to investigators at greatly reduced costs. Because T cells are central to virtually all adaptive immune responses, this technology is applicable to studies in many areas, including autoimmune disorders.

- **New Imaging Technologies for Autoimmune Diseases** Under the leadership of NIAID, with cosponsorship of multiple NIH Institutes, a FY 1999 research initiative was started to develop new methods of in vivo imaging of the immune system in small animal models of human autoimmune diseases. The development of high-resolution imaging technologies will provide new, powerful, noninvasive methods to visualize ongoing normal and deleterious immune responses. Further adaptation of high-resolution imaging for use in humans holds promise for noninvasive detection, diagnosis, and monitoring of immunologic diseases and a new approach for evaluating the efficacy of therapies and vaccines.

- **Imaging Pancreatic Beta Cell Mass, Function, or Inflammation** The NIDDK is sponsoring an initiative in FY 2000 to stimulate the development of techniques or reagents leading to the ability to image or otherwise noninvasively detect pancreatic beta cells in vivo and measure their function, mass, or evidence of inflammation.
- **Transplant Registries** NIAID, NCI, and NHLBI support the International Bone Marrow Transplant Registry (IBMTR) and the Autologous Blood and Marrow Transplant Registry (AMBTR). The IBMTR/ABMTR have collected data on blood cell and bone marrow transplantation for more than 20 years from more than 290 institutions worldwide. Studies address questions regarding short- and long-term outcomes in defined patient groups, relevant prognostic factors, the efficacy of different transplant approaches, and the economic impact of bone marrow transplantation. Both registries serve as a national resource for patients and patient advocacy groups, physicians, researchers, and the NIH. These registries have been collecting data on stem cell transplants performed for autoimmune diseases since early 1998.
- **Pancreas Transplant Registry** Supported by the NIDDK, this registry at the University of Minnesota has collected data on nearly 10,000 pancreas transplants from more than 200 institutions. Based on analysis of data from the registry, the Health Care Financing Administration and some third-party payors now cover the costs of pancreas transplants for individuals who are also undergoing kidney transplant as a result of diabetes.

- **Specialized Centers of Research (SCOR)** Currently, NIAMS SCORs are targeted for RA, SLE, and scleroderma, among other diseases. A SCOR brings together basic and clinical researchers to provide mutually supportive research interactions to (1) advance basic research on disease causation and (2) expedite transfer of these advances into clinical applications and improved patient care. Present studies at the SCORs include a focus on the genetics of SLE and scleroderma.

SCIENTIFIC SYMPOSIA, WORKSHOPS, AND PUBLICATIONS

NIH Institutes, Centers, and Offices cosponsor a variety of scientific, programmatic, educational, and informational activities, often in collaboration with nonfederal partners. Recent (FY 1999 and FY 2000) examples include:

- **Infectious Etiologies of Chronic Diseases** This workshop focused on causative roles for infectious agents in chronic disease, e.g., herpes and human papilloma viruses in Kaposi's sarcoma and cervical cancer, respectively. Workshop participants evaluated preliminary data implicating additional agents in chronic disease, including autoimmune diseases, and identified key components and resource needs of a targeted research effort for future discovery of such agents. (NCI, NIAID)
- **Discovery of Human Immune Response Genes** This workshop focused on resource needs (e.g., patient and normal control cohorts, registries, DNA repositories, cDNA, sequencing, and bioinformatics capabilities) to identify, characterize, and determine the functions of novel genes involved in autoimmune disorders. (NIAID, NIH Office of Rare Diseases [ORD])
- **Linking Environmental Agents and Autoimmune Diseases** This workshop defined the state of the art, future directions, and research needs to understand the mechanistic links between environmental agents and development or exacerbation of autoimmune diseases. (NIEHS, NIAMS, NIAID, NIDDK, ORD, ORWH, Environmental Protection Agency, JDFI,

American Autoimmune Related Diseases Association [AARDA])

- **Basic Research Conference of the American College of Rheumatology** For the second year, this meeting has been cosponsored by NIAMS and NIAID. The focus of the 1999 conference, which had a record attendance of approximately 600 participants, was the basic biology of B cells and their role in autoimmune diseases.

- **New Immunotherapies for Autoimmune Diseases** This unique, dual-track symposium highlighted research advances and opportunities in autoimmune diseases for a combined audience of lay and scientific participants. (NIAID, NIEHS, NIAMS, NIDDK, NINDS, ORWH, ORD, AARDA, JDFI, Arthritis Foundation (AF), Crohn's & Colitis Foundation of America [CCFA], Myositis Foundation, Sjögren's Syndrome Foundation, National Pemphigus Foundation)

- **Institute of Medicine (IOM) Study on Safety of Silicone Breast Implants** In 1997, Congress expressed concerns about fragmentation of research on the safety and health effects of silicone and instructed the Department of Health and Human Services (DHHS) to commission an IOM expert review of research on the association of silicone implants with "autoimmune-like" syndromes (http://www.nap.edu/books/0309065321/html/). (NIAMS, NCI, NIAID, ORWH, FDA Office of Women's Health, CDC, DHHS Office of Public Health and Science, DHHS Office of the Assistant Secretary for Science Policy and Evaluation)

- **Second Annual Arthritis Research Conference** This conference brings together the NIH and privately supported trainees and their mentors to highlight ongoing research in rheumatologic diseases. (NIAMS, NIAID, AF, American College of Rheumatology)

- **Workshop on Accelerated Atherosclerosis in Systemic Lupus Erythematosus** The goals of the conference were to (1) identify and establish potential interventions aimed at reducing mortality and morbidity from accelerated atherosclerosis in SLE and (2) identify research opportunities to establish the pathogenesis of accelerated atherosclerosis in SLE. (NIAMS, NHLBI)

- **Neuropsychiatric Manifestations of Systemic Lupus Erythematosus** The goals of the meeting were to (1) address current conceptual and evaluative tools in rheumatology, neurology, psychiatry, and psychology and their applications to the problem of nervous system involvement in SLE and (2) identify research opportunities using the approaches and tools described for the purpose of facilitating diagnosis and treatment of patients with neuropsychiatric manifestations of SLE. (NIAMS)

- **Gene Therapy Approaches for Diabetes and Its Complications** This workshop assessed the current understanding of the pathogenesis of diabetes and its complications and identified strategies that use gene therapy to intervene in the induction and progression of diabetes. Investigators described their results using gene therapy approaches to treat diabetes in both animal models and patients. (NIDDK, NCRR, NIAID, NHLBI, JDFI, ADA)

- **Stem Cells and Pancreatic Development** The objective of this workshop is to bring together investigators from multiple disciplines doing state-of-the-art research in stem cell biology and development biology of the pancreas to develop methods for stimulating growth or regeneration of beta cells. (NIDDK, ADA, JDFI)

OPPORTUNITIES

In the 21st century, there will be unprecedented opportunities to understand autoimmune diseases at the molecular and genetic levels. A major goal of NIH research in this area is to forge a conceptual and mechanism-based understanding that emphasizes features shared among these disorders. This will enable scientists and clinicians to more rapidly translate new knowledge into more effective treatments for a wide range of autoimmune diseases. Many of these opportunities are outlined in detail in the strategic plans of the individual NIH Institutes located on the World Wide Web (http://www.nih.gov). Individually, these plans pave the way for significant scientific and clinical advances in selected areas, many of which are outlined below. Taken together, the continued success of these efforts will require leadership at the federal level and a high degree of coordination at the NIH.

To begin to address these needs, in November 1999, members of the Autoimmune Diseases Coordinating Committee established nine work groups to foster scientific collaborations and to develop research initiatives in the following areas: (1) vaccines for autoimmune diseases, (2) functional genomics of autoimmunity, (3) gender and autoimmunity, (4) autoimmunity across the life span, (5) environment's role in autoimmunity, (6) neuropsychiatric manifestations of SLE, (7) clinical registries for autoimmune diseases, (8) basic and clinical research in scleroderma, and (9) ankylosing spondyloarthropathies. Opportunities in several of these and other highly promising areas include:

IMMUNE TOLERANCE

Tolerance induction is a major therapeutic goal for the three major disease-related areas of modern immunology: autoimmunity, transplantation, and allergy/asthma. Furthermore, understanding the basic processes that control immune recognition will facilitate new approaches to augment protective immunity, including the design of improved vaccines. Thus, findings generated from this research will be highly relevant to many NIH components. In autoimmunity, efforts to induce tolerance have focused largely on oral administration of antigen. To date, it has not been possible to duplicate in humans several very encouraging studies of oral tolerance in animal models. Through the research programs described above and in collaboration with industry, NIH-supported scientists are now poised to explore a variety of other promising approaches, including (1) costimulatory blockade, (2) T cell depleting recombinant immunotoxins, (3) small peptide inhibitors of T cell activation, (4) stem cell transplantation, and (5) gene transfer-based approaches for cytokine modulation. The development of improved animal models, including nonhuman primate models of autoimmune diseases, will be key to the success of these efforts.

IMPROVED DIAGNOSIS AND PATIENT MANAGEMENT

Autoimmune diseases present many complex challenges to the clinician. Prominent among these are the difficulties in establishing a diagnosis early in the course of disease and the lack of surrogate markers to monitor therapy and predict clinical outcomes. Thus, new tools are needed to ensure that the most promising experimental approaches will lead to better clinical outcomes. Examples include technologies for (1) whole body imaging and imaging immune activation at the cellular level in vivo; (2) tracking numbers and functional activation of antigen-specific immune cells; (3) staging disease, measuring responses to therapy, and predicting clinical outcomes; and (4) profiling disease susceptibility through low-cost, high-throughput, sensitive, and specific screening measures suitable for large-scale prevention trials. The NIH is providing the research infrastructures to support these endeavors through repositories, reagent facilities, and a wealth of recently initiated cooperative clinical programs. Examples of the latter include the Autoimmunity Centers of Excellence, the Immune Tolerance Network, Pilot Trials on Innovative Therapies for Rheumatic and Skin Diseases, Clinical Trials and Clinical Markers in Immunologic Diseases, the Immunohistocompatibility Working Group, the Diabetes Prevention Trial-Type 1, and the proposed Diabetes TrialNet.

GENETICS

As the sequencing of the human genome approaches completion, it will be possible to define autoimmune diseases by focusing on individual genes and the proteins they encode. For example, it will be possible to rapidly, systematically, and at low cost determine the functional state of activation of immune cells and target tissues through a variety of DNA-based technologies, such as DNA microarrays. Similarly, advances in these technologies will enable rapid, low-cost profiling to measure the risks of developing disease in healthy individuals. A major challenge for the NIH will be to establish the bioinformatics capacity to link a variety of disease- and organ-specific databases for hypothesis generation and clinical profiling in a cross-disciplinary manner. A number of NIH Institutes are currently collaborating in this area. In particular, the Genetics Working Group of the Autoimmune Diseases Coordinating Committee is exploring options for a common autoimmune disease genetics database to facilitate data mining and identification of overlapping genetic regions controlling autoimmunity. The NIH currently supports the collection of clinical data and samples from families with various autoimmune diseases for use in research studies. Examples include the Multiple Autoimmune Disease Genetics Consortium, North American Rheumatoid Arthritis Consortium, Lupus Registry and Repository, and Juvenile Rheumatoid Arthritis Study.

GENDER AND AUTOIMMUNITY

Autoimmune diseases disproportionately affect women. For certain autoimmune diseases, incidence rates in females are two to nine times higher than in matched male populations. Many of these diseases increase in frequency after puberty or flare during pregnancy, suggesting a role for sex hormones in their pathogenesis. Recent findings of increased numbers of long-lived cells of fetal origin in patients with certain autoimmune diseases, however, suggest the increased female incidence may be related to factors other than hormones. Thus, both hormonal and nonhormonal factors may contribute to gender-based differences in immune responses.

NIAID sponsored a meeting on gender and autoimmunity and recently participated in a task force on sexual dimorphism in autoimmune disease organized by the National Multiple Sclerosis Society, the latter of which resulted in a major review article titled "A Gender Gap in Autoimmunity," published in *Science* in 1999. The ORWH report titled "Agenda for Research on Women's Health for the 21st Century: A Report of the Task Force on NIH Women's Health Research Agenda for the 21st Century" highlighted the importance of determining the differences in the immune responses of men and women. Each of the groups recommended increased support for basic and clinical research on sex-based differences in the immune response. Recently, NIAID and the National Multiple Sclerosis Society have begun discussion of approaches to collaboratively target this important gap in our knowledge, to provide wider visibility of the problem and the opportunities, and to allow increased support for high-quality and relevant gender-based research. Other NIH Institutes,

Centers, and Offices have expressed interest in this effort by joining the Autoimmune Diseases Coordinating Committee work group on gender and autoimmunity.

VACCINES FOR AUTOIMMUNE DISEASES

The 1999 IOM report titled "Vaccines for the 21st Century" identified vaccines for autoimmune diseases as level-one priorities based on potential medical, social, and economic benefits to society. Vaccines for autoimmune diseases will be distinct from vaccines given to generate immunity to infectious agents. Instead, vaccines for autoimmunity will turn off a destructive immune response directed at the body's own tissues. Although there are currently no vaccines against any autoimmune disease, successes in animal models and increased understanding of autoimmunity indicate the feasibility of developing preventive vaccines for these diseases. Distinct vaccines for each disease will likely be required. Whether general population vaccination or targeted vaccines based on genetic risk will be necessary, however, is not clear. NIAID, with its long history of vaccine development for infectious diseases, is aware of the extensive collaboration of academia, government, industry, and the public required for success. Through the Autoimmune Diseases Coordinating Committee, several institutes and organizations are beginning to work toward this goal.

INFECTIOUS AGENTS AND ENVIRONMENTAL FACTORS

Because identical twins are not concordant for development of autoimmune disease, an environmental or infectious factor, in addition to genetic background, may be necessary. Multiple infectious agents have been suggested, but a definitive mechanism or association has been elusive. Recently, animal studies have elucidated several possible mechanisms, and human studies have focused on several particular agents. It is not likely that a single agent will be involved in each disease, but these new leads might elucidate the role of foreign organisms or compounds in the triggering of these diseases. This knowledge should lead to new approaches to treatment and prevention.

CONCLUSIONS

The U.S. investment in biomedical research has yielded major advances in health and quality of life for Americans. However, each advance brings a new set of challenges. The major challenges facing research in autoimmune diseases today are (1) development of a mechanism-based, conceptual understanding of autoimmune disease; (2) translation of this knowledge into new, broadly applicable strategies for treatment and prevention of multiple diseases; and (3) development of sensitive tools for early and definitive diagnosis, disease staging, and identification of at-risk individuals. Through a wealth of individual, coordinated, and collaborative programs outlined in this report, NIH-supported scientists are vigorously pursuing these goals.

Source: Report of the Autoimmune Diseases Coordinating Committee, National Institutes of Health, October 2000.

BIBLIOGRAPHY
BOOKS

Asherson, Ronald A., Ricard Cervera, and Steven Abramson, eds. *Vascular Manifestations of Systemic Autoimmune Diseases.* Boca Raton, Fla.: CRC Press, 2001.

Cohen, Irun R., and Ariel Miller, eds. *Autoimmune Disease Models: A Guidebook.* New York: Academic Press, 1994.

Cook, Allan R., ed. *Immune System Disorders Sourcebook: Basic Information About Lupus, Multiple Sclerosis, Guillain-Barré Syndrome, Chronic Granulomatous Disease, and More.* Detroit: Omnigraphics, Inc., 1997.

Farid, Nadir R., ed. *Immunogenetics of Autoimmune Disease.* Boca Raton, Fla.: CRC Press, 1991.

Fathman, C. G. *Biologic and Gene Therapy of Autoimmune Disease,* Vol. 2, *Current Directions in Autoimmunity.* Basel, Switzerland: S. Karger Publishing, 2000.

Isenberg, David, and John Morrow. *Friendly Fire: Explaining Autoimmune Disease.* New York: Oxford University Press, 1995.

Leffell, Mary S., ed. *Handbook of Human Immunology.* Boca Raton, Fla.: CRC Press, 1997.

Santamaria, Pere. *Cytokines and Chemokines in Autoimmune Disease,* Vol. 30, *Medical Intelligence Unit.* Austin, Tex.: Eurekah.Com Inc., 2002.

ADDISON'S DISEASE

Soderbergh, Annika. *Organ-Specific Autoantibodies in Addison's Disease & Autoimmune Polyendocrine Syndrome Type I.* Uppsala, Sweden: Uppsala Universitet, 2000.

ALLERGIC ASTHMA

American Lung Association Asthma Advisory Group with Norman H. Edelman, M.D. *Family Guide to Asthma and Allergies.* Boston, Mass.: Little Brown & Co., 1997.

Berger, William. *Allergies and Asthma For Dummies.* Foster City, Calif.: Hungry Minds, 2000.

Fox, Romy. *25 Natural Ways To Relieve Allergies and Asthma.* New York: McGraw-Hill Professional Publishing, 2001.

Marone, Gianni, K. F. Austen, Stephen T. Holgate, and L. M. Lichtenstein, eds. *Asthma and Allergic Diseases:* *Physiology, Immunopharmacology and Treatment.* Chestnut Hill, Mass.: Academic Press, 1998.

Rosenwasser, Lanny J., et al., eds. *The Year Book of Allergy, Asthma, and Clinical Immunology.* St. Louis: Mosby-Year Book, 2001.

Simon, Hans-Uwe. *CRC Desk Reference for Allergy and Asthma.* Boca Raton, Fla.: CRC Press, 2000.

ALLERGIC RHINITIS

Filderman, Ronald B., ed. *Allergic Rhinitis: Diagnosis and Treatment in Family Practice,* Disease Management Series. London: Grosvenor Books, 1998.

Mygind, Niels, and Glenis K. Scadding. *Allergic Rhinitis.* Santa Fe, N. Mex.: Health, 2001.

Van Cauwenberge, C. Paul, et al. *Allergic Rhinitis.* London: Martin Dunitz Ltd., 2002.

ALOPECIA AREATA

Bruning, Nancy. *What You Can Do About Chronic Hair Loss.* New York: Dell, 1993.

Melas, Elizabeth Murphy. *The Girl With No Hair: Alopecia Areata.* Santa Fe, N. Mex.: Health, 2001.

Raquepaw, Jayne. "Psychological and Behavioral Affects of Alopecia" Dissertation. College Station: Texas A&M University, 1990.

Thompson, Wendy J., and Jerry Shapiro. *Alopecia Areata: Understanding and Coping With Hair Loss.* Baltimore, Md.: Johns Hopkins University Press, 1996.

ANKYLOSING SPONDYLITIS

Asherson, Ronald A., Ricard Cervera, and Jean-Charl Piette, eds. *The Antiphospholipid Syndrome.* Boca Raton, Fla.: CRC Press, 1996.

Calin, Andrei, and Joel D. Taurog, eds. *The Spondylarthritides.* New York: Oxford University Press, 1998.

Espinoza, Luis R., and Marta Lucia Cuellar. *Molecular Pathogenic Mechanisms of Spondyloarthropathies (Medical Intelligence Unit).* Austin, Tex.: R. G. Landes Co., 1995.

ANTIPHOSPHOLIPID SYNDROME (APS)

Khamashta, Munther A., ed. *Hughes Syndrome: Antiphospholipid Syndrome.* Berlin: Springer Verlag, 2000.

BEHÇET'S DISEASE

Lee, Sungnack, et al., eds. *Behçet's Disease: A Guide to Its Clinical Understanding.* Berlin: Springer Verlag, 2001.

O'Duffy, J. Desmond, and Emre Kokmen, eds. *Behçet's Disease.* New York: Marcel Dekker, 1991.

Plotkin, Gary R., John J. Calabro, and J. Desmond O'Duffy, eds. *Behçet's Disease: A Contemporary Synopsis.* Armonk, N.Y.: Futura Pub. Co., 1988.

Wechsler, Bertrand, and Pierre Godeau, ed. *Behçet's Disease.* Almere, The Netherlands: Excerpta Medica, 1993.

Zeis, Joanne. *You Are Not Alone: 15 People With Behçet's.* Upbridge, Mass.: Joanne Zeis, 1997.

CARDIOMYOPATHY

Florence Meeting on Advances on Cardiomyopathies. *Advances in Cardiomyopathies: Proceedings of the II Florence Meeting on Advances on Cardiomyopathies, April 24–26, 1997.* Berlin: Springer Verlag, 1998.

Maron, Barry J., with Lisa Salberg. *Hypertrophic Cardiomyopathy: For Patients, Their Families, and Interested Physicians.* Armonk, N.Y.: Futura Media Services, 2001.

Nava, Andrea, Lino Rossi, and Gaetano Thiene, eds. *Arrhythmogenic Right Ventricular Cardiomyopathy/Dysplasia.* Almere, The Netherlands: Excerpta Medica, 1997.

Sasayama, Shigetake, ed. *New Horizons for Failing Heart Syndrome.* Berlin: Springer Verlag, 2000.

Schultheiss, H. P., and P. Schwimmbeck, eds. *The Role of Immune Mechanisms in Cardiovascular Disease.* Berlin: Springer Verlag, 1997.

CELIAC DISEASE

Auricchio, S., and J. Visakorpi, eds. *Common Food Intolerances 1: Epidemiology of Coeliac Disease,* Vol. 2, *Dynamic Nutrition Research.* Basel, Switzerland: S. Karger Publishing, 1992.

Bennett, Aileen M. *Coping With Celiac, The Great Masquerader.* Oxford, Miss.: A&G Publishing, 1998.

Branski, D., P. Rozen, and M. F. Kagnoff, eds. *Gluten-Sensitive Enteropathy,* no. 19 of *Frontiers of Gastrointestinal Research.* Basel, Switzerland: S. Karger Publishing, 1991.

Korn, Danna. *Kids with Celiac Disease: A Family Guide to Raising Happy, Healthy, Gluten-Free Children.* Bethesda, Md.: Woodbine House, 2001.

Marsh, Michael N., ed. *Celiac Disease: Methods and Protocols,* 41 of *Methods in Molecular Medicine.* Totowa, N.J.: Humana Press, 2000.

Mearin, M. L., and C. J. J. Mulder. *Coeliac Disease: 40 Years Gluten-Free,* Vol. 13, *Developments in Gastroenterology.* Dordrecht, The Netherlands: Kluwer, 1991.

CHAGAS' DISEASE

Bastien, Joseph William. *The Kiss of Death: Chagas' Disease in the Americas.* Salt Lake City: University of Utah Press, 1998.

Perleth, Matthias. *Historical Aspects of American Trypanosomiasis (Chagas' Disease),* bd. 43 of *Medizin in Entwicklungslandern.* Berlin: Peter Lang Publishing, 1997.

Tentori, Maria Christina, Elsa L. Segura, and David L. Hayes, eds. *Arrhythmia Management in Chagas' Disease.* Armonk, N.Y.: Futura Pub Co., 2000.

CHRONIC FATIGUE SYNDROME

Campling, Frankie, and Michael Sharpe. *Chronic Fatigue Syndrome (CFS/ME): The Facts.* New York: Oxford University Press, 2000.

Demitrack, Mark A., and Susan E. Abbey, eds. *Chronic Fatigue Syndrome.* New York: Guilford Press, 1999.

Englebienne, Patrick, ed. *Chronic Fatigue Syndrome: A Biological Approach.* Boca Raton, Fla.: CRC Press, 2002.

Jackson, Alastair. *Understanding Chronic Fatigue Syndrome.* Crows Nest, Australia: Allen & Unwin, 2001.

Jacobs, Gill. *M. E.: Chronic Fatigue Syndrome: A Practical Guide.* London: Harper Collins—UK, 2001.

Moss-Morris, Rona, and Keith J. Petrie. *Chronic Fatigue Syndrome (The Experience of Illness).* New York: Routledge, 2001.

Munson, Peggy, ed. *Stricken: Voices from the Hidden Epidemic of Chronic Fatigue Syndrome.* Binghamton, N.Y.: Haworth Press, 2000.

Patarca-Montero, Roberto. *Chronic Fatigue Syndrome and the Body's Immune Defense System.* Binghamton, N.Y.: Haworth Press, 2002.

Patarca-Montero, Roberto. *Treatment of Chronic Fatigue Syndrome in the Antiviral Revolution Era.* Binghamton, N.Y.: Haworth Press, 2002.

Redman, George L. *Energy For Life: How to Overcome Chronic Fatigue.* Bloomingdale, Ill.: Vital Health Publishing, 2000.

CHURG-STRAUSS SYNDROME

Meron, Mietta, Graziana Battini, and Adalberto Sessa. *Renal Involvement in Systemic Vasculitis: Seminar, 1st, Vimercate, September 22, 1990.* Basel, Switzerland: S. Karger Publishers, 1991.

Watt, Ben. *Patient.* New York: Grove/Atlantic, Inc., 1997.

CROHN'S DISEASE

Harper, Virginia M., and Tom Monte. *Controlling Crohn's Disease: The Natural Way.* New York: Kensington Pub Corp., 2002.

Prantera, Cosimo, and Burton I. Korelitz, eds. *Crohn's Disease.* New York: Marcel Dekker, 1996.

Saibil, Fredric G. *Crohn's Disease & Ulcerative Colitis.* Buffalo, N.Y.: Firefly Books, 1997.

Salt II, William B., and Neil F. Neimark. *Irritable Bowel Syndrome and the MindBodySpirit Connection: 7 Steps for Living a Healthy Life With a Functional Bowel Disorder, Crohn's Disease or Colitis.* Columbus, Ohio: Parkview Publishing Co., 2002.

Scala, James. *The New Eating Right for a Bad Gut: The Complete Nutritional Guide to Ileitis, Colitis, Crohn's Disease, and Inflammatory Bowel Disease.* New York: Plume, 2000.

Sklar, Jill, and Manuel Sklar. *The First Year Crohn's Disease and Ulcerative Colitis: An Essential Guide for the Newly Diagnosed (The First Year Series).* New York: Marlowe & Co., 2002.

Thompson, W. Grant. *The Angry Gut: Coping With Colitis and Crohn's Disease.* Cambridge, Mass.: Perseus Publishing, 1993.

Trachter, Amy B., and Henry Wodnicki. *Coping with Crohn's Disease: Manage Your Physical Symptoms and Overcome the Emotional Challenges.* Berkeley, Calif.: Publishers Group West, 2001.

Zonderman, Jon, Ronald S. Vender, and Bernardo Bertolucci. *Understanding Crohn Disease and Ulcerative Colitis.* Jackson, Miss.: University Press of Mississippi, 2000.

COXSACKIE MYOCARDITIS

Tracy, Steven, B. W. Mahy, and N. M. Chapman, eds. *The Coxsackie B Viruses, Vol. 223.* New York: Springer-Verlag New York, Incorporated, 2001.

CREST SYNDROME

(See Scleroderma)

DERMATITIS HERPETIFORMIS (DH)

Rawcliffe, Peter, and Ruth Rolph. *Gluten-Free Diet Book: A Guide to Gluten-Sensitive Enteropathy, Dermatitis Herpetiformis and Gluten-Free Cookery.* Foster City, Calif.: Hungry Minds, Incorporated, 1985.

ENDOMETRIOSIS

Henderson, Lorraine, and Ros Wood. *Explaining Endometriosis,* 2nd ed. Crows Nest, Australia: Allen & Unwin, 2001.

Hoshiai, H., Y. Taketani, and N. Terakawa, eds. *Current Perspectives on Endometriosis and Infertility.* Basel, Switzerland: Karger Publishing, 2002.

Lewis, Jennifer Marie. *Endometriosis—One Woman's Journey.* Glendale, Calif.: Griffin Publishing, 1998.

Mears, Jo. *Endometriosis: A Natural Approach.* Berkeley, Calif.: Ulysses Press, 1998.

Overton, Caroline, L. MacMillan, C. Davis, and R. W. Shaw. *An Atlas of Endometriosis,* 2nd ed. Boca Raton, Fla.: CRC Press-Parthenon Publishers, 2002.

Phillips, Robert H., and Glenda Motta. *Coping With Endometriosis: Sound, Compassionate Advice for Alleviating the Physical and Emotional Symptoms of This Frequently Misunderstood Illness.* New York: Avery Penguin Putnam, 2000.

Venturini, Pier Luigi, and Johannes Leonardus Evers, eds. *Endometriosis: Basic Research and Clinical Practice.* Boca Raton, Fla.: CRC Press-Parthenon Publishers, 1999.

Vernon, Michael. *Endometriosis: A Key to Healing Through Nutrition.* San Francisco: Thorsons Pub., 2002.

FIBROMYALGIA

Baldry, P. E., Muhammad B. Yunus, and Brian Hazleman. *Myofascial Pain and Fibromyalgia Syndromes: A Clinical Guide to Diagnosis and Management.* New York: Churchill Livingstone, 2001.

Cabrera, Chanchal. *Fibromyalgia.* New York: McGraw-Hill, 2002.

Digeronimo, Theresa Foy, and Joseph E. Scherger. *New Hope for People with Fibromyalgia.* Rocklin, Calif.: Prima Publishing, 2001.

Goldenberg, Don. L. *Fibromyalgia: Fact Vs. Fiction: As Explained by an American Authority.* New York: Perigee, 2002.

Lowe, John C., and Jackie G. Yellin. *Speeding Up to Normal: Metabolic Solutions to Fibromyalgia.* Boulder, Colo.: McDowell Publishing Company, 2002.

McIlwain, Harris H., and Debra Fulghum Bruce. *The Fibromyalgia Handbook,* 2nd ed. New York: Owl Books, 1999.

Patarca-Montero, Roberto. *The Concise Encyclopedia of Fibromyalgia and Myofascial Pain.* Binghamton, N.Y.: Haworth Medical Press, 2002.

Selfridge, Nancy, and Franklynn Peterson. *Freedom from Fibromyalgia: The 5-Week Program Proven to Conquer Pain.* New York: Three Rivers Press, 2001.

Starlanyl, Devin J., and Mary Ellen Copeland. *Fibromyalgia and Chronic Myofascial Pain: A Survival Manual,* 2nd ed. Oakland, Calif.: New Harbinger Publications, 2001.

Wallace, Daniel J., and Janice Brock Wallace. *All About Fibromyalgia.* New York: Oxford University Press, 2002.

GRAVES' DISEASE

Bahn, Rebecca S., ed. *Thyroid Eye Disease,* Vol. 14 of *Endocrine Updates.* Dordrecht, The Netherlands: Kluwer Academic Publishers, 2001.

Flax, Katie. *Healing Options: A Report on Graves' Disease Treatments,* 2nd ed. Sparkill, N.Y.: Sally Breer, 2001.

Moore, Elaine A., with Lisa Moore. *Graves' Disease: A Practical Guide.* Jefferson, N.C.: McFarland & Company, 2001.

Rapoport, Basil, and Sandra M. McLachlan, eds. *Graves' Disease: Pathogenesis and Treatment.* Dordrecht, The Netherlands: Kluwer Academic Publishers, 2000.

GUILLAIN-BARRÉ SYNDROME (GBS)

Hatrick, Gloria. *Masks.* London: Orchard Books, 1996.

Heller, Joseph, and Speed Vogel. *No Laughing Matter.* 1966. Reprint. New York: Donald I. Fine, 1995.

Parry, Gareth J., and J. D. Pollard. *Guillain-Barré Syndrome.* New York: Thieme Medical Pub., 1993.

Riley, Jane. *Solomon's Porch: The Story of Ben and Rose.* Frederick, Md.: AmErica House Book Publishers, 2001.

Wilcox, Dorris R. *No Time for Tears: Transforming Tragedy into Triumph.* Mt. Pleasant, S.C.: Corinthian Books, 2000.

HASHIMOTO'S THYROIDITIS

Dirgo, Robert T., comp., and Mary Dirgo, ed. *How I Reversed My Hashimoto's Thyroiditis Hypothyroidism.* Falls Church, Va.: Writers Club Ltd., 2001.

HEPATITIS (AUTOIMMUNE)

Dienes, Hans Peter. *Viral and Autoimmune Hepatitis: Morphologic and Pathogenetic Aspects of Cell Damage in Hepatitis With Potential Chronicity (Progress in Pathology).* Weinheim, Germany: VCH Publishing, 1989.

Krawitt, Edward L., Russell H. Wiesner, and Mikio Nishioka. *Autoimmune Liver Diseases.* New York: Elsevier Science, 1998.

McFarlane, Ian G., and Roger Williams. *Molecular Basis of Autoimmune Hepatitis.* Georgetown, Tex.: Landes Bioscience, 1996.

Nishioka, Mikio, Mikio Zeniya, and Gotaro Toda. *Autoimmune Hepatitis.* New York: Elsevier Science, 1994.

IGA NEPHROPATHY

Coppo, Rosanna, and Licia Peruzzi, eds. *Moderately Proteinuric IgA Nephropathy in the Young.* Amsterdam: IOS Press, 2000.

Tomino, Yasuhiko. *IgA Nephropathy: Pathogenesis and Treatment,* Vol. 126 of *Contributions to Nephrology.* Basel, Switzerland: S. Karger Publishing, 1999.

INCLUSION BODY MYOSITIS (IBM)

Askanas, Valerie, George Serratrice, and W. King Engel, eds. *Inclusion-Body Myositis and Myopathies.* New York: Cambridge University Press, 1998.

Kilpatrick, James R., comp. *Coping with a Myositis Disease.* Kilpatrick Publishing Company, 2000.

INSULIN-DEPENDENT DIABETES (TYPE 1)

Brand-Miller, Jennie, Kaye Foster-Powell, and Wolever Thomas. *The Glucose Revolution Pocket Guide to Children with Type 1 Diabetes.* New York: Marlowe & Company, 2001.

Chase, H. Peter. *Understanding Insulin-Dependent Diabetes.* Denver, Colo.: Children's Diabetes Foundation, 2000.

Hanas, Ragnar. *Insulin-Dependent Diabetes in Children, Adolescents and Adults—How To Become an Expert on Your Own Diabetes.* Uddevalla, Sweden: Piara Publishing, 1998.

Johnson, Patricia D. *Teenagers With Type 1 Diabetes: A Curriculum for Adolescents, Families, and Health Professionals.* New York: McGraw Hill, 2000.

Sosin, Allan E., and Sheila Sobell. *The Doctor's Guide to Diabetes and Your Child: New Therapies for Type 1 and 2.* New York: Kensington Publishing Corporation, 2000.

Stenstrom, Ulf. *Psychological Factors & Metabolic Control in Insulin-Dependent Diabetes Mellitus.* Philadelphia, Pa.: Coronet Books, 1997.

INTERSTITIAL CYSTITIS

Moldwin, Robert M. *The Interstitial Cystitis Survival Guide: Your Guide to the Latest Treatment Options and Coping Strategies.* Oakland, Calif.: New Harbinger Publications, 2000.

Sandler, Gaye Grissom, and Andrew B. Sandler. *Patient to Patient: Managing Interstitial Cystitis & Overlapping Conditions.* Bon Ange LLC, 2001. ISBN: 0-9705590-0-3

Sant, Grannum, ed. *Interstitial Cystitis.* Philadelphia, Pa.: Lippincott Williams & Wilkins Publishers, 1997.

Simone, Catherine M. *Along the Healing Path: Recovering from Interstitial Cystitis.* Cleveland, Ohio: IC Hope, 2000.

Simone, Catherine M. *To Wake in Tears: Understanding Interstitial Cystitis.* Cleveland, Ohio: IC Hope, 1998.

Willis, Amirit K. *Solving the Interstitial Cystitis Puzzle: My Story of Discovery and Recovery.* Beverly Hills, Calif.: Holistic Life Enterprises, 2001.

JUVENILE ARTHRITIS

Aldape, Virginia Tortorica. *Nicole's Story: A Book About a Girl With Juvenile Rheumatoid Arthritis.* Minneapolis, Minn.: Lerner Publications Company, 1996.

Fall, Guy. *Everything You Need to Know About Juvenile Arthritis,* The Need to Know Library. New York: Rosen Publishing Group, 2002.

Murphy Melas, Elizabeth. *Keeping A Secret: A Story About Juvenile Rheumatoid Arthritis.* Santa Fe, N. Mex.: Health, 2001.

Peacock, Judith. *Juvenile Arthritis, (Perspectives on Disease and Illness).* Mankato, Minn.: Lifematters Press, 2000.

MÉNIÈRE'S DISEASE

Arenberg, I. Kaufman, and Malcolm D. Graham. *Treatment Options for Ménière's Disease: Endolymphatic Sac Surgery: Do It or Don't Do It and Why?* Clifton Park, N.Y.: Singular Pub Group, 1998.

Barton, V. K. *Ménière's Disease: An Information Book for People with Ménière's Disease.* New York: Hyperion, 1991.

Harris, Jeffrey P., ed. *Ménière's Disease.* Amsterdam: Kugler Pubns B V (Medical), 1999.

Wilmot, Tom. *Ménière's and Its Management.* Springfield, Ill.: Charles C Thomas Pub Ltd., 1984.

MULTIPLE SCLEROSIS

Bashir, Khurram, John N. Whitaker, Leon Shargel, and Medi-Sim Adelman. *Handbook of Multiple Sclerosis.* Philadelphia, Pa.: Lippincott Williams & Wilkins Publishers, 2002.

Burgess, Megan. *Multiple Sclerosis: Theory and Practice for Nurses.* London: Whurr Pub Ltd., 2002.

Clanet, Michel. *Advances in Multiple Sclerosis: Clinical Research and Therapy.* Boston: Boston Medical Pub Inc., 2002.

Gold, Susan Dudley. *Multiple Sclerosis, (Health Watch).* Berkeley Heights, N.J.: Enslow Publishers, Inc., 2001.

Halper, June, and Nancy J. Holland, eds. *Comprehensive Nursing Management of Multiple Sclerosis,* 2nd ed. New York: Demos Medical Publishing, 2002.

Holland, Nancy J., T. Jock Murray, and Stephen C. Reingold. *Multiple Sclerosis: A Guide for the Newly Diagnosed,* 2nd ed. New York: Demos Medical Publishing, 2001.

Joy, Janet E., and Richard B. Johnston, eds. *Multiple Sclerosis: Current Status and Strategies for the Future.* Washington, D.C.: National Academy Press, 2001.

Matthews, W. B., and Margaret Rice-Oxley. *Multiple Sclerosis: The Facts,* 4th ed. New York: Oxford University Press, 2002.

Neutze, Diana. *As For Tomorrow, I Cannot Say: 33 Years with Multiple Sclerosis.* Boca Raton, Fla.: New Paradigm Books, 2002.

Rumrill, Phillip D., Jr. *Multiple Sclerosis: A Guide for Rehabilitation and Health Care Professionals.* Springfield, Ill.: Charles C. Thomas Pub Ltd., 2001.

Trubo, Richard. *Courage: The Story of the Mighty Effort to End the Devastating Effects of Multiple Sclerosis.* Chicago: Ivan R Dee, Inc., 2001.

MYASTHENIA GRAVIS

Christadoss, Premkumar, ed. *Myasthenia Gravis: Disease Mechanism and Immunointervention.* Dordrecht, The Netherlands: Kluwer Academic Publishers, 2000.

Conti-Fine, Bianca M., ed. *Myasthenia Gravis: The Immunobiology of an Autoimmune Disease (Neuroscience Intelligence Unit).* Austin, Tex.: R G Landes Co., 1997.

Lisak, Robert P., ed. *Handbook of Myasthenia Gravis and Myasthenic Syndromes.* New York, N.Y.: Marcel Dekker, 1994.

Richman, David P., ed. *Myasthenia Gravis and Related Diseases: Disorders of the Neuromuscular Junction,* Vol. 841 of *Annals of the New York Academy of Sciences.* New York Academy of Sciences, 1998.

MYOSITIS

Kilpatrick, James R., comp., *Coping with a Myositis Disease.* Kilpatrick Publishing Company, 2000. ISBN: 0970167105

NEUTROPENIA

Hadley, Andrew, and Peter Soothill, eds. *Alloimmune Disorders of Pregnancy: Anaemia, Thrombocytopenia, and Neutropenia in the Fetus and Neonate.* New York: Cambridge University Press, 2002.

PERIPHERAL NEUROPATHY (PN)

Bril, V., and G. Said, eds. *Emerging Opportunities in Peripheral Neuropathy: Ens Satellite Symposium, Nice, June 8, 1998.* Basel, Switzerland: S. Karger Publishing, 1999.

Cros, Didier, ed. *Peripheral Neuropathy: A Practical Approach to Diagnosis and Management.* Philadelphia, Penn.: Lippincott Williams & Wilkins Publishers, 2001.

Dyck, Peter James, and P. K. Thomas, eds. *Peripheral Neuropathy.* Philadelphia, Pa.: W B Saunders Co., 1993.

Midroni, Gyl, Juan M. Bilbao, and Sandra M. Cohen. *Biopsy Diagnosis of Peripheral Neuropathy.* Newton, Mass.: Butterworth-Heinemann Medical, 1995.

Ouvrier, Robert A., J. D. Pollard, and James G. McLeod. *Peripheral Neuropathy in Childhood,* 2d ed., International Review of Child Neurology Series. New York: Cambridge University Press, 1999.

Senneff, John A. *Numb Toes and Aching Soles: Coping with Peripheral Neuropathy.* San Antonio, Tex.: Medpress, 1999.

Senneff, John A. *Numb Toes and Other Woes: More on Peripheral Neuropathy.* Washington, D.C.: National Academy Press, 2001.

PRIMARY BILIARY CIRRHOSIS

Lindor, Keith D., E. Jenny Heathcote, and Raoul E. Poupon, eds. *Primary Biliary Cirrhosis: From Pathogenesis to Clinical Treatment.* Dordrecht, The Netherlands: Kluwer Academic Publishers, 1998.

PSORIASIS

Baker, Barbara S. *Recent Advances in Psoriasis: The Role of the Immune System.* River Edge, N.J.: World Scientific Publishing Company, 2000.

Bower, H. *Psoriasis.* Quebec: Modus Vivendi Pub Inc., 2000.

Camisa, Charles. *Handbook of Psoriasis.* Malden, Mass.: Blackwell Science Inc., 1998.

Cram, David Lee. *Coping with Psoriasis: A Patient's Guide to Treatment.* Omaha, Nebr.: Addicus Books, 2000.

Davison, Simon, Jonathon Barker, and Thomas F. Poyner. *Pocket Guide to Psoriasis.* Malden, Mass.: Blackwell Science Inc., 2000.

Farber, Eugene M. *Conquering Psoriasis: An Illustrated Guide to the Understanding and Control of Psoriasis.* Hamilton, Ontario: B C Decker Inc., 2002.

Griffiths, C., ed. *Key Advances in the Effective Management of Psoriasis.* London: Royal Society of Medicine, 2000.

Roenigk Jr., Henry H., and Howard I. Maibach, eds. *Psoriasis,* 3d ed. New York: Marcel Dekker, 1998.

Van de Kerkhof, Petrus, and C. Mari. *Textbook of Psoriasis.* Malden, Mass.: Blackwell Science Inc., 1999.

PSORIATIC ARTHRITIS

Gerber, Lynn H., and Luis R. Espinoza. *Psoriatic Arthritis.* New York: Grune & Stratton, 1985.

RAYNAUD'S PHENOMENON

Coffman, Jay D. *Raynaud's Phenomenon.* New York: Oxford University Press, 1989.

RHEUMATIC FEVER

English, Peter C. *Rheumatic Fever in America and Britain: A Biological, Epidemiological, and Medical History.* New Brunswick, N.J.: Rutgers University Press, 1999.

Massell, Benedict F. *Rheumatic Fever and Streptococcal Infection: Unraveling the Mysteries of a Dread Disease.* Cambridge, Mass.: Harvard University Press, 1997.

RHEUMATOID ARTHRITIS

Firestein, Gary S., Gabriel S. Panayi, and Frank A. Wollheim. *Rheumatoid Arthritis: Frontiers in Pathogenesis and Treatment.* New York: Oxford University Press, 2001.

Gabriel, Sherine. *Rheumatoid Arthritis: Epidemiology, Pathogenesis and Treatment.* London: Remedica, 2002.

Goronzy, J. J., and C. M. Weyand, eds. *Rheumatoid Arthritis,* Vol. 3, *Current Directions in Autoimmunity.* Basel, Switzerland: S. Karger Publishing, 2000.

Koehn, Cheryl, Taysha Palmer, and John Esdaile. *Rheumatoid Arthritis: Plan to Win.* New York: Oxford University Press, 2002.

Lahita, Robert G. *Arthritis Solution: The Newest Treatments to Help You Live Pain-Free.* New York: Wholecare, 1999.

Lahita, Robert G. *Rheumatoid Arthritis: Everything You Need to Know.* New York: Avery Penguin Putnam, 2001.

Lee, Thomas F. *Conquering Rheumatoid Arthritis: The Latest Breakthroughs and Treatments.* Amherst, N.Y.: Prometheus Books, 2001.

Llewellyn, Claire. *The Facts About Arthritis.* Mankato, Minn.: Thameside Press, 2001.

Mason, Mary-Claire, and Elaine Smith. *Rheumatoid Arthritis: Your Medication Explained,* Overcoming Common Problems Series. London: Sheldon Press, 2001.

Paget, Stephen A., Michael D. Lockshin, and Suzanne Loebl. *The Hospital for Special Surgery Rheumatoid Arthritis Handbook.* New York: John Wiley & Sons, 2001.

SARCOIDOSIS

Conroy, Sandra. *Sarcoidosis Resource Guide and Directory.* Piscataway, N.J.: PC Publications, 1992.

Duffy, Karen. *Model Patient: My Life As an Incurable Wise-Ass.* New York: Cliff Street Books, 2000.

James, D. Geraint, ed. *Sarcoidosis and Other Granulomatous Diseases.* New York: Marcel Dekker, 1994.

Scadding, J. G., and D. N. Mitchell. *Sarcoidosis,* 2nd ed. Philadelphia, Pa.: Lippincott Williams & Wilkins Publishers, 1985.

SCLERITIS

Foster, C. Stephen, and Maite Sainz De La Maza. *The Sclera.* Berlin: Springer Verlag, 1994.

McCluskey, Peter, and Susan Lightman, eds. *Scleritis.* London: BMJ Books, 2001.

Watson, Peter G., and Joseph M. Ortiz. *Color Atlas of Scleritis.* St. Louis, Mo.: Mosby-Year Book, 1995.

SCLERODERMA

Clements, Philip J., and Daniel E. Furst, eds. *Systemic Sclerosis*. Philadelphia, Pa.: Lippincott, Williams & Wilkins, 1996.

Mayes, Maureen D. *The Scleroderma Book: A Guide for Patients and Families*. New York: Oxford University Press, 1999.

Melvin, Jeanne L. *Scleroderma: Caring for Your Hands & Face*. Bethesda, Md.: American Occupational Therapy Association, Inc., 1994.

Scammell, Henry. *Scleroderma: The Proven Therapy That Can Save Your Life*. New York: M Evans & Co., 1998.

SJÖGREN'S SYNDROME

Carsons, Steven, and Elaine K. Harris, eds. *The New Sjögren's Syndrome Handbook*. New York: Oxford University Press, 1998.

Dauphin, Sue. *Understanding Sjögren's Syndrome*. New York: Pixel Press, 1993.

SYSTEMIC LUPUS ERYTHEMATOSUS (SLE)

Aladjem, Henrietta. *The Challenges of Lupus: Insights & Hope*. New York: Avery Penguin Putnam, 1999.

Henry, Sara J. *New Hope for People with Lupus: Your Friendly, Authoritative Guide to the Latest in Traditional and Complementary Solutions*. Rockllin, Calif.: Prima Publishing, 2002.

Hughes, Graham R. V. *Lupus: The Facts*. New York: Oxford University Press, 2000.

Lahita, Robert G., ed. *Systemic Lupus Erythematosus*. Chestnut Hill, Mass.: Academic Press, 1999.

Lahita, Robert G., and Robert H. Phillips. *Lupus: Everything You Need to Know*. New York: Avery Penguin Putnam, 1998.

Maraux, Andre. *Everything You Need to Know About Lupus*, Need to Know Library. New York: Rosen Publishing Group, 2000.

Phillips, Robert H., Ronald I. Carr, and Harry Spiera. *Coping With Lupus: A Practical Guide to Alleviating the Challenges of Systemic Lupus Erythematosus*, 3d ed. New York: Avery Penguin Putnam, 2001.

Schur, Peter H., ed. *The Clinical Management of Systemic Lupus Erythematosus*. Philadelphia, Pa.: Lippincott Williams & Wilkins Publishers, 1996.

Wallace, Daniel J. *The Lupus Book: A Guide for Patients and Their Families*. New York: Oxford University Press, 2000.

Wallace, Daniel J., and Bevra Hannahs Hahn. *DuBois' Lupus Erythematosus*, 6th ed. Philadelphia, Pa.: Lippincott Williams & Wilkins, 2002.

ULCERATIVE COLITIS

O'Morain, Colm A., ed. *Ulcerative Colitis*. Boca Raton, Fla.: CRC Press, 1991.

Saibil, Fredric G. *Crohn's Disease & Ulcerative Colitis*. Buffalo, N.Y.: Firefly Books, 1997.

Sklar, Jill. *The First Year Crohn's Disease and Ulcerative Colitis: An Essential Guide for the Newly Diagnosed*, The First Year Series. New York: Marlowe & Co., 2002.

Thompson, W. Grant. *The Angry Gut: Coping With Colitis and Crohn's Disease*. Cambridge, Mass.: Perseus Press, 1993.

Zonderman, Jon, and Ronald S. Vender. *Understanding Crohn Disease and Ulcerative Colitis*. Jackson, Miss.: University Press of Mississippi, 2000.

UVEITIS

Benezra, David, ed. *Uveitis Update*, Vol. 31 of *Developments in Ophthalmology*. Basel, Switzerland: S. Karger Publishing, 1999.

Foster, C. Stephen. *Diagnosis and Treatment of Uveitis*. Philadelphia, Pa.: W B Saunders Co., 2002.

Jones, Nicholas P. *Uveitis: An Illustrated Manual*. Newton, Mass.: Butterworth-Heinemann, 2001.

Lightman, Susan, and Hamish Towler, eds. *Uveitis*. Chicago: Login Brothers Book Company, 1999.

Nussenblatt, Robert B., Scott M. Whitcup, and Alan G. Palestine. *Uveitis: Fundamentals and Clinical Practice*, 2nd ed. St. Louis, Mo.: Mosby-Year Book, 1996.

Ohno, Shigeaki, ed. *Uveitis Today*. Almere, The Netherlands: Excerpta Medica, 1998.

Opremcak, E. Mitchel. *Uveitis: A Clinical Manual for Ocular Inflammation*. Berlin: Springer Verlag, 1995.

VASCULITIS

Ball, Eugene, and S. Louis Bridges Jr., eds. *Vasculitis*. New York: Oxford University Press, 2001.

VITILIGO

Hann, Seung-Kung, and James Nordlund, eds. *Vitiligo: A Monograph on the Basic and Clinical Science*. Malden, Mass.: Blackwell Science Inc., 2000.

WEGENER'S GRANULOMATOSIS

Gross, Wolfgang L. *ANCA-Associated Vasculitides: Immunological and Clinical Aspects*. Dordrecht, The Netherlands: Kluwer Academic Publishers, 1993.

BIBLIOGRAPHY
ARTICLES

Cooper, G. S., F. W. Miller, and D. R. Germolec. "Occupational Exposures and Autoimmune Diseases." *International Immunopharmacology* 2, nos. 2–3 (February 2002): 303–313.

Fathman, C. G., and C. M. Seroogy. "Application of Gene Therapy in Autoimmune Disease." *Current Directions in Autoimmunity* 2 (2000): 189–202.

Garren, H., and L. Steinman. "DNA Vaccination in the Treatment of Autoimmune Disease." *Current Directions in Autoimmunity* 2 (2000): 203–216.

La Cava, A., and N. Sarvetnick. "The Role of Cytokines in Autoimmunity." *Current Directions in Autoimmunity* 1 (1999): 56–71.

Zinkernagel, R. M. "Maternal Antibodies, Childhood Infections, and Autoimmune Diseases." *New England Journal of Medicine* 345, no. 8 (November 2001): 1,331–1,335.

ADDISON'S DISEASE

Baker, S., D. Kenward, and K. G. White. "Addison's Disease: After 40 Years Much Remains the Same." *BMJ* 322, no. 7284 (February 24, 2001): 494.

Betterle, C., C. Dalpra, N. Greggio, M. Volpato, and R. Zanchetta. "Autoimmunity in Isolated Addison's Disease and in Polyglandular Autoimmune Diseases Type 1, 2 and 4." *Annals of Endocrinology* (Paris) 62, no. 2 (April 2001): 193–201.

Gradden, C., D. Lawrence, P. M. Doyle, and C. R. Welch. "Uses of Error: Addison's Disease in Pregnancy." *Lancet* 357, no. 9263 (April 2001): 1,197.

Jakobi, J. M., D. W. Killinger, B. M. Wolfe, J. L. Mahon, and C. L. Rice. "Quadriceps Muscle Function and Fatigue in Women with Addison's Disease." *Muscle Nerve* 24, no. 8 (August 2001): 1,040–1,049.

Robinson, S., and A. Grossman. "Addison's Disease Should be Diagnosed Biochemically." *BMJ* 323, no. 7303 (July 7, 2001): 51.

Zargar, A. H., B. A. Laway, S. R. Masoodi, M. I. Bashir, A. I. Wani, and M. Salahuddin. "A Critical Evaluation of Signs and Symptoms in the Diagnosis of Addison's Diseases." *Journal of the Association of Physicians of India* 49 (May 2001): 523–556.

ALLERGIC ASTHMA

Alvarez, D., R. E. Wiley, and M. Jordana. "Cytokine Therapeutics for Asthma: An Appraisal of Current Evidence and Future Prospects." *Current Pharmaceutical Design* 7, no. 11 (July 2001): 1,059–1,081.

Busse, W. W., and R. F. Lemanske. "Advances in Immunology: Asthma." *New England Journal of Medicine* 344 (February 2001): 350–362.

Creticos, P. S. "The Consideration of Immunotherapy in the Treatment of Allergic Asthma." *Annals of Allergy, Asthma, and Immunology* 87, Supp. 1 (July 1987): 13–27.

Leong, K. P., and D. P. Huston. "Understanding the Pathogenesis of Allergic Asthma Using Mouse Models." *Annals of Allergy, Asthma, and Immunology* 87, no. 2 (August 2001): 96–110.

Mazer, B. "Omalizumab Reduced Inhaled Corticosteroid Use and Exacerbations in Childhood Allergic Asthma." *ACP Journal Club* 136, no. 1 (January–February 2002): 16.

Milgrom, H., W. Berger, A. Nayak, N. Gupta, S. Pollard, M. McAlary, A. F. Taylor, and P. Rohane. "Treatment of Childhood Asthma with Anti-Immunoglobulin E Antibody (Omalizumab)." *Pediatrics* 108, no. 2 (August 2001): E36.

Platts-Mills, T. A. "The Role of Immunoglobulin E in Allergy and Asthma." *American Journal of Respiratory and Critical Care Medicine* 164, Part 2 (October 2001): S1–5.

Robert, J. "Advice for Those with Children with Allergic Asthma: Results of Forty Studies." *Archives of Pediatrics and Adolescent Medicine* 8, no. 10 (October 2001): 1,042–1,044.

Yssel, H., S. Lecart, and J. Pene. "Regulatory T Cells and Allergic Asthma." *Microbes and Infection* 3, no. 11 (September 2001): 899–904.

ALLERGIC RHINITIS

Crystal-Peters, J., C. Neslusan, W. H. Crown, and A. Torres. "Treating Allergic Rhinitis in Patients with Comorbid Asthma: The Risk of Asthma-Related Hospitalizations and Emergency Department Visits." *Journal of Allergy and Clinical Immunology* 109, Part 1 (January 2002): 57–62.

Guzman, Susanna E. "Diagnosis and Management of Allergic Rhinitis." *American Family Physician* Monograph, no. 3 (2001).

Hayden, M. L. "Allergic Rhinitis: A Growing Primary Care Challenge." *Journal of the American Academy of Nurse Practitioners* 13, no. 12 (December 2001): 545–554.

Macchia, L., M. F. Caiaffa, R. Di Paola, G. De Michelle, G. Bariletto, A. Iudice, and A. Tursi. "Second Generation Antihistamines in the Treatment of Seasonal Allergic Rhinitis Due to Parietaria and Cypress Pollen." *Pharmacological Research* 44, no. 6 (December 2001): 461–466.

May, J. R. "Allergic Rhinitis: Nothing to Sniffle At." *Journal of the American Pharmaceutical Association* (Wash) 41, no. 6 (November–December 2001): 891–892.

Palma-Carlos, A. G., A. Spinola-Santos, M. B. Ferreira, M. C. Santos, and M. L. Palma-Carlos. "Immunotherapy in Allergic Rhinitis." *Allergie et Immunologie* (Paris) 33, no. 8 (October 2001): 323–326.

Sly, R. M. "Epidemiology of Allergic Rhinitis." *Clinical Reviews in Allergy & Immunology* 22, no. 1 (February 2002): 67–103.

ALOPECIA AREATA

Cipriani, R., G. I. Perini, and S. Rampinelli. "Paroxetine in Alopecia Areata." *International Journal of Dermatology* 40, no. 9 (September 2001): 600–601.

Duvic, M., A. Nelson, and M. de Andrade. "The Genetics of Alopecia Areata." *Clinics in Dermatology* 19, no. 2 (March–April 2001): 135–139.

Epstein, E. "Evidence-Based Treatment of Alopecia Areata." *Journal of the American Academy of Dermatology* 45, no. 4 (October 2001): 640–642.

Freyschmidt-Paul, P., R. Hoffmann, E. Levine, J. P. Sundberg, R. Happle, and K. J. McElwee. "Current and Potential Agents for the Treatment of Alopecia Areata." *Current Pharmaceutical Design* 7, no. 3 (February 2001): 213–230.

Hordinsky, M. K. "Alopecia Areata: Pathophysiology and Latest Developments." *Journal of Cutaneous Medicine and Surgery* 3, Supp. 3 (November 1999): S28–S30.

MacDonald, N., M. C. Wiseman, and J. Shapiro. "Alopecia Areata: Topical Immunotherapy—Application and Practical Problems." *Journal of Cutaneous Medicine and Surgery* 3, Supp. 3 (November 1999): S36–S40.

McDonagh, A. J., and A. G. Messenger. "Alopecia Areata." *Clinics in Dermatology* 19, no. 2 (March–April 2001): 141–147.

Papadopoulos, A. J., R. A. Schwartz, and C. K. Janniger. "Alopecia Areata: Pathogenesis, Diagnosis, and Therapy." *American Journal of Clinical Dermatology* 1, no. 2 (March–April 2000): 101–105.

Randall, V. A. "Is Alopecia Areata an Autoimmune Disease." *Lancet* 358, no. 9,297 (December 2001): 1,922–1,924.

Wiseman, M. C., and J. Shapiro. "Therapeutic Approach to Alopecia Areata." *Journal of Cutaneous Medicine and Surgery* 3, Supp. 3 (November 1999): S31–S35.

Wiseman, M. C., J. Shapiro, N. MacDonald, and H. Lui. "Predictive Model for Immunotherapy of Alopecia Areata with Diphencyprone." *Archives of Dermatology* 137, no. 8 (August 2001): 1,063–1,068.

ANKYLOSING SPONDYLITIS (AS)

Aggarwal, A. N., D. Gupta, A. Wanchu, and S. K. Jindal. "Use of Static Lung Mechanics to Identify Early Pulmonary Involvement in Patients with Ankylosing Spondylitis." *Journal of Postgraduate Medicine* 24, no. 2 (April–June 2001): 89–94.

Barlow, J. H., C. C. Wright, B. Williams, and A. Keat. "Work Disability Among People with Ankylosing Spondylitis." *Arthritis and Rheumatism* 45, no. 5 (October 2001): 424–429.

Chou, C. T. "Factors Affecting the Pathogenesis of Ankylosing Spondylitis." *Chinese Medical Journal (Engl)* 114, no. 2 (February 2001): 211–212.

Dougados, M. "Treatment of Spondylarthropathies: Recent Advances and Prospects in 2001." *Joint, Bone, Spine: Revue du Rhumatisme* 68, no. 6 (December 2001): 557–563.

Stafford, L., and P. P. Youssef. "Spondylarthropathies: An Overview." *Internal Medicine Journal* 32, no. 1–2 (January–February 2002): 40–46.

Ward, M. M. "Functional Disability Predicts Total Costs in Patients with Ankylosing Spondylitis." *Arthritis and Rheumatism* 46, no. 1 (January 2002): 223–231.

ANTIGLOMERULAR BASEMENTAL MEMBRANE (ANTI-GBM) DISEASE

Ara, J., J. Robert, E. Mirapeix, A. Botey, and A. Darnell. "High Prevalence of Antithyroid Antibodies in Anti-Glomerular Basement Membrane Antibody-Mediated Disease." *Journal of Nephrology* 13, no. 1 (January–February 2000): 65–67.

Herody, M., C. Duvic, L. H. Noel, G. Nedelec, and J. P. Grunfeld. "Cigarette Smoking and Other Inhaled Toxins in anti-GBM Disease." *Contributions to Nephrology* 130 (2000): 94–102.

Kluth, D. C., and A. J. Rees. "Anti-Glomerular Basement Membrane Disease." *Journal of the American Society of Nephrology* 10, no. 11 (November 1999): 2,446–2,453.

Saurina, A., J. Ara, E. Mirapeix, E. Coll, M. Vera, and A. Darnell. "Anti-Glomerular Basement Membrane Disease: A New Disease Causing Fever of Unknown Origin?" *Nefrologia* 20, no. 1 (January–February 2000): 79–82.

ANTIPHOSPHOLIPID SYNDROME (APS)

Aron, A. L., A. E. Gharavi, and Y. Shoenfeld. "Mechanisms of Action of Antiphospholipid Antibodies in the Antiphospholipid Syndrome." *International Archives of Allergy and Immunology* 106 (1995): 8–12.

Biller, J. "Antiphospholipid Antibodies and Stroke." *American Academy of Neurology* Annual Meeting (1999).

Brey, R. L., and B. M. Coull. "Antiphospholipid Antibodies: Origin, Specificity, and Mechanism of Stroke." *Stroke* 23, Supp. (1992): I15.

Hinchey, J. A., and C. A. Sila. "Cerebrovascular Complications of Rheumatic Disease." *Rheumatic Diseases Clinics of North America* 23, no. 2 (May 1997): 317–332.

Khamashta, M. A., M. J. Cuadrado, F. Mujic, et al. "The Management of Thrombosis in the Antiphospholipid-Antibody Syndrome." *The New England Journal of Medicine* 332 (1995): 993.

Meroni, P. L., and P. Riboldi. "Pathogenic Mechanisms Mediating Antiphospholipid Syndrome." *Current Opinion in Rheumatology* 13, no. 5 (September 2001): 377–382.

Petri, M. "Pathogenesis and Treatment of the Antiphospholipid Antibody Syndrome." *The Medical Clinics of North America* 81, no. 1 (January 1997): 151–177.

Pisetsky, D. S., G. Gilkeson, and E. G. St. Clair. "Systemic Lupus Erythematosus." *The Medical Clinics of North America* 81, no. 1 (January 1997): 113–128.

Thiagarajan, P., and S. S. Shapiro. "Lupus Anticoagulants and Antiphospholipid Antibodies." *Hematology/Oncology Clinics of North America* 12, no. 6 (December 1998): 1,167–1,192.

AUTOIMMUNE HEMOLYTIC ANEMIA (AIHA)

Petz, L. D. "Treatment of Autoimmune Hemolytic Anemias." *Current Opinion in Hematology* 8, no. 6 (November 2001): 411–416.

Quartier, P., B. Brethon, P. Philippet, J. Landman-Parker, F. Le Deist, and A. Fischer. "Treatment of Childhood Autoimmune Haemolytic Anaemia with Rituximab." *Lancet* 358, no. 9,292 (November 2001): 1,511–1,513.

Smith, L. A. "Autoimmune Hemolytic Anemias: Characteristics and Classification." *Clinical Laboratory Sciences* 12, no. 2 (March–April 1999): 110–114.

AUTOIMMUNE INNER EAR DISEASE (AIED)

Boulassel, M. R., N. Deggouj, J. P. Tomasi, and M. Gersdorff. "Inner Ear Autoantibodies and Their Targets in Patients with Autoimmune Inner Ear Diseases." *Acta Oto-Laryngologica* 121, no. 1 (January 2001): 28–34.

Campbell, K. C., and J. J. Klemens. "Sudden Hearing Loss and Autoimmune Inner Ear Disease." *Journal of the American Academy of Audiology* 11, no. 7 (July–August 2000): 361–367.

Hirose, K., M. H. Wener, and L. G. Duckert. "Utility of Laboratory Testing in Autoimmune Inner Ear Disease." *Laryngoscope* 109, no. 11 (November 1999): 1,749–1,754.

Lasak, J. M., R. T. Sataloff, M. Hawkshaw, T. E. Carey, K. M. Lyons, and J. R. Spiegel. "Autoimmune Inner Ear Disease: Steroid and Cytotoxic Drug Therapy." *Ear, Nose, & Throat Journal* 80, no. 11 (November 2001): 808–811, 815–816, 818.

Roland, J. T. "Autoimmune Inner Ear Disease." *Current Rheumatology Reports* 2, no. 2 (April 2000): 171–174.

AUTOIMMUNE LYMPHOPROLIFERATIVE SYNDROME (ALPS)

Blessing, J. J., M. R. Brown, S. E. Straus, J. K. Dale, R. M. Siegel, M. Johnson, M. J. Lenardo, J. M. Puck, and T. A. Fleisher. "Immunophenotypic Profiles in Families with Autoimmune Lymphoproliferative Syndrome." *Blood* 98, no. 8 (October 2001): 2,466–2,473.

Blessing, J. J., S. E. Straus, and T. A. Fleisher. "Autoimmune Lymphoproliferative Syndrome. A Human Disorder of Abnormal Lymphocyte Survival." *Pediatric Clinics of North America* 47, no. 6 (December 2000): 1,291–1,310.

Chun, H. J., and M. J. Lenardo. "Autoimmune Lymphoproliferative Syndrome: Types I, II and Beyond." *Advances in Experimental Medicine and Biology* 490 (2001): 49–57.

Fleisher, T. A., J. M. Puck, W. Strober, J. K. Dale, M. J. Lenardo, R. M. Siegel, S. E. Straus, and J. J. Blessing. "The Autoimmune Lymphoproliferative Syndrome. A Disorder of Human Lymphocyte Apoptosis." *Clinical Reviews in Allergy & Immunology* 20, no. 1 (February 2001): 109–120.

BEHÇET'S DISEASE

Bang, D. "Clinical Spectrum of Behçet's Disease." *Journal of Dermatology* 28, no. 11 (November 2001): 610–613.

Calikoglu, E., M. Onder, B. Cosar, and S. Candansayar. "Depression, Anxiety Levels, and General Psychological Profile in Behçet's Disease." *Dermatology* 203, no. 3 (2001): 238–240.

Gul, A. "Behçet's Disease: An Update on the Pathogenesis." *Clinical and Experimental Rheumatology* 19, Supp. 24 (September–October 2001): S6–S12.

Meador, R., G. Ehrlich, and J. M. Von Feldt. "Behçet's Disease: Immunopathologic and Therapeutic Aspects." *Current Rheumatology Reports* 4, no. 1 (February 2002): 47–54.

Yazici, H. "Behçet's Syndrome: Where Do We Stand?" *American Journal of Medicine* 112, no. 1 (January 2002): 75–76.

BULLOUS PEMPHIGOID

Anderson, C. K., C. M. Mowad, M. E. Goff, and M. T. Pelle. "Bullous Pemphigoid Arising in Surgical Wounds." *British Journal of Dermatology* 145, no. 4 (October 2001): 670–672.

Ghohestani, R. F., J. Novotney, M. Chaudhary, and R. S. Agah. "Bullous Pemphigoid: From the Bedside to the Research Laboratory." *Clinics in Dermatology* 19, no. 6 (November–December 2001): 690–696.

Joly, P., J. C. Roujeau, J. Benichou, C. Picard, B. Dreno, E. Delaporte, L. Vaillant, M. D'Incan, P. Plantin, C. Bedane, P. Young, and P. Bernard. "A Comparison of Oral and Topical Corticosteroids in Patients with Bullous Pemphigoid." *The New England Journal of Medicine* 346, no. 5 (January 2002): 321–327.

Liu, Z., and L. A. Diaz. "Bullous Pemphigoid: End of the Century Overview." *Journal of Dermatology* 23, no. 11 (November 2001): 647–650.

Stern, R. S. "Bullous Pemphigoid Therapy—Think Globally, Act Locally." *The New England Journal of Medicine* 346, no. 5 (January 2002): 364–367.

CARDIOMYOPATHY

Baba, A., T. Yoshikawa, H. Mitamura, M. Akaishi, and S. Ogawa. "Autoantibodies Against Sarcolemnal Na-K-ATPase in Patients with Dilated Cardiomyopathy: Autoimmune Basis for Ventricular Arrhythmias in Patients with Congestive Heart Failure." *Journal of Cardiology* 39, no. 1 (January 2002): 50–51.

Lokhandwala, Y. "Hypertrophic Cardiomyopathy: The Elusive Terrorist?" *Journal of Postgraduate Medicine* 47, no. 3 (July–September 2001): 163–164.

Mahon, N. G., B. P. Madden, A. L. Caforio, P. M. Elliott, A. J. Haven, B. E. Keogh, M. J. Davies, and W. J. McKenna. "Immunohistologic Evidence of Myocardial Disease in Apparently Healthy Relatives of Patients with Dilated Cardiomyopathy." *Journal of the American College of Cardiology* 39, no. 3 (February 2002): 455–462.

Pahlevan, I., H. Lonergan-Thomas, S. Ande, J. Burks, E. Robin, T. Petropulos, and M. A. Silver. "Difficult Cases in Heart Failure: Familial Dilated Cardiomyopathy." *Congestive Heart Failure* 7, no. 3 (May–June 2001): 163–165.

Silver, M. A. "Familial Dilated Cardiomyopathy—More Than Meets the Eye." *Congestive Heart Failure* 7, no. 3 (May–June 2001): 162.

CELIAC DISEASE

Abdulkarin, A. S., and J. A. Murray. "Celiac Disease." *Current Treatment Options in Gastroenterology* 5, no. 1 (February 2002): 27–38.

Book, L., S. Neuhausen, and J. Zone. "How Should We Define Celiac Disease?" *Journal of Pediatrics Gastroenterology and Nutrition* 34, no. 1 (January 2002): 92.

da Rosa Utiyama, S. R., L. M. da Silva Kotze, R. M. Nisihara, R. F. Carvalho, E. G. de Carvalho, M. G. de Sena, and I. J. de Messias Reason. "Spectrum of Autoantibodies in Celiac Patients and Relatives." *Digestive Diseases and Sciences* 46, no. 12 (December 2001): 2,624–2,630.

Farrell, R. J., and C. P. Kelly. "Celiac Sprue." *The New England Journal of Medicine* 346, no. 3 (January 2002): 180–188.

Farrell, R. J., and C. P. Kelly. "Diagnosis of Celiac Sprue." *American Journal of Gastroenterology* 96, vol. 12 (December 2001): 3,237–3,246.

Lohiniemi, S. "Coeliac Disease. Tricky to Find, Hard to Treat, Impossible to Cure." *Lancet* 358, Supp. (December 2001): S14.

Sollid, L. M., and K. E. Lundin. "Coeliac Disease. An Inappropriate Immune Response." *Lancet* 358, Supp. (December 2001): S13.

Storch, W. B., and U. Schloeder. "A New Autoantibody in Celiac Disease." *Clinical Laboratory* 48, no. 1–2 (2002): 19–23.

CHAGAS' DISEASE

Engman, D. M., and J. S. Leon. "Pathogenesis of Chagas' Heart Disease: Role of Autoimmunity." *Acta Tropica* 81, no. 2 (February 2002): 123–132.

Ferber, D. "Infectious Disease. New Weapons in the Battle of the Bugs." *Science* 295, no. 5,554 (January 2002): 433–434.

Hagar, J. M., and S. H. Rahimtoola. "Chagas' Heart Disease." *Current Problems in Cardiology* 20 (1995): 825–924.

Herwaldt, B. L., and D. D. Juranek. "Laboratory-Acquired Malaria, Leishmaniasis, Trypanosomiasis, and Toxoplasmosis." *American Journal of Tropical Medicine and Hygiene* 48 (1993): 313–323.

Kirchhoff, L. V. "American Trypanosomiasis (Chagas' Disease)." *Gastroenterology Clinics of North America* 25 (1996): 517–532.

Kirchhoff, L. V. "American Trypanosomiasis (Chagas' Disease)—A Tropical Disease now in the United States." *The New England Journal of Medicine* 329 (1993): 639–644.

CHRONIC FATIGUE SYNDROME

Clark, C., D. Buchwald, A. MacIntyre, M. Sharpe, and S. Wessely. "Chronic Fatigue Syndrome: A Step Towards Agreement." *Lancet* 359, no. 9,301 (January 2002): 97–98.

Creswell, C., and T. Chalder. "Defensive Coping Styles in Chronic Fatigue Syndrome." *Journal of Psychosomatic Research* 51, no. 4 (October 2001): 607–610.

Dendy, C., M. Cooper, and M. Sharpe. "Interpretation of Symptoms in Chronic Fatigue Syndrome." *Behaviour Research and Therapy* 39, no. 11 (November 2001): 1,369–1,380.

Hamilton, W. "Chronic Fatigue Syndrome." *British Journal of General Practice* 51, no. 473 (December 2001): 1,015.

Hammond, D. C. "Treatment of Chronic Fatigue with Neurofeedback and Self-Hypnosis." *NeuroRehabilitation* 16, no. 4 (2001): 295–300.

Jason, L. A., H. Eisele, and R. R. Taylor. "Assessing Attitudes Toward New Names for Chronic Fatigue Syndrome." *Evaluation & the Health Professionals* 24, no. 4 (December 2001): 424–435.

Jason, L. A., S. R. Torres-Harding, A. W. Carrico, and R. R. Taylor. "Symptom Occurrence in Persons with Chronic Fatigue Syndrome." *Biological Psychology* 59, no. 1 (February 2002): 15–27.

Murdoch, J. C. "Chronic Fatigue Syndrome." *British Journal of General Practice* 51, no. 470 (September 2001): 758.

Sachs, L. "From a Lived Body to a Medicalized Body: Diagnostic Transformation and Chronic Fatigue Syndrome." *Medical Anthropology* 19, no. 4 (2001): 299–317.

Straus, S. E. "Caring for Patients with Chronic Fatigue Syndrome. Conclusions in CMO's Report Are Shaped by Anecdote Not Evidence." *BMJ* 324, no. 7,330 (January 2002): 124–125.

CHRONIC INFLAMMATORY DEMYELINATING POLYNEUROPATHY (CIDP)

Hughes, R. A. "Chronic Inflammatory Demyelinating Polyradiculoneuropathy." *Annals of Neurology* 50, no. 3 (September 2001): 281–282.

Kuwabara, S., K. Ogawara, S. Misawa, M. Mori, and T. Hattori. "Distribution Patterns of Demyelination Correlate with Clinical Profiles in Chronic Inflammatory Demyelinating Polyneuropathy." *Journal of Neurology, Neurosurgery, and Psychiatry* 72, no. 1 (January 2002): 37–42.

Lindenbaum, Y., J. T. Kissel, and J. R. Mendell. "Treatment Approaches for Guillain-Barré Syndrome and Chronic Inflammatory Demyelinating Polyradiculoneuropathy." *Neurologic Clinics* 19, no. 1 (February 2001): 187–204.

Nevo, Y., and H. Topaloglu. "88th ENMC International Workshop: Childhood Chronic Inflammatory Demyelinating Polyneuropathy (Including Revised Diagnostic Criteria). Naarden, The Netherlands, December 8–10, 2000." *Neuromuscular Disorders* 12, no. 2 (February 2002): 195–200.

Nicolas, G., T. Maisonobe, N. Le Forestier, J. M. Leger, and P. Bouche. "Proposed Revised Electrophysiological Criteria for Chronic Inflammatory Demyelinating Polyradiculoneuropathy." *Muscle Nerve* 25, no. 1 (January 2002): 26–30.

Vermeulen, M., and M. H. Van Oers. "Successful Autologous Stem Cell Transplantation in a Patient with Chronic Inflammatory Demyelinating Polyneuropathy." *Journal of Neurology, Neurosurgery, and Psychiatry* 72, no. 1 (January 2002): 127–128.

CHURG-STRAUSS SYNDROME

Alvarez, C., V. Asensi, A. Rodriguez-Guardado, L. Casado, P. Ablanedo, and C. Alvarez-Navascues. "Unusual Complications in the Churg-Strauss Syndrome." *Annals of the Rheumatic Diseases* 61, no. 1 (January 2002): 94–95.

Churg, A. "Recent Advances in the Diagnosis of Churg-Strauss Syndrome." *Modern Pathology* 14, no. 12 (December 2001): 1,284–1,293.

Gross, W. L. "Churg-Strauss Syndrome: Update on Recent Developments." *Current Opinion in Rheumatology* 14, no. 1 (January 2002): 11–14.

Harrison, B. D., and D. G. Scott. "Churg-Strauss Syndrome." *Thorax* 56, no. 10 (October 2001): 818–819.

Ishiyama, A., and R. F. Canalis. "Otological Manifestations of Churg-Strauss Syndrome." *Laryngoscope* 111, no. 9 (September 2001): 1,619–1,624.

Lilly, C. M., A. Churg, M. Lazarovich, R. Pauwels, L. Hendeles, L. J. Rosenwasser, D. Ledford, and M. E. Wechsler. "Asthma Therapies and Churg-Strauss Syndrome." *Journal of Allergy and Clinical Immunology* 109, no. 1 (January 2002): S1–19.

Morishita, M. "Allergy and Angiitis: Two Aspects of Churg-Strauss Syndrome." *Internal Medicine* 40, no. 2 (February 2001): 77.

Ramakrishna, G., and D. E. Midthun. "Churg-Strauss Syndrome." *Annals of Allergy, Asthma, and Immunology* 86, no. 6 (June 2001): 603–613.

Sabio, J. M., J. Jimenez-Alonso, and F. Gonzalez-Crespo. "More About Churg-Strauss Syndrome and Montelukast Treatment." *Chest* 120, no. 6 (December 2001): 2,116.

Wiik, A. "Laboratory Diagnostics in Vasculitis Patients." *Israel Medical Association Journal* 3, no. 4 (April 2001): 275–277.

CICATRICIAL PEMPHIGOID (CP)

Cheng, Y. S., T. D. Rees, J. M. Wright, and J. M. Plemons. "Childhood Oral Pemphigoid: A Case Report and Review of the Literature." *Journal of Oral Pathology and Medicine* 30, no. 6 (July 2001): 372–377.

Doan, S., J. F. Lerouic, H. Robin, C. Prost, M. Savoldelli, and T. Hoang-Xuan. "Treatment of Ocular Cicatricial Pemphigoid with Sulfasalazine." *Ophthalmology* 108, no. 9 (September 2001): 1,565–1,568.

Megahed, M., S. Schmiedeberg, J. Becker, and T. Ruzicka. "Treatment of Cicatricial Pemphigoid with Mycophenolate Mofetil as a Steroid-Sparing Agent." *Journal of the American Academy of Dermatology* 45, no. 2 (August 2001): 256–259.

Miserocchi, E., S. Baltatzis, M. R. Roque, A. R. Ahmed, and C. S. Foster. "The Effect of Treatment and Its Related Side Effects in Patients with Severe Ocular Cicatricial Pemphigoid." *Ophthalmology* 109, no. 1 (January 2002): 111–118.

Mutasim, D. F., and B. B. Adams. "Cicatricial Pemphigoid Diagnosed by the Use of Indirect Immunofluorescence." *Journal of Cutaneous Medicine and Surgery* 4, no. 4 (October 2000): 205–207.

Razzaque, M. S., C. S. Foster, and A. R. Ahmed. "Tissue and Molecular Events in Human Conjunctival Scarring in Ocular Cicatricial Pemphigoid." *Histology and Histopathology* 16, no. 4 (October 2001): 1,203–1,212.

Sacher, C., A. Rubbert, C. Konig, K. Scharffetter-Kochanek, T. Krieg, and N. Hunzelmann. "Treatment of Recalcitrant Cicatricial Pemphigoid with the Tumor Necrosis Factor Alpha Antagonist Etanercept." *Journal of the American Academy of Dermatology* 46, no. 1 (January 2002): 113–115.

CROHN'S DISEASE

Byrne, M. F., M. A. Farrell, S. Abass, A. Fitzgerald, J. C. Varghese, F. Thornton, F. E. Murray, and M. J. Lee. "Assessment of Crohn's Disease Activity by Doppler Sonography of the Superior Mesenteric Artery, Clinical Evaluation and the Crohn's Disease Activity Index: A Prospective Study." *Clinical Radiology* 56, no. 12 (December 2001): 973–978.

Chen, G. I., F. Saibil, and I. Morava-Protzner. "Two for One: Coexisting Ulcerative Colitis and Crohn's Disease." *Canadian Journal of Gastroenterology* 16, no. 1 (January 2002): 29–34.

Greenberg, G. R. "Infliximab as First-Line Therapy for Crohn's Disease is Premature." *Inflammatory Bowel Diseases* 8, no. 1 (January 2002): 60–65.

Freeman, H. J. "Spontaneous Free Perforation of the Small Intestine in Crohn's Disease." *Canadian Journal of Gastroenterology* 16, no. 1 (January 2002): 23–27.

Reddy, S. I., and J. L. Wolf. "Management Issues in Women with Inflammatory Bowel Disease." *The Journal of the American Osteopathic Association* 101, Supp. (December 2001): S17–S23.

Shanahan, F. "Crohn's Disease." *Lancet* 359, no. 9, 300 (January 2002): 62–69.

van Deventer, S. J. "Immunomodulation of Crohn's Disease." *Current Directions in Autoimmunity* 2 (2000): 150–166.

COGAN'S SYNDROME

Albayram, M. S., R. Wityk, D. M. Yousem, and S. J. Zinreich. "The Cerebral Angiographic Findings in Cogan Syndrome." *AJNR American Journal of Neuroradiology* 22, no. 4 (April 2001): 751–754.

Chynn, E. W., and F. A. Jakobiec. "Cogan's Syndrome: Ophthalmic, Audiovestibular, and Systemic Manifestations and Therapy." *International Ophthalmology Clinics* 36, no. 1 (Winter 1996): 61–72.

Garcia Berrocal, J. R., J. A. Vargas, M. Vaquero, S. Ramon y Cajal, and R. A. Ramirez-Camacho. "Cogan's Syndrome: An Oculo-Audiovestibular Disease." *Postgraduate Medical Journal* 75, no. 883 (May 1999): 262–264.

Gaubitz, M., B. Lubben, M. Seidel, H. Schotte, F. Gramley, and W. Domschke. "Cogan's Syndrome: Organ-Specific Autoimmune Disease or Systemic Vasculitis? A Report of Two Cases and Review of the Literature." *Clinical and Experimental Rheumatology* 19, no. 4 (July–August 2001): 463–469.

Gittinger, J. W. "The Legacy of David G. Cogan, M.D." *Survey of Ophthalmology* 45, no. 3 (November–December 2000): 254–258.

Helmchen, C., V. Arbusow, L. Jager, M. Strupp, W. Stocker, and P. Schulz. "Cogan's Syndrome: Clinical

Significance of Antibodies Against the Inner Ear and Cornea." *Acta Oto-laryngologica* 119, no. 5 (1999): 528–536.

Olfat, M., and S. M. Al-Mayouf. "Cogan's Syndrome in Childhood." *Rheumatology International* 20, no. 6 (August 2001): 246–249.

St. Clair, E. W., and R. M. McCallum. "Cogan's Syndrome." *Current Opinions in Rheumatology* 11, no. 1 (January 1999): 47–52.

Van Doornum, S., G. McColl, M. Walter, I. Jennens, P. Bhathal, and I. P. Wicks. "Prolonged Prodrome, Systemic Vasculitis, and Deafness in Cogan's Syndrome." *Annals of the Rheumatic Diseases* 60, no. 1 (January 2001): 69–71.

COLD AGGLUTININ DISEASE

Dacie, S. J. "The Immune Haemolytic Anaemias: A Century of Exciting Progress in Understanding." *British Journal of Haematology* 114, no. 4 (September 2001): 770–785.

Havouis, S., G. Dumas, P. Ave, O. Pritsch, M. Huerre, G. Dighiero, and C. Pourcel. "A Murine Transgenic Model of Human Cold Agglutinin Disease." *Haematologica* 84 Suppl. EHA (June 1999): 67–69.

Lauchli, S., L. Widmer, and S. Lautenschlager. "Cold Agglutinin Disease—The Importance of Cutaneous Signs." *Dermatology* 202, no. 4 (2001) 356–8.

Layios, N., E. Van Den Neste, E. Jost, V. Deneys, J. M. Scheiff, and A. Ferrant. "Remission of Severe Cold Agglutinin Disease After Rituximab Therapy." *Leukemia* 15, no. 1 (January 2001): 187–188.

Li, Z., Z. Shao, Y. Xu, L. Shen, G. Chen, and Y. Zhang. "Subclasses of Warm Autoantibody IgG in Patients With Autoimmune Hemolytic Anemia and Their Clinical Implications." *Chinese Medical Journal* (Engl) 112, no. 9 (September 1999): 805–808.

Ulvestad, E., S. Berentsen, and T. E. Mollnes. "Acute Phase Haemolysis in Chronic Cold Agglutinin Disease." *Scandinavian Journal of Immunology* 54, no. 1–2 (July–August 2001): 239–242.

Zaja, F., D. Russo, G. Fuga, T. Michelutti, A. Sperotto, R. Fanin, and M. Baccarani. "Rituximab in a Case of Cold Agglutinin Disease." *British Journal of Haematology* 115, no. 1 (October 2001): 232–233.

CONGENITAL HEART BLOCK

Borda, E., and L. Sterin-Borda. "Autoantibodies Against Neonatal Heart M1 Muscarinic Acetylcholine Receptor in Children with Congenital Heart Block." *Journal of Autoimmunity* 16, no. 2 (March 2001): 143–150.

Boutjdir, M. "Molecular and Ionic Basis of Congenital Complete Heart Block." *Trends in Cardiovascular Medicine* 10, no. 3 (April 2000): 114–122.

Buyon, J. P., M. Y. Kim, J. A. Copel, and D. M. Friedman. "Anti-Ro/SSA Antibodies and Congenital Heart Block: Necessary But Not Sufficient." *Arthritis and Rheumatism* 44, no. 8 (August 2001): 1,723–1,727.

Eronen, M., P. Heikkila, and K. Teramo. "Congenital Complete Heart Block in the Fetus: Hemodynamic Features, Antenatal Treatment, and Outcome in Six Cases." *Pediatric Cardiology* 22, no. 5 (September–October 2001): 385–392.

Julkunen, H., and M. Eronen. "The Rate of Recurrence of Isolated Congenital Heart Block: A Population-Based Study." *Arthritis and Rheumatism* 44, no. 2 (February 2001): 487–488.

Klassen, L. R. "Complete Congenital Heart Block: A Review and Case Study." *Neonatal Network: NN* 18, no. 3 (April 1999): 33–42.

Moak, J. P., K. S. Barron, T. J. Hougen, H. B. Wiles, S. Balaji, N. Sreeram, M. H. Cohen, A. Nordenberg, G. F. Van Hare, R. A. Friedman, M. Perez, F. Cecchin, D. S. Schneider, R. A. Nehgme, and J. P. Buyon. "Congenital Heart Block: Development of Late-Onset Cardiomyopathy, a Previously Underappreciated Sequela." *Journal of the American College of Cardiology* 37, no. 1 (January 2001): 238–242.

Qu, Y., G. Q. Xiao, L. Chen, and M. Boutjdir. "Autoantibodies From Mothers of Children With Congenital Heart Block Downregulate Cardiac L-type Ca Channels." *Journal of Molecular and Cellular Cardiology* 33, no. 6 (June 2001): 1,153–1,163.

Yoshida, H., M. Iwamoto, H. Sakakibara, H. Shigeta, F. Hirahara, and K. Sato. "Treatment of Fetal Congenital Complete Heart Block With Maternal Administration of Beta-Sympathomimetics (Terbutaline): A Case Report." *Gynecologic and Obstetric Investigation* 52, no. 2 (2001): 142–144.

COXSACKIE MYOCARDITIS

Goren, A., M. Kaplan, J. Glaser, and M. Isacsohn. "Chronic Neonatal Coxsackie Myocarditis." *Archives of Disease in Childhood* 64, no. 3 (March 1989): 404–406.

Rozkovec, A., G. Cambridge, M. King, and K. A. Hallidie-Smith. "Natural History of Left Ventricular Function in Neonatal Coxsackie Myocarditis." *Pediatric Cardiology* 6, no. 3 (1985): 151–156.

Suckling, P. V., and L. Vogelpoel. "Coxsackie Myocarditis of the Newborn." *Lancet* 2, no. 7669 (August 22, 1970): 421.

Wells, R. G., J. A. Ruskin, and J. R. Sty. "Myocardial Imaging. Coxsackie Myocarditis." *Clinical Nuclear Medicine* 11, no. 9 (September 1986): 661–662.

CREST SYNDROME

Akiyama, Y., M. Tanaka, M. Takeishi, D. Adachi, A. Mimori, and T. Suzuki. "Clinical, Serological and Genetic Study in Patients With CREST Syndrome." *Internal Medicine* 39, no. 6 (June 2000): 451–456.

Chaffee, N. R. "CREST Syndrome: Clinical Manifestations and Dental Management." *Journal of Prosthodontics: Official Journal of the American College of Prosthodontists* 7, no. 3 (September 1998): 155–160.

Jimenez-Balderas, F., A. Zonana-Nacach, M. E. Fonseca-Yerena, A. Ruiz-Chaparro, and D. Pascoe-Lira. "Epidermal Growth Factor and Gastrin in Scleroderma/CREST Syndrome." *Archives of Medical Research* 29, no. 1 (Spring 1998): 51–55.

Kambara, C., I. Kinoshita, T. Amenomori, K. Eguchi, and T. Yoshimura. "Myasthenia Gravis Associated With Limited Scleroderma (CREST Syndrome)." *Journal of Neurology* 247, no. 1 (January 2000): 61–62.

Kondo, H. "CREST Syndrome; a Changing Clinical Significance." *Internal Medicine* 39, no. 6 (June 2000): 437.

Terajima, K., T. Shimohata, M. Watanabe, T. Suzuki, A. Hasegawa, H. Ishiguro, T. Minakawa, and K. Hirota. "Cerebral Vasculopathy Showing Moyamoya-Like Changes in a Patient With CREST Syndrome." *European Neurology* 46, no. 3 (2001): 163–165.

DERMATITIS HERPETIFORMIS (DH)

Caproni, M., C. Cardinali, D. Renzi, A. Calabro, and P. Fabbri. "Tissue Transglutaminase Antibody Assessment in Dermatitis Herpetiformis." *British Journal of Dermatology* 144, no. 1 (January 2001): 196–197.

Cotell, S., N. D. Robinson, and L. S. Chan. "Autoimmune Blistering Skin Diseases." *American Journal of Emergency Medicine* 18, no. 3 (May 2000): 288–299.

Hervonen, K., M. Hakanen, K. Kaukinen, P. Collin, and T. Reunala. "First-Degree Relatives Are Frequently Affected in Coeliac Disease and Dermatitis Herpetiformis." *Scandinavian Journal of Gastroenterology* 37, no. 1 (January 2002): 51–55.

Horvath, K. and D. I. Mehta. "Celiac Disease – A Worldwide Problem." *Indian Journal of Pediatrics* 67, no. 10 (October 2000): 757–763.

Koop, I., R. Ilchmann, L. Izzi, A. Adragna, H. Koop, and H. Barthelmes. "Detection of Autoantibodies Against Tissue Transglutaminase in Patients With Celiac Disease and Dermatitis Herpetiformis." *American Journal of Gastroenterology* 95, no. 8 (August 2000): 2,009–2,014.

Reunala, T. L. "Dermatitis Herpetiformis." *Clinics in Dermatology* 19, no. 6 (November–December 2001): 728–736.

Schmidt, E., and D. Zillikens. "Autoimmune and Inherited Subepidermal Blistering Diseases: Advances in the Clinic and the Laboratory." *Advances in Dermatology* 16 (2000): 16:113–157; discussion 158.

Wills, A. J., B. Turner, R. J. Lock, S. L. Johnston, D. J. Unsworth, and L. Fry. "Dermatitis Herpetiformis and Neurological Dysfunction." *Journal of Neurology, Neurosurgery, and Psychiatry* 72, no. 2 (February 2002): 259–261.

DISCOID LUPUS

Goyal, S., and H. C. Nousari. "Treatment of Resistant Discoid Lupus Erythematosus of the Palms and Soles With Mycophenolate Mofetil." *Journal of the American Academy of Dermatology* 45, no. 1 (July 2001): 142–144.

Gupta, S. "Epidermal Grafting for Depigmentation Due to Discoid Lupus Erythematosus." *Dermatology* 202, no. 4 (2001): 320–323.

Jessop, S., D. Whitelaw, and F. Jordaan. "Drugs for Discoid Lupus Erythematosus." *Cochrane Database of Systematic Reviews* 1 (2001): CD002954.

Kuhn, A., P. M. Becker-Wegerich, T. Ruzicka, and P. Lehmann. "Successful Treatment of Discoid Lupus Erythematosus With Argon Laser." *Dermatology* 201, no. 2 (2000): 175–177.

Letellier, E., H. Longhurst, S. J. Diaz-Cano, and D. D'Cruz. "Polyarteritis Nodosa Developing After Discoid Lupus Erythematosus." *Clinical and Experimental Rheumatology* 19, no. 6 (November–December 2001): 738–739.

Magana, M., and R. Vazquez. "Discoid Lupus Erythematosus in Childhood." *Pediatric Dermatology* 17, no. 3 (May–June 2000): 241–242.

Toro, J. R., D. Finlay, X. Dou, S. C. Zheng, P. E. LeBoit, and M. K. Connolly. "Detection of Type 1 Cytokines in Discoid Lupus Erythematosus." *Archives of Dermatology* 136, no. 12 (December 2000): 1,497–1,501.

DRESSLER'S SYNDROME

Cheng, T. O. "Disappearance of the Dressler Syndrome." *Cardiology* 86, no. 5 (1995): 444.

"Clinical Conferences at the Johns Hopkins Hospital. The Dressler Syndrome." *The Johns Hopkins Medical Journal* 148, no. 4 (April 1981): 179–182.

Jerjes-Sanchez, C., A. Ramirez-Rivera, and C. Ibarra-Perez. "The Dressler Syndrome After Pulmonary Embolism." *American Journal of Cardiology* 78, no. 3 (August 1, 1996): 343–345.

Levin, E. J., and D. Bryk. "Dressler Syndrome (Postmyocardial Infarction Syndrome)." *Radiology* 87, no. 4 (October 1966): 731–736.

ENDOMETRIOSIS

Amso, N. N. "Endometriosis. Clinicians and Patients Should Be Aware of Association Between Endometriosis and Malignancies." *BMJ* 324, no. 7329 (January 12, 2002): 115

Gazvani, R., and A. Templeton. "New Considerations for the Pathogenesis of Endometriosis." *International Journal of Gynaecology and Obstetrics* 76, no. 2 (February 2002): 117–126.

Jones, K. D., and C. Sutton. "Endometriosis. Emphasis on Medical Treatment is Misleading." *BMJ* 324, no. 7329 (January 12, 2002): 115.

Redwine, D. B. "Diaphragmatic Endometriosis: Diagnosis, Surgical Management, and Long-Term Results of Treatment." *Fertility and Sterility* 77, no. 2 (February 2002): 288–296.

Witz, C. A. "Pathogenesis of Endometriosis." *Gynecologic and Obstetric Investigation* 53, Suppl. 1 (2002): 52–62.

ESSENTIAL MIXED CRYOGLOBULINEMIA

Monti, G., F. Saccardo, G. Rinaldi, M. R. Petrozzino, A. Gomitoni, and F. Invernizzi. "Colchicine in the Treatment of Mixed Cryoglobulinemia." *Clinical and Experimental Rheumatology* 13, Suppl. 13 (November–December 1995): S197–199.

Pioltelli, P., P. Maldifassi, A. Vacca, C. Mazzaro, C. Mussini, S. Migliaresi, A. Gabrielli, M. Pietrogrande, A. Monteverde, and G. Monti. "GISC Protocol Experience in the Treatment of Essential Mixed Cryoglobulinaemia." *Clinical and Experimental Rheumatology* 13, Suppl. 13 (November–December 1995): S187–190.

Tavoni, A., M. Mosca, C. Ferri, L. Moriconi, L. La Civita, F. Lombardini, and S. Bombardieri. "Guidelines for the Management of Essential Mixed Cryoglobulinemia." *Clinical and Experimental Rheumatology* 13, Suppl. 13 (November–December 1995): S191–195.

Zaja, F. "Fludarabine in the Treatment of Essential Mixed Cryoglobulinaemia." *European Journal of Haematology* 57, no. 3 (September 1996): 259–260.

EVANS SYNDROME

Maiz, L., A. Munoz, S. Maldonado, A. Pacheco, A. Lamas, and L. Fogue. "Bronchiolitis Obliterans Organizing Pneumonia Associated With Evans Syndrome." *Respiration* 68, no. 6 (2001): 631–634.

Mathew, P., G. Chen, and W. Wang. "Evans Syndrome: Results of a National Survey," *Journal of Pediatric Hematology/Oncology* 19, no. 5 (September–October 1997): 433–437.

McLeod, A. G., M. Pai, R. F. Carter, J. Squire, and R. D. Barr. "Familial Evans Syndrome: A Report of an Affected Sibship." *Journal of Pediatric Hematology/Oncology* 21, no. 3 (May–June 1999): 244–247.

Muwakkit, S., R. Rachid, A. Bazarbachi, T. Araysi, and G. S. Dbaibo. "Treatment-Resistant Infantile Evans Syndrome." *Pediatrics International: Official Journal of the Japan Pediatric Society* 43, no. 5 (October 2001): 502–504.

Oyama, Y., E. B. Papadopoulos, M. Miranda, A. E. Traynor, and R. K. Burt. "Allogeneic Stem Cell Transplantation for Evans Syndrome." *Bone Marrow Transplantation* 28, no. 9 (November 2001): 903–905.

Ozsoylu, S. "Megadose Methylprednisolone for Evans Syndrome." *Pediatric Hematology and Oncology* 17, no. 8 (December 2000): 725–726.

Savasan, S., I. Warrier, and Y. Ravindranath. "The Spectrum of Evans' Syndrome." *Archives of Disease in Childhood* 77, no. 3 (September 1997): 245–248.

EXPERIMENTAL ALLERGIC ENCEPHALOMYELITIS

Boullerne, A. I., J. J. Rodriguez, T. Touil, B. Brochet, S. Schmidt, N. D. Abrous, M. Le Moal, J. R. Pua, M. A. Jensen, W. Mayo, B. G. Arnason, and K. G. Petr. "Anti-S-nitrosocysteine Antibodies Are a Predictive Marker for Demyelination in Experimental Autoimmune Encephalomyelitis: Implications for Multiple Sclerosis." *The Journal of Neuroscience: The Official Journal of the Society for Neuroscience* 22, no. 1 (January 2002): 123–132.

Encinas, J. A., and V. K. Kuchroo. "Genetics of Experimental Autoimmune Encephalomyelitis." *Current Directions in Autoimmunity* 1 (1999): 247–272.

Polfliet, M. M., F. van de Veerdonk, E. A. Dopp, E. M. van Kesteren-Hendrikx N. van Rooijen, C. D. Dijkstra, and T. K. van den Berg. "The Role of Perivascular and Meningeal Macrophages in Experimental Allergic Encephalomyelitis." *Journal of Neuroimmunology* 122, no. 2 (January 2002): 1–8.

Singh, A. K., M. T. Wilson, S. Hong, D. Olivares-Villagomez, C. Du, A. K. Stanic, S. Joyce, S. Sriram, Y. Koezuka, and L. Van Kaer, "Natural Killer T Cell Activation Protects Mice Against Experimental Autoimmune Encephalomyelitis." *The Journal of Experimental Medicine* 194, no. 12 (December 2001): 1,801–1,811.

FIBROMYALGIA

Chester, A. C. "Surgery for Fibromyalgia." *Cleveland Clinic Journal of Medicine* 69, no. 1 (January 2002): 89; discussion 91.

Fors, E. A., and H. Sexton. "Weather and the Pain in Fibromyalgia: Are They Related?" *Annals of the Rheumatic Diseases* 61, no. 3 (March 2002): 247–250.

Gur, A., M. Karakoc, K. Nas Remzi, A. Cevik. A. Denli, and J. Sarac. "Cytokines and Depression in Cases With Fibromyalgia." *Journal of Rheumatology* 29, no. 2 (February 2002): 358–361.

Klein, R., and P. A. Berg. "Diagnostic Relevance of Antibodies to Serotonin and Phospholipids in Fibromyalgia Syndrome." *Journal of Rheumatology* 29, no. 2 (February 2002): 395–396.

Kurtze, N., and S. Svebak. "Fatigue and Patterns of Pain in Fibromyalgia: Correlations With Anxiety, Depression and Co-Morbidity in a Female County Sample." *The British Journal of Medical Psychology* 74, part 4 (December 2001): 523–537.

McGurk, C., D. Wilson, and W. Henry. "Diagnosing Fibromyalgia." *Practitioner* 245, no. 1629 (December 2001): 1,026–1,030.

Paulson, M., E. Danielson, and S. Soderberg. "Struggling for a Tolerable Existence: The Meaning of Men's Lived Experiences of Living With Pain of Fibromyalgia Type." *Qualitative Health Research* 12, no. 2 (February 2002): 238–249.

Raak, R., and L. K. Wahren. "Background Pain in Fibromyalgia Patients Affecting Clinical Examination of the Skin." *Journal of Clinical Nursing* 11, no. 1 (January 2002): 58–64.

Staud, R. "Somatization Does Not Fit All Fibromyalgia Patients: Comment On the Article by Winfield." *Arthritis and Rheumatism* 46, no. 2 (February 2002): 564–565.

Wassem, R., M. McDonald, and J. Racine. "Fibromyalgia: Patient Perspectives on Symptoms, Symptom Management, and Provider Utilization." *Clinical Nurse Specialist CSN* 16, no. 1 (January 2002): 24–28.

GOODPASTURE'S SYNDROME

Avella, P., and M. Walker. "Goodpasture's Syndrome: A Nursing Challenge." *Dimensions of Critical Care Nursing: DCCM* 18, no. 2 (March–April 1999): 2–12.

Borza, D. B., K. O. Netzer, A. Leinonen, P. Todd, J. Cervera, J. Saus, and B. G. Hudson. "The Goodpasture Autoantigen. Identification of Multiple Cryptic Epitopes on the NCI Domain of the Alpha3(IV) Collagen Chain." *Journal of Biological Chemistry* 275, no. 8 (February 2000): 6,030–6,037.

Elson, C. J., and R. N. Barker. "Helper T Cells In Antibody-Mediated, Organ-Specific Autoimmunity." *Current Opinion in Immunology* 12, no. 6 (December 2000): 664–669.

Gunnarsson, A., T. Hellmark, and J. Wieslander. "Molecular Properties of the Goodpasture Epitope." *The Journal of Biological Chemistry* 275, no. 40 (October 2000): 30,844–30,848.

Laczika, K., S. Knapp, K. Derfler, A. Soleiman, W. H. Horl, and W. Druml. "Immunoadsorption in Goodpasture's Syndrome." *American Journal of Kidney Diseases* 36, no. 2 (August 2000): 392–395.

Lettieri, C., and J. Pina "Goodpasture's Syndrome: A Case of Delayed Appearance of Autoantibodies and Renal Disease." *Military Medicine* 166, no. 9 (September 2001): 827–830.

Phelps, R. G. "Immune Recognition of Glomerular Antigens." *Experimental Nephrology* 8, no. 4–5 (July–October 2000): 226–234.

Reisli, I., A. Ozel, U. Caliskan, M. Cakir, and O. Tulunay. "Pathological Case of the Month. Goodpasture Disease." *Archives of Pediatrics and Adolescent Medicine* 155, no. 12 (December 2001): 1,383–1,384.

Salama, A. D., J. B. Levy, L. Lightstone, and C. D. Pusey. "Goodpasture's Disease." *Lancet* 358, no. 9285 (September 15, 2001): 917–920.

Turner, A. N. "Goodpasture's disease." *Nephrology Dialysis Transplantation* 16, no. Suppl. 6 (2001): 52–54.

GRAVES' DISEASE

Antonelli, A., P. Fallahi, C. Nesti, C. Pupilli, P. Marchetti, S. Takasawa, H. Okamoto, and E. Ferrannini. "Anti-CD38 Autoimmunity in Patients With Chronic Autoimmune Thyroiditis or Graves' Disease." *Clinical and Experimental Immunology* 126, no. 3 (December 2001): 426–431.

Bower, B. F. "Therapies for Graves' disease – Choices, Outcomes, and Variations: The Role of the Clinical Endocrinologist." *Endocrine Practice* 7, no. 6 (November–December 2001): 484–485.

Clauser, L., M. Galie, E. Sarti, and V. Dallera. "Rationale of Treatment in Graves Ophthalmopathy." *Plastic and Reconstructive Surgery* 108, no. 7 (December 2001): 1,880–1,894.

Guma, M., A. Olive, M. Juan, and I. Salinas. "ANCA Antibodies in Graves' Disease." *Annals of the Rheumatic Diseases* 61, no. 1 (January 2002): 90–91.

Hao, S. T., C. A. Reasner 2nd, and R. A. Becker. "Use of Cold Iodine in Patients With Graves' Disease: Observations From a Clinical Practice." *Endocrine Practice* 7, no. 6 (November–December 2001): 438–442.

Noth, D., M. Gebauer, B. Muller, U. Burgi, and P. Diem. "Graves' Ophthalmopathy: Natural History and Treatment Outcomes." *Swiss Medical Weekly* 131, no. 41–42 (October 20, 2001): 603–609.

Pijl, H., P. H. de Meijer, J. Langius, C. I. Coenegracht, A. H. van den Berk, P. K. Chandie Shaw, H. Boom, R. C. Schoemaker, A. F. Cohen, J. Burggraaf, and A. E. Meinder. "Food Choice in Hyperthyroidism: Potential Influence of the Autonomic Nervous System and

Brain Serotonin Precursor Availability." *The Journal of Clinical Endocrinology and Metabolism* 86, no. 12 (December 2001): 5,848–5,853.

Schwartz, K. M., V. Fatourechi, D. D. Ahmed, and G. R. Pond. "Dermopathy of Graves' Disease (Pretibial Myxedema): Long-Term Outcome." *The Journal of Clinical Endocrinology and Metabolism* 87, no. 2 (February 2002): 438–446.

Smith, B. R. "Thyroid Autoantibodies." *Scandinavian Journal of Clinical and Laboratory Investigation. Supplementum* 235 (2001): 45–52.

Wall, J. R. "Graves' Disease is a Multi-System Autoimmune Disorder in Which Extra Ocular Muscle Damage and Connective Tissue Inflammation are Variable Features." *Thyroid* 12, no. 1 (January 2002): 35–36.

GUILLAIN-BARRÉ SYNDROME

Bansal, R., J. Kalita, and U. K. Misra. "Pattern of Sensory Conduction in Guillain-Barre Syndrome." *Electromyography and Clinical Neurophysiology* 41, no. 7 (October–November 2001): 433–437.

Chalela, J. A. "Pearls and Pitfalls in the Intensive Care Management of Guillain-Barre Syndrome." *Seminars in Neurology* 21, no. 4 (December 2001): 399–405.

Dattilio, F. M., and J. E. Castaldo. "Differentiating Symptoms of Panic From Relapse of Guillain-Barre Syndrome." *Harvard Review of Psychiatry* 9, no. 5 (September–October 2001): 260–265.

Dziewas, R., B. Kis, F. H. Grus, and C. W. Zimmermann. "Antibody Pattern Analysis in the Guillain-Barre Syndrome and Pathologic Controls." *Journal of Neuroimmunology* 119, no. 2 (October 1, 2001): 287–296.

Govoni, V., and E. Granieri. "Epidemiology of the Guillain-Barre Syndrome." *Current Opinion in Neurology* 14, no. 5 (October 2001): 605–613.

Hartung, H. P., B. C. Kieseier, and R. Kiefer. "Progress in Guillain-Barre Syndrome." *Current Opinion in Neurology* 14, no. 5 (October 2001): 597–604.

Lyu, R. K., L. M. Tang, W. C. Hsu, S. T. Chen, H. S. Chang, and Y. R. Wu. "A Longitudinal Cardiovascular Autonomic Function Study in Mild Guillain-Barre Syndrome." *European Neurology* 47, no. 2 (2002): 79–84.

Mehndiratta, M. M., D. Chowdhury, and V. Goel. "Efficacy and Cost Effectiveness of Current Therapies in Guillain Barre Syndrome." *The Journal of the Association of Physicians of India* 49 (April 2001): 459–469.

Weiss, H., V. Rastan, W. Mullges, R. F. Wagner, and K. V. Toyka. "Psychotic Symptoms and Emotional Distress in Patients with Guillain-Barre Syndrome." *European Neurology* 47, no. 2 (February 2002): 74–78.

Winer, J. B. "Guillain Barre Syndrome." *Molecular Pathology: MP* 54, no. 6 (December 2001): 381–385.

HASHIMOTO'S THYROIDITIS

Degner, D., J. Meller, S. Bleich, V. Schlautmann, and E. Ruther. "Affective Disorders Associated With Autoimmune Thyroiditis." *The Journal of Neuropsychiatry and Clinical Neurosciences* 13, no. 4 (Fall 2001): 532–533.

Hoogenberg, K., and K. M. van Tol. "Hashimoto's Thyroiditis Presenting as a Functioning Adenoma." *Thyroid* 11, no. 9 (September 2001): 893.

Hunt, P. J., S. E. Marshall, A. P. Weetman, M. Bunce, J. I. Bell, J. A. Wass, and K. I. Welsh. "Histocompatibility Leucocyte Antigens and Closely Linked Immunomodulatory Genes in Autoimmune Thyroid Disease." *Clinical Endocrinology (Oxford)* 55, no. 4 (October 2001): 491–499.

Legakis, I., V. Petroyianni, A. Saramantis, and G. Tolis. "Elevated Prolactin to Cortisol Ratio and Polyclonal Autoimmune Activation in Hashimoto's Thyroiditis." *Hormone and Metabolic Research* 33, no. 10 (October 2001): 585–589.

Takao, T., W. Nanamiya, R. Matsumoto, K. Asaba, T. Okabayashi, and K. Hashimoto. "Antipituitary Antibodies in Patients With Lymphocytic Hypophysitis." *Hormone Research* 55, no. 6 (2001): 288–292.

Thieblemont, C., A. Mayer, C. Dumontet, Y. Barbier, E. Callet-Bauchu, P. Felman, F. Berger, X. Ducottet, C. Martin, G. Salles, J. Orgiazzi, and B. Coiffier. "Primary Thyroid Lymphoma is a Heterogeneous Disease." *Journal of Clinical Endocrinology and Metabolism* 87, no. 1 (January 2002): 105–111.

Tomer, Y., D. A. Greenberg, E. Concepcion, Y. Ban, and T. F. Davies. "Thyroglobulin is a Thyroid Specific Gene for the Familial Autoimmune Thyroid Diseases." *Journal of Clinical Endocrinology and Metabolism* 87, no. 1 (January 2002): 404–407.

Tonacchera, M., P. Agretti, G. De Marco, A. Perri, A. Pinchera, P. Vitti, and L. Chiovato. "Thyroid Resistance to TSH Complicated by Autoimmune Thyroiditis." *Journal of Clinical Endocrinology and Metabolism* 86, no. 9 (September 2001): 4,543–4,546.

HEPATITIS (AUTOIMMUNE)

Al-Khalidi, J. A., and A. J. Czaja. "Current Concepts in the Diagnosis, Pathogenesis, and Treatment of Autoimmune Hepatitis." *Mayo Clinic Proceedings* 76, no. 12 (December 2001): 1,237–1,252.

Ben-Ari, Z., and A. J. Czaja. "Autoimmune Hepatitis and Its Variant Syndromes." *Gut* 49, no. 4 (October 2001): 589–594.

Gish, R. G., and A. Mason. "Autoimmune Liver Disease. Current Standards, Future Directions." *Clinics in Liver Disease* 5, no. 2 (May 2001): 287–314.

Heneghan, M., and I. G. McFarlane. "Current and Novel Immunosuppressive Therapy for Autoimmune Hepatitis." *Hepatology* 35, no. 1 (January 2002): 7–13.

Lim, K. N., R. L. Casanova, T. D. Boyer, and C. J. Bruno. "Autoimmune Hepatitis in African Americans: Presenting Features and Response to Therapy." *American Journal of Gastroenterology* 96, no. 12 (December 2001): 3,390–3,394.

McFarlane, I. G. "Autoimmune Liver Diseases." *Scandinavian Journal of Clinical and Laboratory Investigation Supplementum* (2001): 53–60.

Muratori, L., P. Muratori, D. Zauli, A. Grassi, G. Pappas, L. Rodrigo, F. Cassani, M. Lenzi, and F. B. Bianchi. "Antilactoferrin Antibodies in Autoimmune Liver Disease." *Clinical and Experimental Immunology* 124, no. 3 (June 2001): 470–473.

Par, A. "Pathogenesis and Treatment of Autoimmune Hepatitis and Chronic Viral Hepatitis B and C." *Acta Physiologica Hungarica* 87, no. 4 (2000): 373–395.

Shackel, N. A., P. H. McGuinness, C. A. Abbott, M. D. Gorrell, and G. W. McCaughan. "Insights Into the Pathobiology of Hepatitis C Virus-Associated Cirrhosis: Analysis of Intrahepatic Differential Gene Expression." *American Journal of Pathology* 160, no. 2 (February 2002): 641–654.

Yachha, S. K., A. Srivastava, K. Chetri, V. A. Saraswat, and N. Krishnani. "Autoimmune liver disease in children." *Journal of Gastroenterology and Hepatology* 16, no. 6 (June 2001): 674–677.

HERPES GESTATIONIS

Black, M. M. "New Observations on Pemphigoid 'Herpes' Gestationis." *Dermatology* 189, Suppl. 1 (1994): 50–51.

Borrego, L., E. A. Peterson, L. I. Diez, P. de Pablo Martin, J. M. Gleich, and K. M. Leiferman. "Polymorphic Eruption of Pregnancy and Herpes Gestationis: Comparison of Granulated Cell Proteins in Tissue and Serum." *Clinical and Experimental Dermatology* 24, no. 3 (May 1999): 213–225.

Chen, S. H., K. Chopra, T. Y. Evans, S. S. Raimer, M. L. Levy, and S. K. Tyring. "Herpes Gestationis in a Mother and Child." *Journal of the American Academy of Dermatology* 40 no. 5 Pt. 2 (May 1999): 847–849.

Hashimoto, T., M. Amagai, H. Murakami, M. Higashiyama, K. Hashimoto, and T. Nishikawa. "Specific Detection of Anti-Cell Surface Antibodies in Herpes Gestationis Sera." *Experimental Dermatology* 5, no. 2 (April 1996): 96–101.

Lin, M. S., L. A. Arteaga, and Diaz, L. A. "Herpes Gestationis." *Clinics in Dermatology* 19, no. 6 (November–December 2001): 697–702.

Lin, M. S., Gharia, M. A., S. J. Swartz, L. A. Diaz, and G. J. Giudice. "Identification and Characterization of Epitopes Recognized by T Lymphocytes and Autoantibodies From Patients With Herpes Gestationis." *Journal of Immunology* 162, no. 8 (April 15, 1999): 4,991–4,997.

Paternoster, D. M., G. Bruno, and P. V. Grella. "New Observations on Herpes Gestationis Therapy." *International Journal of Gynaecology and Obstetrics* 56, no. 3 (March 1997): 277–278.

Satoh, S., M. Seishima, Y. Sawada, T. Izumi, K. Yoneda, and Y. Kitajima. "The Time Course of the Change in Antibody Titres in Herpes Gestationis." *British Journal of Dermatology* 140, no. 1 (January 1999): 119–123.

Tanzi, P., A. Lojacono, M. Tarantin, and D. Faden. "Herpes Gestationis." *International Journal of Gynaecology and Obstetrics* 45, no. 1 (April 1994): 47–49.

Uncu, G., H. Ozan, S. Tatlikazan, Y. Kimya, and C. Cengiz. "Gestational Herpes: 3 Cases." *Journal of Obstetrics and Gynaecology* 21, no. 4 (August 1995): 381–384.

IDIOPATHIC PULMONARY FIBROSIS (IPF)

Allen, J. T., and M. A. Spiteri. "Growth Factors in Idiopathic Pulmonary Fibrosis: Relative Roles." *Respiratory Research* 3, no. 1 (2002): 13.

Fumeaux, T., C. Rothmeier, and P. Jolliet. "Outcome of Mechanical Ventilation for Acute Respiratory Failure in Patients With Pulmonary Fibrosis." *Intensive Care Medicine* 27, no. 12 (December 2001): 1,868–1,874.

Gauldie, J., M. Kolb, and P. J. Sime. "A New Direction in the Pathogenesis of Idiopathic Pulmonary Fibrosis?" *Respiratory Research* 3, no. 1 (2002): 1.

Hadi, H. A., and A. G. Arnold. "Malaise, Weight Loss, and Respiratory Symptoms." *Postgraduate Medical Journal* 78, no. 915 (January 2002): 55, 58.

King Jr., T. E., M. I. Schwarz, K. Brown, J. A. Tooze, T. V. Colby, J. A. Waldron Jr., A. Flint, W. Thurlbeck, and R. M. Cherniack. "Idiopathic Pulmonary Fibrosis: Relationship Between Histopathologic Features and Mortality." *American Journal of Respiratory and Critical Care Medicine* 164, no. 6 (September 15, 2001): 1,025–1,032.

Lasky, J. A., and L. A. Ortiz. "Antifibrotic Therapy for the Treatment of Pulmonary Fibrosis." *The American Journal of the Medical Sciences* 322, no. 4 (October 2001): 213–221.

Ogushi, F., K. Tani, T. Endo, H. Tada, T. Kawano, T. Asano, L. Huang, Y. Ohmoto, M. Muraguchi, H. Moriguchi, and S. Sone. "Autoantibodies to IL-1 Alpha in Sera From Rapidly Progressive Idiopathic Pulmonary Fibrosis." *The Journal of Medical Investigation: JMI* 48, no. 3–4 (August 2001): 181–189.

Selman, M., and A. Pardo. "Idiopathic Pulmonary Fibrosis: An Epithelial/Fibroblastic Cross-Talk Disorder." *Respiratory Research* 3, no. 1 (2002): 3.

Taylor, D. A., and R. M. du Bois. "Idiopathic Interstitial Pneumonias: A Re-appraisal of Idiopathic Pulmonary Fibrosis." *The International Journal of Tuberculosis and Lung Disease* 5, no. 12 (December 2001): 1,086–1,098.

Verleden, G. M., R. M. du Bois, D. Bouros, M. Drent, A. Millar, J. Muller-Quernheim, G. Semenzato, S. Johnson, G. Sourvino, D. Olivier, A. Pietinalho, and A. Xaubet. "Genetic Predisposition and Pathogenetic Mechanisms of Interstitial Lung Diseases of Unknown Origin." *The European Respiratory Journal Supplement* 32 (September 2001): 17s–29s.

IDIOPATHIC THROMBOCYTOPENIC PURPURA (ITP)

Djulbegovic, B., and Y. Cohen. "The Natural History of Refractory Idiopathic Thrombocytopenic Purpura." *Blood* 98, no. 7 (October 1, 2001): 2,282–2,283.

Dutta, T. K., A. Goel, L. H. Ghotekar, A. Hamide, B. A. Badhe, and D. Basu. "Dapsone in Treatment of Chronic Idiopathic Thrombocytopenic Purpura in Adults." *The Journal of the Association of Physicians of India* 49 (April 2001): 421–425.

Emilia, G., M. Morselli, M. Luppi, G. Longo, R. Marasca, G. Gandini, L. Ferrara, N. D'Apollo, L. Potenza, M. Bertesi, and G. Torelli. "Long-Term Salvage Therapy With Cyclosporin A in Refractory Idiopathic Thrombocytopenic Purpura." *Blood* 99, no. 4 (February 15, 2002): 1,482–1,485.

Kuhne, T., P. Imbach, P. H. Bolton-Maggs, W. Berchtold, V. Blanchette, and G. R. Buchanan. "Newly Diagnosed Idiopathic Thrombocytopenic Purpura in Childhood: An Observational Study." *Lancet* 358, no. 9299 (December 22–29, 2001): 2,122–2,125.

Newland, A. C. "Treatment of Adults With Autoimmune Thrombocytopenic Purpura." *Lancet* 359, no. 9300 (January 5, 2002): 4–5.

Webber, N. P., J. O. Mascarenhas, M. K. Crow, J. Bussel, and E. J. Schattner. "Functional Properties of Lymphocytes in Idiopathic Thrombocytopenic Purpura." *Human Immunology* 62, no. 12 (December 2001): 1,346–1,355.

Zaja, F., I. Iacona, P. Masolini, D. Russo, A. Sperotto, S. Prosdocimo, F. Patriarca, S. De Vita, M. Regazzi, M. Baccarani, and R. Fanin. "B-cell Depletion With Rituximab as Treatment for Immune Hemolytic Anemia and Chronic Thrombocytopenia." *Haematologica* 87, no. 2 (February 2002): 189–195.

IGA NEPHROPATHY

Kaneko, Y., K. Nakazawa, M. Higuchi, K. Hora, and H. Shigematsu. "Glomerular Expression of Alpha-Smooth Muscle Actin Reflects Disease Activity of IgA Nephropathy." *Pathology International* 51, no. 11 (November 2001): 833–844.

Koselj-Kajtna, M., A. Kandus, M. Koselj, T. Rott, A. Vizjak, and A. Bren. "Outcome of Renal Transplants in Patients With IgA Nephropathy." *Transplantation Proceedings* 33, no. 7–8 (November 2001): 3,429–3,430.

Matsumoto, K., and K. Kanmatsuse. "Increased Production of Macrophage Migration Inhibitory Factor By T Cells In Patients With IgA Nephropathy." *American Journal of Nephrology* 21, no. 6 (November–December 2001): 455–464.

Mustonen, J., J. Syrjanen, I. Rantala, and A. Pasternack. "Clinical Course and Treatment of IgA Nephropathy." *Journal of Nephrology* 14, no. 6 (November–December 2001): 440–446.

Schena, F. P., and L. Gesualdo. "Markers of Progression in IgA Nephropathy." *Journal of Nephrology* 14, no. 6 (November–December): 554–574.

Schena, F. P., G. Cerullo, M. Rossini, S. G. Lanzilotta, C. D'Altri, and C. Manno. "Increased Risk of End-Stage Renal Disease in Familial IgA Nephropathy." *Journal of the American Society of Nephrology* 13, no. 2 (February 2002): 453–460.

Syrjanen, J., M. Hurme, T. Lehtimaki, J. Mustonen, and A. Pasternack. "Polymorphism of the Cytokine Genes and IgA Nephropathy." *Kidney International* 61, no. 3 (March 2002): 1,079–1,085.

Wakai, K., S. Nakai, S. Matsuo, T. Kawamura, N. Hotta, K. Maeda, and Y. Ohno. "Risk Factors For IgA Nephropathy: A Case-Control Study With Incident Cases In Japan." *Nephron* 90, no. 1 (January 2002): 16–23.

INCLUSION BODY MYOSITIS (IBM)

Barohn, R. J., and A. A. Amato. "Inclusion Body Myositis." *Current Treatment Options in Neurology* 2, no. 1 (January 2000): 7–12.

Dabby, R., D. J. Lange, W. Trojaborg, A. P. Hays, R. E. Lovelace, T. H. Brannagan, and L. P. Rowland. "Inclusion Body Myositis Mimicking Motor Neuron Disease." *Archives of Neurology* 58, no. 8 (August 2001): 1,253–1,256.

Fam, A. G. "Recent Advances in the Management of Adult Myositis." *Expert Opinion on Investigative Drugs* 10, no. 7 (July 2001): 1,265–1,277.

Jaworska-Wilczynska, M., G. M. Wilczynski, W. K. Engel, D. K. Strickland, K. H. Weisgraber, and V. Askanas.

"Three Lipoprotein Receptors and Cholesterol In Inclusion-Body Myositis Muscle." *Neurology* 58, no. 3 (February 12, 2002): 438–445.

Lawson, Mahowald M. "The Benefits and Limitations of a Physical Training Program in Patients With Inflammatory Myositis." *Current Rheumatology Reports* 3, no. 4 (August 2001): 317–324.

Oldfors, A., and I. M. Fyhr. "Inclusion Body Myositis: Genetic Factors, Aberrant Protein Expression, and Autoimmunity." *Current Opinion in Rheumatology* 13, no. 6 (November 2001): 469–475.

Phillips, B. A., L. A. Cala, G. W. Thickbroom, A. Melsom, P. J., and F. L. Mastaglia. "Patterns of Muscle Involvement in Inclusion Body Myositis: Clinical and Magnetic Resonance Imaging Study." *Muscle & Nerve* 24, no. 11 (November 2001): 1,526–1,534.

Reddy, H., D. Bendahan, M. A. Lee, H. Johansen-Berg, M. Donaghy, D. Hilton-Jones, and P. M. Matthews. "An Expanded Cortical Representation For Hand Movement After Peripheral Motor Denervation." *Journal of Neurology, Neurosurgery, and Psychiatry* 72, no. 2 (February 2002): 203–210.

Rose, M. R., M. P. McDermott, C. A. Thornton, C. Palenski, W. B. Martens, and R. C. Griggs. "A Prospective Natural History Study of Inclusion Body Myositis: Implications For Clinical Trials." *Neurology* 57, no. 3 (August 14, 2001): 548–550.

Sultan, S. M., Y. Ioannou, K. Moss, and D. A. Isenberg. "Outcome in Patients With Idiopathic Inflammatory Myositis: Morbidity and Mortality." *Rheumatology* (Oxford) 41, no. 1 (January 2002): 22–26.

INSULIN-DEPENDENT DIABETES

Acerini, L., M. Williams, and B. Dunger. "Metabolic Impact of Puberty on the Course of Type 1 Diabetes." *Diabetes & Metabolism* 27, no. 4 part 2 (September 2001): S19–25.

Adorini, L., S. Gregori, and L. C. Harrison. "Understanding Autoimmune Diabetes: Insights From Mouse Models." *Trends in Molecular Medicine* 8, no. 1 (January 2002): 31–38.

Field, L. L. "Genetic Linkage and Association Studies of Type I Diabetes: Challenges and Rewards." *Diabetologia* 45, no. 1 (January 2002): 21–35.

Gottlieb, P. A., and G. S. Eisenbarth. "Insulin-Specific Tolerance in Diabetes." *Clinical Immunology* 102, no. 1 (January 2002): 2–11.

Karlsen, A. E., T. Sparre, K. Nielsen, J. Nerup, and F. Pociot. "Proteome Analysis—A Novel Approach to Understand the Pathogenesis of Type 1 Diabetes Mellitus." *Disease Markers* 17, no. 4 (2001): 205–216.

La Cava, A., and N. Sarvetnick. "The Role of Cytokines in Autoimmunity." *Current Directions in Autoimmunity* 1 (1999): 56–71.

Oberholzer, J., C. Toso, F. Ris, P. Bucher, F. Triponez, A. Demirag, J. Lou, and P. Morel. "Beta Cell Replacement for the Treatment of Diabetes." *Annals of the New York Academy of Sciences* 944 (2001): 373–387.

Schilling, L. S., M. Grey, and K. A. Knafl. "The Concept of Self-Management of Type 1 Diabetes in Children and Adolescents: An Evolutionary Concept Analysis." *Journal of Advanced Nursing* 37, no. 1 (January 2002): 87–99.

Shapiro, A. M., E. A. Ryan, and J. R. Lakey. "Diabetes. Islet Cell Transplantation." *Lancet* 358, Suppl. (2001): S21.

Yoon, J. W., and H. S. Jun. "Cellular and Molecular Pathogenic Mechanisms of Insulin-Dependent Diabetes Mellitus." *Annals of the New York Academy of Sciences* 928 (April 2001): 200–211.

INTERSTITIAL CYSTITIS

Agarwal, M., P. H. O'Reill, and R. A. Dixon. "Interstitial Cystitis—A Time For Revision Of Name and Diagnostic Criteria in the New Millennium?" *BJU International* 88, no. 4 (September 2001): 348–350.

Brody, Jane. "Interstitial Cystitis: Help For a Puzzling Illness." *New York Times,* January 25, 1995.

Driscoll, A., and J. M. Teichman. "How Do Patients With Interstitial Cystitis Present?" *The Journal of Urology* 166, no. 6 (December 2001): 2,118–2,120.

Falvey, H. M. "Facilitating a Conceptual Shift: Psychological Consequences of Interstitial Cystitis." *BJU International* 88, no. 9 (December 2001): 863–867.

Hanus, T., L. Zamecnik, M. Jansky, L. Jarolim, C. Povysil, and R. Benett. "The Comparison of Clinical and Histopathologic Features of Interstitial Cystitis." *Urology* 57, no. 6 Suppl. 1 (June 2001): 131.

Metts, J. F. "Interstitial Cystitis: Urgency and Frequency Syndrome." *American Family Physician* 64, no. 7 (October 2001): 1,199–1,206.

Ratner, V. "Interstitial Cystitis: A Chronic Inflammatory Bladder Condition." *World Journal of Urology* 19, no. 3 (June 2001): 157–159.

Warren, J. W. and S. K. Keay. "Interstitial Cystitis." *Current Opinion in Urology* 12, no. 1 (January 2002): 69–74.

Weiss, J. M. "Pelvic Floor Myofascial Trigger Points: Manual Therapy for Interstitial Cystitis and the Urgency-Frequency Syndrome." *Journal of Urology* 166, no. 6 (June 2001): 2,226–2,231.

Yamada, T., and T. Murayama. "Prognosis of Conservative Therapy of Advanced Interstitial Cystitis: Experience of Five Cases." *International Journal of Urology* 8, no. 12 (December 2001): 669–674.

JUVENILE ARTHRITIS

Bloom, B. J. "New Drug Therapies For the Pediatric Rheumatic Diseases." *Current Opinion in Rheumatology* 13, no. 5 (September 2001): 410–414.

Bloom, B. J., J. A. Owens, M. McGuinn, C. Nobile, L. Schaeffer, and A. J. Alario. "Sleep and Its Relationship To Pain, Dysfunction, and Disease Activity in Juvenile Rheumatoid Arthritis." *Journal of Rheumatology* 29, no. 1 (January 2002): 169–173.

Chen, C. Y., C. H. Tsao, L. S. Ou, M. H. Yang, M. L. Kuo, and J. L. Huang. "Comparison of Soluble Adhesion Molecules in Juvenile Idiopathic Arthritis Between the Active and Remission Stages." *Annals of the Rheumatic Diseases* 61, no. 2 (February 2002): 167–170.

Dempster, H., M. Porepa, N. Young, and B. M. Feldman. "The Clinical Meaning of Functional Outcome Scores in Children With Juvenile Arthritis." *Arthritis and Rheumatism* 44, no. 8 (August 2001): 1,768–1,774.

Edelsten, C., V. Lee, C. R. Bentley, J. J. Kanski, and E. M. Graham. "An Evaluation of Baseline Risk Factors Predicting Severity in Juvenile Idiopathic Arthritis Associated Uveitis and Other Chronic Anterior Uveitis in Early Childhood." *British Journal of Ophthalmology* 86, no. 1 (January 2002): 51–56.

Hamilton, J., and H. Capell. "The Treatment of Juvenile Arthritis." *Expert Opinion on Pharmacotherapy* 2, no. 7 (July 2001): 1,085–1,092.

Hashkes, P. J., O. Friedland, and Y. Uziel. "New Treatments For Juvenile Idiopathic Arthritis." *The Israel Medical Association Journal* 4, no. 1 (January 2002): 39–43.

Hull, R. G. "Guidelines for Management of Childhood Arthritis." *Rheumatology* (Oxford) 40, no. 11 (November 2001): 1,309–1,312.

Kulas, D. T., and L. Schanberg. "Juvenile Idiopathic Arthritis." *Current Opinion in Rheumatology* 13, no. 5 (September 2001): 392–398.

Meazza, C., P. Travaglino, P. Pignatti, S. Magni-Manzoni, A. Ravelli, A. Martini, B. F. De. "Macrophage Migration Inhibitory Factor in Patients With Juvenile Idiopathic Arthritis." *Arthritis and Rheumatism* 46, no. 1 (January 2002): 232–237.

LAMBERT-EATON SYNDROME

Carpentier, A. F., and J. Y. Delattre. "The Lambert-Eaton Myasthenic Syndrome." *Clinical Reviews in Allergy & Immunology* 20, no. 1 (February 2001): 155–158.

Itoh, H., K. Shibata, and S. Nitta. "Neuromuscular Monitoring In Myasthenic Syndrome." *Anaesthesia* 56, no. 6 (June 2001): 562–567.

Katz, J., and R. J. Barohn. "Update On the Evaluation and Therapy of Autoimmune Neuromuscular Junction Disorders." *Physical Medicine and Rehabilitation Clinics of North America* 12, no. 2 (May 2001): 381–397.

Motomura, M., S. Hamasaki, S. Nakane, T. Fukuda, and Y. K. Nakao. "Apheresis Treatment in Lambert-Eaton Myasthenic Syndrome." *Therapeutic Apheresis* 4, no. 4 (August 2000): 287–290.

Satoh, K., M. Motomura, H. Suzu, Y. Nakao, T. Fujimoto, T. Fukuda, S. Nakane, T. Nakamura, and K. Eguchi. "Neurogenic Bladder in Lambert-Eaton Myasthenic Syndrome and Its Response to 3,4-diaminopyridine." *Journal of the Neurological Sciences* 183, no. 1 (January 2001): 1–4.

Tyagi, A., S. Connolly, and M. Hutchinson. "Lambert-Eaton Myaesthenic Syndrome: A Possible Association With Hodgkin's Lymphoma." *Irish Medical Journal* 94, no. 1 (January 2001): 18–19.

Wirtz, P. W., R. J. de Keizer, M. de Visser, A. R. Wintzen, and J. J. Verschuuren. "Tonic Pupils in Lambert-Eaton Myasthenic Syndrome." *Muscle & Nerve* 24, no. 3 (March 2001): 444–445.

Wirtz, P. W., B. O. Roep, G. M. Schreuder, P. A. van Doorn, B. G. van Engelen, J. B. Kuks, A. Twijnstra, M. de Visser, L. H. Visser, J. H. Wokke, A. R. Wintzen, and J. J. Verschuuren. "HLA Class I and II in Lambert-Eaton Myasthenic Syndrome Without Associated Tumor." *Human Immunology* 62, no. 8 (August 2001): 809–813.

LICHEN PLANUS

Blanco, A., J. M. Gandara, A. Rodriguez, A. Garcia, and L. Rodriguez. "Biochemical Alterations and Their Clinical Correlation to Oral Lichen Planus." *Medicina Oral* 5, no. 4 (August–October 2000): 238–249.

Eisen, D. "The Clinical Features, Malignant Potential, and Systemic Associations of Oral Lichen Planus: A Study of 723 Patients." *Journal of the American Academy of Dermatology* 46, no. 2 Part 1 (February 2002): 207–214.

Jose, M., A. R. Raghu, and N. N. Rao. "Evaluation of Mast Cells in Oral Lichen Planus and Oral Lichenoid Reaction." *Indian Journal of Dental Research* 12, no. 3 (July–September 2001): 175–179.

Neppelberg, E., A. C. Johannessen, and R. Jonsson. "Apoptosis in Oral Lichen Planus." *European Journal of Oral Sciences* 109, no. 5 (October 2001): 361–364.

Scully, C., D. Eisen, and M. Carrozzo. "Management of Oral Lichen Planus." *American Journal of Clinical Dermatology* 1, no. 5 (September–October 2000): 287–306.

Thornhill, M. H. "Immune Mechanisms In Oral Lichen Planus." *Acta Odontologica Scandinavica* 59, no. 3 (June 2001): 174–177.

Tosti, A., B. M. Piraccini, S. Cambiaghi, and M. Jorizzo. "Nail Lichen Planus in Children: Clinical Features, Response to Treatment, and Long-Term Follow-Up." *Archives of Dermatology* 137, no. 8 (August 2001): 1,027–1,032.

Ukleja, A., K. R. DeVault, M. E. Stark, and S. R. Achem. "Lichen Planus Involving the Esophagus." *Digestive Diseases and Sciences* 46, no. 10 (October 2001): 2,292–2,297.

Vallejo, M. J., G. Huerta, R. Cerero, and J. M. Seoane. "Anxiety and Depression as Risk Factors for Oral Lichen Planus." *Dermatology* 203, no. 4 (2001): 303–307.

Wright, J. M. "A Review and Update of Intraoral Lichen Planus." *Texas Dental Journal* 118, no. 6 (June 2001): 450–454.

MÉNIÈRE'S DISEASE

Akagi, H., K. Yuen, Y. Maeda, K. Fukushima, S. Kariya, Y. Orita, Y. Kataoka, T. Ogawa, and K. Nishizaki. "Ménière's Disease in Childhood." *International Journal of Pediatric Otorhinolaryngology* 61, no. 3 (December 1, 2001): 259–264.

Anderson, J. P. and J. P. Harris. "Impact of Meniere's Disease on Quality of Life." *Otology & Neurotology* 22, no. 6 (November 2001): 888–894.

Ballester, M., P. Liard, D. Vibert, and R. Hausler. "Meniere's Disease in the Elderly." *Otology & Neurotology* 23, no. 1 (January 2002): 73–78.

Barbara, M., C. Consagra, S. Monini, G. Nostro, A. Harguindey, A. Vestri, and R. Filipo. "Local Pressure Protocol, Including Meniett, in the Treatment of Meniere's Disease: Short-Term Results During the Active Stage." *Acta Oto-laryngologica* 121, no. 8 (December 2001): 939–944.

Barrs, D. M., J. S. Keyser, C. Stallworth, and J. T. McElveen Jr. "Intratympanic Steroid Injections for Intractable Meniere's Disease." *Laryngoscope* 111, no. 12 (December 2001): 2,100–2,104.

Di Girolamo, S., P. Picciotti, B. Sergi, A. D'Ecclesia, and W. Di Nardo. "Postural Control and Glycerol Test in Meniere's Disease." *Acta Oto-laryngologica* 121, no. 7 (October 2001): 813–817.

Green, K., and S. Saeed. "Accurate Diagnosis of Meniere's Disease." *Practitioner* 246, no. 1630 (January 2002): 26, 29–32.

Hoffer, M. E., R. D. Kopke, P. Weisskopf, K. Gottshall, K. Allen, D. Wester, and C. Balaban. "Use of the Round Window Microcatheter in the Treatment of Ménière's Disease." *Laryngoscope* 111, no. 11 Part 1 (November 2001): 2,046–2,049.

Kotimaki, J., M. Sorri, and A. Muhli. "Prognosis of Hearing Impairment in Ménière's Disease." *Acta Otolaryngology Supplementum* 545 (2001): 14–18.

Mateijsen, D. J., P. W. Van Hengel, W. M. Van Huffelen, H. P. Wit, and F. W. Albers. "Pure-Tone and Speech Audiometry in Patients With Meniere's Disease." *Clinical Otolaryngology and Allied Sciences* 26, no. 5 (October 2001): 379–387.

MIXED CONNECTIVE TISSUE DISEASE (MCTD)

Greenberg, S. A., and A. A. Amato. "Inflammatory Myopathy Associated With Mixed Connective Tissue Disease and Scleroderma Renal Crisis." *Muscle & Nerve* 24, no. 11 (November 2001): 1,562–1,566.

Kondo, H. "Vascular Disease in Mixed Connective Tissue Disease (MCTD)." *Internal Medicine* 40, no. 12 (December 2001): 1,176.

Ling, T. C., and B. T. Johnston. "Esophageal Investigations in Connective Tissue Disease: Which Tests Are Most Appropriate?" *Journal of Clinical Gastroenterology* 32, no. 1 (January 2001): 33–36.

Nadeau, S. E. "Neurologic Manifestations of Connective Tissue Disease." *Neurologic Clinics* 20, no. 1 (February 2002): 151–178.

Nedumaran, C., P. Rajendran, R. Porkodi, and R. Parthiban. "Mixed Connective Tissue Disease—Clinical and Immunological Profile." *The Journal of the Association of Physicians of India* 49 (April 2001): 412–414.

Uzu, T., H. Iwatani, M. Ko, M. Yamato, K. Takahara, and A. Yamauchi. "Minimal-Change Nephrotic Syndrome Associated With Mixed Connective-Tissue Disease." *Nephrology, Dialysis, Transplantation* 16, no. 6 (June 2001): 1,299–1,300.

Wang, S. J., J. L. Lan, D. Y. Chen, Y. H. Chen, T. Y. Hsieh, and W. Y. Lin. "Solid Phase Radionuclide Esophageal Transit in Mixed Connective Tissue Disease." *Abdominal Imaging* 27, no. 1 (January–February 2002): 6–8.

MOOREN'S ULCER

Chow, C. Y. and C. S. Foster. "Mooren's Ulcer." *International Ophthalmology Clinics* 36, no. 1 (Winter 1996): 1–13.

Gottsch, J. D., S. H. Liu, J. B. Minkovitz, D. F. Goodman, M. Srinivasan, and W. J. Stark. "Autoimmunity To a Cornea-Associated Stromal Antigen in Patients With Mooren's Ulcer." *Investigative Ophthalmology & Visual Science* 36, no. 8 (July 1995): 1,541–1,547.

Sangwan, V. S., P. Zafirakis, and C. S. Foster. "Mooren's Ulcer: Current Concepts in Management." *Indian Journal of Ophthalmology* 45, no. 1 (March 1997): 7–17.

Seino, J. Y., and S. F. Anderson. "Mooren's Ulcer." *Optometry and Vision Science* 75, no. 11 (November 1998): 783–790.

Taylor, C. J., S. L. Smith, C. H. Morgan, S. F. Stephenson, T. Key, M. Srinivasan, E. Cunningham Jr., and P. G. Watson. "HLA and Mooren's Ulceration." *British Journal of Ophthalmology* 84, no. 1 (January 2000): 72–75.

Wagoner, M. D., S. I. Islam, and F. Riley. "Intracorneal Hematoma in Mooren Ulceration." *American Journal of Ophthalmology* 129, no. 2 (February 2000): 251–253.

Watanabe, H., C. Katakami, Y. Tsukahara, and A. Negi. "Cataract Surgery in Patients With Advanced Mooren's Ulcer." *Japanese Journal of Ophthalmology* 45, no. 5 (September–October 2001): 543–546.

Watson, P. G. "Management of Mooren's Ulceration." *Eye* 11, part 3 (1997): 349–356.

Zegans, M. E., and M. Srinivasan. "Mooren's Ulcer." *International Ophthalmology Clinics* 38, no. 4 (Fall 1998): 81–88.

Zhao, J. C., and X. Y. Jin. "Etiopathological Investigation of Mooren's Ulcer." *Chinese Medical Journal (English)* 106, no. 1 (January 1993): 57–60.

MULTIPLE SCLEROSIS

Ben-Zacharia, A. B., and F. D. Lublin. "Palliative Care in Patients With Multiple Sclerosis." *Neurologic Clinics* 19, no. 4 (November 2001): 801–827.

Chard, D. T., C. M. Griffin, G. J. Parker, R. Kapoor, A. J. Thompson, and D. H. Miller. "Brain Atrophy in Clinically Early Relapsing-Remitting Multiple Sclerosis." *Brain* 125, part 2 (February 2002): 327–337.

Filippi, M., M. A. Rocca, B. Colombo, A. Falini, M. Codella, G. Scotti, and G. Comi. "Functional Magnetic Resonance Imaging Correlates of Fatigue in Multiple Sclerosis." *Neuroimage* 15, no. 3 (March 2002): 559–567.

Flechter, S., E. Kott, B. Steiner-Birmanns, P. Nisipeanu, and A. D. Korczyn. "Copolymer 1 (Glatiramer Acetate) in Relapsing Forms of Multiple Sclerosis: Open Multicenter Study of Alternate-Day Administration." *Clinical Neuropharmacology* 25, no. 1 (January–February 2002): 11–15.

Giordana, M. T., P. Richiardi, E. Trevisan, A. Boghi, and L. Palmucci. "Abnormal Ubiquitination of Axons in Normally Myelinated White Matter in Multiple Sclerosis Brain." *Neuropathology and Applied Neurobiology* 28, no. 1 (February 2002): 35–41.

Hoffmann, V., D. Pohlau, H. Przuntek, J. T. Epplen, and C. Hardt. "A Null Mutation Within the Ciliary Neurotrophic Factor (CNTF)-Gene: Implications for Susceptibility and Disease Severity in Patients With Multiple Sclerosis." *Genes and Immunity* 3, no. 1 (February): 53–55.

Inglese, M., A. Ghezzi, S. Bianchi, S. Gerevini, M. P. Sormani, V. Martinelli, G. Comi, and M. Filippi. "Irreversible Disability and Tissue Loss in Multiple Sclerosis: A Conventional and Magnetization Transfer Magnetic Resonance Imaging Study of the Optic Nerves." *Archives of Neurology* 59, no. 2 (February 2002): 250–255.

Rossier, P., and D. T. Wade. "The Guy's Neurological Disability Scale in Patients With Multiple Sclerosis: A Clinical Evaluation of Its Reliability and Validity." *Clinical Rehabilitation* 16, no. 1 (February 2002): 75–95.

Ruprecht, K., M. Warmuth-Metz, W. Waespe, and R. Gold. "Symptomatic Hyperekplexia in a Patient With Multiple Sclerosis." *Neurology* 58, no. 3 (February 12, 2002): 503–504.

Stuifbergen, A. K., and H. Becker. "Health Promotion Practices in Women With Multiple Sclerosis: Increasing Quality and Years of Healtly Life." *Physical Medicine and Rehabilitation Clinics of North America* 12, no. 1 (February 2001): 9–22.

MYASTHENIA GRAVIS

Abel, M. and J. B. Eisenkraft. "Anesthetic Implications of Myasthenia Gravis." *The Mount Sinai Journal of Medicine New York* 69, no. 1–2 (January–March 2002): 31–37.

de Perrot, M., M. Licker, and A. Spiliopoulos. "Factors Influencing Improvement and Remission Rates After Thymectomy for Myasthenia Gravis." *Respiration* 68, no. 6 (2001): 601–605.

Roberts, M. E., M. J. Steiger, and I. K. Hart. "Presentation of Myasthenia Gravis Mimicking Blepharospasm." *Neurology* 58, no. 1 (January 2002): 150–151.

Romi, F., N. E. Gilhus, J. E. Varhaug, A. Myking, G. O. Skeie, and J. A. Aarli. "Thymectomy and Anti-Muscle Autoantibodies in Late-Onset Myasthenia Gravis." *European Journal of Neurology* 9, no. 1 (January 2002): 55–61.

Ronager, J., M. Ravnborg, I. Hermansen, and S. Vorstrup. "Immunoglobulin Treatment Versus Plasma Exchange in Patients With Chronic Moderate to Severe Myasthenia Gravis." *Artificial Organs* 25, no. 12 (December 2001): 967–973.

Tripathi, M., K. Srivastava, S. K. Misra, and G. D. Puri. "Peri-operative Management of Patients for Video Assisted Thoracoscopic Thymectomy in Myasthenia Gravis." *Journal of Postgraduate Medicine* 47, no. 4 (October–December 2001): 258–261.

Uchiyama, A., S. Shimizu, H. Murai, S. Kuroki, M. Okido, and M. Tanaka. "Infrasternal Mediastinoscopic Thymectomy in Myasthenia Gravis: Surgical Results in 23 Patients." *The Annals of Thoracic Surgery* 72, no. 6 (December 2001): 1,902–1,905.

Wang, X. B., M. Kakoulidou, Q. Qiu, R. Giscombe, D. Huang, R. Pirskanen, and A. K. Lefvert. "CDS1 and Promoter Single Nucleotide Polymorphisms of the CTLA-4 Gene in Human Myasthenia Gravis." *Genes and Immunity* 3, no. 1 (February 2002): 46–49.

MYOCARDITIS, AUTOIMMUNE

Afanasyeva, M., Y. Wang, Z. Kaya, S. Park, M. J. Zilliox, B. H. Schofield, S. L. Hill, and N. R. Rose. "Experimental Autoimmune Myocarditis in A/J Mice Is an Interleukin-4-Dependent Disease With a Th2 Phenotype." *American Journal of Pathology* 159, no. 1 (July 2001): 193–203.

Caturegli, P., M. Hejazi, K. Suzuki, O. Dohan, N. Carrasco, L. D. Kohn, and N. R. Rose. "Hypothyroidism in Transgenic Mice Expressing IFN-Gamma in the Thyroid." *Proceedings of the National Academy of Sciences U.S.A.* 97, no. 4 (February 15, 2000): 1,719–1,724.

Kaya, Z., K. M. Dohmen, Y. Wang, J. Schlichting, M. Afanasyeva, F. Leuschner, and N. R. Rose. "Cutting Edge: A Critical Role for IL-10 in Induction of Nasal Tolerance in Experimental Autoimmune Myocarditis." *Journal of Immunology* 168, no. 4 (February 15, 2002): 1,552–1,556.

Kaya, Z., M. Afanasyeva, Y. Wang, K. M. Dohmen, J. Schlichting, T. Tretter, D. Fairweather, V. M. Holers, and N. R. Rose. "Contribution of the Innate Immune System to Autoimmune Myocarditis: A Role for Complement." *Nature Immunology* 2, no. 8 (August 2001): 739–745.

Rose, N. R. "Viral Damage or 'Molecular Mimicry'—Placing the Blame in Myocarditis." *Nature Medicine* 6, no. 6 (June 2000): 631–632.

Stafford, E. A. and N. R. Rose. "Newer Insights Into the Pathogenesis of Experimental Autoimmune Thyroiditis." *International Reviews of Immunology* 19, no. 6 (2000): 501–533.

Wang, Y., M. Afanasyeva, S. L. Hill, Z. Kaya, and N. R. Rose. "Nasal Administration of Cardiac Myosin Suppresses Autoimmune Myocarditis in Mice." *Journal of the American College of Cardiology* 36, no. 6 (November 15, 2000): 1,992–1,999.

MYOSITIS

Fam, A. G. "Recent Advances in the Management of Adult Myositis." *Expert Opinion on Investigational Drugs* 10, no. 7 (July 2001): 1,265–1,277.

NEUTROPENIA

Altclas, J., A. Requejo, G. Jaimovich, V. Milovic, and L. Feldman. "Clostridium Difficile Infection in Patients with Neutropenia." *Clinical Infectious Diseases* 34, no. 5 (March 1, 2002): 723.

Corey, L., and M. Boeckh. "Persistent Fever in Patients with Neutropenia." *New England Journal of Medicine* 346, no. 2 (January 24, 2002): 222–224.

Kanagasegar, S., R. Cimaz, B. T. Kurien, A. Brucato, and R. H. Scofield. "Neonatal Lupus Manifests As Isolated Neutropenia and Mildly Abnormal Liver Functions." *Journal of Rheumatology* 29, no. 1 (January 2002): 187–191.

Lehrnbecher, T., and K. Welte. "Haematopoietic Growth Factors in Children With Neutropenia." *British Journal of Haematology* 116, no. 1 (January 2002): 28–56.

OCULAR CICATRICIAL PEMPHIGOID (OCP)

Chan, R. Y., K. Bhol, N. Tesavibul, E. Letko, R. K. Simmons, C. S. Foster, and A. R. Ahmed. "The Role of Antibody to Human Beta4 Integrin in Conjunctival Basement Membrane Separation: Possible In Vitro Model For Ocular Cicatricial Pemphigoid." *Investigative Ophthalmology and Visual Science* 40, no. 10 (September 1999): 2,283–2,290.

Doan, S., J. F. Lerouic, H. Robin, C. Prost, M. Savoldelli, and T. Hoang-Xuan. "Treatment of Ocular Cicatricial Pemphigoid With Sulfasalazine." *Ophthalmology* 108, no. 9 (September 2001): 1,565–1,568.

Geerling, G., and J. K. Dart. "Management and Outcome of Cataract Surgery in Ocular Cicatricial Pemphigoid." *Graefe's Archive for Clinical and Experimental Ophthalmology* 238, no. 2 (February 2000): 112–118.

Hoang-Xuan, T., H. Robin, P. E. Demers, M. Heller, M. Toutblanc, L. Dubertret, and C. Prost. "Pure Ocular Cicatricial Pemphigoid. A Distinct Immunopathologic Subset of Cicatricial Pemphigoid." *Ophthalmology* 106, no. 2 (February 1999): 355–361.

Holsclaw, D. S. "Ocular Cicatricial Pemphigoid." *International Ophthalmology Clinics* 38, no. 4 (Fall 1998): 89–106.

Koizumi, N., T. Inatomi, T. Suzuki, C. Sotozono, and S. Kinoshita. "Cultivated Corneal Epithelial Stem Cell Transplantation in Ocular Surface Disorders." *Ophthalmology* 108, no. 9 (September 2001): 1,569–1,574.

Letko, E., A. R. Ahmed, and C. S. Foster. "Treatment of Ocular Cicatricial Pemphigoid With Tacrolimus (FK 506)." *Graefe's Archive for Clinical and Experimental Ophthalmology* 239, no. 6 (July 2001): 441–444.

Miserocchi, E., S. Baltatzis, M. R. Roque, A. R. Ahmed, and C. S. Foster. "The Effect of Treatment and Its Related Side Effects in Patients With Severe Ocular Cicatricial Pemphigoid." *Ophthalmology* 109, no. 1 (January 2002): 111–118.

Razzaque, M. S., C. S. Foster, and A. R. Ahmed. "Tissue and Molecular Events in Human Conjunctival Scarring in Ocular Cicatricial Pemphigoid." *Histology and Histopathology* 16, no. 4 (October 2001): 1,203–1,212.

PEMPHIGUS VULGARIS (PV)

Brenner, S., E. Tur, J. Shapiro, V. Ruocco, M. D'Avino, E. Ruocco, N. Tsankov, S. Vassileva, K. Drenovska, P. Brezoev, M. A. Barnadas, M. J. Gonzalez, G. Anhalt, H. Nousari, M. R. Silva, K. T. Pinto, and M. F. Miranda. "Pemphigus Vulgaris: Environmental Factors. Occupational, Behavioral, Medical, and Qualitative Food Frequency Questionnaire." *International Journal of Dermatology* 40, no. 9 (September 2001): 562–569.

Casiglia, J., S. B. Woo, and A. R. Ahmed. "Oral Involvement in Autoimmune Blistering Diseases." *Clinics in Dermatology* 19, no. 6 (November–December 2001): 737–741.

Davenport, S., S. Y. Chen, and A. S. Miller. "Pemphigus Vulgaris: Clinicopathologic Review of 33 Cases in the Oral Cavity." *The International Journal of Periodontics & Restorative Dentistry* 21, no. 1 (February 2001): 85–90.

Grando, S. A., M. R. Pittelkow, L. D. Shultz, M. Dmochowski, and V. T. Nguyen. "Pemphigus: An Unfolding Story." *The Journal of Investigative Dermatology* 117, no. 4 (October 2001): 990–995.

Hertl, M., and C. Veldman. "Pemphigus—Paradigm of Autoantibody-Mediated Autoimmunity." *Skin Pharmacology and Applied Skin Physiology* 14, no. 6 (November–December 2001): 408–418.

Kim, S. C., Y. L. Chung, J. Kim, N. J. Cho, and M. Amagai. "Pemphigus Vulgaris With Autoantibodies to Desmoplakin." *British Journal of Dermatology* 145, no. 5 (November 2001): 838–840.

Korman, N. J. "New Immunomodulating Drugs in Autoimmune Blistering Diseases." *Dermatologic Clinics* 19, no. 4 (October 2001): 637–648, viii.

Ohyama, M., M. Amagai, K. Tsunoda, T. Ota, S. Koyasu, J. Hata Ji, A. Umezawa, and T. Nishikawa T. "Immunologic and Histopathologic Characterization of an Active Disease Mouse Model for Pemphigus Vulgaris." *The Journal of Investigative Dermatology* 118, no. 1 (January 2002): 199–204.

Toth, G. G., and M. F. Jonkman. "Therapy of Pemphigus." *Clinics in Dermatology* 19, no. 6 (November–December 2001): 761–767.

Tsunoda, K., T. Ota, H. Suzuki, M. Ohyama, T. Nagai, T. Nishikawa, M. Amagai, and S. Koyasu. "Pathogenic Autoantibody Production Requires Loss of Tolerance Against Desmoglein 3 in Both T and B Cells in Experimental Pemphigus Vulgaris." *European Journal of Immunology* 32, no. 3 (March 2002): 627–633.

PERIPHERAL NEUROPATHY (PN)

Cohen, J. S. "Peripheral Neuropathy Associated With Fluoroquinolones." *The Annals of Pharmacotherapy* 35, no. 12 (December 2001): 1,540–1,547.

Hughes, R. A. "Peripheral Neuropathy." *BMJ* 324, no. 7335 (February 2002): 466–469.

Mizobuchi, K., S. Kuwabara, S. Toma, Y. Nakajima, K. Ogawara, and T. Hattori. "Properties of Human Skin Mechanoreceptors in Peripheral Neuropathy." *Clinical Neurophysiology* 113, no. 2 (February 2002): 310–315.

Roy, M. K. "Familial Parkinsonism With Peripheral Neuropathy." *The Journal of the Association of Physicians in India* 49 (September 2001): 944.

Vinik, A. I. "Neuropathy: New Concepts in Evaluation and Treatment." *Southern Medical Journal* 95, no. 1 (January 2002): 21–23.

PERIVENOUS ENCEPHALOMYELITIS

Hynson, J. L., A. J. Kornberg, L. T. Coleman, L. Shield, A. S. Harvey, and M. J. Kean. "Clinical and Neuroradiologic Features of Acute Disseminated Encephalomyelitis in Children." *Neurology* 56, no. 10 (May 2001): 1,308–1,312.

Inglese, M., F. Salvi, G. Iannucci, G. L. Mancardi, M. Mascalchi, and M. Filippi. "Magnetization Transfer and Diffusion Tensor MR Imaging of Acute Disseminated Encephalomyelitis." *AJNR American Journal of Neuroradiology* 23, no. 2 (February 2002): 267–272.

Khong, P. L., H. K. Ho, P. W. Cheng, V. N. Wong, W. Goh, and F. L. Chan. "Childhood Acute Disseminated Encephalomyelitis: The Role of Brain and Spinal Cord MRI." *Pediatric Radiology* 32, no. 1 (January 2002): 59–66.

Matsuda, M., J. Miki, K. Tabata, and S. Ikeda. "Severe Depression as an Initial Symptom in an Elderly Patient With Acute Disseminated Encephalomyelitis." *Internal Medicine* 40, no. 11 (November 2001): 1,149–1,153.

Tateishi, K., K. Takeda, and T. Mannen. "Acute Disseminated Encephalomyelitis Confined to Brainstem." *Journal of Neuroimaging* 12, no. 1 (January 2002): 67–68.

Tselis, A. "Acute Disseminated Encephalomyelitis." *Current Treatment Options in Neurology* 3, no. 6 (November 2001): 537–542.

PERNICIOUS ANEMIA

Aydogdu, I., R. Sari, R. Ulu, and A. Sevinc. "The Frequency of Gallbladder Stones in Patients With Pernicious Anemia." *The Journal of Surgical Research* 101, no. 2 (December 2001): 120–123.

Chanarin, I. "Historical Review: A History of Pernicious Anaemia." *British Journal of Haematology* 111, no. 2 (November 2000): 407–415.

Junca, J., A. Flores, M. L. Granada, O. Jimenez, and J. M. Sancho. "The Relationship Between Idiopathic Thrombocytopenic Purpura and Pernicious Anaemia." *British Journal of Haematology* 111, no. 2 (November 2000): 513–516.

POLYATERITIS NODOSA

Bakkaloglu, A., S. Ozen, E. Baskin, N. Besbas, A. Gur-Guven, O. Kasapcopur, and K. Tinaztepe. "The Significance of Antineutrophil Cytoplasmic Antibody in Microscopic Polyangitis and Classic Polyarteritis Nodosa." *Archives of Disease in Childhood* 85, no. 5 (November 2001): 427–430.

Bonsib, S. M. "Polyarteritis Nodosa." *Seminars in Diagnostic Pathology* 18, no. 1 (February 2001): 14–23.

Kroiss, M., U. Hohenleutner, C. Gruss, A. Glaessl, M. Landthaler, and W. Stolz. "Transient and Partial Effect of High-Dose Intravenous Immunoglobulin in Polyarteritis Nodosa." *Dermatology* 203, no. 2 (2001): 188–189.

Kruithof, E., D. Elewaut, J. M. Naeyaert, H. Praet, H. Mielants, E. M. Veys, and F. De Keyser F. "Polyarteritis Nodosa Mimicking Polymyalgia Rheumatica." *Clinical Rheumatology* 18, no. 3 (1999): 257–260.

Langford, C. A. "Treatment of Polyarteritis Nodosa, Microscopic Polyangiitis, and Churg-Strauss Syndrome: Where Do We Stand?" *Arthritis & Rheumatism* 44, no. 3 (March 2001): 508–512.

Letellier, E., H. Longhurst, S. J. Diaz-Cano, and D. D'Cruz. "Polyarteritis Nodosa Developing After Discoid Lupus Erythematosus." *Clinical and Experimental Rheumatology* 19, no. 6 (November–December 2001): 738–739.

Matteson, E. L. "Historical Perspective of Vasculitis: Polyarteritis Nodosa and Microscopic Polyangiitis." *Current Rheumatology Reports* 4, no. 1 (February 2002): 67–74.

Viguier, M., L. Guillevin, and L. Laroche. "Treatment of Parvovirus B19-Associated Polyarteritis Nodosa With Intravenous Immune Globulin." *New England Journal of Medicine* 344, no. 19 (May 2001): 1,481–1,482.

POLYCHONDRITIS

Alissa, H., R. Kadanoff, and E. Adams. "Does Mechanical Insult to Cartilage Trigger Relapsing Polychondritis?" *Scandinavian Journal of Rheumatology* 30, no. 5 (2001): 311.

Behar, J. V., Y. W. Choi, T. A. Hartman, N. B. Allen, and H. P. McAdams. "Relapsing Polychondritis Affecting the Lower Respiratory Tract." *AJR American Journal of Roentgenology* 178, no. 1 (January 2002): 173–177.

Daniel, L., B. Granel, B. Dussol, P. J. Weiller, and J. F. Pellissier. "Recurrent Glomerulonephritis in Relapsing Polychondritis." *Nephron* 87, no. 2 (February 2001): 190–191.

Frances, C., R. el Rassi, J. L. Laporte, M. Rybojad, T. Papo, J. C. Piette. "Dermatologic Manifestations of Relapsing Polychondritis. A Study of 200 Cases At a Single Center." *Medicine (Baltimore)* 80, no. 3 (May 2001): 173–179.

Greenstone, M., and E. Baguley. "Images In Medicine. Large Airway Involvement In Relapsing Polychondritis." *Hospital Medicine* 62, no. 9 (September 2001): 574.

Mark, K. A., and A. G. Franks Jr. "Colchicine and Indomethacin For the Treatment of Relapsing Polychondritis." *Journal of the American Academy of Dermatology* 46, #2 part 2 (February 2002): S22–24.

Selim, A. G., L. G. Fulford, R. H. Mohiaddin, and M. N. Sheppard. "Active Aortitis in Relapsing Polychondritis." *Journal of Clinical Pathology* 54, no. 11 (November 2001): 890–892.

Yamazaki, K., T. Suga, and K. Hirata. "Large Vessel Arteritis in Relapsing Polychondritis." *The Journal of Laryngology and Otology* 115, no. 10 (October 2001): 836–838.

POLYGLANDULAR AUTOIMMUNE SYNDROMES (PGAS)

Baker Jr., J. R. "Autoimmune Endocrine Disease." *JAMA: The Journal of the American Medical Association* 278, no. 22 (December 10, 1997): 1,931–1,937.

Bunnag, P., and R. Rajatanavin. "Polyglandular Autoimmune (PGA) Syndromes: Report of Three Cases and Review of the Literature." *Journal of the Med Association of Thailand* 77, no. 6 (June 1994): 327–333.

Cicchinelli, M., M. Mariani, and F. Scuderi. "Polyglandular Autoimmune Syndrome Type II and Rheumatoid Arthritis." *Clinical and Experimental Rheumatology* 15, no. 3 (May–June 1997): 336–337.

Creutzfeldt, W. "Malabsorption Due to Cholecystokinin Deficiency In a Patient With Autoimmune Polyglandular Syndrome Type I." *New England Journal of Medicine* 345, no. 1 (July 5, 2001): 64–65; discussion 65–66.

Obermayer-Straub, P., and M. P. Manns. "Autoimmune Polyglandular Syndromes." *Bailliere's Clinical Gastroenterology* 12, no. 2 (June 1998): 293–315.

Riley, W. J. "Autoimmune Polyglandular Syndromes." *Hormone Research* 38, supplement 2 (1992): 9–15.

Wang, C. Y., A. Davoodi-Semiromi, W. Huang, E. Connor, J. D. Shi, and J. X. She. "Characterization of

Mutations in Patients With Autoimmune Polyglandu-lar Syndrome Type 1 (APS1)." *Human Genetics* 103, no. 6 (December 1998): 681–685.

POLYMYALGIA RHEUMATICA

Barilla-LaBarca, M. L., D. J. Lenschow, and R. D. Bras-ington. "Polymyalgia Rheumatica/Temporal Arteritis: Recent Advances." *Current Rheumatology Reports* 4, no. 1 (February 2002): 39–46.

Cohen, M. D., and A. Abril. "Polymyalgia Rheumatica Revisited." *Bulletin on the Rheumatic Diseases* 50, no. 8 (2001): 1–4.

Gran, J. T., G. Myklebust, T. Wilsgaard, and B. K. Jacob-sen. "Survival in Polymyalgia Rheumatica and Tem-poral Arteritis: A Study of 398 Cases and Matched Population Controls." *Rheumatology* (Oxford). 40, no. 11 (November 2001): 1,238–1,242.

Kennedy-Malone, L. M., and G. L. Enevold. "Assessment and Management of Polymyalgia Rheumatica in Older Adults." *Geriatric Nursing* 22, no. 3 (May–June 2001): 152–155; quiz 155.

Loeslie, V. "Pain In the Elderly: Polymyalgia Rheumat-ica." *Clinical Excellence for Nurse Practitioners* 4, no. 6 (November 2000): 345–348.

Narvaez, J., J. M. Nolla-Sole, J. Valverde-Garcia, and D. Roig-Escofet. "Sex Differences in Temporal Arteritis and Polymyalgia Rheumatica." *Journal of Rheumatology* 29, no. 2 (February 2002): 321–325.

Salvarini, C., F. Cantini, I. Olivieri, and G. G. Hunder. "Magnetic Resonance Imaging and Polymyalgia Rheumatica." *Journal of Rheumatology* 28, no. 4 (April 2001): 918–919.

Shintani, S., T. Shiigai, and Y. Matsui. "Polymyalgia Rheumatica (PMR): Clinical, Laboratory, and Immu-nofluorescence Studies in 13 Patients." *Clinical Neu-rology and Neurosurgery* 104, no. 1 (January 2002): 20–29.

Siebert, S., T. M. Lawson, M. H. Wheeler, J. C. Martin, and B. D. Williams. "Polymyalgia Rheumatica: Pitfalls in Diagnosis." *Journal of the Royal Society of Medicine* 94, no. 5 (May 2001): 242–244.

Suskovic, T., and D. Vukicevic-Baudoin. "Polymyalgia Rheumatica—an Underdiagnosed Disease." *Acta Med-ica Croatica* 54, no. 4–5 (2000): 199–202.

POLYMYOSITIS

Cherin, P., S. Pelletier, A. Teixeira, P. Laforet, T. Genereau, A. Simon, T. Maisonobe, B. Eymard, and S. Herson. "Results and Long-Term Followup of Intra-venous Immunoglobulin Infusions in Chronic, Refrac-tory Polymyositis: An Open Study With Thirty-Five

Adult Patients." *Arthritis and Rheumatism* 46, no. 2 (February 2002): 467–474.

Choy, E. H., and D. A. Isenberg. "Treatment of Dermato-myositis and Polymyositis." *Rheumatology* (Oxford) 41, no. 1 (January 2002): 7–13.

George, B., D. Danda, M. Chandy, A. Srivastava, and V. Mathews. "Polymyositis—An Unusual Manifestation of Chronic Graft-Versus-Host Disease." *Rheumatology International* 20, no. 4 (May 2001): 169–170.

Golding, E. M., and R. M. Golding. "An Insight Into Cortisol and Polymyositis Control With Steroid Ther-apy." *Medical Hypotheses* 57, no. 1 (July 2001): 76–86.

Marie, I., E. Hachulla, P. Y. Hatron, M. F. Hellot, H. Levesque, B. Devulder, and H. Courtois. "Polymyosi-tis and Dermatomyositis: Short Term and Longterm Outcome, and Predictive Factors of Prognosis." *Jour-nal of Rheumatology* 28, no. 10 (October 2001): 2,230–2,237.

Wenzel, J., and T. Bieber. "Cyclosporin A in Treatment of Refractory Adult Polymyositis/Dermatomyositis." *Journal of Rheumatology* 28, no. 9 (September 2001): 2,139.

Yang, Y., J. Fujita, M. Tokuda, S. Bandoh, H. Dobashi, T. Okada, M. Okahara, T. Kishimoto, T. Ishida, and J. Takahara. "Clinical Features of Polymyositis/Dermato-myositis Associated With Silicosis And a Review of the Literature." *Rheumatology International* 20, no. 6 (August 2001): 235–238.

POSTMYOCARDIAL INFARCTION SYNDROME

Crispell, K. A., J. N. Maran, and E. C. Warren. "Postmy-ocardial Infarction Syndrome: A Case Study." *Focus on Critical Care* 14, no. 5 (October 1987): 67–73.

Khan, A. H. "The Postcardiac Injury Syndromes." *Clinical Cardiology* 15, no. 2 (February 1992): 67–72.

Kossowsky, W. A., and A. F. Lyon. "The Postmyocardial Infarction Syndrome—Vanished or Vanquished? A Twenty-Five-Year Follow-up. A Case Report." *Angiol-ogy* 47, no. 1 (January 1996): 83–85.

Timmis, A. D. "Postmyocardial Infarction Syndrome." *British Medical Journal (Clinical Research Edition)* 289, no. 6446 (September 15, 1984): 636–637.

Williams, R. K., R. E. Nagle, and R. A. Thompson. "Post-coronary Pain and the Postmyocardial Infarction Syn-drome." *British Heart Journal* 51, no. 3 (March 1984): 327–329.

POSTPERICARDIOTOMY SYNDROME

Bajaj, B. P., K. E. Evans, and P. Thomas. "Postpericar-diotomy Syndrome Following Temporary and Perma-nent Transvenous Pacing." *Postgraduate Medical Journal* 75, no. 884 (June 1999): 357–358.

Charitos, C. E., D. A. Kontoyannis, and J. N. Nanas. "Postpericardiotomy Syndrome During Intensive Immunosuppression After Cardiac Transplantation." *Acta Cardiologica* 55, no. 2 (April 2000): 95–97.

Doshi, A. V., K. S. Gupta, and J. M. Joshi. "Post Cardiac Injury Syndrome—One More Cause of False Positive IgG, IgM Antibodies in Pleural Fluid Against Antigen-60 of Mycobacterium Tuberculosis." *Journal of the Association of Physicians of India* 46, no. 8 (August 1998): 734–735.

Kocazeybek, B., S. Erenturk, M. K. Calyk, and F. Babacan. "An Immunological Approach to Postpericardiotomy Syndrome Occurrence and Its Relation With Autoimmunity." *Acta Chirurgica Belgica* 98, no. 5 (October 1998): 203–206.

Preston, I., and A. O'Brien. "Clues to an Elusive Effusion. Postpericardiotomy Syndrome." *Postgraduate Medicine* 109, no. 5 (May 2001): 131–132.

Spindler, M., G. Burrows, P. Kowallik, G. Ertl, and W. Voelker. "Postpericardiotomy Syndrome and Cardiac Tamponade as a Late Complication After Pacemaker Implantation." *Pacing and Clinical Electrophysiology: PACE* 24, no. 9 part 1 (September 2001): 1,433–1,434.

Tarnok, A., and P. Schneider. "Pediatric Cardiac Surgery With Cardiopulmonary Bypass: Pathways Contributing to Transient Systemic Immune Suppression." *Shock* 16, supplement 1 (September 2001): 24–32.

Webber, S. A., N. J. Wilson, A. K. Junker, S. K. Byrne, A. Perry, E. E. Thomas, L. Book, M. Tipple, M. W. Patterson, and G. G. Sandor. "Postpericardiotomy Syndrome: No Evidence For a Viral Etiology." *Cardiology in the Young* 11, no. 1 (January 2001): 67–74.

PRIMARY AGAMMAGLOBULINEMIA

Futatani, T., C. Watanabe, Y. Baba, S. Tsukada, and H. D. Ochs. "Bruton's Tyrosine Kinase is Present in Normal Platelets and Its Absence Identifies Patients With X-linked Agammaglobulinaemia and Carrier Females." *British Journal of Haematology* 114, no. 1 (July 2001): 141–149.

Jones, A. M., and H. B. Gaspar. "Immunogenetics: Changing the Face of Immunodeficiency." *Journal of Clinical Pathology* 53, no. 1 (January 2000): 60–65.

Kainulainen, L., M. Varpula, K. Liippo, E. Svedstrom, J. Nikoskelainen, and O. Ruuskanen. "Pulmonary Abnormalities in Patients With Primary Hypogammaglobulinemia." *The Journal of Allergy and Clinical Immunology* 104, no. 5 (November 1999): 1,031–1,036.

Korpi, M., J. Valiaho, and M. Vihinen. "Structure-Function Effects in Primary Immunodeficiencies."

Scandinavian Journal of Immunology 52, no. 3 (September 2000): 226–232.

Manson, D. E., S. Sikka, B. Reid, and C. Roifman. "Primary Immunodeficiencies: A Pictorial Immunology Primer for Radiologists." *Pediatric Radiology* 30, no. 8 (August 2000): 501–510.

PRIMARY BILIARY CIRRHOSIS

Dohmen, K. "Primary Biliary Cirrhosis and Pernicious Anemia." *Journal of Gastroenterology and Hepatology* 16, no. 12 (December 2001): 1,316–1,318.

Holtmeier, J., and U. Leuschner. "Medical Treatment of Primary Biliary Cirrhosis and Primary Sclerosing Cholangitis." *Digestion* 64, no. 3 (2001): 137–150.

Ikuno, N., I. R. Mackay, J. Jois, K. Omagari, and M. J. "Antimitochondrial Autoantibodies in Saliva and Sera From Patients With Primary Biliary Cirrhosis." *Journal of Gastroenterology and Hepatology* 16, no. 12 (December 2001): 1,390–1,394.

Marzioni, M., S. S. Glaser, G. Alpini, and G. D. LeSage. "Role of Apoptosis in Development of Primary Biliary Cirrhosis." *Digestive and Liver Disease* 33, no. 7 (October 2001): 531–533.

Mason, A., and S. Nair. "Primary Biliary Cirrhosis: New Thoughts on Pathophysiology and Treatment." *Current Gastroenterology Reports* 4, no. 1 (February 2002): 45–51.

Neuberger, J. "Antibodies and Primary Biliary Cirrhosis—Piecing Together the Jigsaw." *Journal of Hepatology* 36, no. 1 (January 2002): 126–129.

Tinmouth, J., G. Tomlinson, E. J. Heathcote, and L. Lilly. "Benefit of Transplantation in Primary Biliary Cirrhosis Between 1985–1997." *Transplantation* 73, no. 2 (January 27, 2002): 224–227.

PSORIASIS

Asadullah, K., H. D. Volk, and W. Sterry. "Novel Immunotherapies for Psoriasis." *Trends in Immunology* 23, no. 1 (January 2002): 47–53.

Barbagallo, J., C. T. Spann, W. D. Tutrone, and J. M. Weinberg. "Narrowband UVB Phototherapy for the Treatment of Psoriasis: A Review and Update." *Cutis; Cutaneous Medicine for the Practitioner* 68, no. 5 (November 2001): 345–347.

Cowen, P. "Management of Psoriasis." *Australian Family Physician* 30, no. 11 (November 2001): 1,033–1,037.

Griffiths, C. E. "Immunotherapy for Psoriasis: From Serendipity to Selectivity." *Lancet* 359, no. 9393 (January 26, 2002): 279–280.

Kaur, I., A. Saraswat, B. Kumar. "Nail Changes in Psoriasis: A Study of 167 Patients." *International Journal of Dermatology* 40, no. 9 (September 2001): 601–603.

Krueger, J. G. "The Immunologic Basis for the Treatment of Psoriasis With New Biologic Agents." *Journal of the American Academy of Dermatology* 46, no. 1 (January 2002): 1–23; quiz 23–26.

Spann, C. T., J. Barbagallo, and J. M. Weinberg. "A Review of the 308-nm Excimer Laser in the Treatment of Psoriasis." *Cutis; Cutaneous Medicine for the Practitioner* 68, no. 5 (November 2001): 351–352.

Travis, L. B., and N. B. Silverberg. "Psoriasis in Infancy: Therapy with Calcipotriene Ointment." *Cutis; Cutaneous Medicine for the Practitioner* 68, no. 5 (November 2001): 341–344.

Tutrone, W. D., M. H. Kagen, J. Barbagallo, and J. M. Weinberg. "Biologic Therapy for Psoriasis: A Brief History, I." *Cutis; Cutaneous Medicine for the Practitioner* 68, no. 5 (November 2001): 331–336.

Tutrone, W. D., M. H. Kagen, J. Barbagallo, and J. M. Weinberg. "Biologic Therapy for Psoriasis: A Brief History, II." *Cutis; Cutaneous Medicine for the Practitioner* 68, no. 6 (December 2001): 367–372.

PSORIATIC ARTHRITIS

Alenius, G. M., B. G. Stegmayr, and S. R. Dahlqvist. "Renal Abnormalities in a Population of Patients With Psoriatic Arthritis." *Scandinavian Journal of Rheumatology* 30, no. 5 (2001): 271–274.

Costello, P., and O. FitzGerald. "Disease Mechanisms in Psoriasis and Psoriatic Arthritis." *Current Rheumatology Reports* 3, no. 5 (October 2001): 419–427.

Gerster, J. C., and D. Hohl. "Nail Lesions in Psoriatic Arthritis: Recovery With Sulfasalazine Treatment." *Annals of the Rheumatic Diseases* 61, no. 3 (March 2002): 277.

Gorter, S., D. M. van der Heijde, S. van der Linden, H. Houben, J. J. Rethans, A. J. Scherpbier, and C. P. van der Vleuten. "Psoriatic Arthritis: Performance of Rheumatologists in Daily Practice." *Annals of the Rheumatic Diseases* 61, no. 3 (March 2002): 219–224.

Hohler, T., and E. Marker-Hermann. "Psoriatic Arthritis: Clinical Aspects, Genetics, and the Role of T Cells." *Current Opinion in Rheumatology* 13, no. 4 (July 2001): 273–279.

Jackson, C. G. "Immunomodulating Drugs in the Management of Psoriatic Arthritis." *American Journal of Clinical Dermatology* 2, no. 6 (2001): 367–375.

Lopez-Montilla, M. D., J. Gonzalez, F. G. Martinez, J. R. Fernandez-Moreno, and E. Collantes. "Clinical Features of Late Onset Psoriatic Arthritis." *Experimental Gerontology* 37, no. 2–3 (January 3, 2002): 441–443.

Salvarani, C., P. Macchioni, I. Olivieri, A. Marchesoni, M. Cutolo, G. Ferraccioli, F. Cantini, F. Salaffi, A. Padula, C. Lovino, L. Dovigo, G. Bordin, C. Davoli, G. Pasero, and O. D. Alberighi. "A Comparison of Cyclosporine, Sulfasalazine, and Symptomatic Therapy in the Treatment of Psoriatic Arthritis." *Journal of Rheumatology* 28, no. 10 (October 2001): 2,274–2,282.

Sokoll, K. B., and P. S. Helliwell. "Comparison of Disability and Quality of Life in Rheumatoid and Psoriatic Arthritis." *Journal of Rheumatology* 28, no. 8 (August 2001): 1,842–1,846.

Taylor, W. J. "Epidemiology of Psoriatic Arthritis." *Current Opinion in Rheumatology* 14, no. 2 (March 2002): 98–103.

RAYNAUD'S PHENOMENON

Benchikhi, H., J. C. Roujeau, M. Levent, M. Gouault-Heilmann, J. Revuz, and A. Cosnes. "Chilblains and Raynaud Phenomenon Are Usually Not a Sign of Hereditary Protein C and S Deficiencies." *Acta Dermato-Venereologica* 78, no. 5 (September 1998): 351–352.

Creutzig, A., L. Caspary, and M. Freund. "The Raynaud Phenomenon and Interferon Therapy." *Annals of Internal Medicine* 125, no. 5 (September 1996): 423.

Fraenkel, L., Y. Zhang, C. E. Chaisson, S. R. Evans, P. W. Wilson, and D. T. Felson. "The Association of Estrogen Replacement Therapy and the Raynaud Phenomenon in Postmenopausal Women." *Annals of Internal Medicine* 129, no. 3 (August 1998): 208–211.

Kroger, K., T. Billen, G. Neuhaus, F. Santosa, C. Buss, E. Kreuzfelder, and K. B. Henneberg-Quester. "Relevance of Low Titers of Cryoglobulins and Cold-Agglutinins in Patients With Isolated Raynaud Phenomenon." *Clinical Hemorheology and Microcirculation* 24, no. 3 (2001): 167–174.

Maricq, H. R., J. R. Jennings, I. Valter, M. Frederick, B. Thompson, E. A. Smith, and R. Hill. "Evaluation of Treatment Efficacy of Raynaud Phenomenon by Digital Blood Pressure Response to Cooling. Raynaud's Treatment Study Investigators." *Vascular Medicine* 5, no. 3 (2000): 135–140.

Maricq, H. R., I. Valter, J. G. Maricq. "An Objective Method to Estimate the Severity of Raynaud Phenomenon: Digital Blood Pressure Response to Cooling." *Vascular Medicine* 3, no. 2 (1998): 109–113.

Spencer-Green, G. "Outcomes In Primary Raynaud Phenomenon: A Meta-Analysis of the Frequency, Rates, and Predictors of Transition to Secondary Diseases." *Archives of Internal Medicine* 158, no. 6 (March 23, 1998): 595–600.

Tan, F. K., and F. C. Arnett. "Genetic Factors in the Etiology of Systemic Sclerosis and Raynaud Phenomenon." *Current Opinion in Rheumatology* 12, no. 6 (November 2000): 511–519.

REITER'S SYNDROME

Amor, B. "Reiter's Syndrome. Diagnosis and Clinical Features." *Rheumatic Diseases Clinics of North America* 24, no. 4 (November 1998): 677–695, vii.

Bryant, G. A. "Reiter's Syndrome." *Orthopedic Nursing* 17, no. 1 (January–February 1998): 57–62.

Connor, B. A., E. J. Johnson, and R. Soave. "Reiter Syndrome Following Protracted Symptoms of Cyclospora Infection." *Emerging Infectious Diseases* 7, no. 3 (May–June 2001): 453–454.

Harootunian, A. M. "Is it Reiter's Syndrome?" *Journal of the American Academy of Nurse Practitioners* 9, no. 9 (September 1997): 427–430.

Hogarth, M. B., S. Thomas, M. H. Seifert, and S. M. Tariq. "Reiter's Syndrome Following Intravesical BCG Immunotherapy." *Postgraduate Medical Journal* 76, no. 902 (December 2000): 791–793.

Kousa, M., P. Saikku, S. Richmond, and A. Lassus. "Frequent Association of Chlamydial Infection With Reiter's Syndrome." *Sexually Transmitted Diseases* 5, no. 2 (April–June 1978): 57–61.

Parker, C. T., and D. Thomas. "Reiter's Syndrome and Reactive Arthritis." *The Journal of the American Osteopathic Association* 100, no. 2 (February 2000): 101–104.

Salaria, M., S. Singh, and L. Kumar. "Reiter's Syndrome." *Indian Pediatrics* 34, no. 10 (October 1997): 943–944.

Shimamoto, Y., H. Sugiyama, and S. Hirohata. "Reiter's Syndrome Associated With HLA-B51." *Internal Medicine* 39, no. 2 (February 2000): 182–184.

Sood, A., V. K. Sharma, T. Garg, M. Nair, and A. K. Dinda. "Amyloidosis in Reiter's Syndrome." *Journal of the Association of Physicians in India* 49 (May 2001): 563–565.

RHEUMATIC FEVER

Carapetis, J. R., and B. J. Currie. "Rheumatic Fever in a High Incidence Population: The Importance of Monoarthritis and Low Grade Fever." *Archives of Disease in Childhood* 85, no. 3 (September 2001): 223–227.

English, P. C. "Emergence of Rheumatic Fever in the Nineteenth Century." *The Milbank Quarterly* 67, supplement 1 (1989): 33–49.

Kurahara, D., A. Tokuda, A. Grandinetti, J. Najita, C. Ho, K. Yamamoto, D. V. Reddy, K. Macpherson, M. Iwamuro, and K. Yamaga. "Ethnic Differences in Risk for Pediatric Rheumatic Illness In a Culturally Diverse Population." *Journal of Rheumatology* 29, no. 2 (February 2002): 379–383.

Markowitz, M. "Susceptibility to Rheumatic Fever." *Circulation* 38, no. 1 (July 1968): 3–4.

Narula, J., and E. L. Kaplan. "Echocardiographic Diagnosis of Rheumatic Fever." *Lancet* 358, no. 9297 (December 2001): 2000.

Rullan, E., and L. H. Sigal. "Rheumatic Fever." *Current Rheumatology Reports* 3, no. 5 (October 2001): 445–452.

Stollerman, G. H. "Rheumatic Fever in the 21st Century." *Clinical Infectious Diseases* 33, no. 6 (September 2001): 806–814.

RHEUMATOID ARTHRITIS

Burr, N., A. L. Pratt, and P. J. Smith. "An Alternative Splinting and Rehabilitation Protocol for Metacarpophalangeal Joint Arthroplasty in Patients With Rheumatoid Arthritis." *Journal of Hand Therapy* 15, no. 1 (January–March 2002): 41–47.

Day, R. "Adverse Reactions to TNF-Alpha Inhibitors in Rheumatoid Arthritis." *Lancet* 359, no. 9306 (February 16, 2002): 540–541.

Fautrel, B., and F. Guillemin. "Cost of Illness Studies in Rheumatic Diseases." *Current Opinion in Rheumatology* 14, no. 2 (March 2002): 121–126.

Feldmann, M., and R. N. Maini. "Discovery of TNF-Alpha as a Therapeutic Target in Rheumatoid Arthritis: Preclinical and Clinical Studies." *Joint, Bone, Spine: Revue du Rhumatisme* 69, no. 1 (January 2002): 12–18.

Gabay, C. "Cytokine Inhibitors in the Treatment of Rheumatoid Arthritis." *Expert Opinion on Biological Therapy* 2, no. 2 (February 2002): 135–149.

Nyman, C. S., and K. Lutzen. "Caring Needs of Patients With Rheumatoid Arthritis." *Nursing Science Quarterly* 12, no. 2 (April 1999): 164–169.

Read, E., C. McEachern, and T. Mitchell. "Psychological Wellbeing of Patients With Rheumatoid Arthritis." *British Journal of Nursing* 10, no. 21 (December 12, 2001): 1,385–1,391.

Reddy, N. P., B. M. Rothschild, E. Verrall, and A. Joshi. "Noninvasive Measurement of Acceleration At the Knee Joint in Patients With Rheumatoid Arthritis and Spondyloarthropathy of the Knee." *Annals of Biomedical Engineering* 29, no. 12 (December 2001): 1,106–1,111.

Robinson, V., L. Brosseau, L. Casimiro, M. Judd, B. Shea, G. Wells, and P. Tugwell. "Thermotherapy For Treating Rheumatoid Arthritis (Cochrane Review)." *Cochrane Database of Systematic Reviews* 1 (2002): CD002826.

Svensson, A., H. Moller, B. Bjorkner, M. Bruze, I. Leden, J. Theander, K. Ohlsson, and C. Linder. "Rheumatoid Arthritis, Gold Therapy, Contact Allergy and Blood Cytokines." *BMC Dermatology* 2, no. 1 (2002): 2.

SARCOIDOSIS

Costabel, U. "Sarcoidosis: Clinical Update." *The European Respiratory Journal Supplement* 32 (September 2001): 56s–68s.

Gullapalli, D., and L. H. Phillips LH 2nd. "Neurologic Manifestations of Sarcoidosis." *Neurologic Clinics* 20, no. 1 (February 2002): 59–83.

Labeck, B., H. Nehoda, C. Kahler, M. Freund, F. Aigner, and H. G. Weiss. "Adjustable Gastric Banding in a Patient With Sarcoidosis." *Surgical Endoscopy* 15, no. 11 (November 2001): 1,361.

Li, S. D., S. Yong, D. Srinivas, and T. Van. "Reactivation of Sarcoidosis During Interferon Therapy." *Journal of Gastroenterology* 37, no. 1 (January 2002): 50–54.

Luisetti, M., A. Beretta, and L. Casali. "Course and Prognosis of Sarcoidosis in African-Americans Versus Caucasians." *The European Respiratory Journal* 18, no. 4 (October 2001): 738.

Miller, A. "Of Time and Experience: Sarcoidosis Revisited." *Chest* 121, no. 1 (January 2002): 3–5.

Motte, G., D. Ducloux, A. Dubiez, E. Justrabo, and J. M. Chalopin. "Renal Involvement After Lung Transplantation for Sarcoidosis." *Clinical Nephrology* 56, no. 5 (November 2001): 411–412.

Quattrocchi, P., D. Bonanno, E. Ferlazzo, G. Marotta, and B. Ferlazzo. "Gastric Angiodysplasia Associated With Sarcoidosis." *Digestive and Liver Disease* 33, no. 9 (December 2001): 804–805.

Rybicki, B. A., M. C. Iannuzzi, M. M. Frederick, B. W. Thompson, M. D. Rossman, E. A. Bresnitz, M. I. Terrin, D. R. Moller, J. Barnard, R. P. Baughman, L. DePalo, G. Hunninghake, C. Johns, M. A. Judson, G. L. Knatterud, G. McLennan, L. S. Newman, D. L. Rabin, C. Rose, A. S. Teirstein, S. E. Weinberger, H. Yeager, and R. Cherniack. "Familial Aggregation of Sarcoidosis. A Case-Control Etiologic Study of Sarcoidosis (ACCESS)." *American Journal of Respiratory and Critical Care Medicine* 164, no. 11 (December 2001): 2,085–2,091.

Tajima, S., Y. Sando, T. Maeno, N. Sagawa, M. Nara, Y. Maeno, J. Nakagawa, T. Ito, Y. Hoshino, T. Suga, M. Arai, and M. Kurabayashi. "Increased Serum Thymidine Kinase Activity in Acute Sarcoidosis." *Internal Medicine* 42, no. 2 (February 2002): 129–132.

SCLERITIS

Afshari, N. A., M. A. Afshari, and C. S. Foster. "Inflammatory Conditions of the Eye Associated With Rheumatic Diseases." *Current Rheumatology Reports* 3, no. 5 (October 2001): 453–458.

Huang, F. C., S. P. Huang, and S. H. Tseng. "Management of Infectious Scleritis After Pterygium Excision." *Cornea* 19, no. 1 (January 2000): 34–39.

Jabs, D. A., A. Mudun, J. P. Dunn, and M. J. Marsh. "Episcleritis and Scleritis: Clinical Features and Treatment Results." *American Journal of Ophthalmology* 130, no. 4 (October 2000): 469–476.

McCluskey, P. J., P. G. Watson, S. Lightman, J. Haybittle, M. Restori, and M. Branley. "Posterior Scleritis: Clinical Features, Systemic Associations, and Outcome in a Large Series of Patients." *Ophthalmology* 106, no. 12 (December 1999): 2,380–2,386.

Rosenbaum, J. T., M. D. Becker, and J. R. Smith. "Toward New Therapies for Ocular Inflammation." *Archivos de la Sociedad Española de Oftalmologia* 75, no. 8 (August 2000): 511–514.

Sahu, D. K., and A. B. Rawoof. "Cilioretinal Artery Occlusion in Posterior Scleritis." *Retina* 20, no. 3 (2000): 303–305.

Sainz de la Maza, M. "Scleritis Immunopathology and Therapy." *Developments in Ophthalmology* 30 (1999): 84–90.

SCLERODERMA

Benrud-Larson, L. M., J. A. Haythornthwaite, L. J. Heinberg, C. Boling, J. Reed, B. White, and F. M. Wigley. "The Impact of Pain and Symptoms of Depression in Scleroderma." *Pain* 95, no. 3 (February 2002): 267–275.

Carbone, L., and L. Myers. "Scleroderma and Body Piercing." *Journal of Pediatrics* 140, no. 2 (February 2002): 241.

Edith Pisa, F., M. Bovenzi, L. Romeo, A. Tonello, D. Biasi, L. M. Bambara, A. Betta, and F. Barbone. "Reproductive Factors and the Risk of Scleroderma: An Italian Case-Control Study." *Arthritis and Rheumatism* 46, no. 2 (February 2002): 451–456.

Gelber, A. C., and F. M. Wigley. "Disease Severity as a Predictor of Outcome in Scleroderma." *Lancet* 359, no. 9303 (January 26, 2002): 277–279.

La Montagna, G., A. Baruffo, R. Tirri, G. Buono, and G. Valentini. "Foot Involvement in Systemic Sclerosis: A Longitudinal Study of 100 Patients." *Seminars in Arthritis and Rheumatism* 31, no. 4 (February 2002): 248–255.

Oikarinen, A., and A. Knuutinen. "Ultraviolet A Sunbed Used for the Treatment of Scleroderma." *Acta Dermato-Venereologica* 81, no. 6 (November–December 2001): 432–433.

Parodi, A., M. Drosera, L. Barbieri, and A. Rebora. "Scleroderma Subsets Are Best Detected by the Simultaneous Analysis of the Autoantibody Profile Using Commercial ELISA." *Dermatology* 204, no. 1 (2002): 29–32.

Sapadin, A. N., and R. Fleischmajer. "Treatment of Scleroderma." *Archives in Dermatology* 138, no. 1 (January 2002): 99–105.

Trojanowska, M. "Molecular Aspects of Scleroderma." *Frontiers in Bioscience* 7 (March 1, 2002): D608–618.

Vijayalakshmi, A. M. "Scleroderma–CREST Syndrome." *Indian Pediatrics* 39, no. 2 (February 2002): 204.

SJÖGREN'S SYNDROME

al-Hashimi, I. "Oral and Periodontal Status in Sjogren's Syndrome." *Texas Dental Journal* 118, no. 10 (October 2001): 932–939.

Amin, K., D. Ludviksdottir, C. Janson, O. Nettelbladt, B. Gudbjornsson, S. Valtysdottir, E. Bjornsson, G. M. Roomans, G. Boman, L. Seveus, and P. Venge. "Inflammation and Structural Changes in the Airways of Patients With Brimary Sjogren's Syndrome." *Respiratory Medicine* 95, no. 11 (November 2001): 904–910.

Bjerrum, K. B. "Primary Sjogren's Syndrome and Keratoconjunctivitis Sicca: Diagnostic Methods, Frequency and Social Disease Aspects." *Acta Ophthalmologica Scandinavica Supplement* 231 (2000): 1–37.

Carsons, S. "A Review and Update of Sjogren's Syndrome: Manifestations, Diagnosis, and Treatment." *American Journal of Managed Care* 7, no. 14 Supplement (September 2001): S433–443.

Fox, R. I. "The Value of Noninvasive Studies of Parotid Glands in Primary Sjogren's Syndrome." *Arthritis and Rheumatism* 45, no. 6 (December 2001): 473–474.

Fox, R. I., Y. Konttinen, and A. Fisher. "Use of Muscarinic Agonists in the Treatment of Sjogren's Syndrome." *Clinical Immunology* 101, no. 3 (December 2001): 249–263.

Kalk, W. W., A. Vissink, B. Stegenga, H. Bootsma, A. V. Nieuw Amerongen, and C. G. Kallenberg. "Sialometry and Sialochemistry: A Non-Invasive Approach for Diagnosing Sjogren's Syndrome." *Annals of the Rheumatic Diseases* 61, no. 2 (February 2002): 137–144.

Kalk, W. W., A. Vissink, F. K. Spijkervet, H. Bootsma, C. G. Kallenberg, and A. V. Nieuw Amerongen. "Sialometry and Sialochemistry: Diagnostic Tools for Sjogren's Syndrome." *Annals of the Rheumatic Diseases* 60, no. 12 (December 2001): 1,110–1,116.

Mulherin, D., J. R. Ainsworth, J. Hamburger, D. Situnayake, B. Speculand, and S. J. Bowman. "Survey of Artificial Tear and Saliva Usage Among Patients With Sjogren's Syndrome." *Annals of the Rheumatic Diseases* 60, no. 11 (November 2001): 1,077.

Niemela, R. K., E. Paakko, I. Suramo, R. Takalo, and M. Hakala. "Magnetic Resonance Imaging and Magnetic Resonance Sialography of Parotid Glands In Primary Sjogren's Syndrome." *Arthritis and Rheumatism* 45, no. 6 (December 2001): 512–518.

SPERM AUTOIMMUNITY

Auer, J., H. Senechal, and M. De Almeida. "Sperm-Associated and Circulating IgA and IgG Classes of Antibodies Recognise Different Antigens on the Human Sperm Plasma Membrane." *Journal of Reproductive Immunology* 34, no. 2 (September 1997): 121–136.

Baker, H. W. "Medical Treatment for Idiopathic Male Infertility: Is It Curative or Palliative?" *Bailliere's Clinical Obstetrics and Gynaecology* 11, no. 4 (December 1997): 673–689.

Diekman, A. B., E. J. Norton, V. A. Westbrook, K. L. Klotz, S. Naaby-Hansen, and J. C. Herr. "Anti-Sperm Antibodies From Infertile Patients and Their Cognate Sperm Antigens: A Review. Identity Between SAGA-1, the H6-3C4 Antigen, and CD52." *American Journal of Reproductive Immunology* 43, no. 3 (March 2000): 134–143.

Hegde, U. C., S. Ranpura, S. D'Souza, and V. P. Raghavan. "Immunoregulatory Pathways in Pregnancy." *Indian Journal of Biochemistry and Biophysics* 38, no. 4 (August 2001): 207–219.

Iborra, A., J. R. Palacio, Z. Ulcova-Gallova, and P. Martinez. "Autoimmune Response in Women With Endometriosis." *American Journal of Reproductive Immunology* 44, no. 4 (October 2000): 236–241.

Lombardo, F., L. Gandini, F. Dondero, and A. Lenzi. "Antisperm Immunity In Natural and Assisted Reproduction." *Human Reproduction Update* 7, no. 5 (September–October 2001): 450–456.

Luckas, M. J., W. M. Buckett, I. A. Aird, P. M. Johnson, and D. I. Lewis-Jones. "Seminal Plasma Immunoglobulin Concentrations in Autoimmune Male Subfertility." *Journal of Reproductive Immunology* 37, no. 2 (February 1998): 171–180.

STIFF-MAN SYNDROME

Dalakas, M. C., M. Fujii, M. Li, B. Lutfi, J. Kyhos, and B. McElroy. "High-Dose Intravenous Immune Globulin for Stiff-Person Syndrome." *New England Journal of Medicine* 345, no. 26 (December 27, 2001): 1,870–1,876.

Dalakas, M. C., M. Li, M. Fujii, and D. M. Jacobowitz. "Stiff Person Syndrome: Quantification, Specificity, and Intrathecal Synthesis of GAD65 Antibodies." *Neurology* 57, no. 5 (September 11, 2001): 780–784.

Fiol, M., A. Cammarota, A. Rivero, A. Pardal, M. Nogues, and J. Correale. "Focal Stiff-Person Syndrome." *Neurologia* 16, no. 2 (February 2001): 89–91.

Gurol, M. E., M. Ertas, H. A. Hanagasi, H. A. Sahin, G. Gursoy, and M. Emre. "Stiff Leg Syndrome: Case Report." *Movement Disorders* 16, no. 6 (November 2001): 1,189–1,193.

Markandeyulu, V., T. P. Joseph, T. Solomon, J. Jacob, S. Kumar, and C. Gnanamuthu. "Stiff-Man Syndrome in Childhood." *Journal of the Royal Society of Medicine* 94, no. 6 (June 2001): 296–297.

Meinck, H. M. "Stiff Man Syndrome." *CNS Drugs* 15, no. 7 (2001): 515–526.

Murinson, B. B., and M. Rizzo. "Improvement of Stiff-Person Syndrome With Tiagabine." *Neurology* 57, no. 2 (July 24, 2001): 366.

Nikhilesh, J., Z. A. Sayeed, P. K. Saravanan, and J. Paul. "Stiff Person Syndrome." *Journal of the Association of Physicians of India* 49 (May 2001): 568–570.

Shariatmadar, S., and T. A. Noto. "Plasma Exchange in Stiff-Man Syndrome." *Therapeutic Apheresis* 5, no. 1 (February 2001): 64–67.

Thompson, P. D. "The Stiff-Man Syndrome and Related Disorders." *Parkinsonism & Related Disorders* 8, no. 2 (October 2001): 147–153.

SUBACUTE BACTERIAL ENDOCARDITIS

Agarwal, A., J. Clements, D. D. Sedmak, D. Imler, N. S. Nahman Jr., D. A. Orsinelli, and L. A. Hebert. "Subacute Bacterial Endocarditis Masquerading As Type III Essential Mixed Cryoglobulinemia." *Journal of the American Society of Nephrology* 8, no. 12 (December 1997): 1,971–1,976.

Darhous, M. S., O. M. Dahab, E. el Atar, and E. el Ghafary. "Dental, Oral and Bacteriological Aspects in Patients At Risk of Subacute Bacterial Endocarditis." *Egyptian Dental Journal* 39, no. 4 (October 1993): 533–539.

Harris, G. D., and J. Steimle. "Compiling the Identifying Features of Bacterial Endocarditis. Vague Clues May Point To This Dangerous Infection." *Postgraduate Medicine* 107, no. 1 (January 2000): 75–76, 79–83.

Hoskins, G. C. "Demonstration of Microorganisms In Subacute Bacterial Endocarditis." *Texas Medicine* 91, no. 6 (June 1995): 11.

Kim, J. E., and D. P. Han. "Premacular Hemorrhage as a Sign of Subacute Bacterial Endocarditis." *American Journal of Ophthalmology* 120, no. 2 (August 1995): 250–251.

Marshall, C., and M. McDonald. "Recurrent Subacute Bacterial Endocarditis As a Presentation of Left Atrial Myxoma." *Australian and New Zealand Journal of Medicine* 28, no. 3 (June 1998): 350.

Martin, L., and C. Gustaferro. "Chronic Cough Associated With Subacute Bacterial Endocarditis." *Mayo Clinic Proceedings* 70, no. 7 (July 1995): 662–664.

Soxman, J. A. "Subacute Bacterial Endocarditis: Considerations For the Pediatric Patient." *Journal of the American Dental Association* 131, no. 5 (May 2000): 668–669.

Subra, J. F., C. Michelet, J. Laporte, F. Carrere, P. Reboul, F. Cartier, J. P. Saint-Andre, and A. Chevailler. "The Presence of Cytoplasmic Antineutrophil Cytoplasmic Antibodies (C-ANCA) In the Course of Subacute Bacterial Endocarditis With Glomerular Involvement, Coincidence or Association?" *Clinical Nephrology* 49, no. 1 (January 1998): 15–18.

SYMPATHETIC OPHTHALMIA

Borkowski, L. M., D. V. Weinberg, C. M. Delany, and L. Milsow. "Laser Photocoagulation for Choroidal Neovascularization Associated With Sympathetic Ophthalmia." *American Journal of Ophthalmology* 132, no. 4 (October 2001): 585–587.

Chan, C. C., and M. Mochizuki. "Sympathetic Ophthalmia: An Autoimmune Ocular Inflammatory Disease." *Springer Seminars in Immunopathology* 21, no. 2 (1999): 125–134.

Das, A., and A. P. Moriarty. "Sympathetic Ophthalmia as a Preoperative Consideration In Adults Having Anterior Segment Revision For Trauma Sustained In Childhood." *Journal of Cataract and Refractive Surgery* 28, no. 1 (January 2002): 6.

Gasch, A. T., C. S. Foster, C. L. Grosskreutz, and L. R. Pasquale. "Postoperative Sympathetic Ophthalmia." *International Ophthalmology Clinics* 40, no. 1 (Winter 2000): 69–84.

Levine, M. R., C. R. Pou, and R. H. Lash. "The 1998 Wendell Hughes Lecture. Evisceration: Is Sympathetic Ophthalmia a Concern In the New Millennium?" *Ophthalmic Plastic and Reconstructive Surgery* 15, no. 1 (January 1999): 4–8.

Sheppard, J. D. "Sympathetic Ophthalmia." *Seminars in Ophthalmology* 9, no. 3 (September 1994): 177–184.

SYSTEMIC LUPUS ERYTHEMATOSUS (SLE)

Ambrus Jr., J. L., V. Contractor, A. Joseph, J. Long, and D. Blumenthal. "A Potential Role for PGE and IL-14 (HMW-BCGF) in B-Cell Hyperactivity of Patients with Systemic Lupus Erythematosus." *American Journal of Therapeutics* 2, no. 12 (December 1995): 933–942.

Bhatia, S., N. B. Silverberg, P. C. Don, and J. M. Weinberg. "Extensive Calcinosis Cutis in Association With Systemic Lupus Erythematosus." *Acta Dermato-Venereologica* 81, no. 6 (November–December 2001): 446–447.

Brunner, H. I., E. D. Silverman, T. To, C. Bombardier, and B. M. Feldman. "Risk Factors For Damage in Childhood-Onset Systemic Lupus Erythematosus: Cumulative Disease Activity and Medication Use Predict Disease Damage." *Arthritis and Rheumatism* 46, no. 2 (February 2002): 436–444.

Dube, G. K., G. S. Markowitz, J. Radhakrishnan, G. B. Appel, and V. D. D'Agati. "Minimal Change Disease in Systemic Lupus Erythematosus." *Clinical Nephrology* 57, no. 2 (February 2002): 120–126.

Gaffney, P. M., K. L. Moser, R. R. Graham, and T. W. Behrens. "Recent Advances in the Genetics of Systemic Lupus Erythematosus." *Rheumatic Diseases Clinics of North America* 28, no. 1 (February 2002): 111–126.

Kiss, E., H. P. Bhattoa, P. Bettembuk, A. Balogh, and G. Szegedi. "Pregnancy in Women With Systemic Lupus Erythematosus." *European Journal of Obstetrics, Gynecology, and Reproductive Biology* 101, no. 2 (March 10, 2002): 129–134.

Lima, D. S., E. I. Sato, V. C. Lima, F. Miranda Jr., and F. H. Hatta. "Brachial Endothelial Function Is Impaired In Patients With Systemic Lupus Erythematosus." *Journal of Rheumatology* 29, no. 2 (February 2002): 292–297.

Nawata, M., N. Seta, M. Yamada, I. Sekigawa, N. Lida, and H. Hashimoto. "Possible Triggering Effect of Cytomegalovirus Infection on Systemic Lupus Erythematosus." *Scandinavian Journal of Rheumatology* 30, no. 6 (2001): 360–362.

Schubert, C., W. Geser, B. Noisternig, P. Konig, G. Rumpold, and A. Lampe. "Stressful Life Events and Skin Diseases: An Additional Perspective From Research on Psychosomatic Dynamics in Systemic Lupus Erythematosus." *Psychotherapy and Psychosomatics* 71, no. 2 (March–April 2002): 123–124.

Stein, C. M., J. M. Olson, C. Gray-McGuire, G. R. Bruner, J. B. Harley, and K. L. Moser. "Increased Prevalence of Renal Disease in Systemic Lupus Erythematosus Families With Affected Male Relatives." *Arthritis and Rheumatism* 46, no. 2 (February 2002): 428–435.

TAKAYASU ARTERITIS

Angeli, E., A. Vanzulli, M. Venturini, G. B. Zoccai, and A. Del Maschio. "The Role of Radiology in the Diagnosis and Management of Takayasu's Arteritis." *Journal of Nephrology* 14, no. 6 (November–December 2001): 514–524.

Filer, A., D. Nicholls, R. Corston, P. Carey, and P. Bacon. "Takayasu Arteritis and Atherosclerosis: Illustrating the Consequences of Endothelial Damage." *Journal of Rheumatology* 28, no. 12 (December 2001): 2,752–2,753.

Kobayashi, Y., and F. Numano F. "3. Takayasu Arteritis." *Internal Medicine* 41, no. 1 (January 2002): 44–46.

Korkmaz, C., I. Zubaroglu, T. Kaya, and O. M. Akay. "Takayasu's Arteritis Associated With Rheumatoid

Arthritis: A Case Report and Review of the Literature." *Rheumatology (Oxford)* 40, no. 12 (December 2001): 1,420–1,422.

Nishiyama, A., S. Matsubara, and J. Toyama. "Takayasu Arteritis With Multiple Cardiovascular Complications." *Heart Vessels* 16, no. 1 (December 2001): 23–27.

Numano, F. "The Story of Takayasu Arteritis." *Rheumatology (Oxford)* 41, no. 1 (January 2002): 103–106.

Nussinovitch, N., B. Morag, and T. Rosenthal. "Takayasu—Pulseless Disease." *Journal of Human Hypertension* 15, no. 7 (July 2001): 503–504.

Ohkawara, M., T. Kuroiwa, and F. Numano. "Immuno-histochemical Studies on Annexin I and II in Takayasu Arteritis." *Annals of the New York Academy of Sciences* 947 (December 2001): 390–393.

Sebnem Kilic, S., O. Bostan, and E. Cil. "Takayasu Arteritis." *Annals of Rheumatic Diseases* 61, no. 1 (January 2002): 92–93.

Sheikhzadeh, A., I. Tettenborn, F. Noohi, M. Eftekharzadeh, and A. Schnabel. "Occlusive Thromboaortopathy (Takayasu Disease): Clinical and Angiographic Features and a Brief Review of Literature." *Angiology* 53, no. 1 (January–February 2002): 29–40.

TEMPORAL ARTERITIS/(GCV)

Bhatti, M. T., and H. Tabandeh. "Giant Cell Arteritis: Diagnosis and Management." *Current Opinion in Ophthalmology* 12, no. 6 (December 2001): 393–399.

Cantini, F., L. Niccoli, C. Salvarani, A. Padula, and I. Olivieri. "Treatment of Longstanding Active Giant Cell Arteritis With Infliximab: Report of Four Cases." *Arthritis and Rheumatism* 44, no. 12 (December 2001): 2,933–2,935.

Cikes, A., M. Depairon, R. M. Jolidon, P. Wyss, and H. J. Lang. "Necrosis of the Tongue and Unilateral Blindness in Temporal Arteritis." *VASA* 30, no. 3 (July 2001): 222–224.

Coors, E. A., and M. Simon Jr. "Bilateral Temporal Arteritis." *Journal of the American Academy of Dermatology* 46, no. 2 Supplement Case Reports (February 2002): S14–15.

Ghosh, C. "Giant Cell Arteritis." *Ophthalmology* 109, no. 2 (February 2002): 221–222.

Kupersmith, M. J., R. Speira, R. Langer, M. Richmond, M. Peterson, H. Speira, H. Mitnick, and S. Paget. "Visual Function and Quality of Life Among Patients With Giant Cell (Temporal) Arteritis." *Journal of Neuro-Ophthalmology* 21, no. 4 (December 2001): 266–273.

Levine, S. M., and D. B. Hellmann. "Giant Cell Arteritis." *Current Opinion in Rheumatology* 14, no. 1 (January 2002): 3–10.

Miller, N. R. "Visual Manifestations of Temporal Arteritis." *Rheumatic Diseases Clinics of North America* 27, no. 4 (November 2001): 781–797, vi.

Schmidt, D., and J. Schulte-Monting. "Giant Cell Arteritis Is More Prevalent In Urban Than In Rural Populations." *Rheumatology (Oxford)* 40, no. 10 (October 2001): 1193.

Smetana, G. W., and R. H. Shmerling. "Does This Patient Have Temporal Arteritis?" *JAMA* 287, no. 1 (January 2, 2002): 92–101.

TRANSVERSE MYELITIS

Andersen, O. "Myelitis." *Current Opinion in Neurology* 13, no. 3 (June 2000): 311–316.

Defresne, P., L. Meyer, M. Tardieu, E. Scalais, C. Nuttin, B. De Bont, G. Loftus, P. Landrieu, H. Kadhim, and G. Sebire. "Efficacy of High Dose Steroid Therapy in Children With Severe Acute Transverse Myelitis." *Journal of Neurology, Neurosurgery, and Psychiatry* 71, no. 2 (August 2001): 272–274.

Ganesan, V., and M. Borzyskowski. "Characteristics and Course of Urinary Tract Dysfunction After Acute Transverse Myelitis in." *Developmental Medicine and Child Neurology* 43, no. 7 (July 2001): 473–475.

Kalita, J., and U. K. Misra. "Neurophysiological Studies in Acute Transverse Myelitis." *Journal of Neurology* 247, no. 12 (December 2000): 943–948.

Laffey, J. G., D. Murphy, J. Regan, and D. O'Keeffe. "Efficacy of Spinal Cord Stimulation For Neuropathic Pain Following Idiopathic Acute Transverse Myelitis: A Case Report." *Clinical Neurology and Neurosurgery* 101, no. 2 (June 1999): 125–127.

Murthy, J. M., J. J. Reddy, A. K. Meena, and S. Kaul. "Acute Transverse Myelitis: MR Characteristics." *Neurology India* 47, no. 4 (December 1999): 290–293.

ULCERATIVE COLITIS

Falasco, G., R. Zinicola, and A. Forbes. "Immunosuppressants in Distal Ulcerative Colitis." *Alimentary Pharmacology and Therapeutics* 16, no. 2 (February 2002): 181–187.

Farrell, R. J., and M. A. Peppercorn. "Ulcerative Colitis." *Lancet* 359, no. 9303 (January 26, 2002): 331–340.

Koch, T. R. "P-ANCA for Ulcerative Colitis Management-Hype or Hope?" *American Journal of Gastroenterology* 97, no. 2 (February 2002): 485.

Langmead, L., and D. S. Rampton. "Plain Abdominal Radiographic Features Are Not Reliable Markers of Disease Extent In Active Ulcerative Colitis." *American Journal of Gastroenterology* 97, no. 2 (February 2002): 354–359.

Matsumoto, T., S. Nakamura, M. Shimizu, and M. Iida. "Significance of Appendiceal Involvement in Patients With Ulcerative Colitis." *Gastrointestinal Endoscopy* 55, no. 2 (February 2002): 180–185.

Okano, A., K. Hajiro, H. Takakuwa, and A. Nishio. "Pseudotumorous Pancreatitis Associated With Ulcerative Colitis." *Internal Medicine* 40, no. 12 (December 2001): 1,205–1,208.

Oxentenko, A. S., E. V. Loftus, J. K. Oh, G. K. Danielson, and T. F. Mangan. "Constrictive Pericarditis in Chronic Ulcerative Colitis." *Journal of Clinical Gastroenterology* 34, no. 3 (March 2002): 247–251.

Seo, M., M. Okada, T. Yao, H. Matake, and K. Maeda. "Evaluation of the Clinical Course of Acute Attacks in Patients With Ulcerative Colitis Through the Use of an Activity Index." *Journal of Gastroenterology* 37, no. 1 (January 2002): 29–34.

Sood, A., V. Midha, N. Sood, V. Kaushal, and G. Awasthi. "Methylprednisolone Acetate Versus Oral Prednisolone in Moderately Active Ulcerative Colitis." *Indian Journal of Gastroenterology* 21, no. 1 (January–February 2002): 11–13.

Xu, C. T., and B. R. Pan. "Current Medical Therapy for Ulcerative Colitis." *World Journal of Gastroenterology* 5, no. 1 (February 1999): 64–72.

UVEITIS

Bakunowicz-Lazarczyk, A., R. Antosiuk, J. Wysocka, and M. Sulkowska. "Cellular Immunity in Pediatric Uveitis." *International Journal of Tissue Reactions* 23, no. 4 (2001): 137–143.

Gonzales, C. A., J. G. Ladas, J. L. Davis, W. J. Feuer, and G. N. Holland. "Relationships Between Laser Flare Photometry Values and Complications of Uveitis." *Archives of Ophthalmology* 119, no. 12 (December 2001): 1,763–1,769.

Lightman, S., and H. Kok. "Developments in the Treatment of Uveitis." *Expert Opinion on Investigational Drugs* 11, no. 1 (January 2002): 59–67.

Manzotti, F., J. G. Orsoni, L. Zavota, L. Cimino, E. Zola, and C. Bonaguri. "Autoimmune Uveitis In Children: Clinical Correlation Between Antinuclear Antibody Positivity and Ocular Recurrences." *Rheumatology International* 21, no. 4 (January 2002): 127–132.

Queiro, R., J. C. Torre, J. Belzunegui, C. Gonzalez, J. R. De Dios, F. Unanue, and M. Figueroa. "Clinical Features and Predictive Factors in Psoriatic Arthritis-Related Uveitis." *Seminars in Arthritis and Rheumatism* 31, no. 4 (February 2002): 264–270.

Rosenbaum, J. T., and J. R. Smith. "Uveitis and Juvenile Arthritis." *British Journal of Ophthalmology* 86, no. 1 (January 2002): 1–2.

Sikic, J., and S. P. Suic. "Surgical Treatment of Uveitis." *Collegium Antropologicum* 25, Supplement (2001): 71–76.

Smith, J. R., and J. T. Rosenbaum. "Management of Uveitis: A Rheumatologic Perspective." *Arthritis and Rheumatism* 46, no. 2 (February 2002): 309–318.

VASCULITIS

Cuchacovich, R. "Immunopathogenesis of Vasculitis." *Current Rheumatology Reports* 4, no. 1 (February 2002): 9–17.

Kodo, K., M. Hida, S. Omori, T. Mori, M. Tokumura, S. Kuramochi, and M. Awazu. "Vasculitis Associated With Septicemia: Case Report and Review of the Literature." *Pediatric Nephrology* 16, no. 12 (December 2001): 1,089–1,092.

Langford, C. A., and G. S. Kerr. "Pregnancy in Vasculitis." *Current Opinion in Rheumatology* 14, no. 1 (January 2002): 36–41.

Savage, C. O., L. Harper, M. Holland. "New Findings in Pathogenesis of Antineutrophil Cytoplasm Antibody-Associated Vasculitis." *Current Opinion in Rheumatology* 14, no. 1 (January 2002): 15–22.

Takeuchi, T., and T. Abe. "2. Role of Adhesion Molecules in Vasculitis Syndrome." *Internal Medicine* 41, no. 1 (January 2002): 41–44.

Yoshida, M. "4. Antineutrophil Cytoplasmic Antibody (ANCA) Associated Vasculitis: From Molecular Analysis to Bedside." *Internal Medicine* 41, no. 1 (January 2002): 47–49.

VITILIGO

Falabella, R. "What's New In the Treatment of Vitiligo." *Journal of the European Academy of Dermatology and Venereology* 15, no. 4 (July 2001): 287–289.

Fesq, H., K. Brockow, K. Strom, M. Mempel, J. Ring, and D. Abeck. "Dihydroxyacetone in a New Formulation—a Powerful Therapeutic Option in Vitiligo." *Dermatology* 203, no. 3 (2001): 241–243.

Kemp, E. H., E. A. Waterman, and A. P. Weetman. "Autoimmune Aspects of Vitiligo." *Autoimmunity* 34, no. 1 (2001): 65–77.

Kim, C. Y., T. J. Yoon, and T. H. Kim. "Epidermal Grafting After Chemical Epilation in the Treatment of Vitiligo." *Dermatologic Surgery* 27, no. 10 (October 2001): 855–856.

Le Poole, I. C., R. Sarangarajan, Y. Zhao, L. S. Stennett, T. L. Brown, P. Sheth, T. Miki, and R. E. Boissy. "'VIT1', a Novel Gene Associated With Vitiligo." *Pigment Cell Research* 14, no. 6 (December 2001): 475–484.

Moretti, S., A. Spallanzani, L. Amato, G. Hautmann, I. Gallerani, and P. Fabbri. "Vitiligo and Epidermal Microenvironment: Possible Involvement of Ker-

atinocyte-Derived Cytokines." *Archives of Dermatology* 138, no. 2 (February 2002): 273–274.

Njoo, M. D., and W. Westerhof. "Vitiligo. Pathogenesis and Treatment." *American Journal of Clinical Dermatology* 2, no. 3 (2001): 167–181.

van Geel, N., K. Ongenae, M. De Mil, and J. M. Naeyaert. "Modified Technique of Autologous Noncultured Epidermal Cell Transplantation For Repigmenting Vitiligo: A Pilot Study." *Dermatologic Surgery* 27, no. 10 (October 2001): 873–876.

Westerhof, W., W. Lontz, W. Vanscheidt, and L. Braathen. "Vitiligo: News in Surgical Treatment." *Journal of the European Academy of Dermatology and Venereology* 15, no. 6 (November 2001): 510–511.

Zaima, H., and M. Koga. "Clinical Course of 44 Cases of Localized Type Vitiligo." *Journal of Dermatology* 29, no. 1 (January 2002): 15–19.

WEGENER'S GRANULOMATOSIS

Abdou, N. I., G. J. Kullman, G. S. Hoffman, G. C. Sharp, U. Specks, T. McDonald, J. Garrity, J. A. Goeken, and N. B. Allen. "Wegener's Granulomatosis: Survey of 701 Patients in North America. Changes In Outcome In The 1990s." *Journal of Rheumatology* 29, no. 2 (February 2002): 309–316.

Brons, R. H., M. C. de Jong, N. K. de Boer, C. A. Stegeman, C. G. Kallenberg, and J. W. Cohen Tervaert. "Detection of Immune Deposits in Skin Lesions of Patients With Wegener's Granulomatosis." *Annals of Rheumatic Diseases* 60, no. 12 (December 2001): 1,097–1,102.

de Groot, K., D. K. Schmidt, A. C. Arlt, W. L. Gross, and E. Reinhold-Keller. "Standardized Neurologic Evaluations of 128 Patients With Wegener Granulomatosis." *Archives of Neurology* 58, no. 8 (August 2001): 1,215–1,221.

Iking-Konert, C., S. Vogt, M. Radsak, C. Wagner, G. M. Hansch, and K. Andrassy. "Polymorphonuclear Neutrophils in Wegener's Granulomatosis Acquire Characteristics of Antigen Presenting Cells." *Kidney International* 60, no. 6 (December 2001): 2,247–2,262.

Inoue, K., Y. Kawahito, H. Sano, and T. Yoshikawa. "Antituberculous Drugs For Wegener's Granulomatosis." *Chest* 120, no. 6 (December 2001): 2,112–2,113.

Neviani, C. B., A. Carvalho Hde, C. Hossamu, S. Aisen, and W. Nadalin. "Radiation Therapy as an Option For Upper Airway Obstruction Due to Wegener's Granulomatosis." *Otolaryngology and Head and Neck Surgery* 126, no. 2 (February 2002): 195–196.

Pleasure, D. "Peripheral Neuropathy As the First Clinical Manifestation of Wegener Granulomatosis." *Archives of Neurology* 58, no. 8 (August 2001): 1,204.

Regan, M. J., D. B. Hellmann, and J. H. Stone. "Treatment of Wegener's Granulomatosis." *Rheumatic Diseases Clinics of North America* 27, no. 4 (November 2001): 863–886, viii.

Schmitt, W. H., R. Linder, E. Reinhold-Keller, and W. L. Gross. "Improved Differentiation Between Churg-Strauss Syndrome and Wegener's Granulomatosis By an Artificial Neural Network." *Arthritis and Rheumatism* 44, no. 8 (August 2001): 1,887–1,896.

Thomas-Golbanov, C., and S. Sridharan. "Novel Therapies in Vasculitis." *Expert Opinion on Investigational Drugs* 10, no. 7 (July 2001): 1,279–1,289.

INDEX

Boldface page numbers indicate major treatment of a subject.

A

AARDA. *See* American Autoimmune Related Diseases Association
absolute neutrophil count 164
absolute risk **1**
ACE. *See* angiotensin-converting enzyme
acetylcholine 159
acetylcholine receptor antibodies 159, 160
Achilles tendinitis, in ankylosing spondylitis 23
acitretin (Soriatane), for psoriasis 184
acquired immunity. *See* immunity
acquired immunodeficiency syndrome. *See* AIDS
ACTH 2
   deficiency of 3
   for multiple sclerosis 153
ACTH stimulation test 3–4
active immunity **1**
acute disseminated encephalomyelitis 138, 169–170. *See also* perivenous encephalomyelitis
acute inflammatory demyelinating polyneuropathy. *See* Guillain-Barré syndrome
acute-phase proteins **1**
ADA. *See* Americans with Disabilities Act
ADCC. *See* antibody-dependent cell-mediated cytotoxicity
Addison, Thomas **1**
addisonian crisis 3, 4–5
Addison's anemia. *See* pernicious anemia
Addison's disease **1–5,** 40

menstrual problems in 147
and polyglandular autoimmune syndromes 173, 174
ADEM. *See* acute disseminated encephalomyelitis
adenocarcinoma, in celiac disease 49
adolescents
   with autoimmune diseases **5–6**
   chronic fatigue syndrome in 5, 53
adrenal insufficiency
   chronic. *See* Addison's disease
   primary 2–3, 4
   secondary 3, 4
adrenocorticotropin. *See* ACTH
African Americans, with autoimmune diseases **6–7,** 203–204
agammaglobulinemia, primary **178–180**
aging, and autoimmune diseases **8**
agranulocytes **8,** 138
AIDS **8–11,** 108
   research on **11**
AIED. *See* autoimmune inner ear disease
AIH. *See* hepatitis (autoimmune)
AIHA. *See* autoimmune hemolytic anemia
air conditioners, in allergy management 16
air filters, in allergy management 16
Alaska Natives, and autoimmune diseases **11**
alcohol
   and autoimmune diseases **11–12**
   and cardiomyopathy 45
   drug interactions with 144
aldosterone
   actions of 2
   deficiency of, in Addison's disease 2–3

allergen(s) **12,** 14
   in asthma 13
   avoidance of 15–16
allergic angiitis. *See* Churg-Strauss syndrome
allergic asthma **12–14**
   in African Americans 6–7
   childhood 121
   economic cost of 77
   in Hispanics/Latinos 108
   hospitalization for 112
allergic granulomatosis. *See* Churg-Strauss syndrome
allergic reaction **14**
   dapsone-related 72
allergic rhinitis 14, **14**
allergy **14–17**
   and chronic fatigue syndrome 55
allergy shots 17
   for asthma 14
allogeneic transplantation 41, 42
allograft **17,** 100
alopecia areata **17–19**
   celebrities with 47
   national registry for 19–20
   and polyglandular autoimmune syndromes 173, 174
   research on **19–20**
alopecia totalis 18
alopecia universalis 18
alpha-blockers, for Raynaud's phenomenon 190
alpha interferon, for multiple sclerosis 154
ALPS. *See* autoimmune lymphoproliferative syndrome
alternative medical treatments **20–22**
   for rheumatoid arthritis 200
   for systemic lupus erythematosus 229
alum 247

CHB. *See* congenital heart block

chemokines **51**

chemotaxis **51**

chemotherapy, for Mooren's ulcer 149

chest X ray
    in sarcoidosis 204–205
    in Wegener's granulomatosis 252

children
    allergic asthma in 12–14
    ankylosing spondylitis in 22
    arthritis in. *See* juvenile arthritis
    with autoimmune disease, and family functioning 90–91
    celiac disease in 121
    Chagas' disease in 121
    chronic fatigue syndrome in 52, 53
        and school attendance 208
    Crohn's disease in 52
    diabetes in. *See* insulin-dependent diabetes (type 1)
    HIV infection (AIDS) in 9, 109–110
    immune-mediated thrombocytopenia in 52
    inflammatory bowel disease in 52
    multiple sclerosis in 52
    myasthenia gravis in, race/ethnicity and 186
    of parents with autoimmune diseases 51–52, 90
    of parents with rheumatoid arthritis 90
    pernicious anemia in 170
    scleroderma in 52
    systemic lupus erythematosus in 52
    thrombocytopenic purpura in 117
    thyroiditis in 52
    ulcerative colitis in 52
    vitiligo in 52

Chlamydia trachomatis, and Reiter's syndrome 190–192

chlorambucil (Leukeran)
    for Behçet's disease 38
    for bullous pemphigoid 44
    for essential mixed cryoglobulinemia 85

cholangitis
    chronic nonsuppurative destructive. *See* primary biliary cirrhosis
    primary autoimmune. *See* primary biliary cirrhosis

chorea, in rheumatic fever 195

chronic active hepatitis
    autoimmune. *See* hepatitis (autoimmune)
    female:male ratio in 254
    idiopathic. *See* hepatitis (autoimmune)

chronic fatigue syndrome **52–59,** 74
    in adolescents 5, 53
    celebrities with 47
    in children 52, 53
        and school attendance 208
    and driving 76
    exercise in 87
    work/employment in 80

chronic inflammatory demyelinating polyneuropathy **59–60**
    sex differences in 145

chronic relapsing polyneuropathy. *See* chronic inflammatory demyelinating polyneuropathy

Churg-Strauss syndrome **60**
    celebrity with 47
    and polyarteritis nodosa 171

cicatricial pemphigoid 40, **60–62.** *See also* ocular cicatricial pemphigoid
    age distribution of 8

CIDP. *See* chronic inflammatory demyelinating polyneuropathy

cladribine (Leustatin), for multiple sclerosis 154

claudication 233

climate, and rheumatoid arthritis 198

clinical studies/research **62**
    advances in (future directions for) xvii–xviii
    on autoimmune disease 33
    managed care and 111

clonal deletion **62**

clonal expansion **62**

clones **62**

coal tar, for psoriasis 183

COBRA 127

coenzymes, for chronic fatigue syndrome 58

Cogan's syndrome 40, **62–63**

cognitive impairment, in multiple sclerosis 151

colchicine, for Behçet's disease 39

cold agglutinin disease 33, **63**
    age distribution of 8

colectomy, in Crohn's disease 68

collagen. *See* scleroderma

colon cancer, ulcerative colitis and 243

colonoscopy 66
    in ulcerative colitis 243

committed progenitors 221

common variable immunodeficiency 179

complement **63,** 231
    in cold agglutinin disease 63
    in myocarditis 162

complementary medicine. *See* alternative medical treatments

complement cascade 64

complement system **63–64**

complete congenital heart block 64

compliance. *See* medication compliance

compression neuropathies 168–169

congenital heart block **64–65,** 121

congenital myasthenic syndrome 159

conjunctivitis
    in Reiter's syndrome 190–193
    in Wegener's granulomatosis 252

connective tissue disease 210. *See also* mixed connective tissue disease
    early 32
    Raynaud's phenomenon in 187–188
    undifferentiated 32. *See also* mixed connective tissue disease

constipation, in multiple sclerosis 158

contracture(s) 169

copolymer I (Copaxone), for multiple sclerosis 155

polymyalgia rheumatica **174–176**
  age distribution of 8
  and giant cell arteritis 235
polymyositis 120, 162, **176**
  Raynaud's phenomenon in
    187–188
postcardiac injury syndrome. *See*
  Dressler's syndrome; postmyocardial infarction syndrome
postcardiotomy pericarditis. *See*
  Dressler's syndrome; postmyocardial infarction syndrome; postpericardiotomy syndrome
postcoital test, for sperm autoimmunity 218
postinfarction syndrome. *See* postmyocardial infarction syndrome
post-MI pericarditis. *See* Dressler's
  syndrome; postmyocardial infarction syndrome
postmyocardial infarction syndrome
  176–177
postpericardiotomy syndrome **177**
pouchitis 244
PPS. *See* postpericardiotomy syndrome
prednisone 143
  adverse effects and side effects
    of 106
  for autoimmune hepatitis
    106–107
  for Behçet's disease 38
  for bullous pemphigoid 44
  for cicatricial pemphigoid 61,
    166
  for dermatomyositis 73
  for idiopathic pulmonary fibrosis
    116
  for Lambert-Eaton myasthenia
    syndrome 137
  for mixed connective tissue dis-
    ease 148
  for Mooren's ulcer 149
  for myasthenia gravis 160
  for polychondritis 172
  for polymyalgia rheumatica
    175
  for polymyositis 176
  for sarcoidosis 206
  for sperm autoimmunity 219
  for systemic lupus erythemato-
    sus 228

for temporal arteritis/GCV 235
for ulcerative colitis 243
for Wegener's granulomatosis
  252–253
pregnancy **177–178**. *See also* herpes
  gestationis
  Addison's disease and 4
  antiphospholipid syndrome and
    28–29, 92
  diabetes and 125, 178
  endometriosis and 82–83
  Graves' disease and 178
  Hashimoto's thyroiditis and 178
  multiple sclerosis and 153
  rheumatoid arthritis and 178,
    201
  sarcoidosis and 205–206
  systemic lupus erythematosus
    and 178, 230
prevalence **178**
prevention, of autoimmune disease
  xi
primary agammaglobulinemia
  178–180
primary biliary cirrhosis **180–181**
  in Alaska Natives 11
  female:male ratio in 254
  liver dysfunction in 11
primary immune response **181**
procainamide 84
programmed cell death. *See* apoptosis
progressive multifocal leukoencephalopathy 152
progressive systemic sclerosis. *See*
  scleroderma
prostatitis, in Reiter's syndrome 191
protease inhibitors, for HIV-infected
  (AIDS) patients 10
protein-antigen feeding, for multiple sclerosis 156
proteins **181**
psoralen photochemotherapy. *See
  also* psoralen with ultraviolet A
  adverse effects and side effects
    of 249
psoralen with ultraviolet A
  for psoriasis 183–184
  for vitiligo 249
psoriasis 31, **181–184**
  economic cost of 78
  erythrodermic 182

guttate 182
hospitalization for 112
inverse 182
pain in 167
plaque 182
pustular 182
treatment of 21
psoriatic arthritis **184**
pulmonary embolism, in antiphospholipid syndrome 28
pulmonary function testing
  in myasthenia gravis 160
  in sarcoidosis 205
pulmonary hypertension 116
purpura. *See also* idiopathic thrombocytopenic purpura
  definition of 117
PUVA. *See* psoralen with ultraviolet
  A
PV. *See* pemphigus vulgaris
pyridostigmine, for myasthenia
  gravis 160

Q

quality of life **185**
  rheumatoid arthritis and 202
  systemic lupus erythematosus
    and 229

R

RA. *See* rheumatoid arthritis
race/ethnicity, and autoimmune
  disease 31, **186**
radioactive iodine, for Graves' disease 101
radioallergosorbent test 15
RAST. *See* radioallergosorbent test
Raynaud's phenomenon **186–190,**
  210
  exercise and 189
  primary 187
  secondary 187–188
  smoking and 189
Rebif. *See* beta interferon
recombinant DNA technology. *See*
  genetic engineering
red blood cells. *See* erythrocytes/red
  blood cells
reduviid bugs 50
reishi 21
Reiter's syndrome **190–193**
  exercise in 192–193
  sex differences in 145